M. Samii W. Draf

Surgery of the Skull Base

An Interdisciplinary Approach

With a Chapter on Anatomy by J. Lang

With 289 Figures in 841 Separate Illustrations

Springer-Verlag Berlin Heidelberg GmbH

Professor Dr. med. Prof. h.c. MADJID SAMII
Medizinische Hochschule Hannover,
Direktor der Neurochirurgischen Klinik am Krankenhaus Nordstadt der Landeshauptstadt Hannover, Haltenhoffstraße 41, D-3000 Hannover 1

Professor Dr. med. WOLFGANG DRAF
Chefarzt der Klinik für HNO-Krankheiten und Plastische Gesichtschirurgie, Städtische Kliniken Fulda, Pacelliallee 4, D-6400 Fulda

Professor Dr. med. JOHANNES LANG
Vorstand des Anatomischen Instituts der Universität, Koellikerstraße 6, D-8700 Würzburg

ISBN 978-3-642-73063-4 ISBN 978-3-642-73061-0 (eBook)
DOI 10.1007/978-3-642-73061-0

Library of Congress Cataloging-in-Publication Data. Samii, Madjid. Surgery of the skull base : an interdisciplinary approach / M. Samii, W. Draf ; with a chapter on Anatomy by J. Lang. p. cm. Includes bibliographical references. ISBN 0-387-18448-1 (U.S. : alk. paper) 1. Skull base—Surgery. I. Draf, Wolfgang, 1940– . II. Lang, Johannes, 1923– . III. Title. [DNLM: 1. Skull—anatomy & histology. 2. Skull—surgery. WE 705 S 188s] RD529.S26 1989 617.5'14059—dc20 DNLM/DLC for Library of Congress 89-21699 CIP

Softcover reprint of the hardcover 1st edition 1989

Illustrations: J. Kühn, R. Himmelhan, H. Konopatzki, and T. Randolph (with the exception of the chapter entitled "Surgical Anatomy of the Skull Base")

Reproduction of figures: Graphische Kunstanstalt G. Dreher, Stuttgart

Typesetting, printing and bookbinding: Universitätsdruckerei H. Stürtz AG, Würzburg
2122/3130-543210 – Printed on acid-free paper

To our families for their support and accepting part-time fathers

Preface

The region of the skull base was long considered a surgical barrier because of its complex anatomy. With few exceptions, the region immediately beyond the dura or bony skull base constituted a "no man's land" for the surgeon working from the other direction. A major reason for this was the high morbidity associated with operative procedures in that area using traditional dissection techniques.

This situation changed with the advent of the operating microscope. Used initially by ear, nose and throat specialists for resective and reconstructive surgery of the petrous bone and paranasal sinuses, the operating microscope was later introduced in other areas, and neurosurgeons began using it in the mid-1960s. With technical equality thus established, the groundwork was laid for taking a new, systematic, and interdisciplinary approach to surgical problems of the skull base.

Intensive and systematic cooperation between ear, nose and throat surgeons and neurologic surgeons had its origins in the departments of the University of Mainz bindly supported by our chairmen Prof. Dr. Dr. hc Kurt Schürmann (Department of Neurosurgery) and Prof. Dr. W. Kley (Department of Ear, Nose and Throat Diseases, Head and Neck Surgery). The experience gained from this cooperation was taught in workshops held in Hannover from 1979 to 1986, acquiring a broader interdisciplinary base through the participation of specialists from the fields of anatomy, pathology, neuroradiology, ophthalmology, and maxillofacial surgery. The present monograph represents a comprehensive account of our own clinical experience and the results of the workshop discussions – a condensation of neurosurgical and otorhinolaryngologic techniques that is intended to advance the state of Skull Base Surgery.

Particular attention is given to surgical approaches and dissection techniques that have proven successful in our hands. We hope to provide the interested surgeon with a basic reference on the practice of skull base surgery. A discussion of the full range of surgical options is not attempted in the interest of didactic clarity.

We wrote this book as a supplement to existing, specialized surgical textbooks so that we could confine our attention to problems of the skull base and refer the reader to the pertinent literature when necessary.

We extend special thanks to Prof. Dr. Johannes Lang, Chairman of the Department of Anatomy of Würzburg University, for describing the normal anatomy of the skull base and its variations. His contribution follows the division of this book into the anterior, middle, and posterior skull base and is a valuable guide to microsurgical procedures in those areas.

We are also grateful to the many radiologists and pathologists here and abroad who kindly placed original photographs and findings at our disposal for inclusion in the Case Reports. This enabled us to demonstrate the practical applications of the various operative techniques described. We are specially indebted to Prof. Dr. R. Bässler, Fulda, Prof. Dr. J.P. Haas, Fulda, Prof. Dr. H.J. Löblich, Hannover, Prof. Dr. Ostertag, Hannover, Dr. L. Osterwald, Hannover, Prof. Dr. Vogelsang†, Hannover, and Prof. Dr. S. Wende, Mainz for their kind support and assistance.

This book would not have been possible without the constant self-sacrifice and understanding of our anesthesiologists, assistants, and nursing staff. We express special thanks to our secretaries, Mrs. Plünnecke, Mrs. Töllner, and Mrs. Schicker, for their tireless work in typing the manuscript, and to our colleagues, Dr. G. Penkert, Dr. W. Bini, Dr. M. Ammirati, and Dr. R. Keerl for their help with proofreading. We thank Mr. T. Telger for undertaking the translation of the German manuscript into English so that our text could be made accessible to an international readership.

We thank our illustrators, Mrs. T. Randolph, Mr. J. Kühn, Mr. R. Himmelhan, and H. Konopatzki, for cooperating in the production of the high-quality drawings that form an essential part of this work.

Springer-Verlag, and especially Mr. Bergstedt and his colleagues, deserve special recognition for their generous help and outstanding production work.

M. Samii, Hannover W. Draf, Fulda

Contents

Surgery of the Anterior Skull Base (AS)

Surgery of the Posterior Skull Base (PS)

Surgery of the Clivus (CL)

Surgery of the Craniocervical Junction (CJ)

Facial Nerve and Skull Base Surgery (FN)

Introduction

Lesions of the skull base pose special problems of diagnosis and treatment, because multiple specialties are involved. Diseases in this region are rarely limited to areas that are assigned to a single specialty, and so an interdisciplinary approach for evaluation and operative treatment is mandatory.

Efforts to surmount the barriers among disciplines led to close cooperation, which in turn formed a basis for the development of a systematic, common diagnostic and surgical strategy for patients with skull base disorders. Leading representatives of ear, nose and throat surgery, neurosurgery, and maxillofacial surgery already have made many fundamental contributions in areas that are relevant to surgery of the skull base (*ENT surgery:* Arena 1974, Boenninghaus 1974, Conley 1964, Denecke 1953, 1959/60, 1969, Fisch 1970, 1976, 1977, Grunert 1894, Guggenheim and Kleitsch 1967, House 1961, 1964, Ketcham et al. 1963, 1966, 1969, Kley 1967, 1968, Krekorian et al. 1969, Seiferth 1954, Seiferth and Wustrow 1977, Voss 1936, H. E. Wullstein 1972; *neurosurgery:* Cushing 1917, Dandy 1922, 1925, 1941, Derome 1972, Dietz 1970, Dott 1958, Drake 1969, 1978, Guiot and Derome 1976, Guiot et al. 1967, Kempe 1968, Krayenbühl and Yasargil 1975, Rand 1969, Tönnis and Schürmann 1951, Yasargil et al. 1976, Yasargil 1978; *maxillofacial surgery:* Schuchardt 1966).

Once these principles had become assimilated into the interdisciplinary field of skull base surgery, it became possible, through microsurgical techniques, to go beyond disease eradication and make progress toward preservation of function and true functional reconstruction.

Lesions of the skull base region may spread caudally to involve extracranial structures, or cranially to involve intracranial structures. With destruction of the bony barrier of the skull base, the pathway is open for the intra- or extracranial extension of disease, bearing in mind that the site of origin of the lesion in any given case may be extra- or intracranial. Through careful history taking, a thorough clinical examination by multiple specialties, and the implementation of all neuroradiologic methods of evaluation, it is possible in most cases to establish the size and extent of the pathological process as a necessary prelude to operative planning. Subdivision of the skull base by topographic-anatomic criteria into anterior, middle, and posterior portions has certain drawbacks in view of the apparent continuity of those areas when viewed from below, but we believe it is useful for purposes of convenience. Special areas, such as surgery of the facial nerve and surgery of the craniocervical junction, are treated separately to facilitate orientation and eliminate the need to search through different chapters.

Years of common surgical activity have repeatedly shown that even techniques that appear to be perfected require ongoing interdisciplinary up-dating in terms of performance and indications. Maintaining an interdisciplinary dialogue on specific problems is essential if progress is to continue. If we do not take the time for this, we may fail to recognize advances in other specialties and miss opportunities for dynamic growth.

References

Arena S (1974) Tumour surgery of the temporal bone. Laryngoscope 84:645

Bonninghaus HG (1974) Die operative Behandlung von Verletzungen der Rhinobasis. In: Naumann HH (Ed) Head and neck surgery, vol 1. Thieme, New York

Conley JJ (1964) Tumors of the infratemporal fossa. Arch Otolaryngol 79:498

Cushing H (1917) Tumors of the nervus acusticus and the syndrome of the cerebellopontine angle. Saunders, Philadelphia

Dandy WE (1922) An operation for the total extirpation of tumors of the cerebellopontine angle: a preliminary report. Bull Hopkins Hosp 33:344–345

Dandy WE (1925) An operation for the total removal of cerebellopontine (acoustic) tumors. Surg Gynecol Obstet 41:129–148

Dandy WE (1941) Results of removal of acoustic tumors by the unilateral approach. Arch Surg 42:1026–1033

Denecke JH (1953) Die otorhinolaryngologischen Operationen. In: Gulecke N, Zenker R (ed) Allgemeine und spezielle chirurgische Operationslehre, vol 5, 2nd edn. Springer, Berlin Göttingen Heidelberg

Denecke HJ (1959/1960) Operationstechnische Probleme bei der Entfernung großer Neurinome im Bereich von Felsenbeinpyramide, N. facialis, Pharynx, Gefäßscheide, Ösophagusmund und Zunge. HNO 8:343

Denecke JH (1969) Surgery of extensive glomus jugulare tumors of the ear. Rev Laryngol 90:265–270

Derome PJ (1972) Les tumeurs spheno-ethmoidales. Neurochirurgie 18 Suppl 1

Dietz H (1970) Die frontobasale Schädelhirnverletzung. Springer, Berlin Heidelberg New York

Dott NM (1958) Facialis paralysis–restitution by extrapetrous nerve graft. Proc R Soc Med 51:900–902

Drake CG (1969) The surgical treatment of vertebral basilar aneurysm. Clin Neurosurg 16:114–169

Drake CG (1978) Treatment of aneurysms of the posterior cranial fossa. Prog Neurol Surg 9:122–194

Fisch U (1970) Transtemporal surgery of the internal auditory canal. Adv Otorhinolaryngol 17:203–240

Fisch U (1976) Chirurgie im inneren Gehörgang und an benachbarten Strukturen. In: Naumann HH (ed) Kopf- und Hals-Chirurgie, vol 3, Thieme, Stuttgart, pp 457–543

Fisch U (1977) Infratemporal fossa approach for extensive tumors of the temporal bone and base of the skull. In: Silverstein H, Norell H (eds) Neurological surgery of the ear. Aesculapius, Birmingham AL, pp 34–53

Grunert KA (1894) Die operative Ausräumung des Bulbus venae jugularis (Bulbusoperation) Arch Ohrenheilkd 36:71

Guggenheim P, Kleitsch WP (1967) Combined craniotomy-rhinotomy for ethmoid cancer. Ann Otol (St. Louis) 76:105

Guiot G, Derome P (1976) Surgical problems of pituitary adenomas. In: Advances and technical standards in neurosurgery, vol 3. Springer, Vienna New York

Guiot G, Bouche J, Oppotu A (1967) Les indications de l'abord transsphenoidal des adenomes hypophysaires. Press Med 75:1563

House WF (1961) Surgical exposure of the internal auditory canal and its contents through the middle cranial fossa. Laryngoscope 71:1363–1385

House WF (1964) Transtemporal bone microsurgical removal of acoustic neuromas. Arch Otolaryngol 80:597–730

Kempe LG (1968) Operative neurosurgery, vol 1. Springer, Berlin Heidelberg New York

Ketcham AS, Wilkins RH, Buren JM van, Smith RR (1963) A combined intracranial facial approach to the paranasal sinusses. Am J Surg 196:699

Ketcham AS, Hoye RC, Buren JM van, Johnson RH, Smith RR (1966) Complications of intracranial facial resection for tumors of the paranasal sinusses. Amer J Surg 112:591

Ketcham AS, Hammond WG, Chretien P, Buren JM van (1969) Treatment of advanced cancer of the ethmoid sinusses. Nobel Symposium 10. Almquist and Wiksell, Stockholm

Kley W (1967) Diagnostik und operative Versorgung von Keilbeinhöhlenfrakturen. Laryngol Rhinol Otol (Stuttg) 46:469–478

Kley W (1968) Die Unfallchirurgie der Schädelbasis und der pneumatischen Räume. Arch Otorhinolaryngol 191:1–216

Krayenbühl H, Yasargil MG (1975) Chondromas. Progr Neurol Surg 6:435–463

Krekorian EA, Kempe LG (1969) The combined otolaryngology-neurosurgery approach to extensive benign tumors. Laryngoscope 79:2086

Rand RW (1969) Microneurosurgery for acoustic tumors. In: Rand RW (ed) Microneurosurgery. Mosby, St. Louis, pp 126–155

Schuchardt K (ed) (1966) Das frische Trauma im Kiefer-Gesichts-Bereich. Thieme, Stuttgart (Fortschr Kiefer- und Gesichtschirurgie, vol 11)

Seiferth LB (1954) Unfallverletzungen der Nase, der Nebenhöhlen und der Basis der vorderen Schädelgrube. Arch Otorhinolaryng 165:1

Seiferth LB, Wustrow F (1977) Verletzungen im Bereich der Nase, des Mittelgesichts und seiner Nebenhöhlen sowie frontobasale Verletzungen. In: Berendes, Link, Zöllner (eds) Hals-Nasen-Ohren-Heilkunde in Praxis und Klinik, vol 1/I/8, 2nd edn. Thieme, Stuttgart

Tönnis W, Schürmann K (1951) Meningeome der Keilbeinflügel. Zentralbl Neurochirur 11:1–13

Voss O (1936) Die Chirurgie der Schädelbasisfrakturen aufgrund 25jähriger Erfahrungen. Barth, Leipzig

Wullstein HL (1972) Hat Terminologie zur Definition unseres Faches eine praktische Bedeutung? HNO 20:259–261

Yasargil MG (1978) Mikrochirurgie der Kleinhirnbrückenwinkel-Tumoren. In: Plester D, Wende S, Nakayama N (eds) Kleinhirnbrückenwinkeltumoren. Springer, Berlin Heidelberg New York, pp 215–257

Yasargil MG, Antic J, Laciga R, Jain KK, Hodosh RM, Smith RD (1976) Microsurgical pterional approach to aneurysm of the basilar bifurcation. Surg Neurol 6:83–91

Surgical Anatomy of the Skull Base (SA)

Johannes Lang

Anatomy of Malformations of the Anterior Skull Base

Nasal Fistulas, Nasal Cysts, Meningoceles

(Figs. SA 1, SA 2)

Various types of cephalocele are recognized. One type, the meningocele, is a cerebrospinal fluid-filled hernial sac that is covered only by skin or surrounding tissue. If the sac also contains brain tissue, it is called a meningoencephalocele. An encephalocele contains brain tissue only, the dura mater usually merging with the outer periosteum at the margin of the bony defect. In an encephalocystocele the sac contains portions of the ventricles in addition to brain. Combined forms may occur. The various malformations cannot always be distinguished clinically, because the tissue in the hernial sac is greatly altered and may even be difficult to identify histologically. The anterior skull base region may be affected by frontoethmoid cephaloceles, which emerge anterior or lateral to the cribriform plate of the ethmoid bone in the area of the foramen cecum. From there the sac may project forward, presenting over the nasal root. This may be associated with a splitting or diastasis of the nasal bones or the frontal process of the maxilla. Nasoethmoid cephaloceles project downward between the ethmoid bone and the frontal or nasal bone and are commonly associated with asymmetries of the anterior fossa. Naso-orbital cephaloceles project forward into the anterior part of the orbit between the frontal, ethmoid, and lacrimal bones (anterior orbital cephalocele). Generally the sac displaces the globe laterally downward while displacing the lacrimal sac medially. Spheno-orbital cephaloceles (rare) may protrude between the orbital surface of the frontal bone and the lesser wing of the sphenoid or may traverse the superior orbital fissure or optic canal to enter the posterior part of the orbit (posterior orbital cephalocele), producing the symptoms of a retrobulbar mass. Some of these lesions remain clinically silent until adulthood. A nasomaxillary cephalocele protrudes through the same opening but then passes through the inferior orbital fissure into the pterygopalatine fossa. Nasopharyngeal cephaloceles may penetrate the cribriform plate or pass between the cribriform plate and the developing anterior border of the sphenoid downwards into the nasopharynx. A sphenopharyngeal cephalocele protrudes into the pharynx through the former synchondrotic zones of the sphenoid.

Dermal Sinus

Dermal sinus is a closure defect resulting from incomplete separation of the neural tube from the skin surface. An epithelium-lined tract may extend to varying depths from the skin surface and may even penetrate the skull through small openings in the bone.

Müsebeck and Karst (1967) reported on a familial occurrence of dermoid fistulas of the nose.

Gliomas and Encephaloceles

Gliomas and encephaloceles can arise from the region of the foramen cecum. Karma et al. (1977) reviewed a series of 138 nasal gliomas that had been reported to that time (mostly in newborns, a few in adults). Sixty percent developed extranasally, 30% intranasally, and 10% involved combined intra- and extranasal forms. Whitaker et al. (1981) described a congenital extracranial nasofrontal glioma in an 11-month-

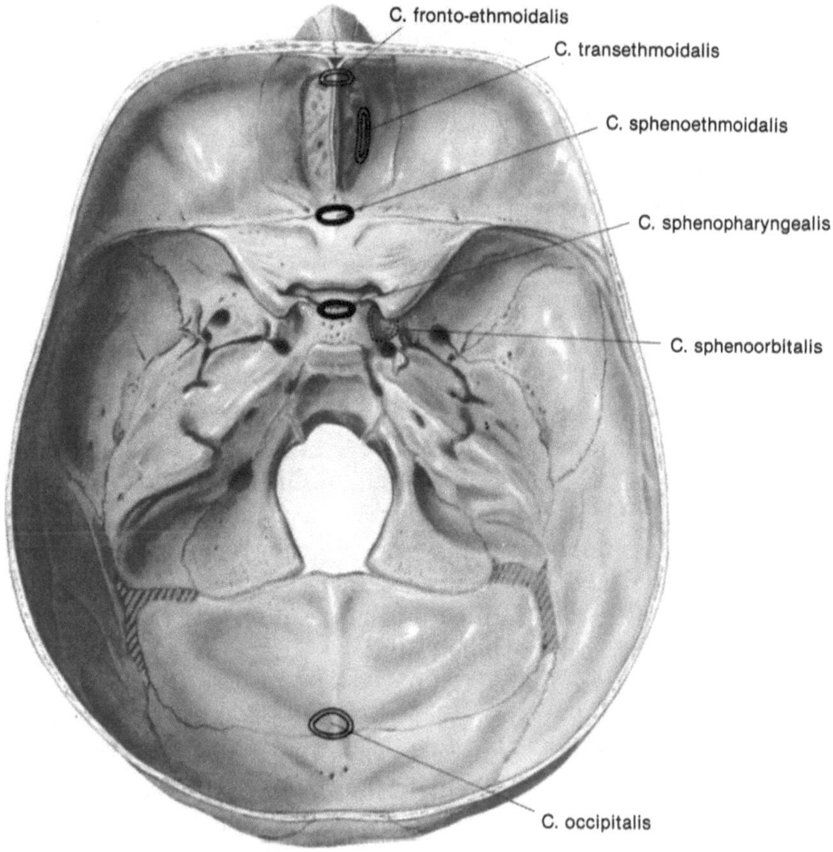

Fig. SA 1. Possible sites of occurrence of encephaloceles and meningoceles in the neonatal skull (modified from Gerlach 1960). *Heavy black lines:* frequent and unfavorable cephaloceles; *double black lines:* frequent and favorable cephaloceles; *double broken lines:* rare cephaloceles with a favorable prognosis

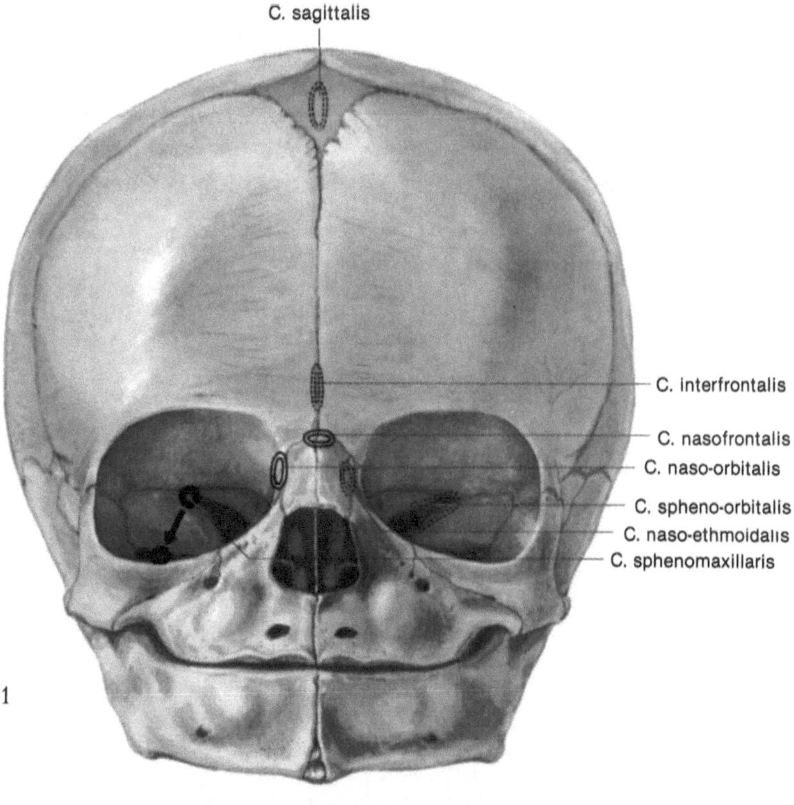

Fig. SA 2. Legend see Fig. 1

old girl. They stated that the lesion resulted from a dural projection through the foramen cecum, thus emulating the pathogenesis of an encephalocele.

In normal skulls the anterior border of the foramen cecum is generally formed by the frontal bone and the posterior and lateral margins of the ethmoid. The foramen cecum always opens into a connective tissue tract which communicates with the nasal cavity and represents a very fine emissary. This led Hyrtl (1885) to suggest the term "porus cranionasalis." Boyd (1931) states that it is very rare for a vein to course within the foramen cecum or the adjacent canal. Generally the foramen cecum contains a dural plug with relatively small blood vessels.

Walker et al. (1952) noted that 37 intranasal encephaloceles had been reported prior to their publication. Spontaneous cerebrospinal fluid leaks are common in this condition, nasal respiration is impaired, and the lesion is apt to be mistaken for a nasal tumor (polyp or neoplasm). With further growth the lesion may encroach upon the naris or project backward toward the pharynx. Nasofrontal cephaloceles are illustrated in Figs. SA 1, SA 2. Additional details may be found in Converse et al. (1973), Pfeifer (1974), and Tessier (1976).

Cephaloceles that form between the two squamae of the frontal bone are called interfrontal cephaloceles. The cranium at this site is still open in fetuses and newborns. A metopic frontal suture persists in 10% (7%–12.5%). A metopic fontanelle may be present for a time.

The "supranasal triangle" is located in the inferior portion of the interfrontal suture (Schwalbe 1901), and adjacent to it is the glabella. Generally this area is ossified from multiple centers in both frontal bones; occasionally a deep groove persists. Zook et al. (1984) note that lesions composed of heterotopic brain tissue have very often been described as "nasal gliomas." The term originates from Schmidt (1900), who reported on rare closure defects in the area of the middle frontal process. Zook et al. note that five cases of ectopic glial tissue in the scalp and two in the face have been reported to date.

Gisselsson (1947) claimed that the rare "transsphenoidal" encephalocele was the result of a congenital malformation. Pollock and Newton (1971) believed that defects of neural tube closure and a transient rise of intraventricular pressure during embryonic development were responsible for the anomaly. Causal importance has also been ascribed to ossification defects in the sphenoid bone and to a persistence of the craniopharyngeal canals. Agenesis of the corpus callosum is frequently reported in association with encephaloceles (Manelfe et al. 1978), and hypertelorism with an abnormally broad nasal root is commonly present in affected individuals. The cystic mass in the upper part of the nasopharynx enlarges when compression is applied to the jugular veins. Complaints relating to the optic chiasm or hypothalamus may also be reported. Rarely the defect extends through the floor of the sella. (Further details may be found in Williamson and Barelli 1951)

Anatomy of the Skin and Scalp in the Frontobasal Approach

In our material the mean thickness of the scalp in the frontal region including the muscles, the subgaleal layer, and the pericranium is 6.7 (2.71–10.67) mm.

Frontal Belly of the Epicranial Muscle

(Figs. SA 3, SA 4)

The frontal belly of the epicranial muscle has no bony attachments, being bound by connective tissue to the area of the eyebrow and glabella. It has several actions such as creasing the forehead and drawing the skin of the glabella upward. The muscle is relatively thin and, according to Eisler (1912), continuous anteroinferiorly with the contralateral homonymous muscle. The paired *corrugator supercilii muscles* arise from the superciliary arch deep to the depressor capitis supercilii. The distance between the two corrugator muscles ranges from 3 to 8 mm.

The *depressor capitis supercilii* arises at the superior end of the maxillary frontal process, above the medial palpebral ligament. Its fibers diverge upward and insert in the medial half of the eyebrow area. They act with the depressor glabellae (just deep to the depressor supercilii) to draw the head (medial part) of the eyebrow downward and medially.

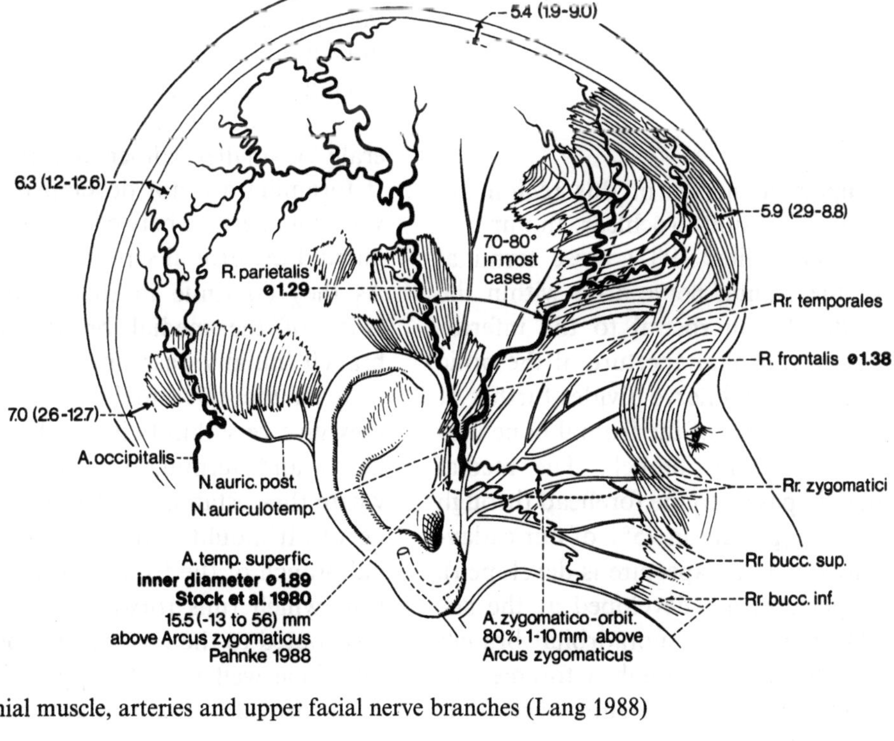

Fig. SA 3. Epicranial muscle, arteries and upper facial nerve branches (Lang 1988)

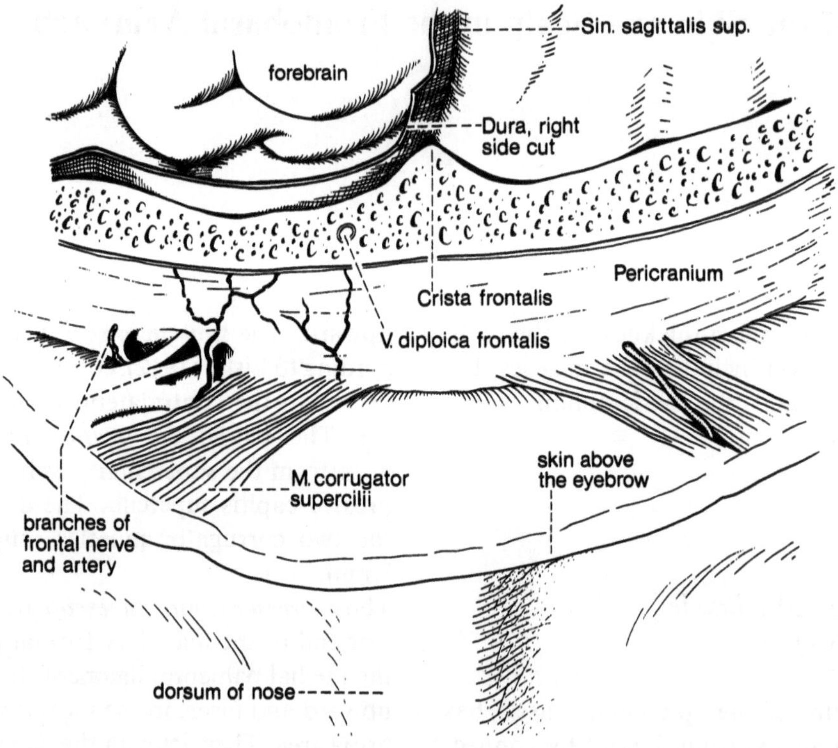

Fig. SA 4. The scalp, mobilized superiorly and reflected forward

A *transverse muscle of the glabella* uniting the orbicular muscles of the eyes at the upper part of the nasal dorsum is present in some individuals.

Nerves (Fig. SA 5)

The most important nerves of this region are the supraorbital and supratrochlear. In our material (Lang and Reiter 1987) these terminal branches of the frontal nerve arise within the orbit 19.59 (0–44) mm rostral to the inferior border of the intraorbital aperture of the optic nerve. The supraorbital nerve divides further at the supraorbital margin of the frontal bone into a medial and a lateral branch. The medial branch generally passes to the forehead through a frontal incisure (present in 75% of our cadavers when only one bony aperture is developed). When two apertures are developed at the superior orbital margin, the supraorbital branch emerges from the orbit through a foramen in 40.6% of cases and through a supraorbital incisure in 49.4%. When only one aperture is developed, its distance from the midline is 22.1 (14.5–32.0) mm; with two apertures, the paramedian distance is 23.7 (14–35) mm for the supraorbital foramen or incisure and 18.8 (8–29) mm for the frontal foramen or incisure. The medial branch of the supraorbital nerve is generally of smaller caliber than the lateral branch. If foramina are not developed, the nerves traverse an aperture between the supraorbital margin and the orbital septum.

As they continue in their course, the largest twigs of the medial branch and the lateral branch initially pass upward below the frontal belly of the epicranial muscle (through which they give very thin twigs to the skin of the forehead) and terminate in the parietal region, where they establish anastomoses with adjacent nerves. It should be noted that the second terminal branch of the frontal nerve, the supratrochlear, which runs forward over the trochlea, is distributed to the root of the nose and the frontal skin as well as to the upper lid. When surgery is performed in the frontal region, it is custom-

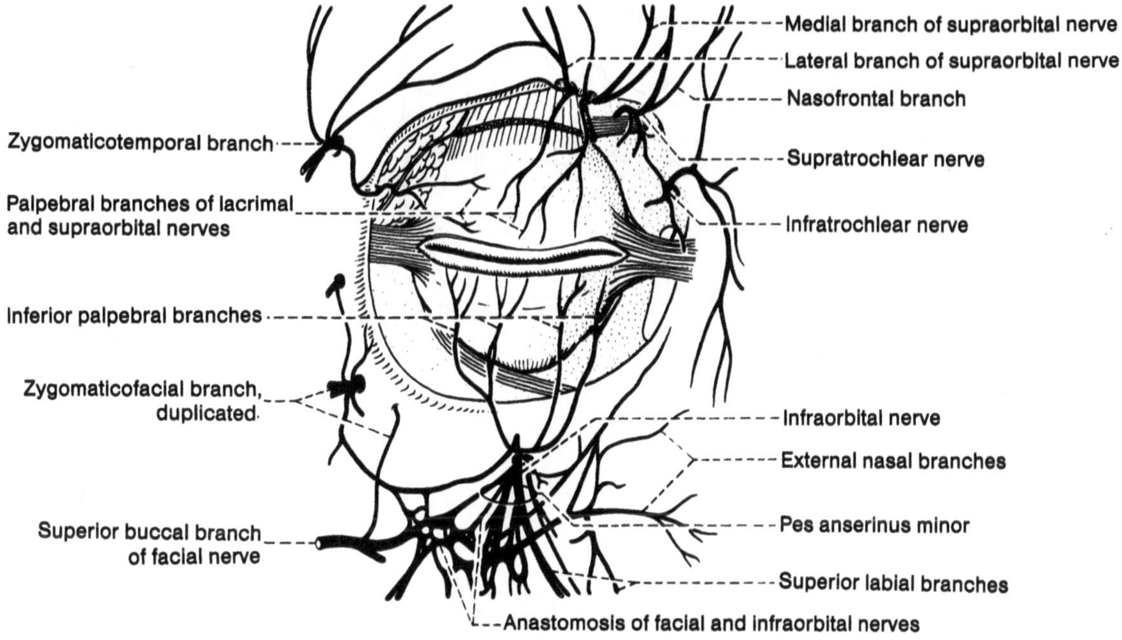

Fig. SA 5. Nerves in the area of the orbital margin and eyelids (from Lang 1988)

ary to divide the scalp in the area of the frontal hairline and then reflect the flap forward and downward. The scalp flap includes the various parts of the epicranial muscle (including its frontal belly) and the rigid attachments of the corium with the galea aponeurotica (tendinous fibers passing chiefly between the frontal and occipital bellies of the epicranius muscle). Reflection of the flap is aided by the presence of loose tissue below the galea aponeurotica consisting of several vascularized connective tissue layers (see Lang and Ricker, 1970, for further details). The pericranial layer, also well endowed with blood vessels, is left on the skull.

Arteries (Fig. SA 6)

The most important terminal branch of the ophthalmic artery is the supraorbital. A branch of that vessel, the supratrochlear artery, accompanies the supraorbital nerve to supply the skin of the forehead, the palpebral apparatus, and the root of the nose. This artery has an outer diameter of 0.67 (0.3–0.75) mm (Lang and Kageyama, in press). Frequently a smaller twig accompanies the branches of the supraorbital nerve itself. These help to supply the frontal belly of the epicranius muscle and the skin of the forehead. The most important vessel in the anterior and lateral portion of the scalp is the superficial temporal artery and its branches. That vessel and its branches have long been utilized for reconstructions in head and neck surgery (Carpue 1816; Gillies 1935; Converse 1942; etc.). Stock et al. (1980) measured the outer diameter of the superficial temporal artery proximal to its division into frontal and parietal branches and reported a value of 2.03 ± 0.33 mm. Angiography indicated a vascular diameter of 1.89 ± 0.68 mm in this area. In the 25 cadavers examined by the authors, the bifurcation of the superficial temporal artery was above the zygomatic arch in 15 cases, level with the zygomatic arch in 8 cases, and below the arch in 2. The superficial temporal artery runs about 9.4 mm anterior to the external acoustic meatus and 13.9 mm anterior to the upper at-

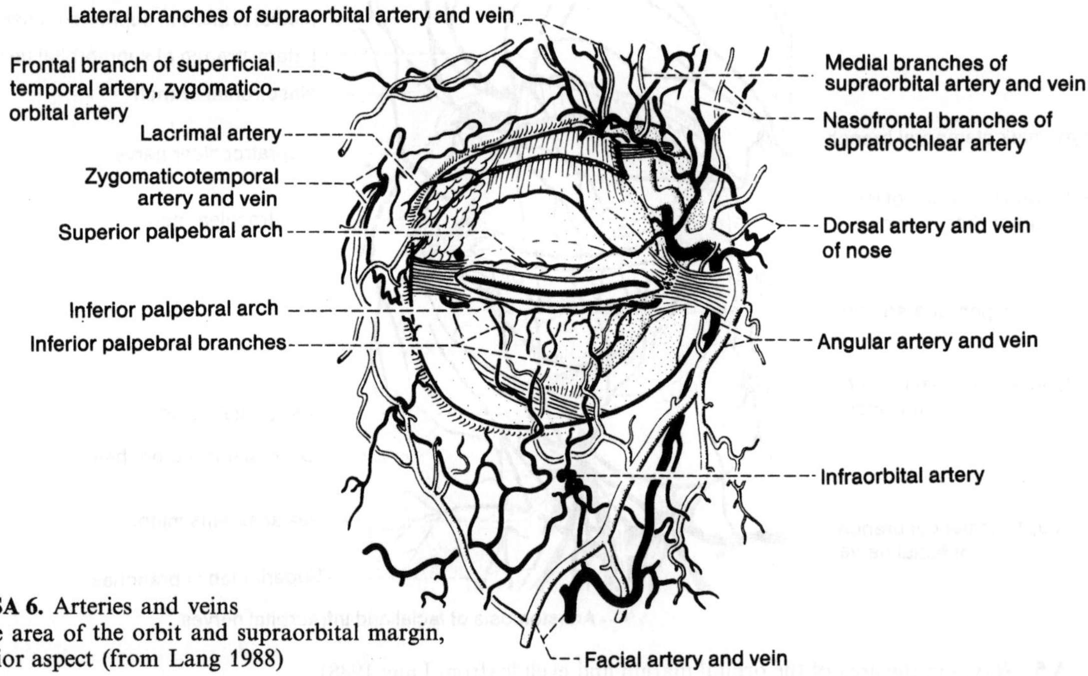

Fig. SA 6. Arteries and veins in the area of the orbit and supraorbital margin, anterior aspect (from Lang 1988)

tachment of the auricle. In our material we found that the two terminal branches of the superficial temporal artery were extremely diverse in their calibers and, not infrequently, were accompanied by a third branch running forward below the frontal branch. Both the frontal and parietal branches of the vessel anastomose with homonymous vessels of the opposite side and with branches of the supraorbital and supratrochlear arteries. The larger branches of the superficial temporal artery are placed deeply in the scalp, the smaller branches more superficially. The vessels course over and beneath homonymous veins. The collagenous structures of the scalp make the vessel walls tense; they account for the frequent failure of physiologic arterial occlusion following injuries to the scalp and for the significant hematomatous swelling that occurs with vascular ruptures. According to Grote (1901) the right superficial temporal artery is more strongly developed than the left artery in 21% of cases, and the left is more strongly developed in 9.3%. In surgical operations on the cranial vault, care should be taken to spare a branch of the superficial temporal artery so that it can be anastomosed to branches of the middle cerebral artery if need be.

According to Mangold et al. (1980), the medial branch of the supratrochlear artery is generally the larger of the two branches that pass to the skin of the forehead. These authors found that the trunk of the supratrochlear artery is placed 16.5 (14–19) mm from the midline, approximately on the plane of the medial canthus. The position of these vessels is of surgical importance in the creation of forehead flaps (Schröder 1967; Pfeifer 1978; etc.).

Veins (Fig. SA 6)

The large-caliber supratrochlear and supraorbital veins course through the anterior scalp region before uniting with the facial vein. The facial vein also receives blood from the superior palpebral veins, the external nasal veins, and other tributaries (see Fig. SA 6 and Lang 1983 for further details).

Frontal Squama and Frontal Sinus

The lower the frontal approach to the anterior cranial fossa, the greater the likelihood of entering the frontal sinus. Like most of the paranasal sinuses, the frontal sinus undergoes most of its development in postnatal life (see Lang 1985 for details). The mean height of the sinus is 24.3 mm, with a range of 5–66 mm (Milosslawski 1903). In our material as well, we found a frontal sinus with a maximum vertical dimension of 60 mm (see Fig. 7 in Lang 1983). It should be noted that the frontal sinus enlarges in both the vertical and sagittal dimensions after middle age. The floor of the frontal sinus may be situated on, above, or below the plane of the cribriform plate (see Figs. 44 and 45 in Lang 1975, Fig. 69 in Lang 1983, and Fig. 7 in Lang 1983). The medial parts of the floor are generally set lower than the lateral parts. Occasionally there may be a third frontal sinus with its own orifice or a single frontal sinus with two orifices (see Fig. 69 in Lang 1983). The surgical approach to the medial part of the anterior cranial fossa (the olfactory fossa) relies on a knowledge of the torus olfactorius. Occasionally the olfactory fossa bulges into a prominently developed frontal sinus just adjacent to the midline. The frontal sinus also may be permeated by septa of varyious sizes. These septa may conduct vessels that establish anastomoses between the ophthalmic artery and the frontal branch of the middle meningeal. Rarely, rarefactions are observed in the orbital aspect of the floor of the frontal sinus (see Fig. 38 in Lang 1983).

Frontal Sinus Mucosa and Blood Vessels

A number of arterial vessels are distributed to the bony wall and mucosa of the frontal sinus: the anterior ethmoidal artery, the meningo-orbital branch, the lateral nasal branches, and others. The rich capillary network of the frontal sinus mucosa may drain along the nasofrontal duct to veins of the nasal cavity, to the trochlear fovea in the orbit (see Fig. 71 in Lang 1983), to frontal diploic veins, to middle meningeal veins, and to other orbital veins (see Fig. 70 in Lang 1983).

Dura Mater of the Anterior Cranial Fossa

(Fig. SA 7)

The dura mater of the cranium is composed of an outer fibrous layer and an inner fibrous layer. The outer layer acts as the inner periosteum of the adjacent cranial bones. In the anterior fossa the fibers of the outer layer radiate from the frontal tuber, passing downward and medially. The dura is thinned in the area of the olfactory fossa, and the dura on the planum sphenoidale consists of transverse fibers grouped into thicker bundles. The inner layer of the dura mater is relatively thin. Between the two layers are the larger branches of the dural vessels, which give off small branches to the cranium and to the dura itself. The major vessels of the cerebral dura mater (and of the bones of the anterior fossa) are the ethmoidal arteries and the frontal branch of the middle meningeal. The ethmoidal arteries anastomose with various nasal arteries, while the frontal branch of the middle meningeal anastomoses with branches of the ethmoidal arteries and also with branches of the ophthalmic artery. In our material we occasionally found a branch of the internal carotid artery entering the most posterior portion of the floor of the anterior cranial fossa (Yasargil et al. 1984 identified this branch consistently). In the frontal midline approach to the skull base, attention must be given to the superior sagittal sinus, which extends only part way to the skull base, and to the falx cerebri. The falx carries a relatively large branch of the anterior ethmoidal artery called the anterior falceal artery. All the dural arteries interanastomose with one another and with the contralateral homonymous vessels. Venous drainage from the dura mater generally follows the course of the dural arteries.

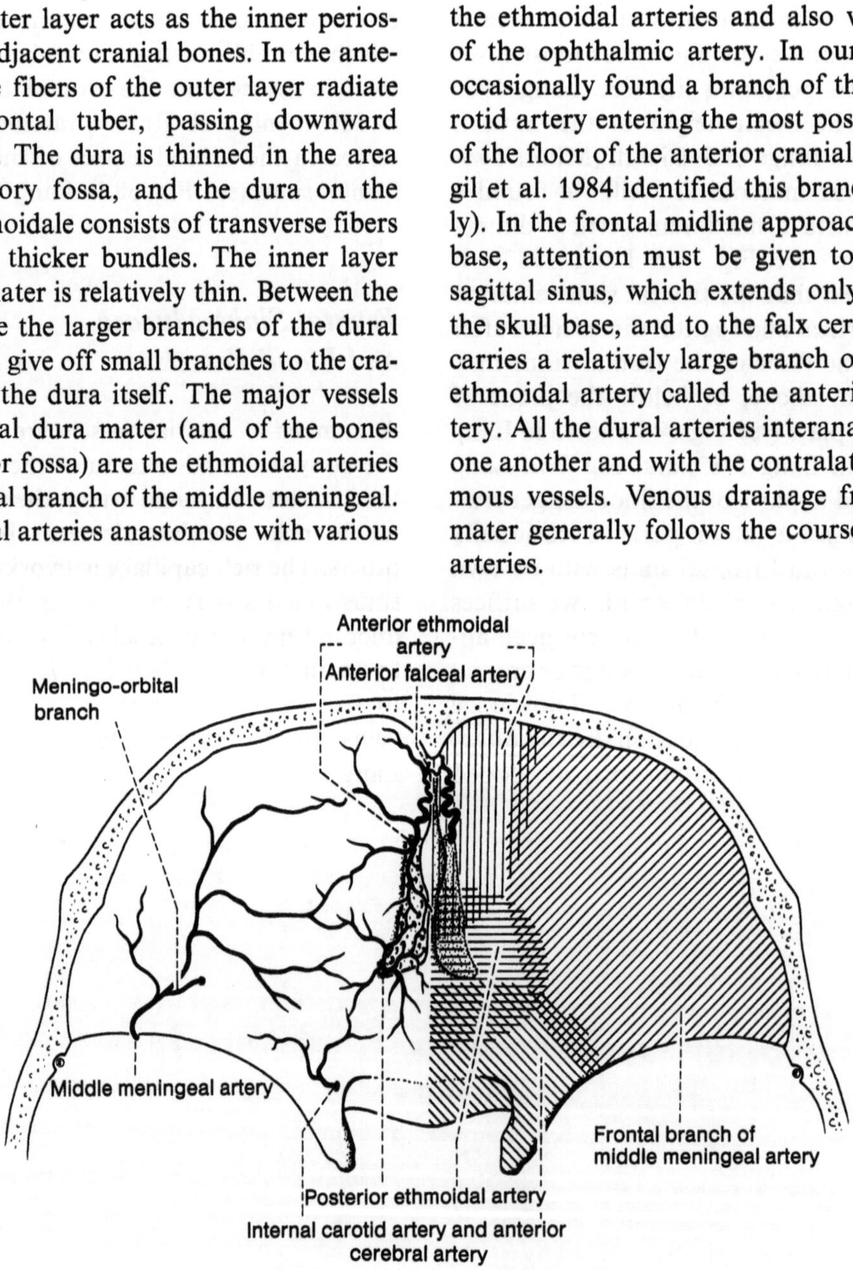

Fig. SA 7. Arteries supplying the dura and bone of the anterior cranial fossa

Floor of the Anterior Cranial Fossa

The floor of the anterior cranial fossa is the part of the interior skull base which supports most of the orbital frontal lobe of the cerebrum, olfactory bulb, and olfactory tract. The posterior part of the floor overhangs the middle fossa somewhat, especially where it relates to the medial portion of the frontal lobe (see Lang 1979). The orbital parts of the frontal bone form the greater portion of the floor of the anterior fossa. Between them is the ethmoid bone with its cribriform plate. The posterior floor region is completed by the lesser wings of the sphenoid, which delimit the optic canals, and by the planum sphenoidale. The lesser wing extends laterally for a variable distance and becomes continuous with the sylvian crest formed by the frontal bone below the greater sphenoid wing. In 30%–60% of the population this area contains a branch

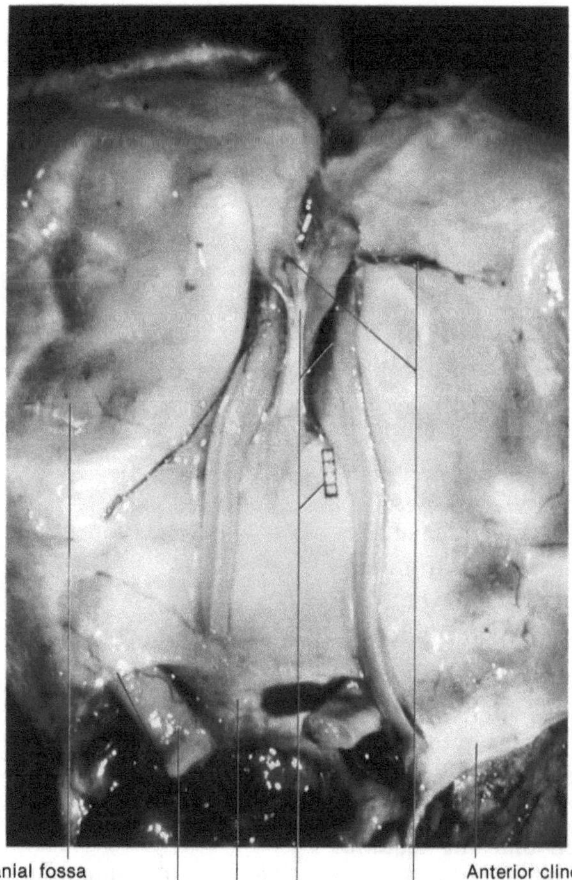

Fig. SA 8. Olfactory bulb and tract and midportion of the anterior cranial fossa

of the meningeal artery, its accompanying veins, and/or the meningeal sinus (e.g., Lang and Tisch-Rottensteiner 1976). The anatomy of this portion of the floor is an important surgical concern in patients with frontobasal fractures, olfactory groove neoplasms, and in surgical approaches to the pituitary region and optic canal.

Olfactory Fossa (Fig. SA 8)

We have found the mean length of the cribriform plate in adults to be 20.78 mm, as compared with a mean length of only 15.8 mm for the olfactory fossa. The width of the dura-lined olfactory fossa is also slightly less than that of the cribriform plate. It is significant that the olfactory fossa generally forms the lowest part of the floor of the anterior cranial fossa. It is bordered medially by the crista galli, which varies in length and thickness. Laterally the ethmoid cells, which generally are covered superiorly by the frontal bone, often project above the olfactory fossa. They enlarge with postnatal growth. By six months of age the sloping cribriform plate has, on average, attained a level 13.5 mm above the FHP (Frankfurt horizontal plane). In nine-year-olds it is 20.4 mm above this reference plane, and in adults 21.2 mm. Being extremely thin, the cribriform plate is commonly involved in skull fractures, resulting in hemorrhage and CSF discharge into the nasal cavity, anosmia, and a portal for ascending infection. The thicker the crista galli, the smaller the volume of the olfactory fossa. In our material the crista galli is pneumatized from the frontal sinus in about 10% of cases. Its mean length in adults is 21.56 (15.1–31.4) mm, its width 4.65 (1.6–9.4) mm. Its mean height is 12.05 (7.2–18.2) mm (Schmidt 1974). The depth of the bony olfactory fossa is 5.85 (1–16) mm in its anterior part and 4.81 (1–10) mm in its posterior third. Keros (1962) reported that the distance between the cribriform plate and the highest point of the ethmoid labyrinth is 6.89 (2–18) mm in the anterior third and 5.8 (2–18) mm in the posterior third. We saw many instances in our material where the cribriform plate sagged toward the nasal cavity in its anterior third. Keros (1962) determined that the olfactory fossa was shallow (1–3 mm) in approximately 12% of cases, moderately deep (4–7 mm) in slightly more than 70%, and deep (8–16 mm) in slightly more than 18%. The lowest point of the cribriform plate in our material is 2.5 mm below the level of the planum sphenoidale on the right side and 2.3 mm on the left side. The level of the cribriform plate was found to be 7.9 mm on average (up to 17 mm) below the nasion or nasofrontal suture (Schmidt 1974). The foramina of the cribriform plate are highly variable in their distribution. Overall, the plate bears an average of 44 foramina on the right side and 43 on the left, their number ranging from 26 to 71 (Schmidt 1974). The foramina transmit a medial and a lateral group of olfacto-

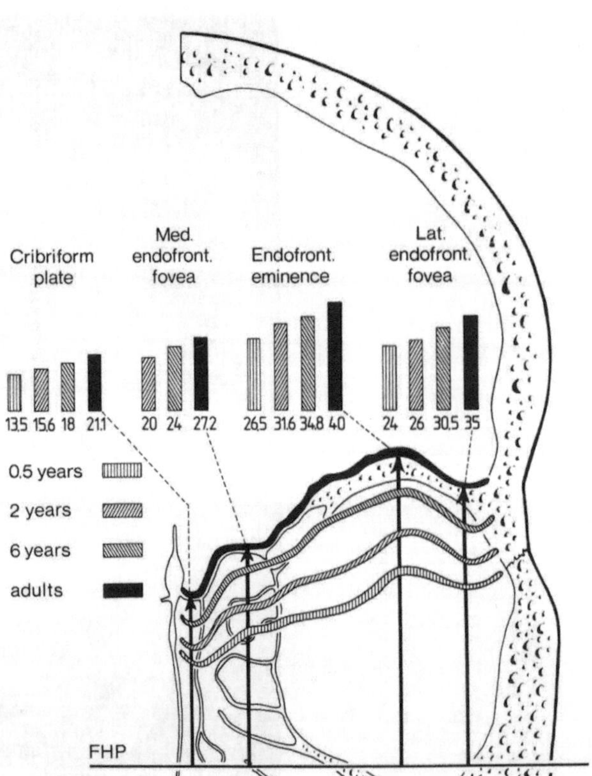

Fig. SA 9. Cribriform plate, medial endofrontal fovea, endofrontal eminence, and lateral endofrontal fovea. Mean height increase in mm during the postnatal period and in adults relative to the Frankfurt horizontal plane (FHP)

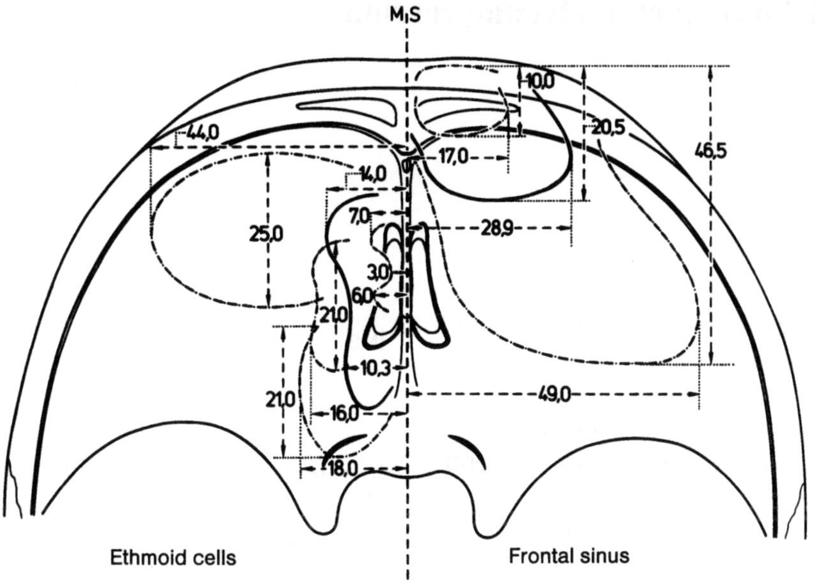

Fig. SA 10. Paranasal sinuses in the orbital roof area. *Heavy lines* indicate mean values in our material (Lang and Haas 1979); *broken lines* indicate maximum and minimum extension. Measurements in mm (extremals)

ry fibers, which are covered by sleevelike prolongations of the dura mater and subarachnoid space. The foramina are also traversed by branches from the ethmoidal arteries.

Endofrontal Foveae and Eminence
(Fig. SA 9)

Figure SA 9 shows how the level of the floor of the anterior fossa varies in relation to the FHP. We determined in 1976 (Lang et al.) how the lateral, depressed part of the floor – the *lateral endofrontal fovea* – varies in elevation during postnatal life. This area is related to the inferior frontal gyrus of the brain. The midportion of the floor generally bears a rounded elevation that we call the *endofrontal eminence*. The floor sinks again in the area of the ethmoid cells to form the *medial endofrontal fovea*. Medial to that depression is the olfactory fossa.

Pneumatization
(Fig. SA 10)

The floor of the anterior cranial fossa is pneumatized not just by prominently developed frontal sinuses but also by the middle and posterior superior ethmoid cells and occasionally by the sphenoid sinus. The mean and extreme extents of the sinuses and superior ethmoid cells are shown in Fig. SA 10. Data on the length and width of the anterior cranial fossa are given in Fig. SA 12.

Anatomy of Optic Nerve Decompression

(Figs. SA 8, SA 11)

The optic canal transmits the optic nerve with its dural and arachnoid coverings and also the ophthalmic artery from the orbit to the cranial cavity. In our material we determined a mean length of 9.8 mm for the upper wall of the optic canal and 4.63 mm for the lower wall. The medial wall of the canal is 11.4 (8–16) mm long, the lateral 10.79 (8.5–15) mm long (Lang and Oehmann 1976; Lang and Reiter 1985). The posterior superior wall of the optic canal is overlapped by a dural layer 2.58 (0.5–8.0) mm long composed of transverse fibers. Bony substance is lost from this area in postnatal life, leaving only the dura mater. We found in our material that the ophthalmic artery, with an outer diameter of 1.47 (0.9–2.1) mm (Lang and Kageyama, in press), can emerge in the subarachnoid space (approx. 47% of cases), at the junction between the dural opening of the internal carotid artery and subdural space (33.3%), or even in the cavernous sinus (approx. 18%) (Engel 1975).

The *thickness of the medial wall* of the optic canal is an important surgical consideration in the *transethmoidal and transsphenoidal approaches* to the canal. If the medial wall of the canal borders on the sphenoid sinus, as is usually the case, then the wall facing the sinus is 0.21 (0.1–0.31) mm thick (Maniscalco and Habal 1978). It is noteworthy that in at least 12% of cases the medial wall of the optic canal is bordered not by the sphenoid sinus but by a posterior superior ethmoid air cell (Onodi's cell). Our material includes specimens in which the posterior part of the medial wall of the optic canal is bordered by the sphenoid sinus and the anterior part by an ethmoid cell, as well as specimens in which two posterior ethmoid cells, one atop the other, border on the medial wall of the canal. The medial wall is slightly thickened in places where septa or sinus walls are present.

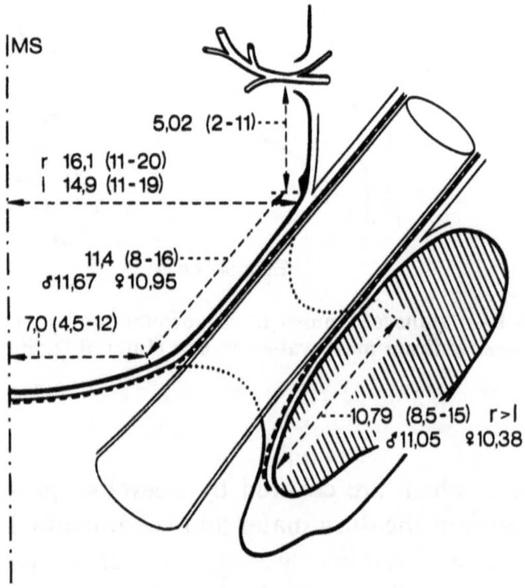

Fig. SA 11. Medial and lateral walls of the optic canal, length values and paramedian distances of the intracranial and intraorbital openings. The location of the posterior ethmoid canal is indicated. Data show the results of our measurements (mean and extreme values in mm), right-left differences, and sex differences. (After Lang and Schlehahn 1978 and Lang and Reiter 1985)

The *inclination angle of the optic canal* relative to its surroundings is a practically important concern. In adults the axis of the optic canal is angled forward and downward by 15.5° (3.2–28.5°) relative to the FHP. The canal is also angled medially to laterally from behind forward, forming an angle of 39.1° (33–44.4°) with the midsagittal plane in adults. (See Lang 1979 for details on postnatal changes in these angular dimensions.) The medial wall of the optic canal is 11.4 (8–16) mm long in our material. The intracranial opening of the canal is set 7.0 (4.5–12) mm from the midline; the anterior opening is 16.1 (11–20) mm from the midline on the right side and 14.9 (11–19) mm on the left (Lang and

Oehmann 1976; Lang and Reiter 1985). The site of entry of the posterior ethmoidal artery can lie 5.02 (1–11) mm from the orbital aperture of the optic canal (Lang and Schlehahn 1978). When the medial wall of the optic canal is opened, a dural-endocranial layer is found to intervene between the cerebral dura mater and periorbita and the dural sheath of the optic nerve. Opening this dural layer exposes the arachnoid of the optic nerve, followed by the subarachnoid space and finally the pia mater of the optic nerve. Deep to the optic nerve is the ophthalmic artery, a variable portion of which is fused to the dura-endocranial layer. We found that in 15.5% of cases the ophthalmic artery enters the orbital cavity on the medial side of the orbital aperture of the optic canal, posing a danger of injury (Engel 1975). The canal itself is constricted in its midportion, forming a passageway 4.63 (4–5.1) mm wide and 5.1 (4.1–6.2) mm high in adults (Lang and Oehmann 1976). The intracranial part of the optic nerve is supplied by branches from the internal carotid and anterior cerebral arteries, and the intraorbital part by branches from the ophthalmic and central retinal arteries. The optic nerve vessels form an arterial boundary zone within the canal. (See Lang 1983 for further details.) It should be noted that anterior origins of the superior oblique muscle can occur in proximity to the posterior ethmoid canal (see Fig. 54 in Lang 1983).

If the frontal sinus is prominently developed, it will be opened in the subfrontal approach to the optic nerve (Fig. SA 12). The frontal lobe is elevated, preserving the olfactory bulb and tract if possible. In our material the distance from the rounded junction of the floor of the anterior cranial fossa and the anterior wall of the fossa to the anterior border of the prechiasmatic sulcus is 44.9 (36–54) mm. Slightly smaller values have been measured on the left side

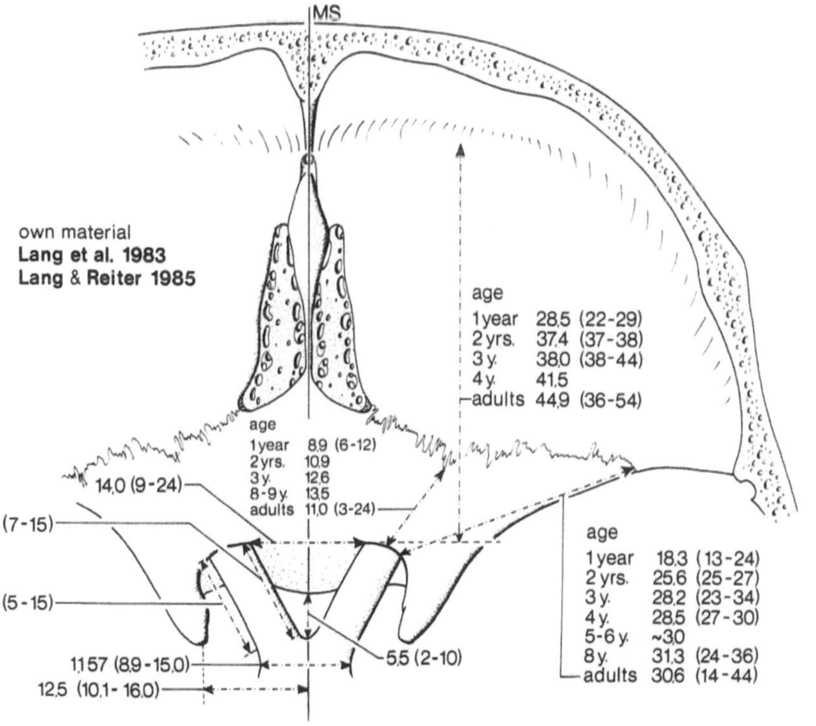

Fig. SA 12. Measured length of the anterior cranial fossa (at floor level), distance between the optic canals (intracranial), lateral and medial length of the intracranial part of the optic nerve, width of the optic chiasm, paramedian distance of the anterior clinoid process, length of the lesser wing of the sphenoid bone and sutures. The distance of the tuberculum sellae from the anterior border of the chiasm is also shown. Mean (and extreme) values are expressed in mm (Lang 1988)

(Lang and Haas 1979). The anterior border of the prechiasmatic sulcus is continuous laterally with the superior border of the intracranial opening of the optic canal. The intracranial superior wall of the optic canal is lost during postnatal life, leaving behind a dural layer which we regard as part of the optic canal: the "membranous part" of the canal. This portion of the dura mater, composed of transverse fibers, is 2.58 (0.5–8.0) mm long in our material (Lang 1973). When the optic nerve is displaced by very large or atheromatous internal carotid arteries or ophthalmic arteries (dolichomegaly), the superior border of the optic nerve may be notched. It is important to note that the portion of the optic nerve in the subarachnoid space is 5.03 (2.5–7.0) mm wide and 3.16 (1.5–5.0) mm high (Lang et al. 1983). Often the nerve still presents a transverse oval shape at the canal inlet. Once inside the canal, the nerve acquires a more rounded cross-section (Lang et al. 1983). In our material the intracranial length of the optic nerve between the dural layer and chiasm is 10.48 (7–15) mm on the medial side of the nerve. A value of 10.14 (5–14.5) mm has been measured on the lateral side (Lang and Reiter 1985). For surgical exposure of the optic canal from above, the dural layer is split first before proceeding to unroof the canal.

Another approach to the anterior skull base besides the bifrontal or frontal approach is the frontolateral. The length of the anterior cranial fossa as far as the anterior margin of the prechiasmatic sulcus was previously discussed. In our material the width of the anterior cranial fossa from the midsagittal plane to the dura mater on the lateral skull wall was 47 (42–54) mm (Lang and Haas 1979). The lateral length of the anterior fossa from the farthest rostral extension of the dura over the lesser wing (2.04 mm thick; range, 1.5–3.0 mm) to the junction of the floor with the front wall of the anterior cranial fossa was determined to be 35.4 (28–43) mm (Lang and Haas 1979). The frontolateral approach begins from the frontotemporal point, representing the "isthmus" of the forehead. This point corresponds to the most medial zone of the temporal line, which in our material lies 17.8 (11–26) mm above the frontozygomatic suture. On the interior aspect of the skull, this zone is placed 11.3 (-4 to +17) mm below the lateral endofrontal fovea (related to the inferior frontal gyrus; Krauss 1987).

Anatomy of the Orbit and Adjacent Skull Base

(Fig. SA 13)

For an *anterior orbitotomy* the skin incisions are placed so that

1) There is minimal destruction of nerves, blood vessels, and important muscles.
2) Good cosmetic results are obtained.

The principal supporting structures of the globe are shown in Fig. SA 13. Because the four rectus muscles of the eye act to displace the globe posteriorly and are opposed only by two oblique muscles which pull the globe forward and mediad, the most important suspensory apparatus of the eye is on the lateral orbital wall. The loop of the superior oblique muscle and the origin of the inferior oblique muscle are shown in Fig. SA 13, which also shows the partition of the lacrimal gland by the aponeurosis of the levator palpebrae superioris. An effort should be made to spare the lacrimal passages when performing an orbitotomy from the medial side. The nerves and blood vessels that should be spared are shown. The eyeball itself can be displaced relatively far laterally for two reasons:

1) The lateral orbital margin is placed a mean distance of 17.3 mm behind a frontal plane at the nasion on the right side, and 16.5 mm on the left side (sutural zone between the nasal bones and frontal bone).
2) The optic nerve has redundant length. We found in our material that the nerve tends to sag downward within the orbit. Its length in the unstretched condition (measured on the superior aspect) is 22.94 (17.5–31.0) mm. With the nerve stretched out, we measured an interorbital length of 26.8 (21–34.5) mm.

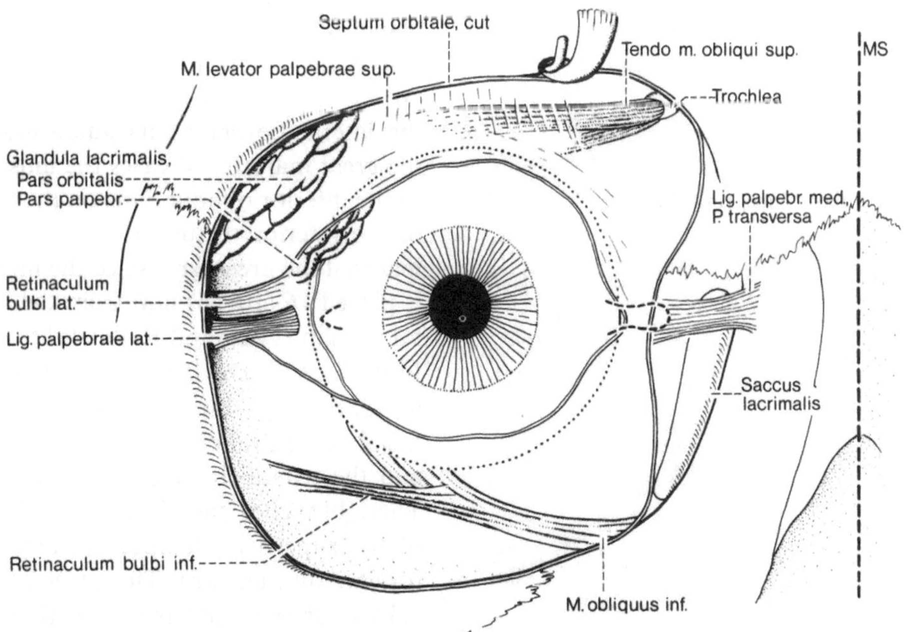

Fig. SA 13. Suspensory apparatus of the eye viewed from the front. Important structures include the lateral retinaculum, the inferior retinaculum, and the trochlear area (Lang 1988)

The difference of almost 4 mm makes it possible to displace the optic nerve laterally along with the globe without causing injury (Lang and Reiter 1985). According to Schürmann (personal communication 1986), the globe can be displaced so far laterally that the region of the orbital apex can be visualized from the medial aspect in an anterior orbitotomy.

The following anatomic points are important when *the orbit is entered from the maxillary sinus* (Fig. SA 14 a,b): In our material the floor of the orbit, or roof of the maxillary sinus, has a mean length of 38.4 (30.1–49.2) mm on the right side and 39.1 (31.1–45.8) mm on the left side (Lang and Papke 1984). The width of the anterior part of the maxillary sinus is 26.2 (16.4–37.9) mm on the right side and 26.9 (16.1–39.8) mm on the left side. The anterior part of the superior wall of the maxillary sinus is thickened. In the Caldwell-Luc procedure and other approaches, attention must be given to the course of the infraorbital sulcus and canal. In our material the infraorbital sulcus and canal have a mean width of 3.2 mm, and the anterior segment of the canal forms an angle of 24.3° with the midsagittal plane. Its outlet, the infraorbital foramen, is 4 (3–5.5) mm across. Medial to the infraorbital sulcus and canal, we determined an orbital floor thickness of about 0.37 (0.07–1.3) mm. A dehiscence in the inferior wall of the infraorbital sulcus or canal 3–11.2 mm long was noted on the right side in 12% of cases and on the left side in 15.4%. The orbital floor lateral to the infraorbital canal-sulcus was found to be 0.5 (0.09–1.1) mm thick (Lang and Papke 1984). The first structure encountered upon opening the orbital floor is the well-vascularized periorbita, followed generally by a thin layer of fat and then the muscles subjacent to the globe. In our material the inferior oblique muscle forms an angle of about 62° (50–78°) with the midsagittal plane. The inferior rectus muscle forms an angle of 21° (12.5–28°) with the midsagittal, while the medial rectus forms an average angle of 1.5° on the right side and 0.7° on the left side. The lateral rectus forms an angle of 44.5° (36–51°) with the midsagittal plane. The nerve to the inferior oblique runs below the inferior rectus in 7.1% of cases, especially on the right side. In 4.7% it follows the lateral border of its guide muscle, and in the great majority of cases the muscular branch to the inferior oblique runs on the upper surface of the inferior rectus to its destination. In our material the area nervosa of the inferior oblique is placed 16 (10–23) mm from the inferior orbital margin (Lang and Reiter 1985).

In the *lateral bony orbitotomy*, an effort is made to spare the orbicularis oculi muscle and the facial nerve branches which supply that muscle and the frontal belly of the epicranius muscle. These branches pass deep to the frontal branch of the superficial temporal artery and diverge forward and upward. The branch to the frontal belly courses within two lines that diverge forward and upward from the earlobe, the upper line passing to the frontal hairline and the lower

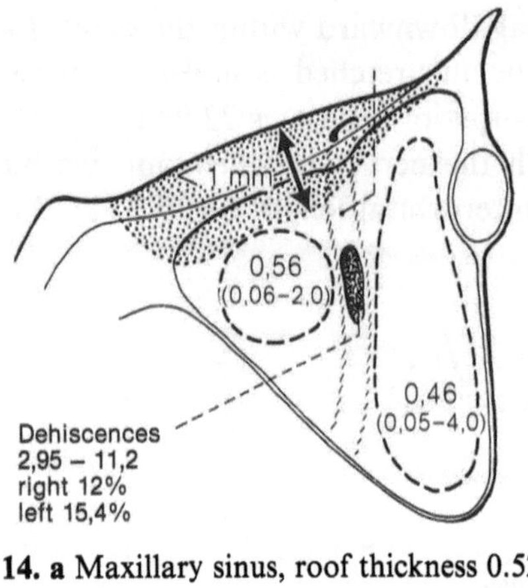

Fig. SA 14. a Maxillary sinus, roof thickness 0.52 (0.05–4.0) mm

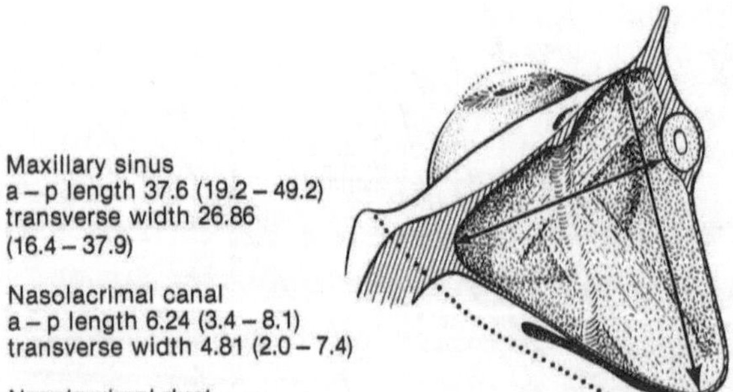

Fig. SA 14. b Length and width of the maxillary sinus, of the nasolacrimal canal, and of the nasolacrimal duct

line to the eyebrow (De Castro Correia and Zani 1973). We feel it is more important to preserve the function of the orbicularis oculi. A portion of its orbital fibers (which produce "laugh lines") enter the muscle superficially. The orbicularis oculi, including its palpebral part, is supplied from below by temporal and zygomatic branches of the facial nerve. These branches reach the zygomatic arch directly in front of the temporomandibular joint, from there diverging toward the outer canthus, lower lid, and inferior orbital margin. In our material we most commonly found 2 or 3 temporal branches and 2 (1–4) zygomatic branches. Besides the orbicularis oculi, the zygomatic branches also supply the greater and lesser zygomatic muscles, the levator labii superioris alaeque nasi, levator labii superioris, and occasionally the levator anguli oris. Like the temporal branches, they anastomose with branches of the trigeminal nerve (lacrimal nerve, zygomaticofacial nerve, infraorbital nerve).

It should be noted that the palpebral part of the orbicularis oculi is not only responsible for blinking and closure of the lids but also permits normal lacrimal drainage. Paralysis of the nerve leads to paralytic ectropion, and lacrimal drainage is impaired because the lacrimal point of the lower lid is no longer in contact with the lacrimal fluid (danger of corneal and conjunctival drying). Spastic ectropion, which is most common in younger patients, refers to a lower lid everted by conjunctival swelling or exophthalmos secondary to tonic spasm of the orbicularis oculi. Spastic entropion (inversion of the eyelid) can also occur, causing the ciliae to brush against the conjunctiva and cornea.

The operation of Krönlein (1889) as modified by Berke (1954) involves the removal of the lateral orbital wall. The skin is opened with an esthetically favorable incision that spares the nerves and vessels, and the periosteum at the lateral orbital margin (together with the orbicularis oculi) is reflected forward over the orbital rim. A saw cut is made into the lateral orbital margin, which is displaced outward and backward. The lateral orbital wall, which is thinned posteriorly, can be removed without difficulty. The temporal muscle is reflected posteriorly. The farther posteriorly the orbit is to be entered, the deeper the space becomes between the zygomatic arch and the lateral orbital wall. In our material the distance from the zygomatic arch to the lateral orbital wall is 14.2 (10.7–19.7) mm in neonates, 17.1 (10.5–29.9) mm in 4- to 5-year-olds, and 21.1 (10.8–35.5) mm in adults (Lang and Götzfried 1982). Fatty tissue is consistently found deep to and below the lateral orbital rim, adjacent to the bone, in our material (elderly individuals). The middle temporal vein and the anterior deep temporal arteries and nerve may be damaged in this approach. The inferior orbital fissure, covered over by the orbital muscle, is at the lower border of the path of the surgical approach. The width of this fissure is greatest anteriorly and laterally and equals 5.2 (1.8–16.3) mm in our adult material (Lang and Schlehahn 1981).

In some cases we observed a transition of intraorbital and temporal fat at the anterior edge of the inferior orbital fissure. Displacements of this fat, which Adachi (1904) termed "fat hernias", can contribute to a reduction of retroorbital fat and to postoperative enophthalmos. On average, the anterior end of the fissure extends to within 9.13 mm of the orbital margin in children 5 months to 2 years of age, and to within 11 mm in 12- to 14-year-olds. Adachi determined that this distance was 17.3 (9–21) mm in adults. Removal of the lateral orbital wall exposes the well-vascularized periorbita, which is most firmly adherent about the bony openings in the orbit. Below the periorbita or within its substance is the branch of the zygomatic nerve, which conveys secretory fibers to the lacrimal gland. We also find frequent anastomoses between the arteries in the region of the orbital floor and lacrimal artery in this area. Removal of the lateral orbital margin necessarily involves the retinaculum bulbi laterale and the area of attachment of the levator palpebrae superioris. The fat-filled premarginal recess lies in front of these structures and behind the orbital septum. The lacrimal gland presents anterosuperiorally along with the lacrimal nerve with its accompanying vessels. The zygomaticotemporal branch and its accompanying arteries may present inferiorly. With division of the periorbita, a thin layer of fat is usually encountered first, followed by the rectus bulbi lateralis. This muscle, supplied by the abducent nerve, is slightly more than 10 (5–15) mm wide at its midportion (Lang et al. 1980). Retraction of the muscle will permit attack upon any lesions that are inside the orbit. The entry zone of the abducent nerve fibers is placed well posteriorly. In our material the most anterior nerve fiber entered the muscle 30 (18–44) mm behind the lateral orbital margin. The nerve entry zone itself is 6.43 (3–10) mm long and lies 15 (8–21) mm from the inferior border of the optic canal (Lang and Reiter 1983). It is noteworthy that the branches of the ophthalmic artery anastomose with each other inside the orbit and also with branches of the middle meningeal artery and extracranial arterial branches.

In the *transfrontal intracranial approach to the orbit*, it is important to consider the vascularization of the dura mater and bony floor of the anterior cranial fossa, which is illustrated in Fig. SA 7. Figure SA 10 is also helpful in that it shows the mean and maximum extents of the paranasal sinuses in the orbital roof. We found in our material that when the orbit is unroofed completely (i.e., between the dacryon and the orbital frontomalar, see below), an area of 907.5 mm^2 (667–1133 mm^2) of the orbital roof region is exposed (Lang and Roth 1984). If the roof is removed only to the supraorbital margin and posteriorly to the center of the orbital opening of the optic canal, an area of 730 mm^2 (423–960 mm^2) is exposed. The distance from the center of the optic canal to the center of the superior orbital margin is 39.53 (32–45) mm in our material. It should be noted that the superior orbital margin is comparatively thick and should be spared due to the close proximity of the supraorbital nerves. For the intracranial approach to the lateral orbital region, we established a tangent between the "orbital frontomalar" (point where the frontozygomatic suture intersects the lateral orbital margin) and the lateral edge of the superior orbital fissure and midsagittal plane. In our material this angle is equal to 35° (25.5–52.0°). The lateral end of the superior orbital fissure is placed 34.32 mm from the orbital frontomalar on the right side and 34 (25–40) mm on the left side. At the junction of the orbital roof with the lateral orbital wall, we found a lateral depression 4.51 mm deep (0–7.5 mm) related to the lacrimal gland and separated from it by periorbita. We identified this area as the fossa of the lacrimal gland. The first structure encountered on removal of the orbital roof is the periorbita. It is composed of collagen fibers, which are arranged most densely around the bony orifices of the orbital cavity (optic canal, superior orbital fissure, etc.). The outer capillary plexus of the periorbita anastomoses with cranial vessels, while its inner plexus consists of a peculiar capillary type having vascular connections with the orbital contents (Lang 1975). In addition, arteries and veins of the orbit traverse the periorbita and skull and anastomose with branches of the meningeal vessels and external carotid artery. Incision of the periorbita exposes a fatty layer of variable thickness that is thought to enhance the mobility of the globe (Lang 1975). This layer may be reflected to uncover the frontal nerve and its branches. It is known that the frontal nerve enters the orbit through the superior orbital fissure above and lateral to the tendinous ring and initially runs forward, usually in a parasagittal direction. In our material the nerve was most commonly found at about the medial third of the levator palpebrae superioris. Generally the first branch of the nerve is the supratrochlear, which arises from its medial side and runs forward above the trochlea of the superior oblique muscle. The supratrochlear nerve originates about 19 (0–44) mm rostral to the plane of the inferior border of the optic canal and is much smaller than the frontal nerve, for which we determined a mean transverse diameter of 2.57 (1.0–5.0) mm (Lang and Reiter 1987) (Fig. SA 15). Distal to the origin of the supratrochlear, the larger prolongation of the frontal nerve continues on as the supraorbital nerve. This divides into a medial branch which passes through the frontal notch or foramen to the skin of the forehead, and a lateral branch which ascends to the scalp through the supraorbital notch or foramen. The mean length of the frontal nerve and supraorbital nerve to its point of initial division into branches, measured from the inferior

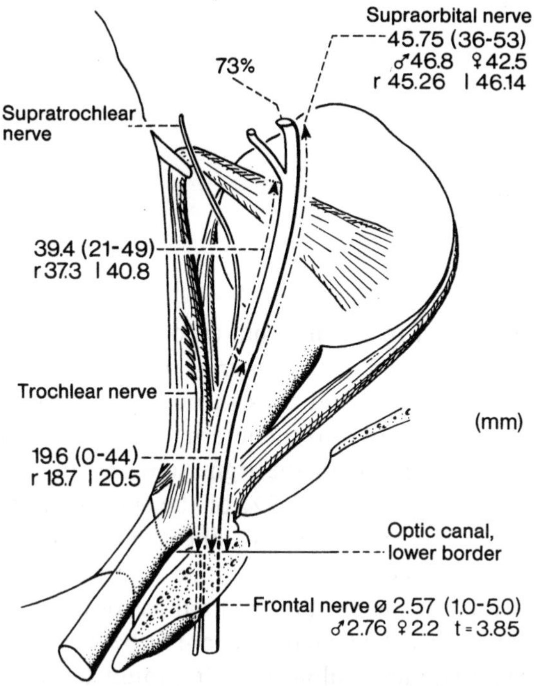

Fig. SA 15. Length of the intraorbital segment of the frontal nerve, origin of the supratrochlear nerve and supraorbital nerve. The trochlear nerve is also pictured. Mean and extreme values are stated in mm along with sex differences and left-right differences. All lengths are measured from the lower border of the optic canal (from Lang and Reiter 1987)

Fig. SA 16. Orbital apex, location of muscular origins, and entry sites of nerves and arteries. The most common exit site for the ophthalmic vein is indicated by *solid lines*; other potential exit sites are indicated by *hatched lines*

border of the orbital opening of the optic canal, is 45.7 (36–53) mm. The textbook pattern of nerve division was confirmed in slightly more than 73% of our specimens. In 22% the supraorbital nerve ramified into three branches, and in 2.3% into four branches. The lacrimal nerve courses in the far lateral part of the superior orbital wall. We determined its length (again measured from the inferior border of the optic canal) to be 37.88 (31–47) mm. This nerve generally arises from the ophthalmic nerve while still in the lateral wall of the cavernous sinus and then enters the orbit lateral to and slightly below the frontal nerve (see Lang 1979). It should be noted that supraorbital and frontal foramina were found as much as 4.5 mm above the supraorbital margin in our youngest material (Lang and Reiter 1987). In several specimens we found nerve exit sites 3 cm above the supraorbital margin.

The trochlear nerve takes an intracisternal course of 32.65 (20–42) mm. Then, accompanied by an arachnoid sheath (Lang 1974), the nerve pierces the dura below the free border of the cerebellar tentorium in 20% and anterior to it in 80%. Then it passes forward and downward in the lateral wall of the cavernous sinus. Before entering the orbit it crosses over the oculomotor nerve and then passes to the upper surface of the superior oblique muscle. Sites of nerve entry and muscle origins at the orbital apex are shown in Fig. SA 16.

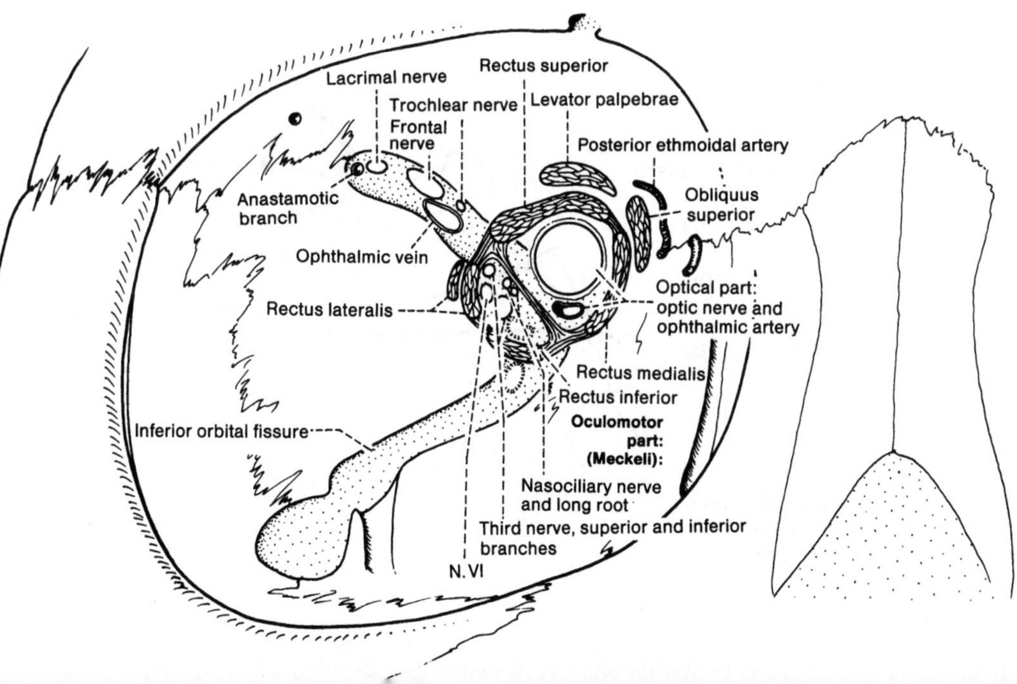

Anatomy of the Cavernous Sinus

(Figs. SA 17, SA 18)

Parkinson (1965) described an approach to the cavernous part of the internal carotid artery through a triangular area ("Parkinson's triangle") bounded superiorly by the trochlear nerve, posteriorly by the rim of the clivus (posterior petroclinoid fold), and inferiorly by the upper border of the ophthalmic nerve. It is noteworthy that the trigeminal ganglion is frequently placed above the upper border of this nerve in our material. The length of artery accessible through Parkinson's triangle will vary somewhat with the individual vascular anatomy. Using the definition of Parkinson's triangle given by Harris and Rhoton (1976), we were able to identify the feature in only 31.4% of our material. Assuming that a safe approach to the internal carotid artery through Parkinson's triangle requires a minimum width of 4 mm between the ophthalmic nerve and trochlear nerve (to avoid damage to adjacent nerves), we found that this criterion was satisfied in 35% of cases on the right side and in 24% on the left side. However, it must be considered that the abducent nerve runs lateral to the internal carotid artery. This nerve passes above the superior pole of the trigeminal ganglion, and thus through the route of surgical approach to the internal carotid artery, in 16% of cases on the right side and in 23% on the left side. In 13.5% of the specimens examined, nerves IV and V_1 and the ophthalmic nerve ran so close together that it appeared impossible to reach the internal carotid artery either below the trochlear nerve or between that nerve and the oculomotor. It should be noted that the position of the cranial nerves may be altered in the presence of an AV shunt or aneurysm in the cavernous sinus. Moreover, attention need not be given to the aforementioned cranial nerves if they are already damaged, and the internal carotid artery may be approached without concern. In cases where the carotid arteries take a relatively straight course in the cavernous sinus (14.7%), Parkinson's triangle may lie well above the internal carotid artery. Finally it should be noted that the internal carotid gives off 2–6 small arteries that may be ruptured in

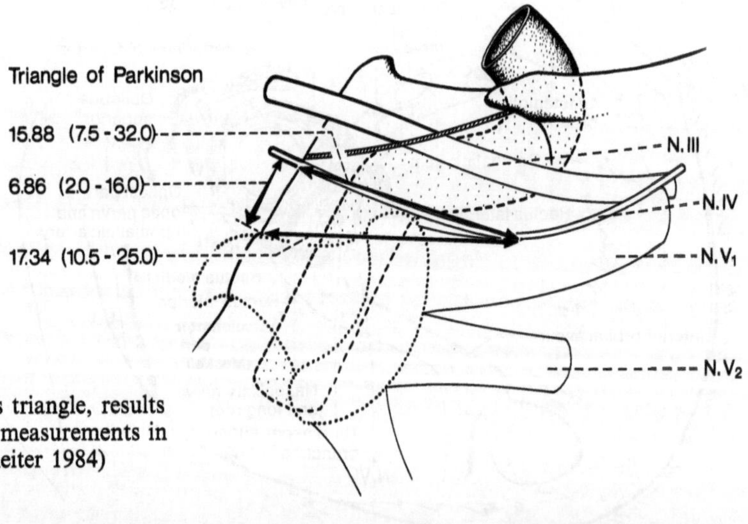

Fig. SA 17. Parkinson's triangle, results of our dissections and measurements in mm (after Lang and Reiter 1984)

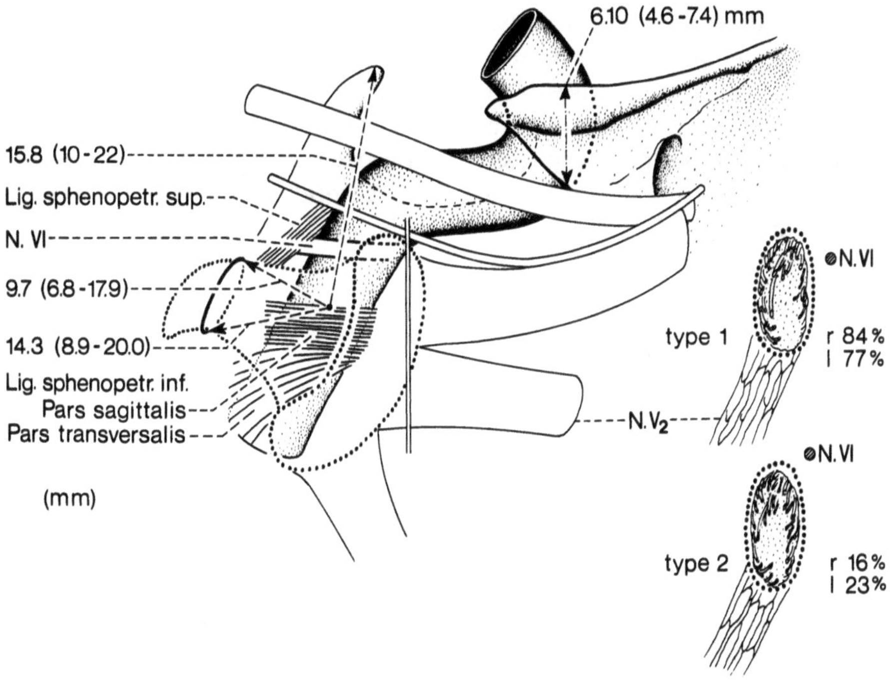

Fig. SA 18. Nerves in the area of Parkinson's triangle and the course of the abducent nerve to the superior pole of the trigeminal ganglion. Dissections and measurements by Lang and Strobel (1978) and Lang and Reiter (1984)

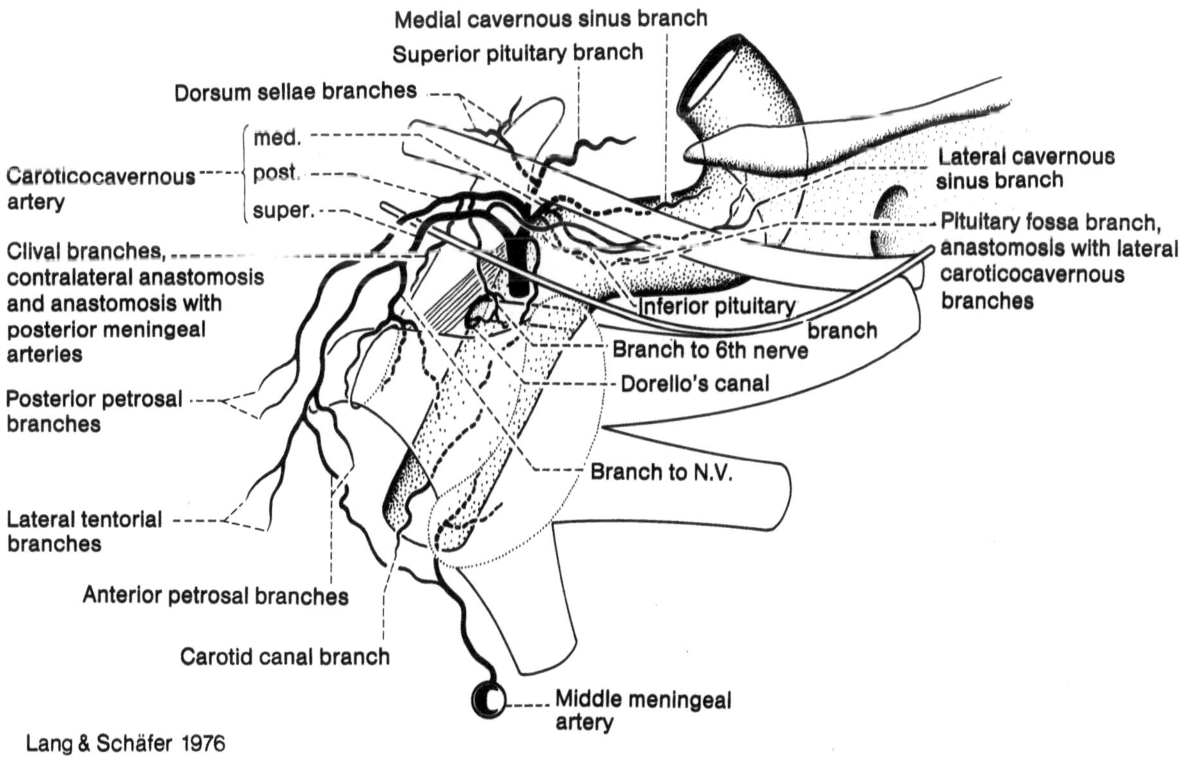

Fig. SA 19. Posterior caroticocavernous trunk and its branches. Branches to the trigeminal ganglion and anastomoses with the middle meningeal artery are shown skull trauma (Lang and Schäfer 1976). However, the vessel that we identified as the posterior caroticocavernous trunk usually arises from the posterior cavernous curvature of the internal carotid artery and gives off the pituitary fossa branches and other branches in addition to the inferior pituitary artery (see Fig. SA 19). The caroticocavernous trunk lies in the path of the surgical approach through Parkinson's triangle. Koos et al. (1985) point out that 14% of "giant aneurysms" (which are rare) involve the internal carotid artery. They described an anterior approach to the anterior sinus genu of the internal carotid artery that involves removing the anterior clinoid process and opening the cavernous sinus in that area.

Anatomy of the Sellar Region

The *transseptal transsphenoidal approach to the pituitary* is made through the nasal septum, whose mucosa and periosteum are stripped on only one side if possible to avoid atrophic rhinopathy. Figure SA 20 (from Lang and Baumeister) presents data on the size of the piriform aperture, at whose lower border the anterior nasal spine can be removed. In several studies we have determined the distance between the zone below the anterior nasal spine (subspinal zone) to the aperture of the sphenoid sinus, finding a mean value of 53.7 (43–64) mm in adults. The arteries of the nasal septum are shown in Fig. SA 21 (from Lang 1985). The anterior inferior part of the nasal septum is generally supplied by the anterior inferior septal branch of the superior labial artery (Lang and Schulz 1985).

Adjacent to that is the area of anastomosis between the posterior septal branch of the sphenopalatine artery and the great palatine artery. The anastomosis passes through the incisive canal to the lateral surface of the septum. In adults this zone lies 11.6 (8–18) mm behind the subspinal zone (see above). The sphenopalatine artery, the terminal branch of the maxillary, gives off septal branches which pass to the nasal septum from behind and above (in the area of the anterior wall of the sphenoid sinus). This zone is consistently located in front of the posterior border of the septum (Lang and Schäfer 1979).

The veins of the nasal septum accompany the nasal arteries to adjacent larger veins. The lymphatics of the nasal septum run backward and laterally in the direction of the lateral pharyngeal wall to the area of the pharyngeal ostium of the auditory tube and to the soft palate (route for metastases!). The nasal septum is supplied by branches of the ethmoidal nerves superiorly and also by the nasopalatine nerve (of Scarpa) from the maxillary. Frequently this nerve occupies a groove in the vomer and, like the posterior septal branches of the sphenopalatine artery, follows a posterosuperior-to-anteroinferior course. The nerve is joined in its course by sympathetic and parasympathetic fibers from the sphenopalatine ganglion. The upper part of the nasal septum includes a portion of the olfactory area, which according to Smith (1941) occupies an area of 133.99 mm^2 on one side. Smith noted that the olfactory area diminishes in size with increasing age.

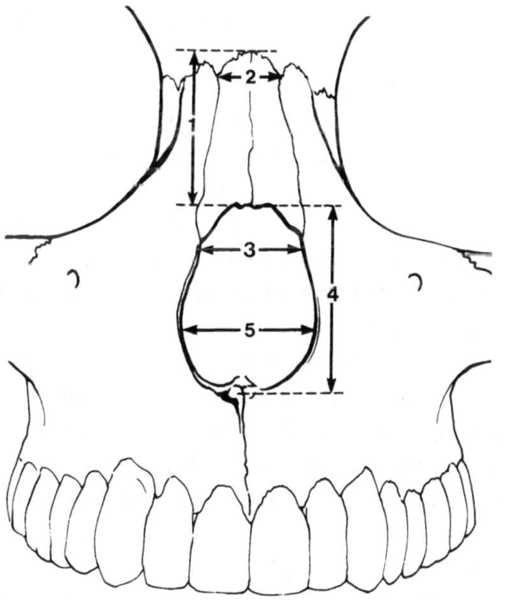

Nasal bones						Piriform aperture			
1 Length		2 Superior width		3 Inferior width		4 Height		5 Maximum width	
Newborn	8.33	Newborn	8.38	Newborn	9.75	Newborn	11.33	Newborn	12.38
2 years	13.63	2 years	11.25	2 years	12.17	2 years	18.14	2 years	17.00
5 years	16.19	5 years	11.42	5 years	13.29	5 years	22.59	5 years	18.20
Adult	24.87	Adult	13.02	Adult	16.30	Adult	29.08	Adult	23.63

Fig. SA 20. Nasal bones and piriform aperture, postnatal growth (mean values in mm from Lang and Baumeister 1982)

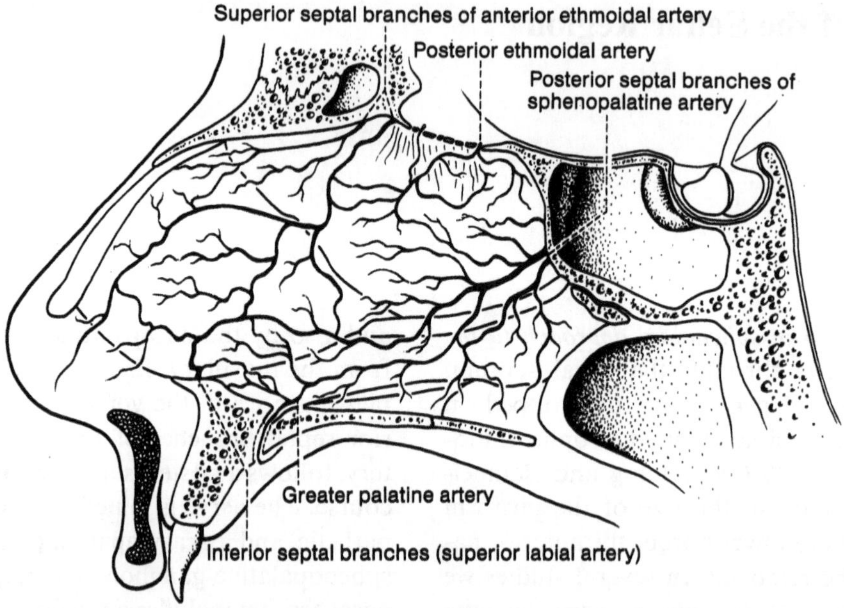

Fig. SA 21. Arteries of the mucosa of the nasal septum, viewed from the medial aspect with the cartilaginous and bony parts of the septum removed (Lang 1988)

In our material we identified a well-developed sphenoethmoidal recess (containing the ostium of the sphenoid sinus) in only 48.3% of adults (Lang and Sakals 1981). We observed rounded sinus apertures with a relatively small diameter in 70% and pinhead-sized apertures in 15%. The apertures were oval in 28%, usually with their greater diameter directed vertically. Fahlbusch (personal communication) states that the aperture is the site of choice for entering the sphenoid sinus.

Numerous studies confirm the variability in the dimensions of the sphenoid sinus (for details see Lang 1985 and Figs. SA 22–SA 25). The sinus is occupied by septa which show extreme variations in their shape, size, and orientation. Fujii et al. (1980) measured the distance between the aperture of the sphenoid sinus and the floor of the sella, finding a mean value of 17.1 (12–23) mm. We determined a value of 14.3 (9–21) mm for this distance in our material. Data on the sinus dimensions are presented in Fig. SA 22. Following removal of the sphenoid sinus mucosa, the anterior part of the floor of the sella (which varies greatly in thickness) is removed. The next structure to be encountered is the endocranial layer of the pituitary fossa. Several branches of the inferior pituitary artery may traverse the floor of the sella and contribute to the vascular supply of the sphenoid body and the sphenoid sinus mucosa. The endocranial layer may be adjoined by blood-filled channels of variable shape (the intercavernous sinuses) that contains branches of the inferior pituitary artery. The last intervening structure before the pituitary itself is the pituitary capsule. Hardy (1969) found that the anterior lobe of the pituitary is enclosed by a potential space between the pituitary capsule and endocranial stratum. In our material we found a two-layered pituitary capsule drained by inferior pituitary veins (Lang 1985). Hardy further determined that the anterior pituitary lobe has a yellowish color and a relatively firm consistency which contrast with the grayish color and softer, gelatinous consistency of the posterior lobe. The posterior lobe is also more firmly attached to the back wall of the pituitary fossa than the anterior lobe is to its surroundings. Hardy states that in operations on the pituitary the posterior lobe can be distinguished from the anterior lobe by the numerous colloidal follicles and venous

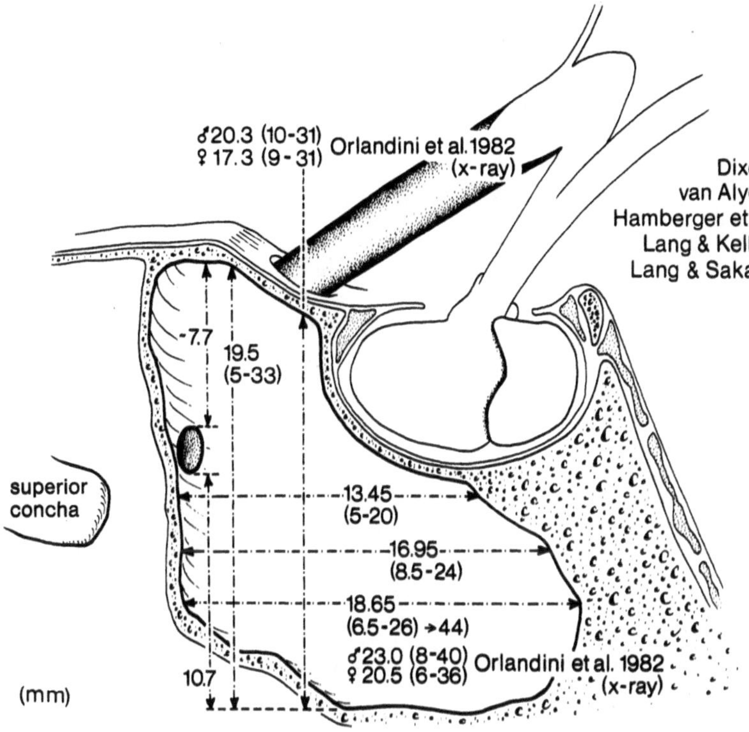

Fig. SA 22. Data from various authors on the dimensions of the sphenoid sinus and the most common location of its aperture

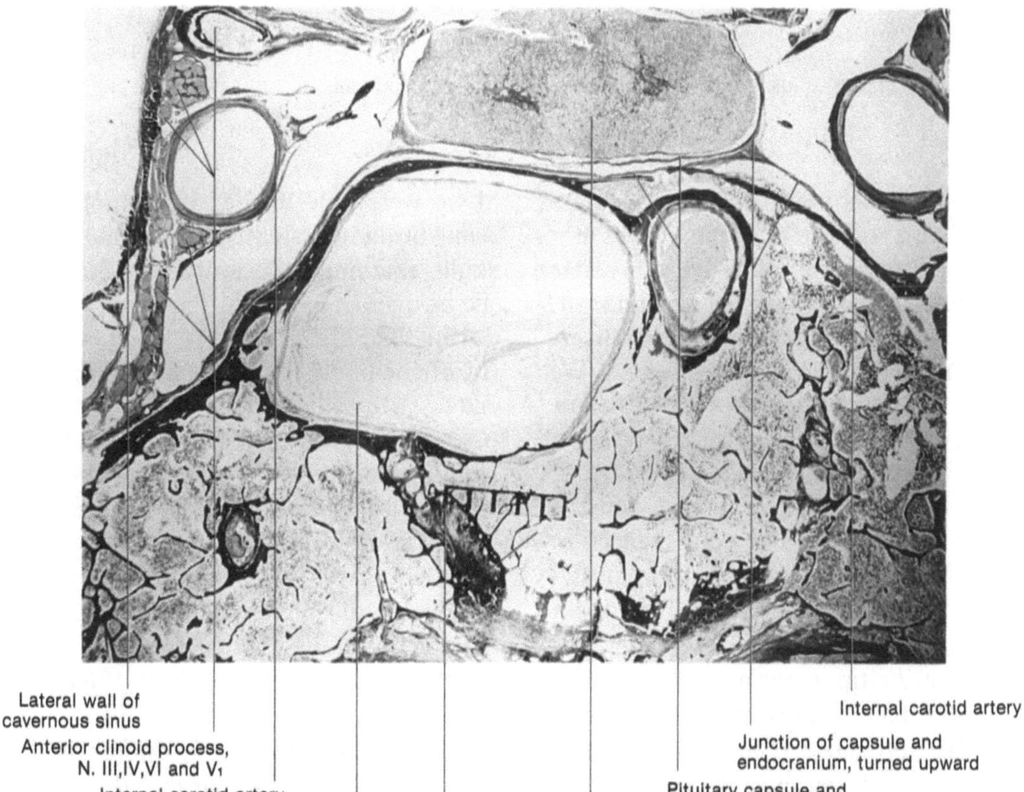

Fig. SA 23. Pituitary and cavernous sinus, coronal section, 50 years of age (Ladewig)

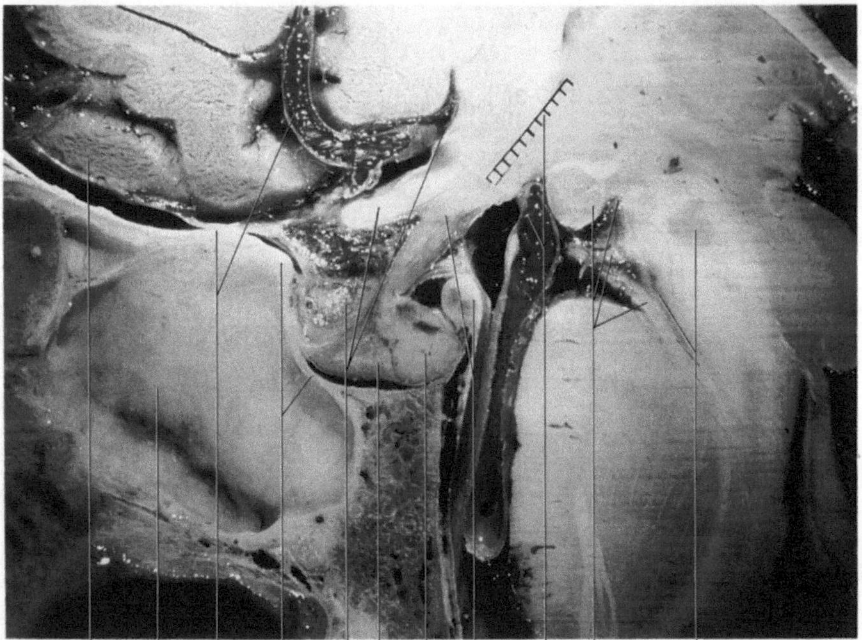

Fig. SA 24. Pituitary region, midsagittal section viewed from the medial side

capillary areas which mark the intermediate lobe of the gland. In our material it was not unusual to find rarefaction of the dorsum sellae as well as connections between the posterior intercavernous sinus (or an inferior intercavernous sinus) and the basilar venous plexus. We also demonstrated penetrating branches of the inferior pituitary artery on the clivus. Rarefaction of the floor of the pituitary fossa is quite rare.

In 1977 we first described a *sellar spine* in the skull of a 23-year-old man. The bony projection was 4.35 mm long and extended from the posterior aspect of the pituitary fossa into the fossa and thence into the gland. The spine was 1.25 mm thick at its tip, tapering posteriorly to 0.6 mm. It may have represented the ossified remains of the notochord (Lang 1977). Sellar bridges (bony bars uniting the anterior and posterior clinoid processes) occur on the lateral border of the pituitary fossa in 5%–7% of cases (Müller 1952; Platzer 1957; etc.). In our material we were able to identify complete, bilateral sellar bridges in slightly more than 2.4% of the skulls examined. Sutural zones in the area of the bridges suggest that the structures appeared during fetal life.

Caroticoclinoid foramina are commonly associated with sellar bridges. They are formed by osseous bridges which pass between the anterior clinoid process and a middle clinoid process, creating apertures for the internal carotid artery that may be complete or interrupted by small clefts (Lang 1977). The angle of these foramina relative to the planes of the head is extremely variable. (Details may be found in Hochstetter 1940; Neiss 1956; Bergerhoff 1960; Reinbach 1963; and Lang 1977.)

According to Arey (1950, quoted in Lowman et al. 1966), a craniopharyngeal canal exists in 0.42% of adults. The superior opening is in the lowest part of the sella turcica and is 1–1.5 mm in diameter.

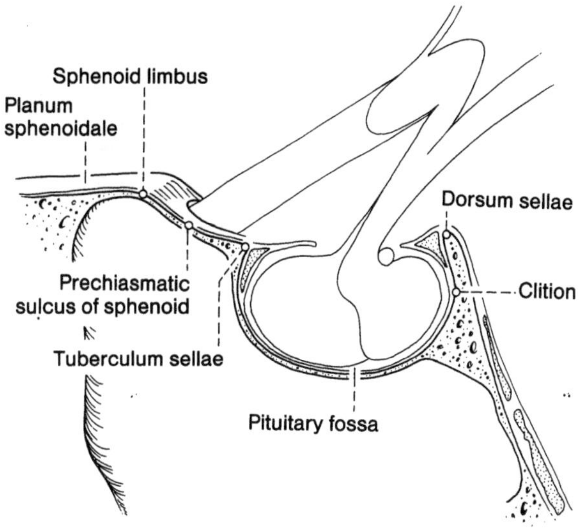

Fig. SA 25. Bony structures of the pituitary region

In the material of Renn and Rhoton (1975), the floor of the sella has a mean width of 14 (10–16) mm. Taveras and Wood (1964) report a range of 10 to 15 mm. In our material the maximum width of the pituitary fossa is 3–7.5 mm behind the tuberculum sellae. The left border of the fossa is lower than the right in 60% of cases, while the right is lower than the left in 35%. In approximately 4% the right and left borders are of equal height (Lang and Tisch-Rottensteiner 1977). In adults the sellar floor is placed 13.2 (−2.3 to +21.3) mm above the Frankfurt horizontal plane (Lang and Schäfer 1977).

In our material (Lang 1973) we identified a *pituitary cistern* (Fig. SA 24) measuring up to 8 mm wide and 3 mm deep, which extended below the sellar diaphragm to the anterior lobe of the pituitary. A dorsal expansion of the cistern was evident in some specimens. Bergland et al. (1968) found pituitary cisterns in about 20% of their material. Shealy et al. (1968) in particular noted the presence of loose arachnoidal tissue in this region.

As the pituitary body becomes smaller (with age), the pituitary cistern increases in volume and size until an "empty sella" appears. Other authors assume that a large diaphragmatic foramen and diaphragma sellae must be present in order for an "empty sella" to occur. A median sagittal section demonstrates some anthropological points (Fig. SA 25).

The *diaphragma sellae* (Fig. SA 26) extends from the tuberculum sellae to the posterior clinoid processes. In our material we observed longitudinal and oblique fibers of dura mater (passing laterally backward) in the anterior and lateral portions of the diaphragma sellae and transverse fibers along its posterior border. The diaphragmatic foramen itself is surrounded by circular fibers. Renn and Rhoton (1975) state that the diaphragma sellae is as thick as the dura in 38% of cases and extremely thin in 62%. In the transsphenoidal approach to the pituitary, it is thin enough to be easily injured in 10% of patients. Shealy et al. (1968) even claimed that the diaphragma sellae consisted only of arachnoidal tissue in 65% of cases, but we dispute this assertion on the basis of studies in our own material. Renn and Rhoton (1975) report that the diaphragma sellae has a mean width of 11 (6–15) mm and a mean length of 8 (5–13) mm.

According to McLachlan et al. (1968), the diaphragma sellae is attached anteriorly to the tuberculum sellae and posteriorly to the forepart of the posterior clinoid process and dorsum sellae. The most common site of attachment is on the anterior border of the dorsum and less commonly on its apex. According to Joplin (1965, quoted in McLachlan 1968) the diaphragma is elevated about 5–8 mm from the bone posterior to the sphenoidal limbus (= anterior border of prechiasmatic sulcus).

Bergland and coworkers (1968) report that the *diaphragmatic foramen* has a diameter of 5 mm or more in older individuals. Renn and Rhoton

Table 1. Mean width of the floor of the sella (mean length = 11.64 mm) (from Lang and Tisch-Rottensteiner 1976)

From the tuberculum sellae to a point – mm behind the tuberculum sellae	1.5 mm	10.33 mm
	1.5–3 mm	11.85 mm
	3.0–4.5 mm	12.73 mm
	4.5–6.0 mm	12.53 mm
	6.0–7.5 mm	12 mm
	7.5–9.0 mm	11.20 mm
	9.0–10.5 mm	11.24 mm
	10.5–12.0 mm	10.70 mm

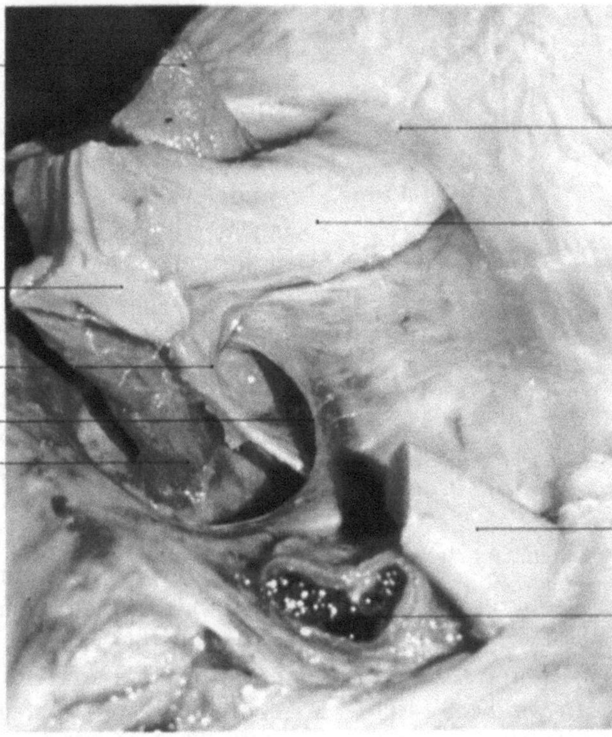

Fig. SA 26. Diaphragma sellae and arachnoid, superior oblique view from the right side

(1975) found that the foramen was round in 54% and had a transverse oval shape in 46%. The foramen enlarges with age. Besides the infundibulum, the diaphragmatic foramen is traversed by the superior pituitary arteries (which rarely may pierce the diaphragma itself) and by arachnoidal tissue. The superior pituitary arteries arise in most cases from the medial aspect of the internal carotid artery in the transition area between the cavernous and the subarachnoid parts. Usually there are two and occasionally one, three, or four of these vessels, which run backward and upward to the undersurface of the optic chiasm and then pass down along the infundibulum to the diaphragma sellae. Generally they form a plexus around the infundibulum. A posterior superior pituitary artery may also be present. In our material we found additional superior pituitary arteries which originated from the posterior communicating artery, supplied the tuber cinereum, and established fairly large anastomoses with the superior pituitary artery or its branches.

Bruneton et al. (1979) determined the morphologic variants of the *tuberculum sellae*-sella turcica junction that are important in the *transcranial intradural approach to the sellar region.* They found that the junction was rounded in 27% of cases and sharp-edged in 24.5%. The tuberculum was rounded in 20.5%, angular in 15.5%, and pointed in 4.5%. Flat junctions were found in 1%. The distance between the anterior border of the *prechiasmatic sulcus* and tuberculum sellae does not increase remarkably during postnatal life. We determined values of 6.14 mm in neonates and 6.8 (3.3–10.3) mm in adults. The distance between the foramen cecum and tuberculum sellae is an important consideration in the frontal route of approach to that region. This distance increased slightly from the neonatal period to adulthood. We measured distances of 37.75 (32–41) mm in one-year-olds as compared with 42.57 (28–50) mm in adults. Age-related changes in the cribriform plate dimensions (Fig. SA 27) are remarkable. This plate has a mean length of 23.2 (21–25.5) mm

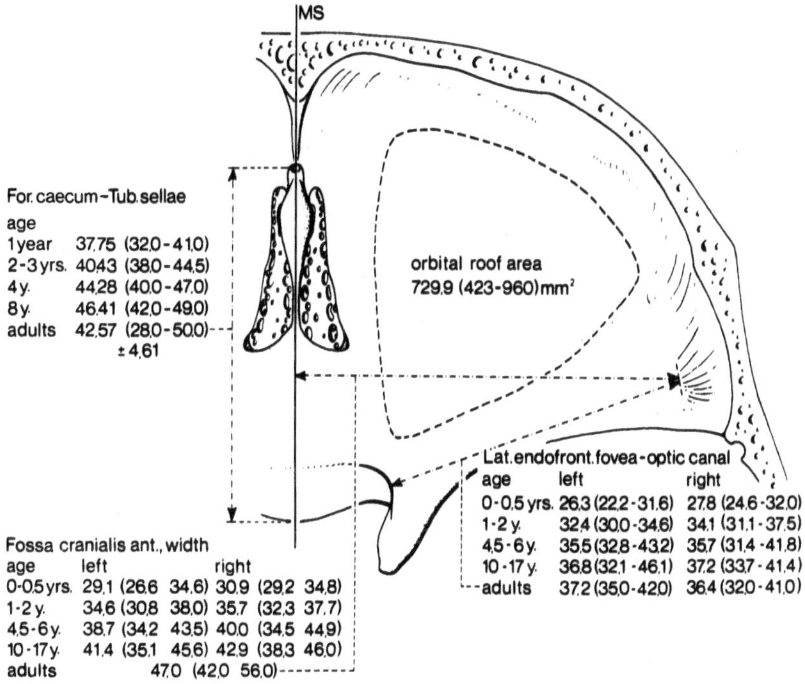

Fig. SA 27. Dimensions of the anterior cranial fossa: postnatal increase in the distance between the foramen cecum and tuberculum sellae, width of the anterior fossa, distance between the lateral border of the optic canal and the lateral endofrontal fovea and orbital roof below the floor of the anterior fossa. All values were taken from measurements in the Wurzburg material and are expressed in mm (range)

up to one year of age and in subsequent years attains a length of up to 27.78 (25–34) mm. By adulthood the mean value is only 20.8 (15.5–25.8) mm. The shortening of the cribriform plate after eight years of age is probably due to the fact that the planum sphenoidale (extending from the posterior rim of the cribriform plate to the anterior edge of the prechiasmatic sulcus) lengthens after the neonatal period and increasingly overlaps the posterior border of the cribriform plate. The courses of nerves and blood vessels (from the posterior ethmoidal artery) lend support to this concept.

In approaching the optic nerve and infundibulum, attention must be given to the relatively thick arachnoid membrane between the intracranial opening of the optic canal and the arachnoid of the anterior cranial fossa. Medially adjacent is the anterior wall of the chiasmatic cistern and farther upward the anterior wall of the cistern of the lamina terminalis. When pituitary neoplasms, craniopharyngiomas, and other lesions in this area are approached surgically, an effort is made to spare the anterior cerebral arteries and the anterior communicating artery and its central branches. The anterior cerebral artery (A1 segment) is 13.5 (8–18.5) mm long in our material and 2.1 (0.75–3.75) mm in diameter. Both vessels show considerable variation in caliber. Wollschläger et al. (1967) reported finding hypoplastic cerebral arteries in 8.6% of their material (about 4% on the left side and more than 3% bilaterally). The anterior cerebral artery may pass above the optic chiasm or optic nerve, and its course may be curved or relatively straight.

The anterior communicating artery (Fig. SA 28) conforms to the textbook description in about 75% of cases (von Mitterwallner 1955). In about 25% of cases the artery is duplicated, V-shaped, or reticulated. Perlmutter and Rhoton (1976) determined a mean length of 2.6 (0.3–7.0) mm for the vessel. We have examined the central branches of the anterior cerebral artery and anterior communicating artery in some detail. The branches arising from the proximal part of the

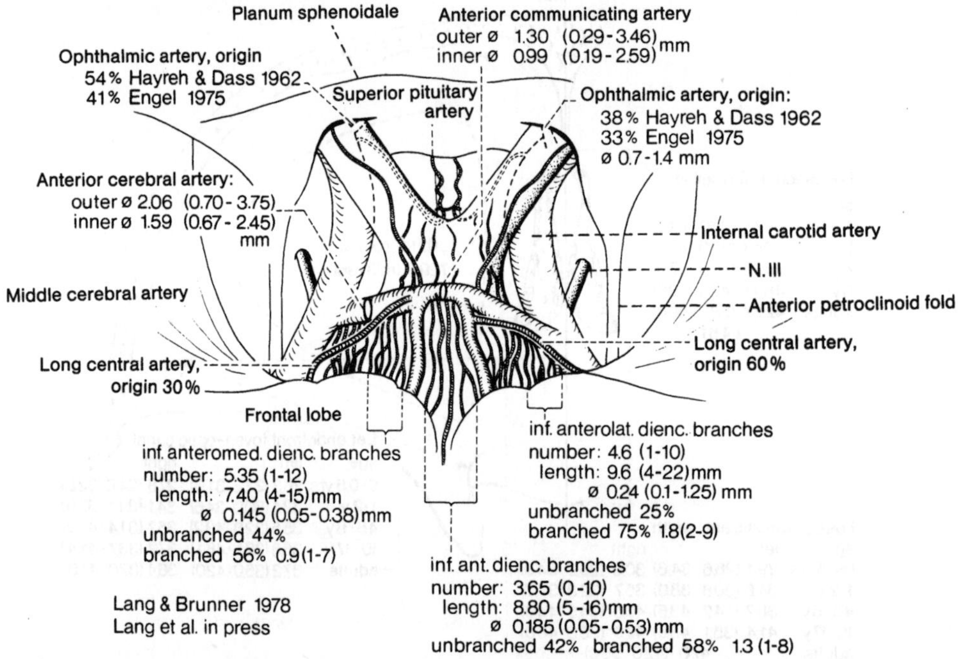

Fig. SA 28. Anterior inferior diencephalic branches, results of our previous and current investigations. The number, extracerebral length, width, and cerebral branching of these small branches are indicated

A1 segment pass to the anterior perforated substance. The smaller branches arising from the distal A1 segment and from the anterior communicating artery supply anterior portions of the diencephalon; we call these the anterior inferior diencephalic branches. The anterior recurrent artery ("long central artery" of Heubner) has a mean width of 0.57 mm in our material and is duplicated in 30%. It arises from the anterior cerebral artery within a zone between 8 mm proximal and 3 mm distal to the anterior communicating artery. On average, the origin of the vessel is 0.4 mm distal to the anterior communicating artery. A distal origin is the rule, occurring in about 60% of cases. The vessel arises at the level of the anterior communicating artery in 30% and proximal to it in 11.3% (Lang and Brunner 1978). Remarkably, we found that the long central artery had a significantly larger diameter on the left side (0.60 mm) than on the right side (0.54 mm).

Besides the frontal approach to the *pituitary region*, the *frontolateral approach* may also be used. The key landmark for this approach is the frontotemporal point or most medial portion of the temporal line. This point cannot be accurately defined from outside the skull, so we determine the level of the lateral endofrontal fovea above the zygomaticofrontal suture, which is always visible. In our material this feature lies 17.8 (11–26) mm above the zygomaticofrontal suture in adults. Burr holes at this site will penetrate the skull just above the floor of the anterior cranial fossa. The distance between the opened part of the anterior fossa and the lateral edge of the intracranial opening of the optic canal is approximately 45 mm in our material. These approaches are used for operations on the anterior communicating artery, the anterior cerebral arteries, and the tumors previously mentioned. In cases where the tumor has grown between the two optic nerves or originates from the pituitary, the spacing of the two intracranial openings of the optic canals becomes an important surgical concern (see Fig. SA 12). Access to the infundibulum and its surroundings is more difficult when the openings are spaced close together than when they are farther apart. The intracranial length of the optic nerve is also significant: the longer the nerve, the more posterior the position of the optic chiasm. Therefore we determined the intracranial length of the optic nerve on both the medial and lateral sides as well as the distance of the optic chiasm from the tuberculum sellae. Additional measurements are shown in Fig. SA 27. In our material the infundibulum forms an angle of 121° (90–160°) with the FHP. It should be added that the extreme values in that range are very uncommon. Unusually large carotid arteries, ophthalmic arteries, or anterior cerebral arteries can cause compressive injury to the optic nerve. Decompression is effected in these cases by dividing the dural layer over the optic canal, which may be up to 8 mm long, and then unroofing the canal.

Anatomy of the Temporal Fossa

(Fig. SA 29)

The temporal fossa is the area on the side of the cranium from which the temporal muscle arises. The skin over this area is relatively thin and derives its blood supply from branches of the superficial temporal artery. It is drained chiefly by the superficial temporal vein. The temporal fossa is relatively flat in its superior portion and deepens inferiorly. Its lower border, which we call the infratemporal crest, is marked by several tubercles. The temporal fossa is bridged by the zygomatic arch, whose posterior (larger) root arises from the temporal squama and whose anterior root is formed by the zygomatic process of the zygoma. The temporal muscle is covered laterally by the temporal fascia, upon which course the superficial temporal vessels and the auriculotemporal nerve and its branches; these are adherent to the outer border of the zygomatic arch. From the area of the articular tubercle of the temporomandibular joint, branches of the facial nerve are distributed to the frontal belly of the epicranius muscle and to the orbicularis oculi (temporal branches of the facial nerve). The bony part of the temporal fossa is formed anteriorly by the zygomatic bone, somewhat more posteriorly by the greater wing of the sphenoid, and still farther posteriorly by the temporal squama. But the upper margin of the temporal muscle is applied to the squama of the frontal bone and to the parietal bone. Its most anterior fibers pass downward and backward at about a 10° angle (to the masticatory plane), and the adjacent fibers descend in an almost vertical line. The posterior fibers of the muscle converge forward and downward, and the most posterior fibers pass almost horizontally to their sites of attachment on the lateral and medial surfaces of the coronoid process. The deep portion of the muscle, which arises partly from the infratemporal plane of the skull, possesses a strong tendon that extends to the retromolar trigone. This tendon is easily palpated from within the oral cavity. Below the temporal fascia is the temporal aponeurosis (deep layer of the temporal fascia), which covers the temporal muscle and is attached to the medial surface of the zygomatic arch. Most of the temporal fibers arise from the temporal plane, and a few (constituting the superficial part) arise from the temporal aponeurosis. This fiber arrangement imparts a plumose structure to the muscle. A deep fiber group arises from the infratemporal plane. Most of the temporal fibers become tendinous while still above the zygomatic arch (see Fig. SA 30). The middle temporal vein, highly variable in its course and caliber, courses upon the muscle fibers which arise from this area and from the temporal aponeurosis. The temporal muscle is innervated by the anterior, middle, and posterior deep temporal nerves. These branches of the trigeminal run laterally in various directions on the infratemporal plane and pass around the infratemporal crest before entering the temporal muscle. It is believed that trauma to the nerves of the temporalis can be minimized by mobilizing the muscle from the anterior aspect. The muscle derives its blood supply from the deep temporal arteries, which spring from various branches on the external carotid and maxillary.

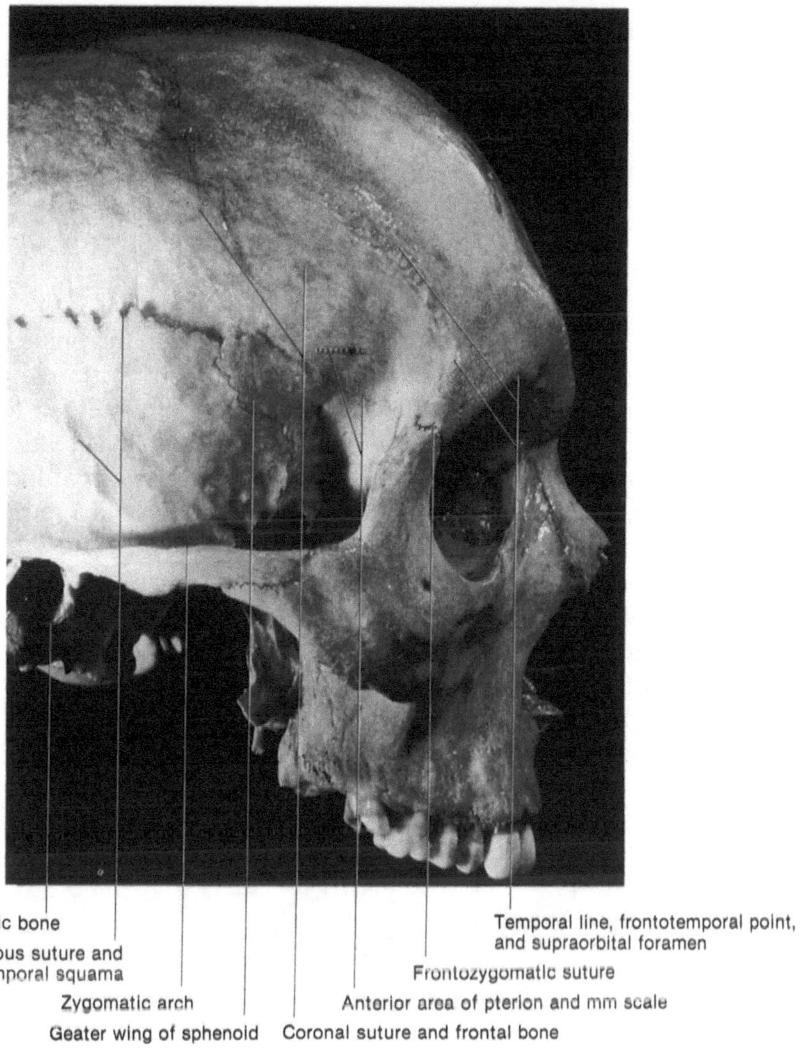

Fig. SA 29. Temporal fossa and surrounding structures

Anatomy of the Infratemporal Fossa and Infratemporal Plane

(Fig. SA 30)

The infratemporal crest, lateral pterygoid plate, and coronoid process of the mandible outline an approximately flat area on the external skull base. Its most anterior portion includes the inferior orbital fissure, the maxillary tuber, and the sphenomaxillary fissure, which marks the lateral approach to the pterygopalatine fossa. The upper margin of the inferior orbital fissure frequently bulges downward. Immediately behind it is a groove, followed fairly consistently by an infratemporal spine that is continuous with a small roof posterolaterally. This area is the infratemporal crest. When the temporal muscle is damaged, it should be considered that the muscle exerts an adducting force of 353 N on the mandible and a retractile force of 98 N (posterior fibers; Schumacher 1961). It exerts only 29.4 N of tension medially and 19.6 N anteriorly (for details see Lang in Lanz/Wachsmuth 1985).

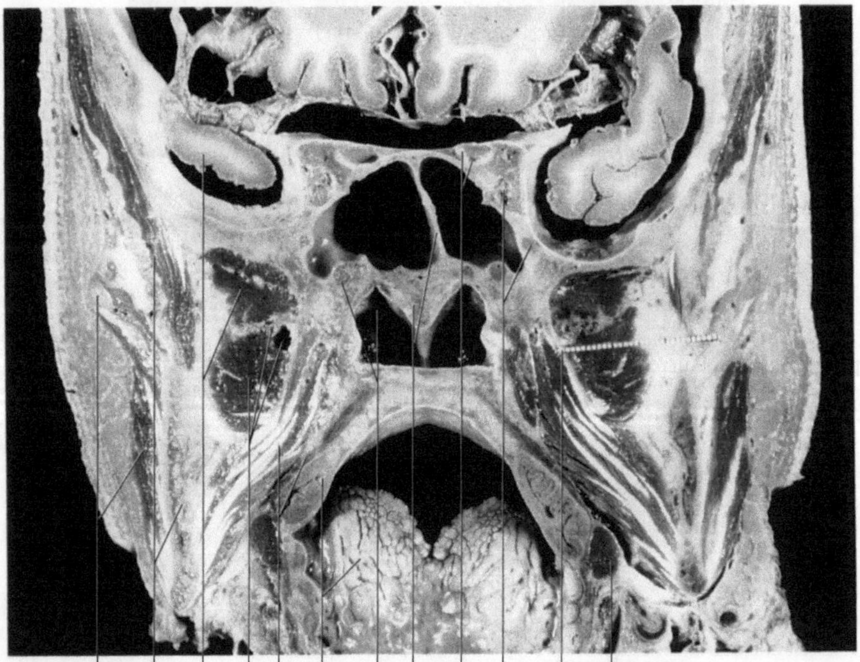

Fig. SA 30. Coronal section through the head, posterior aspect

When the masticatory space is approached from the lateral side, the zygomatic arch may be osteotomized along with the origin of the masseter muscle. The masseter is grossly subdivided into a superficial part and a deep part. The superficial part arises from the anterior part of the lower border of the zygomatic arch and zygomatic bone (often including a masseteric tubercle) and runs obliquely downward and backward to the angle of the mandible and to the masseteric tuberosity on the lateral surface of the base of the mandible. The deep part of the masseter has a more vertical course and arises from the deep surface of the zygomatic process of the temporal bone directly in front of the temporomandibular joint. This part of the muscle has connections with the temporal muscle referred to as the zygomaticomandibular muscle. The zygomaticomandibular muscle arises from the zygomatic arch and is inserted into the coronoid process of the mandible. The muscle is innervated by zygomatic branches from the mandibular nerve which reach the muscle (along with homonymous arteries) through the mandibular notch. It inserts into the posterior one-fourth to one-third of the mandibular body as far as the second molar and into the masseteric tuberosity as far as the base of the coronoid process. It exerts an adductive force of 274.7 N. The deep part can also retract the lower jaw.

When the masticatory space is approached surgically, the zygomatic arch may be osteotomized and the main area of insertion of the temporal muscle removed with the coronoid process almost to the midportion of the mandibular ramus. Attention is given to the course of the inferior alveolar nerve and its accompanying vessels, which should be spared.

Figure SA 31 presents data of the position of the mandibular foramen (the site of entry of the inferior alveolar nerve and its accompanying vessels) in relation to different parts of the mandible. Fat and loose connective tissue can be dissected away to reveal the pterygoid muscles.

Age	Right		Left	
0– 2 years	14,9	(14–16)	14,7	(14–16)
2– 4	15,8	(13–20)	16,0	(13–21)
5– 6	15,4	(14–18)	15,2	(14–17)
7–10	17,7	(14–25)	17,2	(14–22)
adult	22,2	(12–30)	22,7	(15–28)
senium	21,5	(15–26)	21,5	(14–27)

Age	Right		Left	
0– 2 years	13,9	(13–16)	14,0	(13–15)
2– 4	14,8	(13–17)	14,7	(13–17)
5– 6	14,8	(13–17)	14,8	(13–17)
7–10	16,3	(15–19)	16,1	(13–22)
senium	18,3	(11–30)	18,4	(11–28)
adult	16,3	(9–22)	16,8	(12–21)

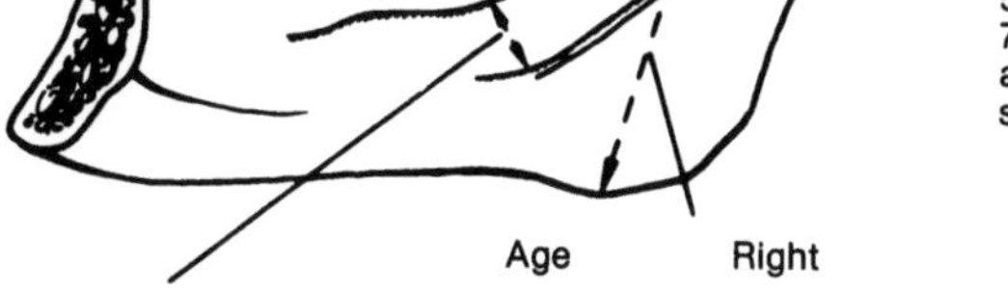

Age	Right		Left	
0– 2 years	10,2	(10–11)	9,9	(9–12)
2– 4	10,9	(9–14)	10,4	(7–13)
5– 6	10,6	(8–13)	10,6	(8–13)
7–10	11,7	(8–18)	11,2	(10–14)
adult	14,3	(11–20	14,9	(11–20)
senium	13,3	(8–18)	13,2	(10–16)

Age	Right		Left	
0– 2 years	14,3	(13–16)	14,9	(14–17)
2– 4	16,1	(14–18)	16,3	(14–19)
5– 6	14,9	(11–19)	15,4	(13–18)
7–10	19,2	(15–26)	19,7	(15–30)
adult	29,5	(15–40)	29,2	(15–41)
senium	28,2	(16–39)	28,7	(17–39)

Age	Right		Left	
0– 2 years	6,3	(6– 7)	6,1	(6– 7)
2– 4	7,4	(6– 9)	7,3	(6– 9)
5– 6	7,4	(7– 8)	7,6	(7– 9)
7–10	9,1	(5–13)	8,6	(7–10)
adult	9,6	(7–13)	9,0	(5–12)
senium	8,5	(6–11)	8,8	(5–13)

Fig. SA 31. Position of the mandibular foramen during postnatal development distances to different areas are expressed in mm (range) (from Lang and Öder 1984)

The lateral pterygoid muscle consists of two heads which we call the infratemporal and the pterygoid. The infratemporal (upper) head arises from the infratemporal plane and infratemporal spine (anterior part of infratemporal crest), passes downward and backward along the plane, and inserts into the articular capsule and pterygoid fovea of the mandible. Its muscular force (anterior pull) is approximately 31.4 N (Zenker 1955; Schumacher 1976). The pterygoid (lower) head arises from the lateral pterygoid plate. Its fibers converge backward toward the pterygoid fovea, where they are inserted. Zenker (1955) states that the muscle can exert about 98 N of force. The lateral pterygoid moves the head of the mandible forward when the mouth is opened.

The medial pterygoid muscle forms the lower part of the muscular floor of the *masticatory space*. Like the lateral pterygoid, this muscle consists of two parts. The thicker pterygoid part arises from the pterygoid fossa of the pterygoid process, while the thinner tuberal part arises from the maxillary tuber. Both groups of fibers unite before passing downward and backward to the pterygoid tuber on the medial surface of the angle and body of the mandible. This muscle exerts an adducting force of 151 N and a protruding force of 26.5 N. The masseter and medial pterygoid together form a muscular sling able to exert a total adducting force of 42.2 N. The infratemporal plane is bounded posterolaterally by the articular tubercle of the temporomandibular joint (often palpable), which gives origin to the most important ligament of the joint, the lateral ligament. The bulk of the collagen fibers of this ligament pass downward and backward from the tubercle to the neck of the mandible. The inferior alveolar artery runs behind the homonymous nerve in 70% of cases, lateral to it in 14%, and anterior to it in 8.3% upon entering the inferior alveolar canal (see Lang and Öder 1984 for further details).

Anatomy of the Temporomandibular Joint

(Fig. SA 32)

The part of the temporomandibular joint (TMJ) surface formed by the temporal squama is 25 (23–29) mm wide and 18.6 (13–23) mm long in our material (Hoffmann 1973). The rounded eminence of the articular tubercle of the temporal bone bounds the articular fossa from the front and helps to retain a normal occlusion and mastication. The articular disc of the TMJ, which moves forward when the mouth is opened, is 3–4 mm thick posteriorly, 1–2 mm thick centrally, and 1.5–2 mm thick anteriorly (where it apposes the articular eminence). A

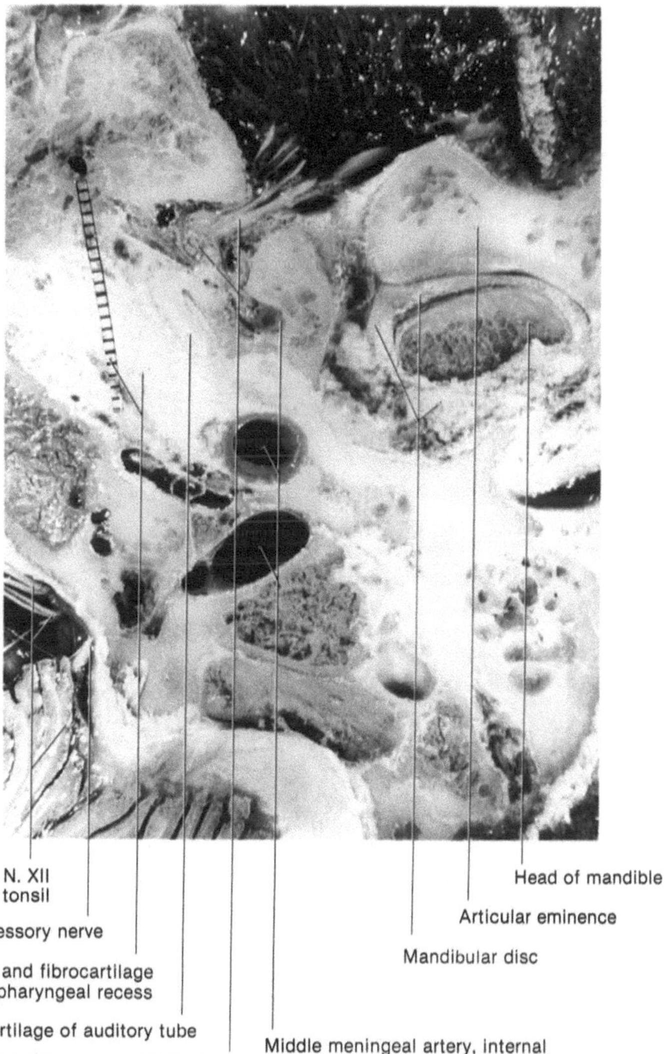

Fig. SA 32. Transverse section through the temporomandibular joint, superior aspect

pars discosquamalis intervenes between the skull base and the articular disc, while a pars discomandibularis is placed between the articular disc and the head of the condyle. In the upper joint space, the articular surface facing the skull base has an area of 581 mm^2; that facing the articular disc has an area of 501 mm^2. In the lower joint space, the articular surface on the disc side has a mean area of 396 mm^2; on the mandibular side, 367 $\bar{x}\,mm^2$ (Lang and Niederfeilner 1975). The nerves of the TMJ are derived from the masseteric branches, the deep temporal branches, the auriculotemporal nerve, and in 50% of cases from the facial nerve (Guerrier and Bolönyi 1948; Kitamura 1974; Schmidt 1976; Thilander 1962; Moffet 1957; Oberbeckmann and Lautenbach 1979; etc.).

Thin articular cartilage covers the head of the mandible on its upper surface and some of its anterior surface (Schiller 1978), producing a slight anteversion of the mandibular joint surface. The cartilage layer is only 0.58 ($\pm$ 0.22) mm thick (Hansson and Nordström 1977).

In 98% of cases the temporal surface of the TMJ is bounded posteriorly by a retroarticular process of variable morphology whose function is to prevent excessive backward displacement of the head of the mandible and the articular disc (Oliveira 1979).

Anatomy of the Pterygoid Process and Pterygoid Fossa

(Fig. SA 33)

The pterygoid process with its lateral and medial plates and the pterygoid fossa on the undersurface of the skull provide surfaces of attachment for the masticatory muscles and give support to the auditory tube. As Zehm (1966) points out, Conley (1956) and Fluur (1964) were the first to redirect serious attention to the operative exposure of this region, which had previously been considered inaccessible. Tumors can develop silently in this area (which Zehm calls the "retromaxillary space") because of their concealed location. The medial surface of the medial pterygoid plate grossly demarcates the retromaxillary space from the nasopharynx. A tubal process no longer listed in current anatomic nomenclature projects sometimes backward from the medial plate and gives support to the cartilaginous part of the auditory tube slightly above its midpoint. The cartilage itself usually projects 2–3 mm past the posterior

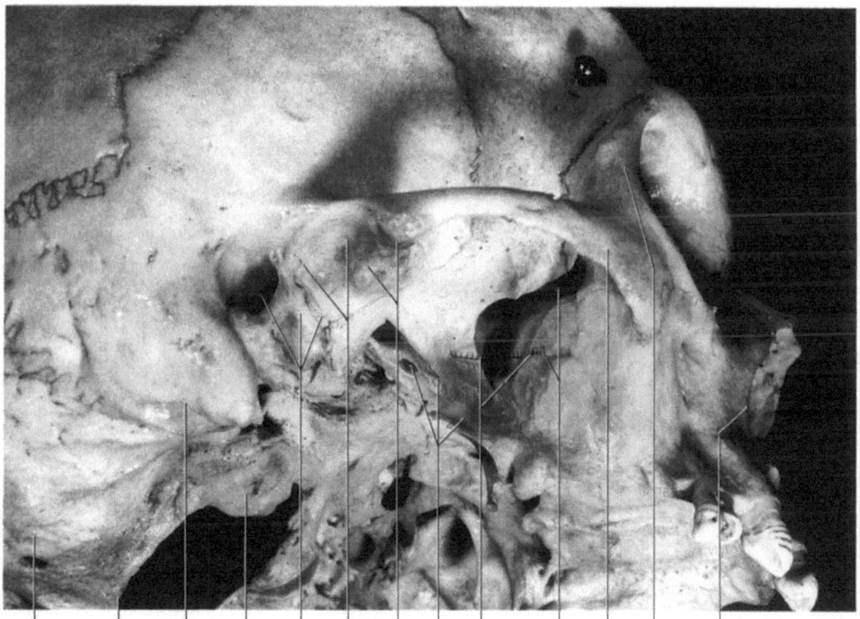

Fig. SA 33. Pterygomaxillary fissure with a bony spine of the pterygoid process. Lamina pterygospinosa extremely wide, viewed from laterally and below

border of the medial pterygoid plate. Perovic (1958) noted that a "tubal impression" could sometimes be identified above the tubal process. Close to the skull base is the scaphoid fossa, which apposes the auditory cartilage and provides a site of origin for the tensor veli palatini. In our material we determined the paramedian distances, lengths, and angulations of the pterygoid plates as well as their distances from the midsagittal plane and the contralateral pterygoid processes (Lang and Hetterich 1983).

If the lateral plate extends as far back as the sphenoid spine, *pterygospinal laminae* are said to be present. These may pass medial as well as lateral to the foramen ovale. If the plate is lateral to the foramen ovale, controlled thermocoagulation of the trigeminal ganglion may prove difficult or impossible. If the plate is medial to the foramen ovale, openings must be present through which the nerves and arteries can pass to the medial pterygoid muscle. This was pointed out more than a century ago by the anatomist Hyrtl (1862). The pterygospinal ligament stretches from the sphenoid spine to the lateral pterygoid plate.

Anatomy of the Pterygopalatine Fossa

(Fig. SA 33, Table 2)

The sphenomaxillary fissure, bounded in front by the maxillary tuber and behind by anterior portions of the pterygoid process, affords lateral access to the pterygopalatine fossa. It should be noted that the lower part of the pterygoid fossa and anterior border of the pterygoid process is formed by the pyramidal process of the palatine bone. That is why the area below the fissure must be termed the maxillopalatine or maxillopyramidal suture (contrary to textbook definitions and those of earlier authors). This suture zone is important in surgical procedures for the treatment of maxillofacial fractures (LeFort fractures). In our material the length of the sphenomaxillary fissure between the infratemporal spine and this suture zone is 19.87 (13–29) mm. The maximum width of the fissure is 5.66 (2–12) mm. The various types of sphenomaxillary fissure are illustrated in Fig. SA 34 (after Fink 1978).

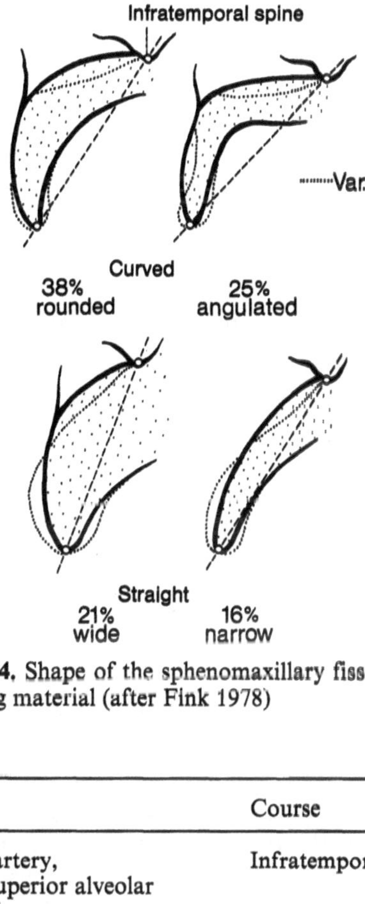

Fig. SA 34. Shape of the sphenomaxillary fissure in the Würzburg material (after Fink 1978)

Table 2. Openings in the pterygopalatine fossa

Openings		Contents	Course
1. Lateral opening	Pterygomaxillary fissure	Maxillary artery, Posterior superior alveolar arteries, veins, nerves	Infratemporal fossa
2. Posterior openings	a. Foramen rotundum, superolateral	Maxillary nerve and artery	Middle cranial fossa
	b. Pterygoid canal, superomedial	Pterygoid nerve, Artery of pterygoid canal	Inferior skull base
	c. Vomerovaginal canal, more medial	Small arteries and nerves	Fornix of pharynx
	d. Palatovaginal canal, medial	Pharyngeal branches of pterygopalatine ganglion and artery	Roof of pharynx
3. Medial opening	Sphenopalatine foramen, superomedial	Posterior nasal branches, sphenopalatine artery	Nasal cavity
4. Anterior opening	Inferior orbital fissure, anterosuperior	Infraorbital artery and nerve, zygomatic nerve	Orbit
5. Inferior opening	Greater palatine canal	Greater and lesser palatine arteries, veins, nerves	Hard and soft palate, nasal cavity

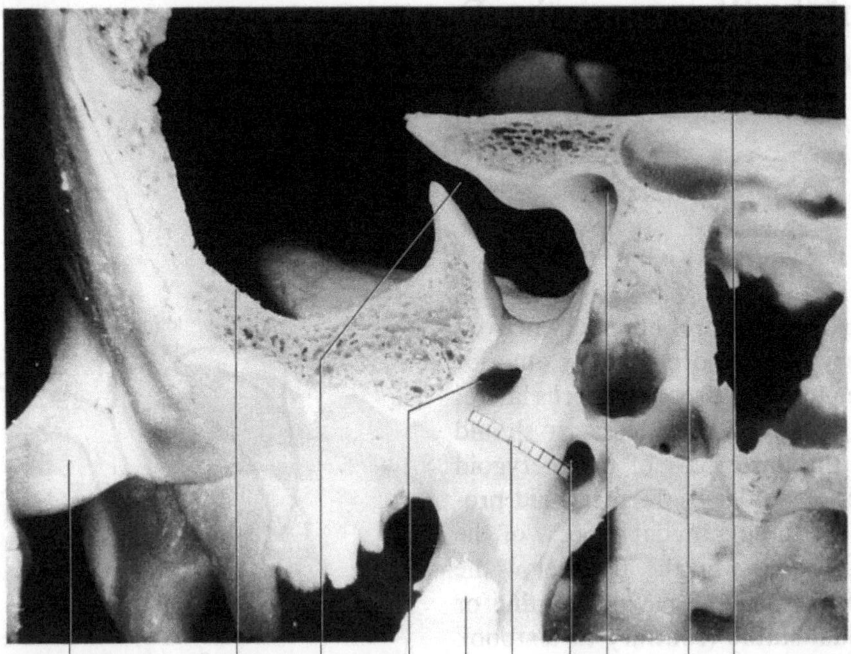

Fig. SA 35. Posterior wall of the pterygopalatine fossa, coronal section, anterior view

The anterior wall of the pterygopalatine fossa is formed by the maxillary tuber, the medial wall by the vertical lamina of the palatine bone, the posterior wall by the pterygoid process. The openings in the pterygopalatine fossa and their contents are listed in Table 2. The pterygopalatine fossa is bounded laterally and anteriorly by the inferior orbital fissure. The maxillary nerve enters the fossa through the foramen rotundum. The nerve may be unifascicular or may contain up to 30 fascicles in the area of the foramen rotundum (Lang and Keller 1978). The foramen is also traversed by two small arteries whose lumina are about 135 µm in size. The posterior boundary of the pterygopalatine fossa and its surroundings are illustrated in Fig. SA 35.

Middle Skull Base and Its Openings Viewed from Below

The mandibular nerve traverses the foramen ovale, which in our material is 7.2 (2.2–9.9) mm long and 3.7 (1.7–6.5) mm wide. Its long axis is generally oblique, being directed from anteromedially to posterolaterally. The distances between the foramina ovale (and other external openings in the skull base) in adults are pictured in Fig. SA 36. The mandibular nerve is surrounded by a venous plexus called the venous plexus of the foramen ovale, which communicates inferiorly with the pterygoid venous plexus and intracranially with the veins accompanying the middle meningeal artery and with the cavernous sinus. In about 30% of cases a foramen of Vesalius is present which transmits a sphenoidal emissary vein. Generally these openings in the external skull base are found about the upper border of the pterygoid fossa.

Behind and lateral to the foramen ovale is the foramen spinosum, which generally is medial to the sphenoid spine. It transmits the middle meningeal artery and its accompanying veins to the middle cranial fossa (see Lang 1979 and Lang 1983 for further details).

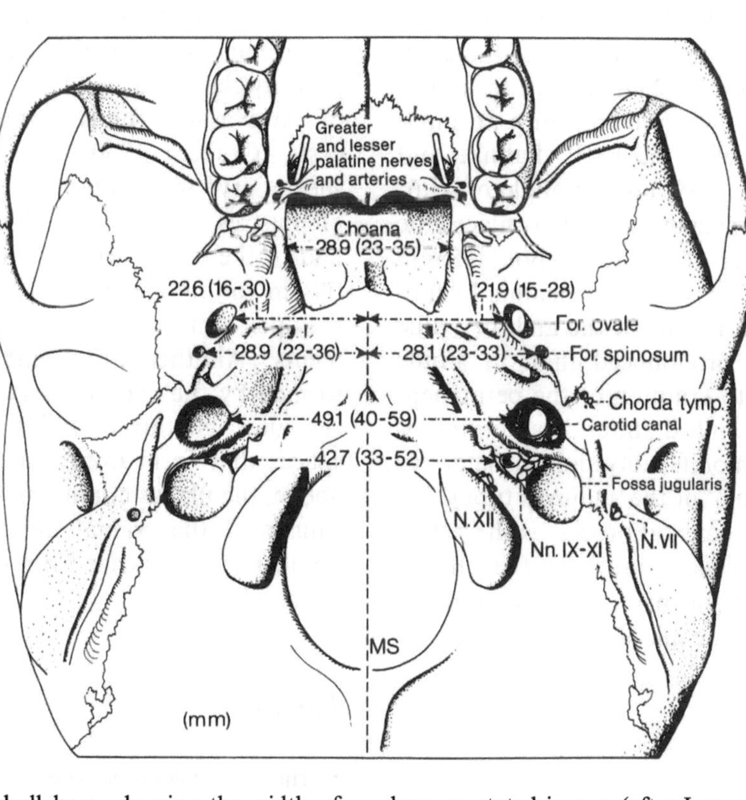

Fig. SA 36. External skull base, showing the width of the choanae in adults, the distances of the foramina ovalia and spinosa from the midline, and the spacing of the medial borders of the carotid canals and anterior portions of the jugular foramina. Mean and extreme values are stated in mm (after Lang and Issing, in press). The inferior orbital fissures, the medial and lateral plates of the pterygoid process, and the sphenosquamous and zygomaticotemporal sutures (on the zygomatic arch) are also shown

Anatomy of the Auditory Tube

The musculotubar canal opens on the undersurface of the skull posteromedial to the foramen spinosum, and directly behind that aperture in children. The end of the bony part of the auditory tube and the lower part of the tensor tympani occur in that area. It should be noted that fibers always pass between the tensor tympani and the tensor veli palatini (both of which are supplied by the trigeminal nerve). The upper canal for the tensor tympani and the lower canal for the auditory tube are separated by a septum which is often perforated. The bony part of the auditory tube is 11–12 mm long in our adult material and forms a 50° angle (42–57°) with the midsagittal plane. The cartilaginous part of the auditory tube is usually 24–25 mm long in adults. It runs medially downward, forming an angle of 34.6° (14–47°) with the FHP (Pahnke and von Lüdinghausen 1989) and an angle of 43.6° (32–52°) with the median plane. This places the pharyngeal opening of the tube about 15 mm below the plane of its tympanic opening. In children, the downward slope of the auditory tube is somewhat less pronounced than in adults (about 10°) prior to eruption of the permanent teeth. The tube is angled about 5° anteroinferiorly at the junction of its bony and cartilaginous parts (the "isthmus" of the auditory tube). Behind the inferior tegmental process is the petrotympanic fissure which transmits the chorda tympani to the lingual nerve and the anterior tympanic artery to the middle ear.

Anatomy of the Masticatory Space and Peripharyngeal Space

(Figs. SA 37, SA 38)

General

The fascial compartments of the infracranial space have long been an object of surgical and anatomic interest. The earliest description was published by Burns (1811), and the fascia were later studied and described by Velpeau (1830), Dittel (1857), Henle (1871), Weber-Liel (1873), Poulsen (1886), Merkel (1892), Bulatnikow (1915), Grodinsky and Holyoke (1938), Hall (1934), Singer (1935), Zenker (1955), and others. The region between the maxilla and mandible anteriorly and the prevertebral muscles posteriorly is occupied by a number of connective tissue membranes which control at least temporarily the spread and the direction of spread of extravasated fluids, abscesses, tumors, and cysts (Casberg 1950). Most of these fascial sheets serve to facilitate the relative movement of muscles, nerves, and blood vessels. The fat pad of the cheek, with its numerous processes, fills in the interspaces between the muscles as they perform their diverse functions and movements. Another important function is performed by the venous pterygoid plexus, which can alter its state of filling to obliterate dead spaces that form during movement. As noted above, the plexus communicates with veins and sinuses of the cranial interior and receives a number of tributaries from the undersurface of the skull.

Fasciae

Earlier we discussed the temporal aponeurosis and temporal fascia covering the outer surface of the temporal muscle. There is also a fascia on the deep surface of the muscle, the *deep temporal fascia*, which attaches to the lateral border

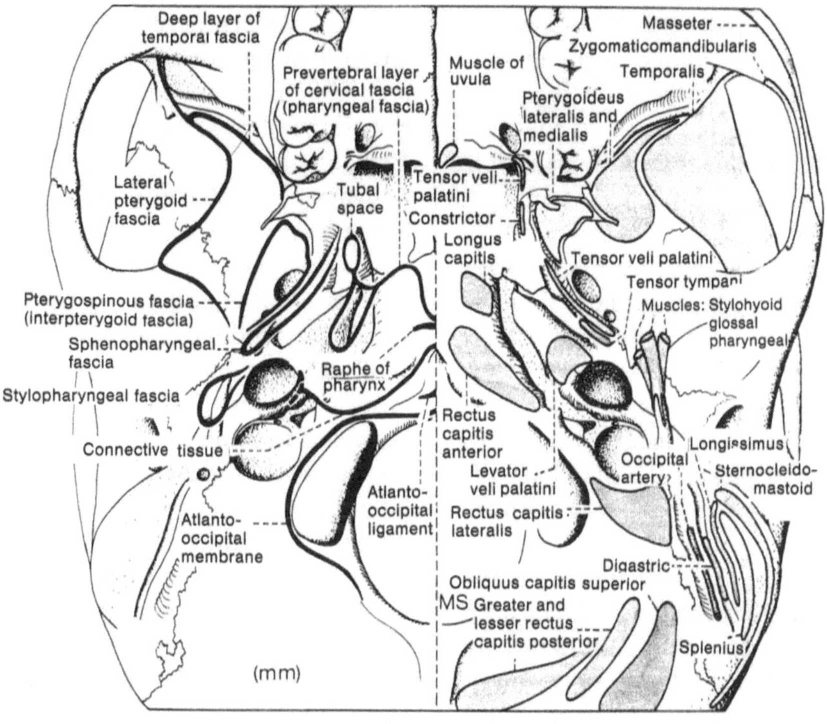

Fig. SA 37. Muscles and fasciae on the inferior surface of the skull base (Lang 1987)

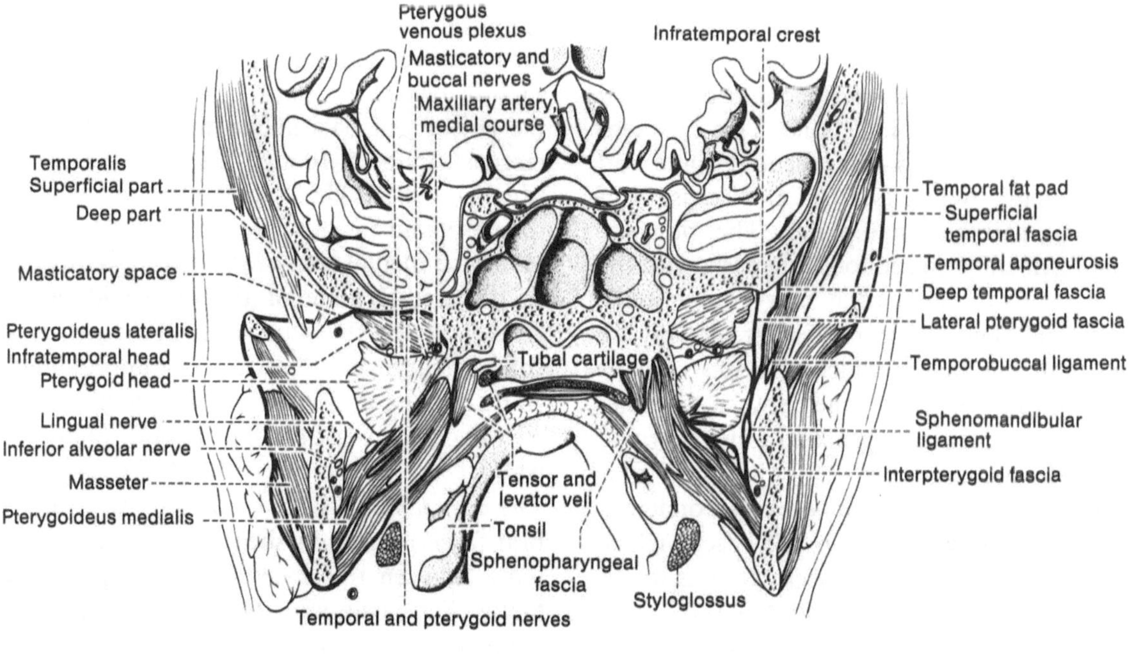

Fig. SA 38. Muscles and fasciae on a coronal section through the head (Lang 1987)

of the infratemporal fossa, the infratemporal crest, and the retromolar trigone of the mandible. The anterior border of the deep temporal fascia is continuous with the cover of the buccinator muscle. The oblique line of the mandible also affords attachment to the deep temporal fascia (Zenker 1955).

The relatively thin *lateral pterygoid fascia* courses on the lateral aspect of the lateral pterygoid muscle (Henle 1871), the inferior orbital fissure, the infratemporal spine and infratemporal crest, terminating posteriorly at the capsule of the TMJ. The fascia incorporates portions of the pterygoid plexus, the maxillary artery and its branches and, in its upper portion, the temporal nerves.

Lateral and anterior to this fascial sheet is the pterygoid process of the *buccal fat pad.* The deep temporal fascia and lateral pterygoid fascia are open anteriorly; posteriorly they interconnect. Farther downward the lateral pterygoid fascia is attached to the lateral plate of the pterygoid process, the posterior margin of the sphenomaxillary fissure, and the maxillary tuber. Anteriorly it blends with the buccinator fascia and more posteriorly with the interpterygoid fascia. It is continuous inferiorly with the retromandibular trigone and has connections with the sphenomandibular ligament.

The *pterygospinal ligament* (interpterygoid fascia) stretches between the posterior border of the lateral plate of the pterygoid process and the spine of the sphenoid bone. This ligament extends posteriorly to the sphenoid spine and petrotympanic fissure (see earlier discussion of the bony pterygospinal plate). The pterygospinal ligament is continuous inferiorly with the lateral cover of the medial pterygoid muscle. The lingual and inferior alveolar nerves are fused with this fascia, which also has connections with the boundary zone between the palatine bone and pterygoid process in the pterygoid fossa and maxillary tuber.

The *temporobuccinator ligament* is a condensation of connective tissue in the fascia which bounds the superficial and deep tendons of the temporal muscle. About 2 cm long by 1 cm wide (Zenker 1955), the ligament runs downward from the medial surface of the superficial tendon of insertion of the temporal muscle and anterior border of the coronoid process of the mandible to the buccinator fascia, slightly anterior to the pterygomandibular raphe (Gaughran 1957).

A ligamentous structure called the *stylopharyngeal fascia* arises anterolateral to the external aperture of the carotid canal, the styloid process and its sheath, and the base of the sphenoid spine. Descending from its attachment on the skull, it splits into two parts which include the levator veli palatini anteriorly and the medial ligamentous apparatus. This apparatus encloses the stylopharyngeal and styloglossus muscles laterally. It has a connection with the stylomandibular ligament, the stylomandibular fascia. This outer layer also forms the inner boundary for the retromandibular process of the parotid gland. Additional connective tissue layers intervene between this fascia and the buccopharyngeal fascia.

The *sphenopharyngeal fascia* (salpingopharyngeal fascia, sphenopterygopharyngeal fascia) arises behind the foramen ovale and foramen spinosum in the area of the greater wing of the sphenoid and unites with the stylopharyngeal fascia anterior and lateral to the external opening of the carotid canal, the styloid process, and the medial border of the tympanic part of the temporal bone. Its medial extensions envelop the tensor veli palatini. A lateral extension arises slightly below the skull base posterolateral to the tensor veli palatini. In most cases the two fasciae unite 5–10 mm behind the muscle (Zenker 1955). The lateral band extends into the pterygoid fossa, while the medial band runs along the medial side of the tensor veli palatini to the medial plate of the pterygoid process. Zenker states that the area of origin of the sphenopharyngeal fascia is approximately 30 mm long and 5 mm wide. Its site of insertion is 1–2 cm lateral to the lateral pharyngeal wall.

The *deep lamina of the cervical fascia* (prevertebral fascia) is a thin sheet of connective tissue lying between the pharynx (lateral pharyngeal fascia) anteriorly and the prevertebral muscles posteriorly. It consists of several vascularized connective tissue layers which impart lateral-medial mobility to the pharynx, the great vessels, and the lower cranial nerves.

Hall (1934) and Grodinsky and Holyoke (1938) state that the deep lamina of the cervical fascia is composed of two layers, the alar fascia and the prevertebral fascia. The alar fascia extends across the midline behind the pharynx and blends with the prevertebral lamina. A prolongation runs forward and medially to form the anterior wall of the carotid sheath, a sleeve of connective tissue enclosing the internal and common carotid arteries, their accompanying nerves, and the internal jugular vein.

The *pharyngeal fascia* (buccopharyngeal fascia) is the thin layer of connective tissue that encloses the pharynx and its nerves and veins.

Spaces

Juvara (1870) was apparently the first to describe the *masticatory space* (Fig. SA 38), so named by Coller and Yglesias (1935). This space contains the masseter and pterygoid muscles and the ramus of the mandible. It is bounded superiorly by the temporal muscle. The space lies anterior and lateral to the lateral parapharyngeal space and in front of the parotid gland. On the outer skull base the masticatory space is bounded by the lateral pterygoid muscle and its fascia and by the pterygospinal ligament and its continuation. It has connections with the tensor veli palatini and the membranous part of the auditory tube.

The *salpingopharyngeal space*, placed posteromedial to the sphenopharyngeal space, contains the auditory tube, the levator veli palatini, and portions of the ascending palatine artery.

The carotid sheath (see above) is also construed as a separate space. The space enclosed by the sheath is posterolateral to the salpingopharyngeal space and contains the internal carotid artery, the internal jugular vein, the ascending pharyngeal artery, the superior pharyngeal veins, and the ninth through twelfth cranial nerves on various planes and at varying locations. The fibrous sheet blends anterolaterally with the stylopharyngeal fascia, and posteriorly it borders on the loose connective tissue of the prevertebral lamina of the cervical fascia.

Parapharyngeal Space

Earlier authors subdivided the parapharyngeal space into an anterior part (containing the lymph nodes and connective tissue between the skull base and angle of the mandible) and a posterior part located behind the pharynx and containing the prevertebral muscles.

The prevertebral lamina of the cervical fascia invests the sympathetic trunk with its ganglia. The superior deep ansa cervicalis (linking C_1 and C_2 with the hypoglossal nerve) is also placed beneath this fascia.

Masticatory Space, Arteries and Nerves

Maxillary Artery (Fig. SA 39)

The maxillary artery is the anterior terminal branch of the external carotid artery (the other branch being the superficial temporal). In our

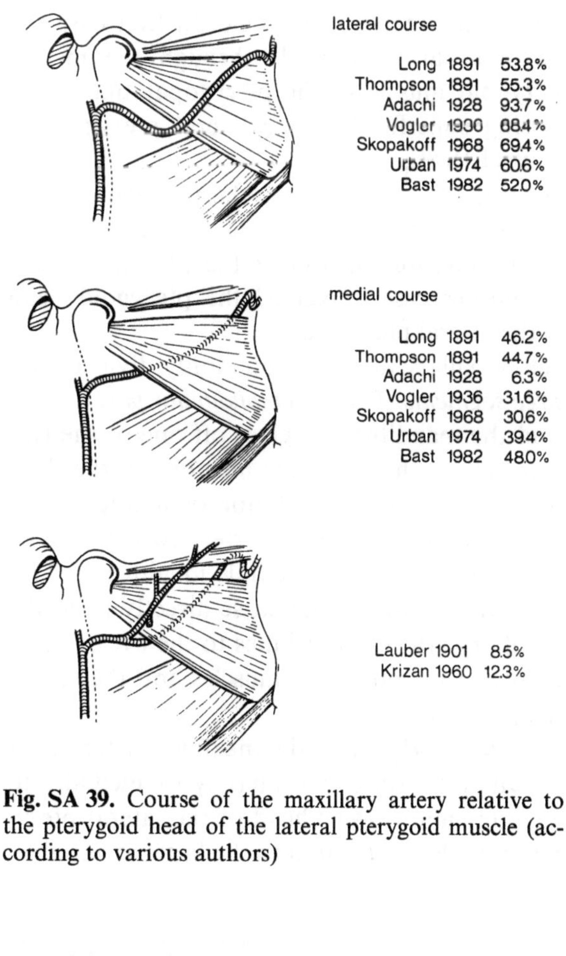

Fig. SA 39. Course of the maxillary artery relative to the pterygoid head of the lateral pterygoid muscle (according to various authors)

material its origin is 24.6 (17–29) mm below the head of the mandible, usually at the posterior border of the neck or ramus (Kagerbauer 1985). Joessel (1878) once found a maxillary artery arising behind the mandibular angle. From its origin the vessel runs forward and mediad, forming an angle of 0°–5° with the FHP in 50% of cases, and ascending at a greater angle (up to 26°) in 35%. In the rest the maxillary artery descends slightly before turning upward (especially when it passes lateral to the pterygoid head of the lateral pterygoid muscle).

Variations of the Maxillary Artery
(Fig. SA 39)

In a specimen of Hyrtl (1859), the maxillary artery was completely absent and was replaced by a prominently developed ascending palatine artery. A similar case is illustrated in Quain's atlas (Plate VIII, Fig. 6).
Very rarely the external carotid artery divides into its two terminal branches while still in the area of the mandibular angle. In that case the maxillary artery ascends through the medial pterygoid muscle to the pterygopalatine fossa, passing superficial to the lateral pterygoideus (Joessel 1878).
In some of our specimens the maxillary artery pierced the deep head of the temporal muscle in the anterior portion of the pterygoid part, in another case it pierced the pterygoid head of the lateral pterygoid.
The maxillary artery is commonly divided into *three segments*. The *retromandibular part* lies behind the mandible and gives off one of the two branches to the tympanic membrane, the deep auricular artery, the anterior tympanic artery, and the middle meningeal artery (which usually gives off the accessory middle meningeal). This thin branch, which may arise directly from the maxillary artery, contributes to the extracranial supply of the pterygoid muscles and the tensor veli palatini.
The *pterygoid part* of the maxillary artery runs obliquely forward and laterally or medially to the pterygoid (lower) head of the lateral pterygoid muscle. Its relation to the latter is variable, as Fig. SA 39 demonstrates. Lauber (1901) showed that a relatively large branch passes to the temporal muscle lateral to the pterygoids in 8.5% of cases, a finding which we can confirm in another case it pierced the pterygoid head of the lateral pterygoid.

Pterygoid Part, Branches

Krizan (1960) noted that the middle meningeal artery generally arises proximal to the inferior alveolar artery when the maxillary artery takes a lateral course, and vice-versa. Branches from this segment also pass to the pterygoid muscles, the masseter muscle, and the deep temporal arteries. The latter pass upward to the temporal muscle along small grooves in the temporal squama.

Maxillary Artery and Adjacent Nerves

In most cases the pterygoid part of the maxillary artery runs lateral to the inferior alveolar and lingual nerves and medial to the buccal nerves. But it may also pass between the inferior alveolar nerve and lingual nerve, medial to both nerves, or through a loop of the inferior alveolar nerve (see Fig. SA 40). Czerwinski (1981) found that a maxillary artery passing medial to the pterygoid head of the lateral pterygoid muscle lies medial to the lingual and inferior alveolar nerves in 3.3% of cases; it runs lateral to these nerves in 20.8%, between them in 5.8%, and through the inferior alveolar nerve in 4.1%.
When the artery runs lateral to the lateral pterygoid muscle, the maxillary artery was found always to pass lateral to the lingual and inferior alveolar nerves. Anastomoses between the lingual nerve and inferior alveolar nerve are not too uncommon. They are most often seen in the area of the pterygoid hiatus. Ernst and Inke (1962) determined the distance between the lower border of the trigeminal ganglion and the division of the mandibular nerve into the inferior alveolar and lingual nerves. The length of the intracranial segment of the mandibular nerve in our material is 6.66 (2.9–11.5) mm (Lang 1981). Based on the findings of Ernst and

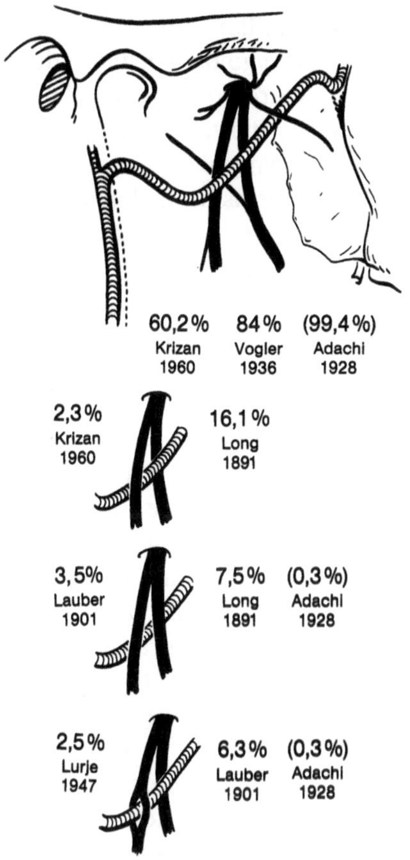

Fig. SA 40. Relation of the maxillary artery to the mandibular and lingual nerves in the masticatory space (according to various authors)

Inke (1962), the bifurcation of the mandibular nerve lies 10–15 mm distal to the ganglion in 40% of cases, 16–20 mm in 26.6%, 6–10 mm in 13.3%, and 21–25 mm in 13.3%. The buccal nerve arises 0–10 mm distal to the trigeminal ganglion, most commonly in the range of 6–10 mm. The auriculotemporal nerve arises 5–10 mm distal to the ganglion in about two-thirds of cases, with extreme values of 0 and 15 mm. It should be noted that the buccal nerve may arise proximal to the auriculotemporal.

Baumel et al. (1971) found two auriculotemporal nerve roots in 75% of cases, three roots in 14%, and four roots in fewer than 1%. In the rest the upper and lower roots appear to divide into two additional fiber bundles. Normally the upper root is about twice as thick as the lower. According to Ernst and Inke (1962), the upper root of the auriculotemporal nerve usually arises from the mandibular nerve 5–10 (3–11) mm distal to the trigeminal ganglion. Krizan (1956) determined an extracranial mandibular nerve length of 7–12 mm. Thus it is not surprising that the lower root of the auriculotemporal nerve occasionally is a branch of the inferior alveolar.

When the nerve arises by two roots, these generally encircle the middle meningeal artery in V-shaped fashion. Usually the lower root is lateral to the artery and the upper root is medial to it, although variations can occur. The nerve then winds around the temporomandibular joint from behind and below, passing between the joint and the external acoustic meatus below the upper part of the parotid gland. There it makes contact with the superficial temporal vessels and initially accompanies them on their posterior aspect as it ascends toward the temporal region. See Lang (1984, 1985) for details on anastomoses with the facial nerve.

Chorda Tympani and Lingual Nerve. The chorda tympani leaves the middle ear cavity through the petrotympanic fissure and, covered by the spine of the sphenoid bone, runs forward and downward. Its length is variable. Ernst and Inke (1962), for example, found that the chorda tympani joins the lingual nerve 2–23 mm distal to the lingual nerve origin and 6–39 mm distal to the trigeminal ganglion. In about two-thirds of cases the lingual nerve courses for 0–10 mm before it is joined by the chorda tympani.

In rare cases a multi-root origin of the lingual nerve has been described. The material of Ernst and Inke (1962) included one case where the auriculotemporal nerve established anastomoses with the buccal nerve.

Inferior Alveolar Artery

In our material it is not unusual to find the inferior alveolar artery arising opposite the origin of the middle meningeal artery from the maxillary. The origin may also lie distal or (more rarely) proximal to the origin of the middle meningeal.

Maxillary Artery, Pterygoid Part

The maxillary artery traverses the sphenomaxillary fissure to enter the pterygopalatine fossa. Turvey and Fonseca (1980) report an arterial diameter of 2.63 (2.5–3.0) mm in this area (in our material this artery has a smaller diameter). Their findings indicate that the vessel enters the pterygopalatine fossa at a level 25 (23–28) mm above the maxillopyramidal suture. This distance is of surgical importance in LeFort III osteotomies, which involve division of the pterygomaxillary connection. The length of the osteotomy may average 15 mm, as the suture is 14.6 (11–18) mm long. According to Navarro et al. (1982), the maxillary artery may traverse the sphenomaxillary suture by two paths: a transverse path along the maxillary tuber, and a more longitudinal path along the lateral plate of the pterygoid process. In our material the pterygoid fossa was located through the opened maxillary sinus by noting the course of the pterygoid part of the maxillary artery and the sequence of its branches (Lang and Urban 1977). If the maxillary artery runs deep to the lateral pterygoid muscle in its distal course, it generally forms a laterally projecting loop; if it runs superficial to the lateral pterygoid, it usually forms an upward bow. When its course is medial, the artery ascends in a laterally convex arc to the upper border of the pterygopalatine fossa.

This segment gives off the posterior superior alveolar artery, the infraorbital artery, and occasionally pharyngeal and meningeal branches. From the upper part of the pterygopalatine fossa, the final segment of the artery usually runs downward and medially, forming an S-shaped loop. We distinguish between an upper and a lower arc, the terminal part of the lower arc being continuous with the sphenopalatine artery. Generally the posterior superior alveolar artery and infraorbital artery spring from the maxillary as it enters the pterygopalatine fossa; pharyngeal and meningeal branches occasionally arise there as well. In our material the posterior superior alveolar artery and infraorbital artery were occasionally found to arise from a common trunk. The greater and lesser palatine arteries arise somewhat farther distally (medially). When the maxillary artery runs superficial to the lateral pterygoid, it usually describes a medially convex arc from which the posterior superior alveolar artery, infraorbital artery, and occasionally pharyngeal branches are derived. The artery then forms an S-shaped loop in the upper part of the pterygopalatine fossa. The descending palatine artery often arises from the upper arc of the maxillary artery when that vessel lies superficial to the lateral pterygoideus. In this situation the pterygopalatine fossa usually contains a longer portion of the sphenopalatine artery. On the whole, we found that the posterior superior alveolar artery in our specimens usually represented the first branch of the pterygoid part of the maxillary artery. With a laterally placed maxillary artery, this vessel has a common origin with the infraorbital artery in 20% of our cases. With a medial course of the maxillary artery relative to the lateral pterygoid, the two vessels displayed a common origin in almost 50% of cases. In this situation the superior alveolar artery often divides into two branches while giving off additional twigs to the periosteum of the maxilla, to the gingiva of the molar teeth, and to the buccal mucosa. It then enters the posterior alveolar foramina of the maxilla, accompanied by the homonymous nerves. In specimens from very elderly individuals, we noted extreme thinning or even abscence of the posterior superior alveolar arteries. In the material of Navarro et al. (1982), the posterior superior alveolar artery sprang directly from the maxillary artery in 55% of cases and from the infraorbital artery in 45%.

In our material the *infraorbital artery* arises from the segment of the maxillary artery that ascends in the pterygopalatine fossa (often in conjunction with the posterior superior alveolar artery). Navarro et al. (1982) state that the vessel arises in conjunction with the artery of the pterygoid canal and the pterygopalatine artery in 1.66% of cases, and with the artery of the canalis rotundus in another 1.66%. In one of their cases (1.66%) the artery pierced the posterior wall of the maxillary sinus.

When the maxillary artery is superficial to the lateral pterygoid, the *descending palatine artery* in our material generally arises from the upper arc of the maxillary at the roof of the pterygopalatine fossa or, less frequently, from the adjacent intervening arterial segment. When the maxillary artery is deep to the lateral pterygoid, the vessel usually arises from the lower arc of the maxillary. In the material of Navarro et al. (1982) the vessel arises at the medial wall of the pterygopalatine fossa – at the bifurcation of the maxillary artery in over 96% of cases and at a trifurcation in 3.3%. In our material the descending palatine artery then runs a short distance mediad before descending through the pterygopalatine canal with the homonymous nerve. One or two lesser palatine arteries are given off while the main trunk continues downward to the palate as the greater palatine artery. Fink (1978) found in our material that the greater palatine artery invariably arises from the maxillary. Accessory palatine arteries (if present) and lesser palatine arteries branch either separately or jointly from the maxillary artery or from the greater palatine. Or one set may arise from the maxillary artery and the other from the greater palatine. In the material of Navarro et al. (1982) the descending palatine artery enters the palatine canal at once in 68.33% of cases, and in 16.66% it runs a short distance outside the palatine canal (q.v.) before entering it. We found the artery giving off various branches in its descent to the palate: at its exit from the pterygopalatine fossa (70%), at its entry into the palatine canal (65%), and at the level of the greater palatine foramen (17.5%).

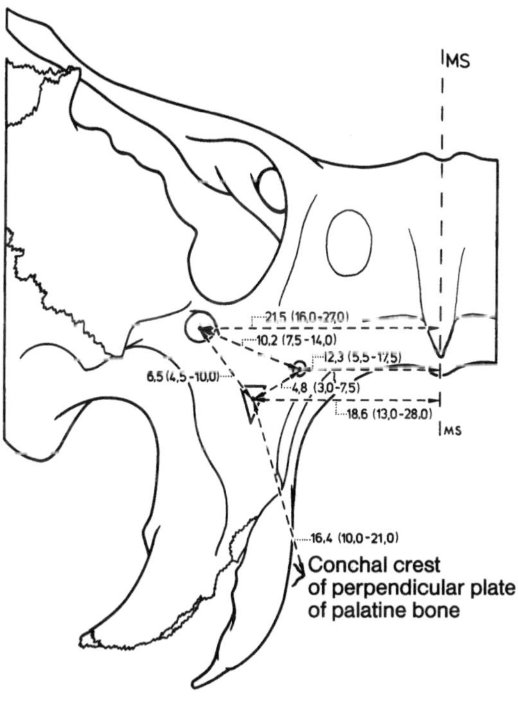

Fig. SA 41. Pterygopalatine ganglion, its distance from the center of the extracranial opening of the foramen rotundum, the anterior opening of the pterygoid canal, and the conchal crest. The figure also shows the paramedian distances of the external openings of the pterygoid canal and foramen rotundum and of the pterygopalatine ganglion (after Lang and Keller 1978) lateral to the midsagittal plane (MS). The sphenoid rostrum and the openings of the sphenoid sinus and optic canal are seen; above is the superior orbital fissure; below are the pterygoid process and the posterior wall of the pterygopalatine fossa

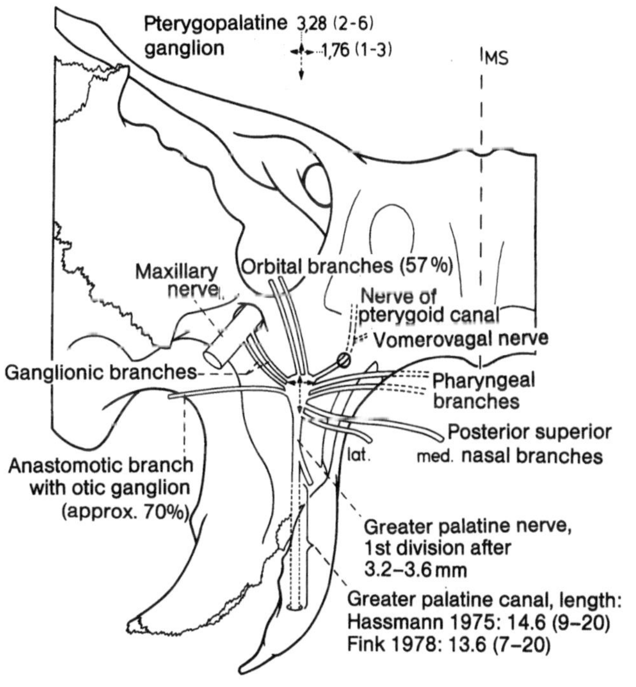

Fig. SA 42. Pterygopalatine ganglion and its branches, anterior aspect. The dimensions of the ganglion and the connections of its branches are shown (after Tanaka 1932 and our material)

Artery of the Pterygoid Canal

In our material (Urban 1974) this artery generally does not arise from the descending palatine artery as most textbooks indicate. It usually takes its origin from the maxillary artery (before the takeoff of the superior alveolar) or proximal to the origin of the infraorbital artery.

Posterior Inferior Nasal Artery

The posterior inferior nasal artery usually arises near the medial wall of the pterygopalatine fossa, crosses the fossa, and passes below the middle nasal concha covered by the mucous membrane of the nasal cavity to the inferior nasal concha.

Pterygopalatine Ganglion
(Figs. SA 41, SA 42)

This ganglion is always behind the pterygopalatine part of the maxillary artery in our material and lies a mean distance of 18.6 (13–28) mm from the midline. It is 6.5 (4.5–10) mm from the foramen rotundum, 4.8 (3.0–7.5) mm from the pterygoid canal, and 16.4 (10–21) mm from the conchal crest (see Lang and Keller 1978 for further details). The ganglion has three roots, conforming to the textbook description. Its parasympathetic root is derived from the greater petrosal nerve and its sympathetic roots from the deep petrosal nerve. The sensory roots originate from the maxillary nerve and are called the pterygopalatine nerves.

Anatomy of the Carotid Canal Region

The first part of the carotid canal runs upward and forward. This segment, which we call the ascending petrous part of the carotid canal (Lang and Schreiber 1983), forms an average angle of 122° with the FHP in neonates and 99.7° (86–114°) in adults. The canal then turns forward and medially at almost a right angle. This bend has been termed the petrous curvature. We found the distance from the external orifice of the carotid canal (lateral wall) to the supramastoid crest to be 17.3 (16–19) mm in neonates, 21.5 (18–23) mm at 3 years of age, 24.67 (24–25) mm at 8 years of age, and 28.4 (23–35) mm in adults (Lang et al. 1983).

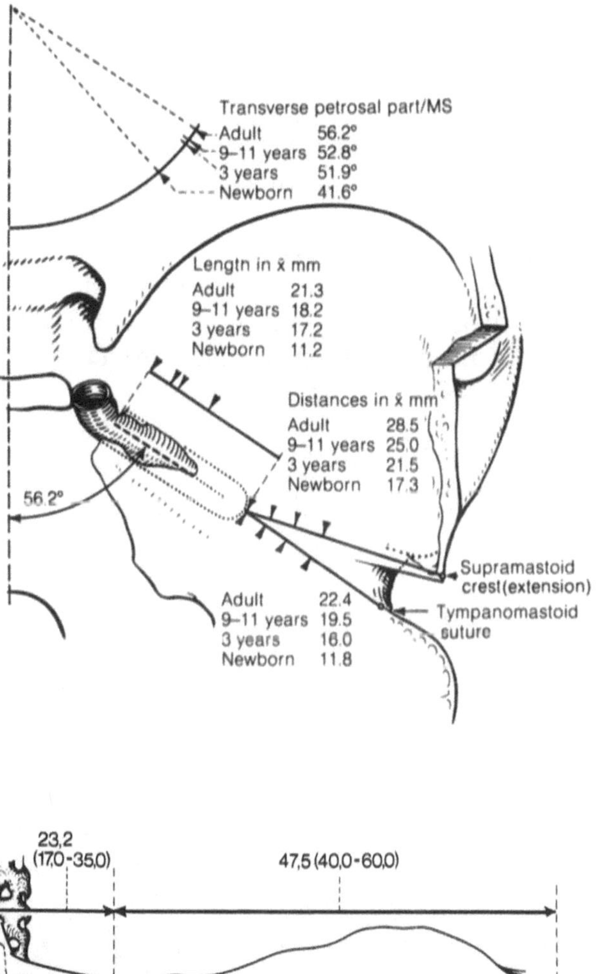

Fig. SA 43. Transverse petrous part of the internal carotid canal, length and angle with respect to the midsagittal plane and distances from the petrous curvature of the canal to the supramastoid crest and tympanomastoid suture. Mean values in mm, postnatal development (after Lang et al. 1983)

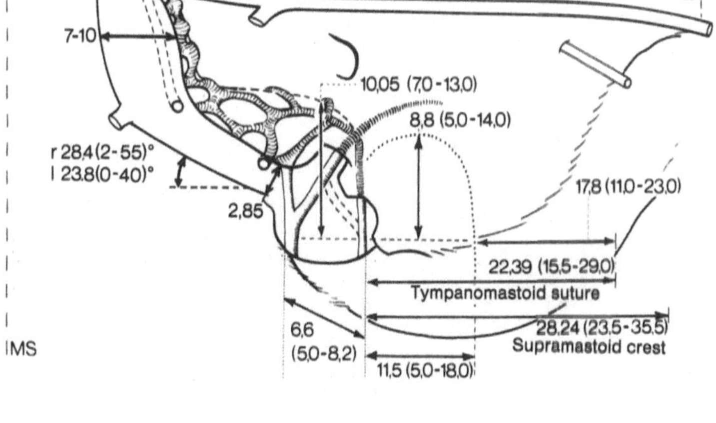

Fig. SA 44. Posterior view of the carotid canal and jugular bulb showing the venous network of the carotid canal and the superior petrosal sinus. Data include the diameter of the jugular bulb and internal jugular vein, the elevation of the bulb above the terminal crest of the sigmoid sinus, the length and diameter of the ascending part of the carotid canal in adults, and distances from landmarks on the lateral skull wall. The bulb of the internal jugular vein is *stippled*, and the venous plexus of the internal carotid artery (canal portion) is *hatched*. Measurements in mm

The lateral border of the carotid canal was found to be 11.8 (10.5–13.5) mm from the tympanomastoid suture in newborns, 17.67 (17–19) mm at 8 years of age, and 22.39 (15.5–29.0) mm in adults. From the petrous curvature the canal runs forward and medially. We measured the angle (open posteriorly) formed by this segment of the canal with the midsagittal plane in adults and obtained values of 56.17° (39.5–72.6°) on the right side and 56.98° (34.5–70.7°) on the left side. It is noteworthy that smaller mean angles were found in neonates and children (see Fig. SA 43 which is from Lang et al. 1983). We determined the length of the carotid canal from the medial edge of the external opening of the canal to the base of the lingula of the sphenoid. The mean length is 14.9 mm in newborns, 23.52 mm at 2 years of age, slightly more than 28 mm at 8 years of age, and 31.51 (20–50) mm in adults on the right side and 31.21 (22–42) mm on the left side. The ascending petrous part of the canal accounts for slightly more than 10 mm of that length in adults, with the transverse petrous part contributing an average of 21.3 mm (see Fig. SA 43). It is noteworthy that the medial portion of the upper wall (lateral to the sphenoid lingula) shows dehiscences of varying size in 96% of our material. Their length in our adult material is 12.5 (6.0–13.8) mm. This portion of the carotid canal is covered by the transverse part of the inferior sphenopetrous ligament, which bounds the trigeminal cavity below. On the medial side this connective tissue membrane is continuous with a more sagittally oriented boundary layer which we call the pars sagittalis (Lang and Strobel 1978). This ligamentous sheet covers the juncture of the internal carotid artery and cavernous sinus from the lateral side.

Anatomy of the Jugular Foramen

In adults the lateral rim of the jugular foramen lies 14.1 (8–19) mm from the inferior margin of the porus acusticus on the right side and 15.5 (9–21) mm on the left side. Hence:

1) The mean distance is shorter on the right side, probably due to the fact that the jugular foramen is better developed on that side.
2) This distance shows a very large range of individual variation.

Distances to the tip of the mastoid process and their postnatal progression have also been described (Lang and Schreiber 1983). The patterns of subdivision of the jugular foramen are illustrated in Fig. SA 45.

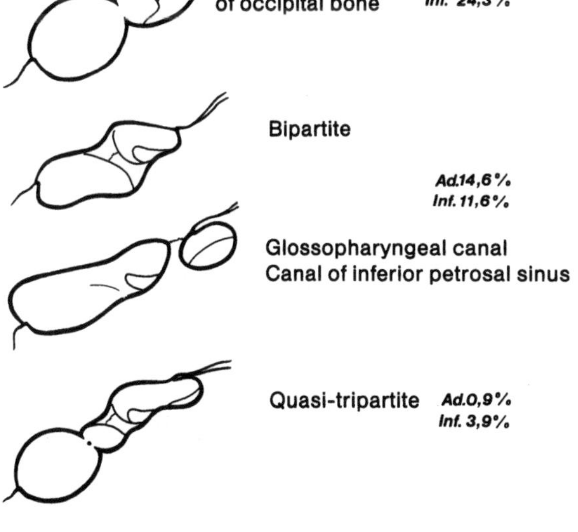

Fig. SA 45. Patterns of subdivision of the jugular foramen (Lang and Schreiber 1983)

Data on the level of the petrous curvature of the carotid canal and the superior bulb of the internal jugular vein relative to the terminal sigmoid margin are given in Fig. SA 44. The intrapetrous veins, the superior and inferior petrosal sinuses, and the carotid venous plexus are also depicted as we found them in our material (Lang and Weigel 1983). It is emphasized that the ninth, tenth, and eleventh cranial nerves may traverse the jugular foramen at various sites. They always run in a connective tissue septum that is continuous with the dura mater of the cranial cavity and with the pericranium exterior to the skull (Lang 1981). This septum contains openings for the inferior petrous sinus. These may pass between the ninth and tenth nerves (48%), in front of the glossopharyngeal nerve (30%). Behind the tenth nerve (16%), or between the tenth and eleventh nerves (6%) (Lang and Weigel 1983) (Fig. SA 46). These openings are variable in number.

In the *extracranial approach to the internal carotid artery and internal jugular vein* from the lateral side, it is customary to release the sternocleidomastoid muscle on its bony mastoid attachment. This may also involve releasing the origin of the splenius capitis and in rare cases the origin of longissimus capitis. The mandible and retromandibular part of the parotid gland are retracted forward, and the *site of emergence and course of the facial nerve* are noted (Fig. SA 47). The stylomastoid foramen in our adult material lies 11.1 (7.2–19.2) mm medial to the tympanomastoid suture on the right side and 11.4 (6.1–17.7) mm on the left side. Hogg and Kratz (1958) state that the nerve runs only 6–8 mm medial to the medial end of the tympanomastoid suture, a measurement later confirmed by Tabb et al. (1973). The first extracranial branches of the facial nerve are as follows:

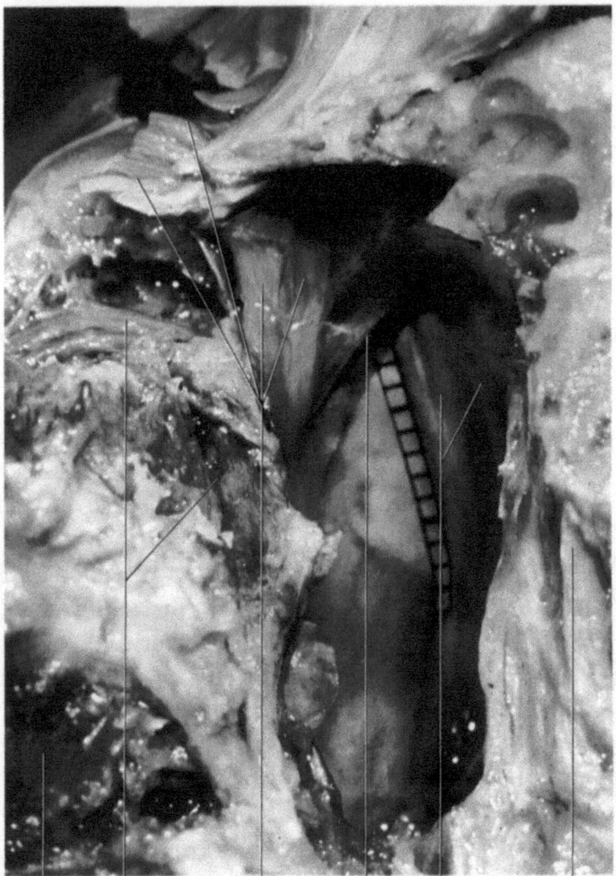

Fig. SA 46. Internal jugular vein, lateral wall removed

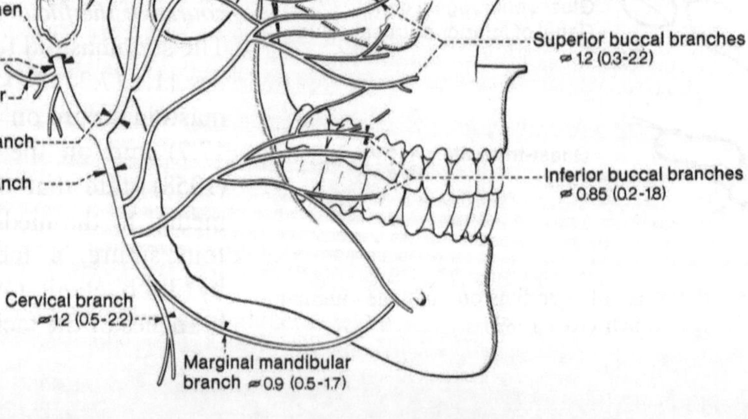

Fig. SA 47. Facial nerve branches and their widths (mm)

1) The posterior auricular nerve, which arises 2.6 (0–6) mm below the stylomastoid foramen in our material. This branch anastomoses with a filament from the auricular branch of the vagus nerve, with the great auricular nerve, and with a branch of the lesser occipital. The nerve runs laterally backward and upward at varying distances from the root of the auricular cartilage. It gives off an auricular branch which supplies the posterior auricular muscle and the muscles on the medial aspect of the auricle. A portion of the superior auricular muscle and a skin area over the mastoid process also receive branches from this nerve. A second, larger branch runs upward behind the auricle and then backward along the superior nuchal line to supply the occipital belly of the epicranius muscle.
2) The second extracranial branch of the facial nerve in our material is the stylohyoid. It arises an average of 6.9 (3–14) mm distal to the stylomastoid foramen and passes as a long, slender nerve to the middle or terminal portion of the stylohyoid muscle, either alone or accompanied by the digastric branch for part of its course.
3) On emerging from the stylomastoid foramen, the main part of the facial nerve runs downward and laterally into the substance of the parotid gland. Generally it bifurcates into two major divisions while still within the gland:
4) An upper division, the temporofacial, and
5) a lower division, the cervicofacial. In our material this surgically important bifurcation is placed 18 (13–27) mm anterior and lateral to the stylomastoid foramen. Denecke (1966) states that the nerve may bifurcate while still in the mastoid portion of the facial canal (see Miehlke 1973 for further details). The bifurcation lies 9.8 (4–17) mm from the posterior border of the ramus of the mandible and 10.8 (9–13) mm from the anterior border of the mastoid process.

Anteromedial to the facial bifurcation in the lateral approach is the styloid process, which varies greatly in its length, and also the muscles that arise from the styloid process and are lateral to the internal jugular vein.

Hypoglossal Nerve

In its course on the external skull base, the hypoglossal nerve runs deep to the internal jugular vein and lateral to the vagus nerve in 92% of cases. It then loops around the occipital artery (58%) or its inferior sternocleidomastoid branch (26%) and runs forward and laterally across all the branches of the external carotid artery. In 8% of cases the nerve passes around the external carotid artery distal to the origin of the occipital (Löwy 1910) and rarely around a sternocleidomastoid branch of the superior thyroid artery. The extracranial part of the hypoglossal nerve in our material is 1.53 (0.8–2.44) mm wide and 0.9 (0.6–2.13) mm thick. It unites with the anterior branches of C_1 and C_2 to form the superior deep ansa cervicalis. The descending branch of the hypoglossal nerve leaves the nerve 14.3 (0–34) mm distal to the ansa. The hypoglossal nerve invariably communicates with the lingual nerve (within the tongue).

Accessory Nerve

The accessory nerve traverses the connective tissue sheet in the jugular foramen just behind the vagus nerve. Almost at once it gives off internal branches to the superior ganglion of the vagus nerve and to a portion of the vagus nerve below the ganglion. The larger nerve trunk becomes the external branch of the accessory nerve, which in our material is 1.28 (0.67–2.44) mm wide and 0.64 (0.18–1.52) mm thick. In our material the external branch of the accessory nerve then runs below the skull base to the sternocleidomastoid, passing in front of the internal jugular vein in about 85% of cases and behind it in 15%. It communicates with the cervical plexus in a highly variable fashion. In several of our specimens the nerve was found passing through a low union of the inferior petrosal sinus with the internal jugular vein. The mastoid branch of the occipital artery accompanies the accessory nerve for a short distance. Besides the sternocleidomastoid, the accessory nerve also supplies the trapezius together with branches of segments C_3 and C_4, although it is not the sole motor supply to that muscle. Paralytic torticollis results from unilateral lesions of the accessory nerve, while spastic torticollis may result from compression of the nerve (Freckmann 1981 in Samii and Jannetta 1981).

Vagus Nerve

The superior ganglion of the vagus nerve occurs at the site of entry of the vagus nerve into the duplication of dura mater in the jugular foramen. The ganglion is up to 4 mm long and is bathed with cerebrospinal fluid from above. In this area we found an average of 1.48 (1–3) anastomoses with the glossopharyngeal nerve. The internal branch (branches) of the accessory nerve arises 11.34 (2–19) mm below the sigmoid terminal margin of the jugular foramen. This branch is 9.75 (3–24) mm long and unites with the vagus nerve. Below that site we found 1.4 (1–3) anastomoses between the tenth and ninth nerves, having a length of 4.94 (2–19) mm (Müller 1985). The *auricular branch of the vagus nerve* also originates from the lower part of the superior vagal ganglion. Generally this branch communicates with branches of the glossopharyngeal. This nerve runs initially in the jugular fossa before passing through a narrow canal in the petrous part of the temporal bone to reach the posterior or anterior part of the mastoid portion of the facial nerve. There it generally anastomoses with the seventh cranial nerve.

Numerous ganglion cells are embedded in the segment of the nerve (within the carotid sheath) that is level with the first and second cervical vertebrae. This is the inferior ganglion of the vagus nerve. At a level 5 mm below the inferior ganglion, the vagus nerve is 2.88 (1.8–5.3) mm wide and 1.5 (0.4–2.44) mm thick in our material. We invariably found anastomoses between the inferior vagal ganglion and the superior cervical ganglion of the sympathetic trunk, and in most cases the ganglion communicated with the ansa between the anterior rami of C_1 and C_2. Anastomoses with the hypoglossal nerve were not a consistent finding: the mean number was 2, with a range from 0 to 9.

The first, pharyngeal branch of the vagus nerve emerges from the area of the inferior ganglion. The next branch of the vagus is the superior laryngeal nerve, which arises 37 (26–52) mm below the terminal sigmoid margin. In most cases it issues from the inferior ganglion of the vagus nerve. The auricular branch of the vagus nerve contains chemoreceptors called glomera (see Glossopharyngeal Nerve and Lang 1981 for further details).

Glossopharyngeal Nerve

The glossopharyngeal nerve (ninth cranial) emerges from the most anterior and medial portion of the jugular foramen (Fig. SA 46).

The superior ganglion of the glossopharyngeal nerve, like that of the vagus nerve, is partially embedded in the dura mater and is bathed with cerebrospinal fluid from above. The perilymphatic aqueduct of the inner ear opens immediately above the superior ganglion (where also the labyrinthine vein runs toward the inferior petrosal sinus or internal jugular vein). A thin branch of the ninth nerve, the tympanic nerve, arises from the area of the superior ganglion or slightly below it. It passes to the middle ear through the tympanic canaliculus, accompanied by a branch of the ascending pharyngeal artery, and then ascends on the promontory. The course of the nerve is marked by the presence of 2–6 glomera (chemoreceptors = intumescentiae in Fig. SA 48), from which glomus tumors can arise (Guild 1941). Another branch of the glossopharyngeal anastomoses with the vagus nerve in this area. Once outside the skull, the ninth nerve descends on the lateral surface of the internal carotid artery, medial to the internal jugular vein. Like these vessels and the vagus nerve, it is embedded in the carotid sheath. At a lower level the nerve and its branches run downward and forward from the internal carotid. The landmark for this nerve is the stylopharyngeus muscle, which the nerve also supplies. The nerve permeates the entire muscle in about 12% of our material (especially on the left side). The ninth nerve establishes anastomoses with:

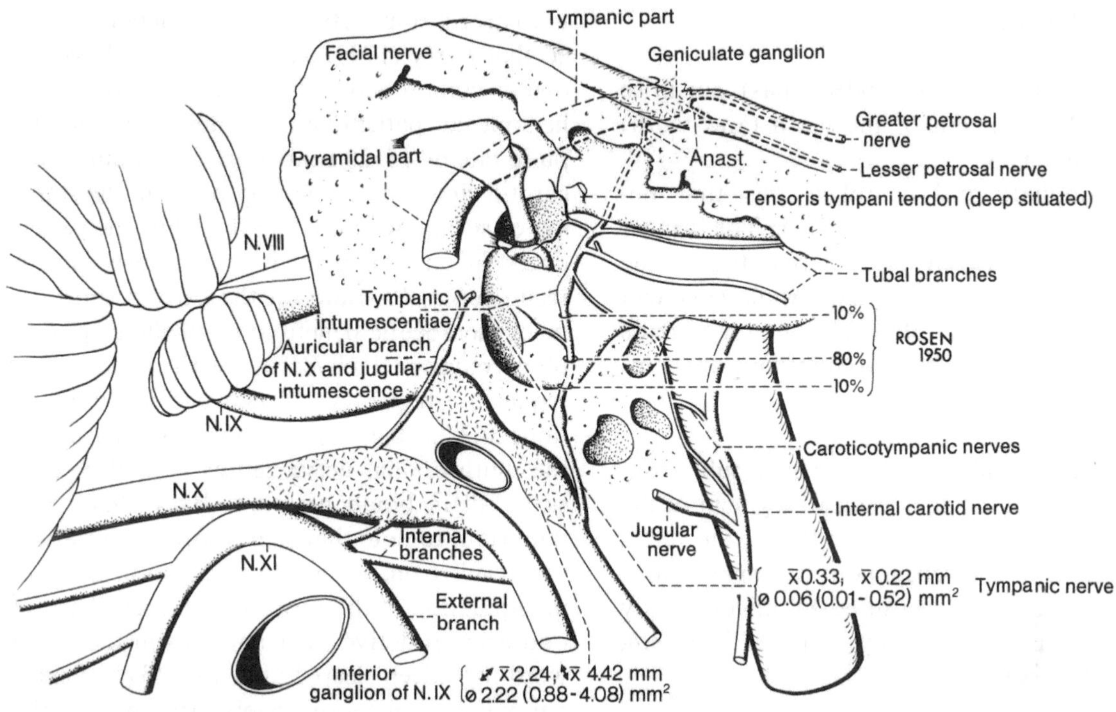

Fig. SA 48. Most frequent course of the tympanic nerve and the auricular branch of the vagus nerve, and most frequent locations of the tympanic intumescentiae. These organs are believed to be chemoreceptors and can form a nidus for chemodectomas (glomus tumors). The connections of the tympanic nerve with the geniculate ganglion, facial nerve, greater and lesser petrosal nerves, and internal carotid artery are also shown (Wurzburg material)

1) The sympathetic plexus of the internal carotid artery.
2) The facial nerve.
3) The tenth and twelfth nerves.

The anastomosis with the seventh nerve reaches the first extracranial segment of the facial nerve or the digastric branch. This anastomosis may transmit sensory fibers from the concha auris to the ninth nerve. Three or four pharyngeal branches from the glossopharyngeal are distributed to the posterior surface of the pharynx, tonsillar branches to the tonsillar capsule, and lingual branches to the pharyngeal part of the tongue, the vallate papillae, the epiglottic vallecula, and the upper surface of the epiglottis. Motor branches of the glossopharyngeal supply the stylopharyngeus and the superior constrictor muscle of the pharynx (in conjunction with the tenth cranial nerve). Sensory fibers (including gustatory) are distributed to the posterior third of the tongue, the posterior portions of the oral cavity, the isthmus faucium, and the pharynx. The sensory innervation of the ninth nerve conducts fibers from the isthmus faucium, the palatine tonsil, the pharyngeal surface of the tongue, the posterior and lateral wall of the pharynx, the tympanic cavity, the auditory tube, and a small area behind the ear. Parasympathetic secretory fibers of the ninth nerve are conducted in the tympanic nerve and then in the lesser petrosal nerve to the otic ganglion and parotid gland. The buccal glands, molar glands, and the glands of the vallate papillae and posterior third of the tongue are also supplied by the ninth nerve.

Surgical Importance

1) Glomus tumors (chemodectomas) can arise from the glomera of the ninth (and tenth) cranial nerves.
2) Glossopharyngeal neuralgia was first described by Weisenburg (1910). The trigger zone lies between the palatine tonsil, the tongue, and the pharynx. Swallowing can precipitate attacks of pain lasting for seconds to minutes and affecting numerous areas including the ear.

Glossopharyngeal neuralgia can result from compression of the glial (central) segment of the glossopharyngeal nerve by the PICA, the vertebral artery, or a cerebellopontine angle tumor. Other attacks may be caused by an unusually long styloid process or by a tumor involving the ninth nerve.

Carotid Sinus Branches

The carotid sinus branches range from one to four in number; Boyd (1937) stated that there are usually two. He reported a length of about 12.7 mm between the first carotid sinus branch and the skull base. Franke (1963) reported on the carotid sinus syndrome and the "hyperactive carotid sinus reflex" in some detail. He noted that Parry (1799) was the first to show that digital compression of the carotid artery in a hemiplegic patient immediately lowered the pulse rate by 15–20 beats/min. The spontaneous carotid sinus syndrome may occur in the standing or sitting position, or even while the patient dozes in an armchair; it is extremely rare in recumbency. Pressure on the carotid sinus can be of therapeutic benefit in controlling episodes of paroxysmal tachycardia with no undesired sequelae (frequency of neurogenic complications 0.22%–0.25%). Intracranial division of the ninth cranial nerve causes a sudden, transient fall in blood pressure (Bucy 1936). It is important to note that significant complications can result from external compression or other manipulation of the carotid sinus area. The carotid arteries derive their name from the Greek word for "deep sleep," after the effect of external pressure on those vessels. Ancient Assyrian physicians used carotid compression as a means of inducing analgesia for circumcisions. Calverley and Millikan (1961) described several instances in which carotid sinus massage (e.g., for stiffness of the neck) produced severe cerebral effects including sudden paralysis of the arm and leg, bleeding into the internal capsule, infarction of the frontoparietal region, hemiplegia, and homonymous hemianopsia.

Parapharyngeal Space

Arteries

Common Carotid Artery

The length of the common carotid artery in our material is 98.8 (81–125) mm on the right side and 121.2 (100–145) mm on the left side (Meuer 1983).

Carotid Bifurcation

Many studies have been done on the level at which the common carotid artery bifurcates into the internal and external carotids. Lippert and Pabst (1985) reviewed the results of many authors and found that the division occurred at the C_4 level in 35% of cases, at the superior border of C_4 in 30%, at C_3 in 12%, at the C_4/C_5 interspace in 12%, at the C_5/C_6 interspace in 5%, at the C_2/C_3 interspace in 4%, at C_2 (lower portion) in 1%, and at the C_5/C_6 interspace in 1%. Shah and Srivastava (1965) found that the bifurcation was level with the superior border of the thyroid cartilage in 63.33% of cases and above it in the remainder. In 20% the bifurcation was 3–4 cm above the thyroid cartilage; it was never found below it. Kantor (1905) cited cases in which the common carotid artery was entirely absent, and the internal and external carotids arose separately from the aorta. He also described a common carotid artery 1 cm long (with a normal origin) giving rise to an internal carotid artery that ascended behind and medial to the external carotid.

Carotid Triangle and Its Relation to the Carotid Bifurcation

The carotid triangle is bounded by the anterior border of the sternocleidomastoid muscle, the posterior belly of the digastric, and the superior belly of the omohyoid. The carotid bifurcation presents within this triangle when viewed strictly from the lateral aspect. With dorsiflexion of the head, the upper part of the sternocleidomastoid muscle moves farther posteriorly while the bifurcation (and the internal and external carotid arteries) moves to a point between the anterior border of the sternocleidomastoid, the inferior border of the digastric, and the superior belly of the omohyoid. Other positional changes occur when the head is rolled, ventrally flexed, or tilted to one side (see Lanz and Wachsmuth 1955, Figs. 86 and 92–96).
Poisel and Golth (1974) studied 156 necks of adults and found that the carotid bifurcation occupied the middle third of the carotid triangle in 67.31%, the upper third in 20.51%, and the lower third in 10.90%. The bifurcation was slightly below the carotid triangle in 1.28%.

Cervical Portions of the Internal and External Carotid Arteries

Jazuta (1928) studied 100 adults and 100 8- to 9-month fetuses and newborns. He determined that the internal carotid artery runs relatively far backward from the external carotid artery in 85% of adults. In 10.5% it runs closely adjacent to the external carotid, and in 2% its medial border projects in front of the external carotid before taking a backward and upward course above the origin of the facial artery. In 2% most of the anterior border of the internal carotid artery curves out in front of the external carotid, and in 0.5% the first part of the internal carotid artery is entirely anterior to the first part of the external carotid. In children the carotid arteries were widely separated in 50% and closely adjacent (with the internal carotid behind the external carotid) in 30%. Minor transpositions were noted in the lower part of the internal carotid artery in 19%.

Smith and Larsen (1979) showed angiographically that the internal carotid artery emerges posteriorly from the common carotid in 46% of cases on the right side and 54% on the left, and posterolaterally in 36% on the right side and 40% on the left. It arises posteromedially in 11% on the right and 5% on the left, and medially in 7% on the right and 1% on the left. Overall, the internal carotid artery ran backward or posterolaterally from the posterior or posterolateral surface of the common carotid artery in 82% of cases on the right side and in 94% on the left side. Posteromedial or medial origins were noted in 18% on the right and 6% on the left. The internal carotid artery usually ascends on the posterolateral wall of the pharynx (in the parapharyngeal space). Very rarely it courses entirely on the posterior wall of the pharynx, and Kelly (1925) observed this pattern unilaterally and bilaterally. In this case the artery produces a pulsating bulge in the pharynx that can be palpated.

Carotid Sinus and Carotid Arteries, Diameters

The diameter of the carotid sinus in our material (older males) is 14.8 (10–21) mm on the right side and 15.2 (11–20) mm on the left side (Meuer 1983). The outer diameter of the internal carotid artery is 5.9 (4.0–7.5) mm on the right side and 6.2 (4.5–8.0) mm on the left; that of the external carotid, 5.9 (4.0–7.5) mm on the right side and 5.8 (4.0–8.0) mm on the left. Czerwinski determined a mean outer diameter of 6.1 mm for the external carotid artery in men and 5.4 mm in women.

Carotid Tortuosity

Rowlands and Swan (1902) and Fisher (1915) were among the first authors to note the presence of loops and coils in the extracranial portion of the internal carotid artery. Kelly (1925) expressed the belief that the tortuosity was of ontogenic origin. It is known that the artery develops from the third aortic arch and the dorsal aorta, and it is at the junction of these two parts that tortuosity is most commonly observed. Cairney (1924) examined 36 cadavers and found 10 in which the internal carotid artery displayed significant tortuosity (bilateral in one case). The second loop was usually directed medially. Weibel and Fields (1965) studied the wall changes associated with kinking and suggested that the stenosis was mechanically induced. Hassler (1961) noted the occurrence of intima proliferation at sites of luminal change (bifurcations, etc.) and suggested that this phenomenon might also occur secondary to coiling or other tortuosity. Lazorthes et al. (1961) devised a system for classifying the course of the internal carotid artery: In their type A (30.5%) the course of the artery is straight or minimally curved toward one side. In type B (48.5%) the artery presents an S-shaped curvature, and in type C (21%) the artery presents irregular kinks or coils. Lazorthes et al. (1971) showed that the internal carotid artery can become compressed by the digastric muscle during ipsilateral movements of the head. As early as 1902, Smith described true coiling of the internal carotid artery below the digastric muscle. McMurtry and Yahr (1966) described a duplication of the posterior belly of the digastric which compressed the internal carotid artery about 1 cm distal to its origin. Francke et al. (1982) determined the length of the cervical part of the internal carotid artery (from the bifurcation to the lower end of the carotid canal), finding a value of 80.2 ± 10 mm on the left side and 82.2 ± 11.6 mm on the right side.

Numerous studies have been done on agenesis and hypoplasia of the internal carotid artery and the possible familial occurrence of those conditions (e.g., Tharp et al. 1965; Smith et al. 1968; Lhermitte et al. 1968; Austin and Stears 1971; consult Lie 1968 and Lang 1986 for further details).

Like other sections of the internal carotid artery, its cervical part is susceptible to aneurysm formation. Aneurysmal bleeding in this area was first observed by Delens (1870, quoted in Hamby 1952). Weaver and Young (1964) note that Todman (1960) described a spontaneous hemorrhage from the internal carotid artery into the retropharyngeal space in a 22-year-old man. Wishart (1923) reported on a similar case with a retropharyngeal abscess. Gross and Holzman (1954) described a peculiar case involving the development of a common carotid artery aneurysm following the ligation of an intracranial aneurysm (in a 25-year-old man). Spallone and Cantore (1981) demonstrated that kinking and coiling of the cervical part of the internal carotid artery is more common in patients with intracranial aneurysms than in controls.

Primitive Hypoglossic Artery, Postoccipital Artery

Batujeff (1889) published the first description of a "primitive hypoglossic artery". In his specimen a vessel branched from the internal carotid artery at the lower end of the carotid canal and entered the skull through the left hypoglossal canal. In the case described by Jackson (1964) the primitive hypoglossic artery arose at C_2, and in the case described by Begg it arose 1.5 cm below the anterior arch of the atlas. Its extracranial course to the hypoglossal canal was approximately 2 cm.

If this artery enters the skull through the foramen magnum rather than the hypoglossal canal, it is referred to as the "postoccipital artery" (Gerlach et al. 1962). These vessels must be spared in the extracranial approach to the internal carotid artery and the craniocervical junction, as they may replace a vertebral artery. In the case of Batujeff (1889) the contralateral vertebral artery fed only the posterior inferior cerebellar artery. In the case of Oertel (1922) the contralateral vertebral artery was extremely thin, as it was in the case of Morris and Moffat.

Ascending Pharyngeal Artery
(Figs. SA 49, SA 50)

The ascending pharyngeal artery is of practical surgical importance, especially for the embolization of glomus tumors. Its branches to the skull base anastomose with caroticocavernous vessels, as Lasjaunias and Moret (1976) described in some detail. Because the ascending pharyngeal artery also gives off the posterior meningeal artery, which traverses various openings to supply the dura mater and bone of the posterior cranial fossa. Attention should be given to this vessel even in procedures which open the posterior fossa. Its small branches accompany the tympanic nerve into the middle ear and constitute the primary vascular supply of the tympanic glomera. A branch of the ascending pharyngeal artery also accompanies the auricular branch of the vagus nerve in most cases. Tumors of the glomera were first described by Keen and Funke (1906) and later by Rosenwasser (1945), who was the first to observe these lesions in the middle ear. Mulligan (1950) introduced the term "chemodectoma" for tumors arising from glomera, since the glomera themselves are believed to be chemoreceptors (especially for blood pH). In our material (Lang and Heilek 1984) the ascending pharyngeal artery arises from the external carotid artery or one of its branches in some 86% of cases. In 55.6% it arises directly, in 11.1% from a trunk that gives off an additional head vessel, and in 12.7% directly from the carotid bifurcation or in close proximity to it. Its origin lies 12.5 (0–36) mm above the bifurcation, ranging between 6 and 20 mm in two-thirds of our cases. In 17.4% the ascending palatine artery and the ascending pharyngeal artery arise from a common trunk. Origins from the area of the bifurcation were noted in 12.7%. In 7.9% the vessel sprang from the occipital artery. It is noteworthy that the artery can arise directly from the internal carotid. As early as 1811, Burns described a case in which all branches of the external carotid artery arose from the internal carotid. Hyrtl (1853) and Matsuda et al. (1977) described cases in which the occipital artery left the cervical segment of the internal carotid artery about 2 cm distal to the bifurcation. In our material the ascending pharyngeal artery emerged from the internal carotid in about 5% of cases, arising 17.7 (17–19) mm distal to the bifurcation. It originated from the facial artery in 1.6%.

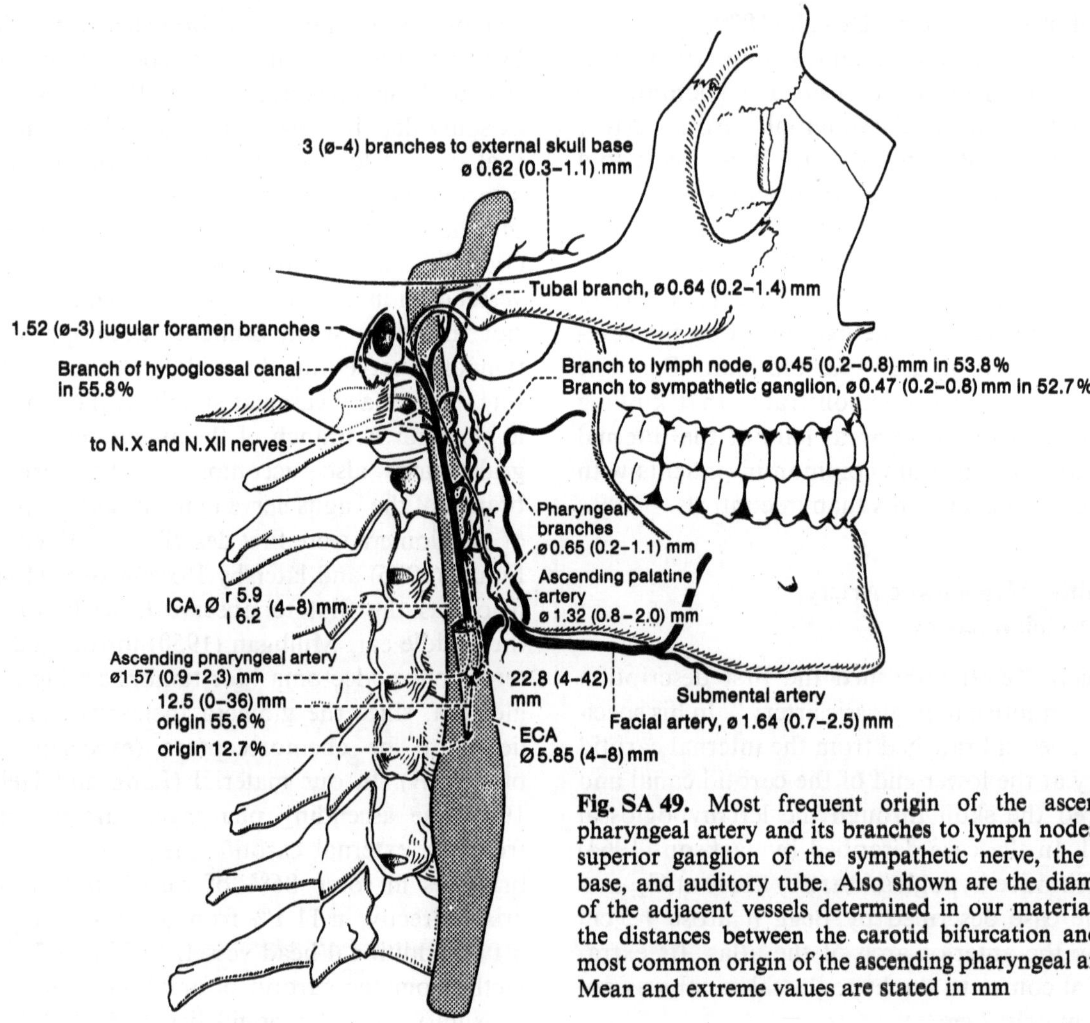

Fig. SA 49. Most frequent origin of the ascending pharyngeal artery and its branches to lymph nodes, the superior ganglion of the sympathetic nerve, the skull base, and auditory tube. Also shown are the diameters of the adjacent vessels determined in our material and the distances between the carotid bifurcation and the most common origin of the ascending pharyngeal artery. Mean and extreme values are stated in mm

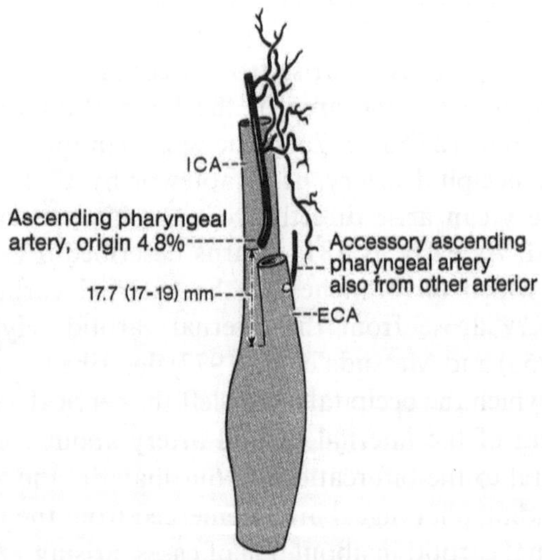

Fig. SA 50. Ascending pharyngeal artery arising from the internal carotid, and accessory pharyngeal arteries

Accessory ascending pharyngeal arteries were also identified. When catheterization is planned, it is important to know the side of the vessel from which the ascending pharyngeal artery arises. The most common site of origin in our material was the medial circumference of the external carotid artery (41.4%), followed in frequency by the posteromedial side of the external carotid (22.7%) and the mediorostral side (15.9%). In 83% the ascending pharyngeal artery arose at a relatively small angle (0°–20°), and in the rest the angle was less acute (maximum of 35°). The mean outer diameter of the ascending pharyngeal artery (10 mm from its origin) was 1.57 (0.9–2.3) mm.

The relationship of the ascending pharyngeal artery to the internal carotid artery (distal to its origin) was medial in 38.9% of our material, mediorostral in 35.2%, rostral and lateral in 9.25%, and lateral in 7.4%. As early as 1925, Kelly noted that the ascending pharyngeal artery may arch toward the pharynx when there is coiling of the internal carotid artery. (Consult Lang and Heilek 1984 for details on the branches of the ascending pharyngeal artery.) The branches of greatest interest are the pharyngeal branches, the lymph node branches, the branches to the sympathetic ganglion, the branches to the vagus and hypoglossal nerves, the muscular branches to the prevertebral musculature, the carotid canal branches, and the inferior tubal artery. Branches to the jugular foramen were always present and averaged 1.52 in number. One such branch was demonstrated in 50% of our cases, 2 in 37.5%, and 3 in 10.5%. These branches generally are closely apposed to the upper cervical part of the internal carotid artery and, embedded in connective tissue, pass directly below the external skull base to the jugular foramen (in slightly more than 4% branches of the occipital artery also enter the jugular foramen). Branches of the ascending pharyngeal artery also are distributed to the external skull base in most cases, and these usually numbered three in our material. We also identified branches to the nasopharynx, and branches to the hypoglossal canal were present in about 56% of cases. As early as 1861, Luschka performed injection studies of the ascending pharyngeal arteries and found that its largest meningeal branch entered the hypoglossal canal and ramified in the wall of the marginal sinus of the foramen magnum. This author also described anastomoses with clival twigs of the caroticocavernous branches in addition to jugular foramen branches and carotid branches (see Lang and Heilek 1984 for further details).

Veins

Internal Jugular Vein (see Fig. SA 44)

Gabrielsen et al. (1968) reported a mean diameter of 9.5 (6–16) mm for the right internal jugular vein and 8 (5–13) mm for the left internal jugular vein. Arnold et al. (1980) reported mean values of 17.3 mm for the right side in lower cervical levels and 14.4 mm for the left side. In our material and at the infrahyoid area, the right jugular vein has a diameter of 12.08 (6–23) mm, the left 10.47 (5–19) mm (Kessler 1989). Cornel (1969) described unilateral absence of the internal jugular vein, and we made a similar observation in our material (left internal jugular vein). It is noteworthy that Schweizer and Leak (1952) observed a rise of cerebrospinal fluid pressure following the removal of both internal jugular veins. In the upper cervical area the internal jugular vein generally runs lateral and slightly posterior to the internal carotid artery.

Tributary Veins and Sinus (Fig. SA 44)

In our material (Lang and Weigel 1983) the inferior petrosal sinus traverses the jugular foramen between the ninth and tenth nerves in about 50% of cases, anterior and medial to the ninth nerve in 30%, anterior to the tenth nerve and behind the ninth nerve in 16%, and between the tenth and eleventh nerves in 6%. We also observed "low drainage" of the inferior petrosal sinus, as did Luschka (1861) more than a century ago.

The inferior petrosal sinus runs below the skull base to the internal jugular vein in only about 10% of our material (Lang and Weigel 1983). In a few cases the inferior petrosal sinus was found as a vein a full 20 mm below the skull base. Luschka (1861) also observed an extracranial vein 2 mm in diameter and 6 mm long that arose from the inferior petrosal sinus and ended in the internal jugular vein.

The anterosuperior aspect of the internal jugular vein generally receives a superior pharyngeal vein, which drains the pharyngeal fornix and the posterior wall of the pharynx and usually receives additional blood from the venous plexus of the hypoglossal canal. This plexus is also known to communicate with the marginal sinus of the foramen magnum, the vertebral plexuses, and the jugular foramen. An inferior pharyngeal vein joins the medial circumference of the internal jugular vein, usually at a low site level with the hyoid bone. The position of the superior

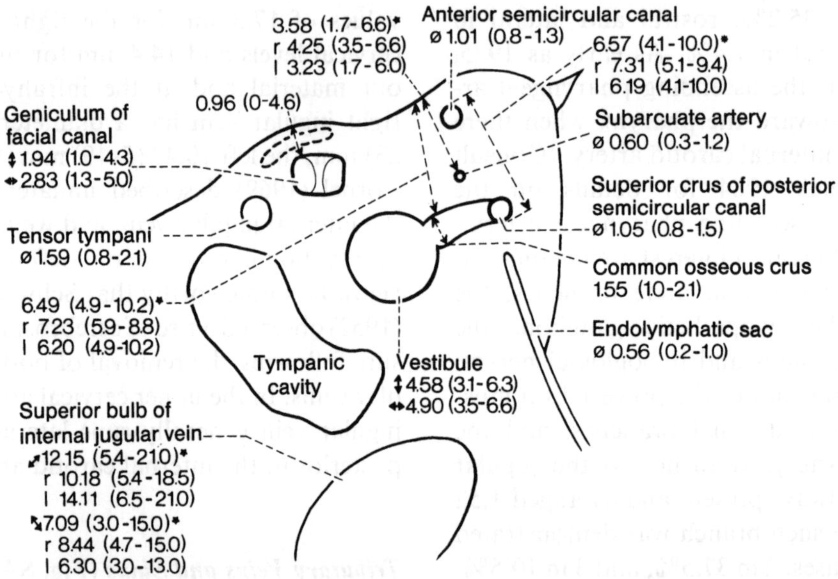

Fig. SA 51. Parasagittal section through the petrous part of the temporal bone, showing the dimensions of various canals and the superior bulb of the internal jugular vein (from Fichtl). Measurements in mm

bulb of the internal jugular vein is illustrated in Figs. SA 44, SA 51, and SA 52. Overton and Ritter (1973) observed "high-placed" jugular bulbs (i.e., above the level of the tympanic ring) in 6% of their material. Similarly, we found in our material that the upper wall of the jugular bulb occasionally bordered directly on the mucosa of the tympanic cavity. We make a distinction between medially and laterally high-placed jugular bulbs. In the latter case the upper wall of the bulb protrudes into the tympanic cavity; in the former the bulb is in contact with the endolymphatic sac (we occasionally found no bony wall between both structures). In some of our specimens the jugular bulb projected up to the level of the internal acoustic meatus.

In the surgical treatment of glomus tumors and other tumors occurring medially and in the region of the jugular foramen and tympanic cavity, it is necessary not only to remove the jugular foramen and superior jugular bulb but also to mobilize the petrous part of the internal carotid artery to gain access to more of the petrous part of the temporal bone and also the clivus. Denecke (1966) showed that glomus tumors have a tendency to spread along adjacent veins. In our material we found a lateral and a medial intrapetrosal vein in 50% of cases and a medial intrapetrosal vein in the remaining 50% (Lang and Weigel 1983) (see Fig. SA 44). When exposing the ascending petrous part of the internal carotid artery, it is important to know the position, caliber, and direction of this section of the canal. The length of the ascending part of the carotid canal in our adult material is 10.05 (7–13) mm on the right side and 10.22 (6.5–13.5) mm on the left side (Lang et al. 1983). Generally the canal runs upward and forward (Lang and Schreiber 1983). It is important to note that the medial wall of this section of the canal (and the inferior wall of the transverse petrous part) may be absent in rare cases, making it possible to visualize the entire petrous part of the internal carotid artery on the inferior skull base. The genu region (petrous curvature of the carotid canal) may be placed extremely high in the tympanic cavity and may occasionally be dehiscent. In these cases the internal carotid artery projects into the anterior part of the tympanic cavity. Paullus et al. (1977) state that, in 2% of cases, portions of the wall of the carotid canal are absent in this area. Anderson et al. (1972) described aneurysms of the internal carotid artery in the lateral part of the carotid canal

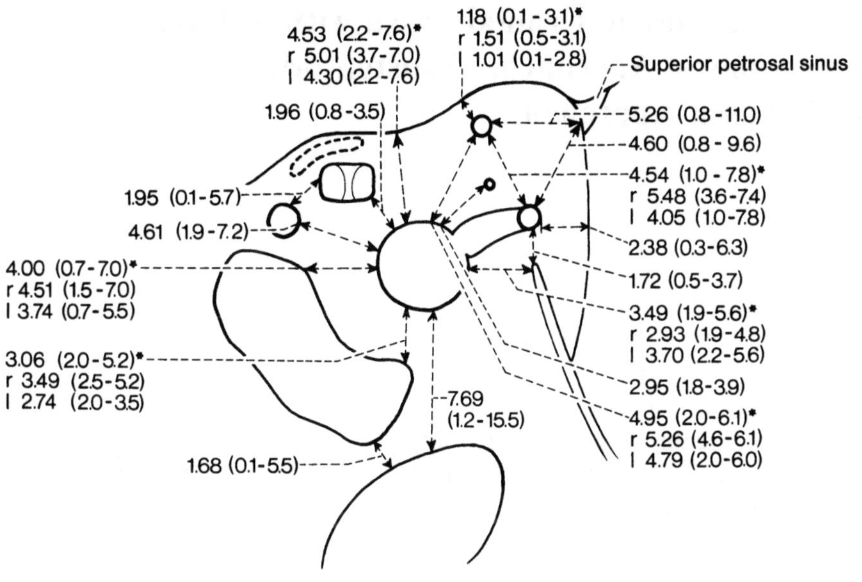

Fig. SA 52. Parasagittal section through the petrous part of the temporal bone, showing the dimensions of various canals and the superior bulb of the internal jugular vein. The distances from the superior bulb to the vestibule and to the tympanic cavity are also shown. Measurements in mm (after researchments from Fichtl)

mimicking the symptoms of a glomus tumor. In two patients they described a pulsating mass below the deformed tympanic membrane. When the inferior wall of the transverse part of the carotid canal (which has a mean length of 21.3 mm in our adult material) is opened with a cutting burr, this section of the internal carotid artery can be exteriorized. The total length of carotid artery within the canal in our adult material is 31.51 (20–50) mm on the right side and 31.21 (22–42) mm on the left side (Lang et al. 1983). It should be emphasized that the internal carotid venous plexus runs within the carotid canal, extending from the lower opening of the canal to the posterior portal region of the cavernous sinus. This venous plexus was first described by Soemmering (1791). Rektorzik (1858) later studied these veins in more detail and described them as a venous sinus in the human carotid canal, as did Teufel (1964). Generally these veins are not encountered in the surgical approach to the carotid canal (Wullstein, personal communication 1985). Besides the veins, the carotid canal contains a layer of endocranium on its wall, a mobile layer between the arteries and adjacent structures, and generally two nerves, often of large caliber, derived from the superior cervical ganglion of the sympathetic trunk. When the transverse petrous part of the internal carotid canal is transposed downward and forward, it is possible to visualize and open the transverse and sagittal parts of the inferior sphenopetrosal ligament from below. The transverse part of this ligament (Lang and Strobel 1978) is developed in 96% of cases, covers the rostral circumference of the wall of the carotid canal, is 12.5 (6–23.5) mm long and 4.6 (2–13.8) mm wide. Removal of this wall, especially of its anterior portions, is apt to damage the greater petrosal nerve (and possibly the lesser petrosal) leading to a disturbance in the secretory functions of the lacrimal and parotid glands. We call the medial, more sagittally oriented part of this ligament the sagittal part of the inferior sphenopetrosal ligament. It is 0.5 (0.3–1.0) mm thick and 3.9 (1–7) mm high and covers the site of entry of the internal carotid artery into the cavernous sinus. Both segments support portions of the triangular part of the trigeminal nerve and possibly of the trigeminal ganglion, which are bounded by the thin inferior wall of the trigeminal cave.

Anatomy of the Middle Cranial Fossa with Reference to the Subtemporal Approach, Transtentorial Approach, and Middle Fossa Approach

In the subtemporal approach to the middle cranial fossa, part of the temporal muscle is usually detached with a piece of the lateral cranial wall (temporal squama, greater wing of sphenoid) and reflected downward. The route of surgical approach, the branches of the superficial temporal artery, the temporal muscle, the middle temporal vein, and the deep temporal arteries are discussed in connection with the pterional approach. The depth of the temporal fossa during postnatal life is illustrated in Fig. SA 53 (from Lang and Götzfried 1982). The lowest point of the middle cranial fossa (and the FHP) is roughly level with the upper border of the zygomatic arch and is slightly posterior to the articular tubercle of the temporomandibular joint. The upper part of the zygomatic arch may be burred away to make room for the necessary downward reflection of muscle and bone (Spetzler, personal communication 1986). The floor of the middle cranial fossa is bounded anteriorly and inferiorly by the greater wing of the sphenoid, by the temporal squama in the area of the surgical approach, and posteriorly by the anterior surface of the petrous part. It should be noted that impressions of the temporal gyri may greatly thin the temporal squama (see Lang 1983 for details). The floor of the middle fossa is also thin:

1) About the articular fossa of the temporomandibular joint.
2) In front of the foramen ovale and lateral to the foramen rotundum.

Generally the thickest part of the floor is the mandibular eminence of the temporomandibular joint; less frequently it is a jugum in the floor of the middle fossa (Lang and Brückner 1981). The bone and dura mater of the middle fossa floor are supplied by branches of the middle meningeal artery and by caroticocavernous branches (see Fig. SA 54 which is from Lang and Schäfer 1976, Lang and Brückner 1981). Earlier we noted that the foramen rotundum, the foramen ovale, the foramen spinosum, and the foramen of Vesalius on the right side of the head are placed closer to the midsagittal plane than on the left side. Furthermore, the foramina on the right are set slightly farther posteriorly than on the left. Overall we may say that the more rostrally the foramina are placed, the more lateral their position; the more posteriorly they are placed, the closer they are to the midsagittal plane (Lang and Tisch-Rottensteiner 1976). A later study confirmed this tendency during postnatal development (Lang et al. 1984). Figure SA 55 shows the distances of these foramina from points on the external surface of the skull and the midsagittal plane. Our material included foramina ovalia that were open posteriorly, foramina spinosa that communicated with the foramen ovale, and foramina ovalia that were partially divided in two.

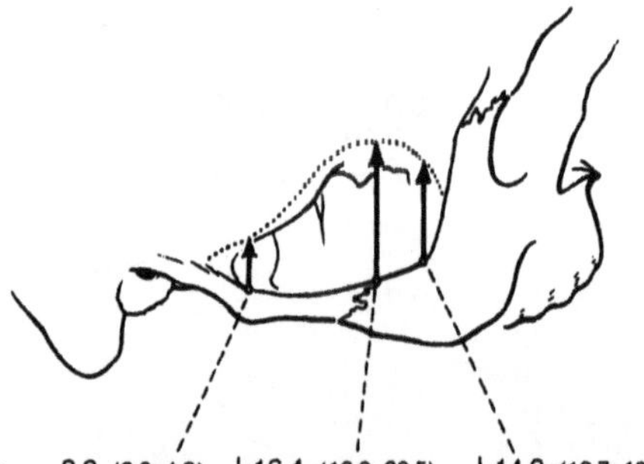

Neonates	3.0 (2.0–4.0)	16.4 (12.3–20.5)	14.2 (10.7–19.7)
1 year	4.1 (3.7–4.6)	22.6 (18.4–24.1)	15.9 (9.6–22.6)
4–5 years	5.7 (3.2–8.5)	26.2 (16.9–46.1)	17.1 (10.5–29.9)
15–17 years	7.6 (6.0–8.9)	26.0 (14.6–34.9)	18.2 (11.0–23.4)
Adult	10.8 (5.3–18.6)	29.2 (19.7–47.2)	21.1 (10.8–35.5)

Fig. SA 53. Postnatal deepening of the temporal fossa (after Lang and Götzfried 1982)

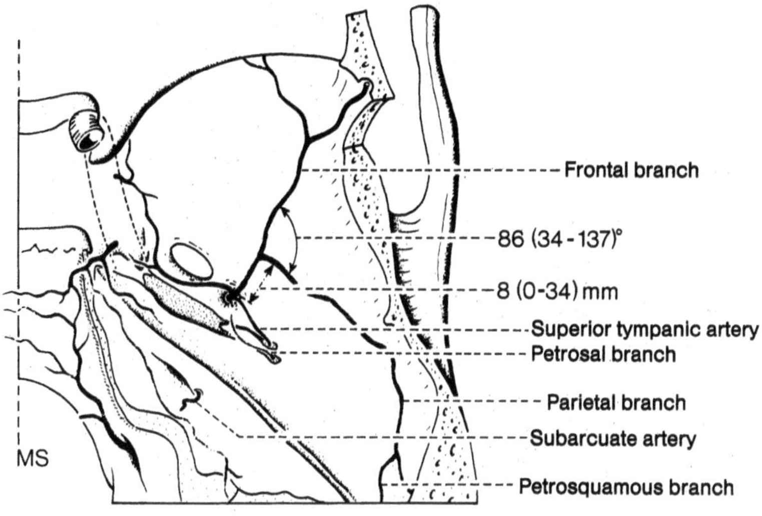

Fig. SA 54. Meningeal arteries in the floor of the middle cranial fossa (after Lang and Schäfer 1976; Lang and Brückner 1981). The branches of the middle meningeal artery and their anastomoses with caroticocavernous trunks are shown

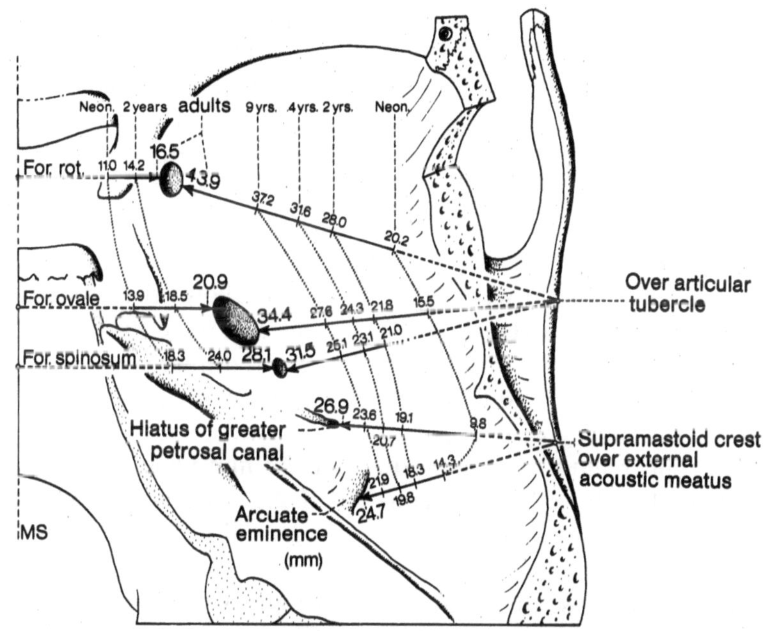

Fig. SA 55. Foramen rotundum, foramen ovale, foramen spinosum, hiatus of the facial canal, and arcuate eminence. Postnatal changes in their distance from points and landmarks on the external skull surface, and their progressive postnatal separation from the midline (after Lang et al. 1983)

The anterior wall of the floor of the middle fossa carries a depression adapted to the pole of the temporal lobe. It is noteworthy that a dural layer with a mean thickness of 2 mm (including the sphenoparietal sinus) overlaps the posterior aspect of the lesser wing of the sphenoid (Lang and Haas 1979). Planimetric measurements in skull sections indicate that the mean depth of the depression is 3.1 (0–7.7) mm laterally, 3.6 (0–9) mm centrally, and 3.6 (0–18.3) mm medially (Lang and Götzfried 1982).

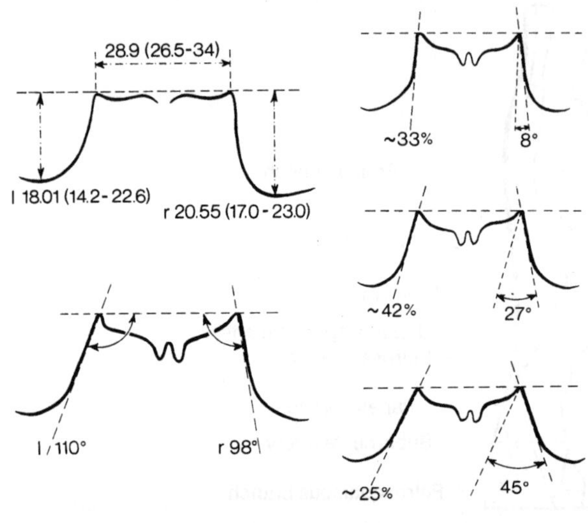

Fig. SA 56. Width of the roof of the cavernous sinus at the level of the foramen diaphragmatis, mean angulation of the right and left walls of the cavernous sinus on this plane, and variability in the orientation of the lateral walls

We determined the maximum width of the roof of the cavernous sinus in the area of the foramen diaphragmatis. Remarkably, we found a mean width of 30 mm in mesocranic skulls, 29.05 mm in brachycranic skulls, and only 28.36 mm in hyperbrachycranic (very broad) skulls (Fig. SA 56). These findings in our material were subsequently rechecked and confirmed (Horn 1978). The superior wall of the cavernous sinus is bordered laterally in this area by the anterior petroclinoid fold, which usually projects upward above the rest of the upper sinus wall. Its mean distance from the lateral skull wall (at the same level) is 39.3 mm on the right side and 37.0 mm on the left. Because the foramina rotundum, ovale, and spinosum are set close to the midline on the right side, the right lateral wall of the cavernous sinus displays a significantly sharper slope than its left wall. The anterior petroclinoid fold forms the anterior extension of the tentorial notch. It is attached in front to the anterior clinoid process. There is also a posterior petroclinoid fold, which extends to the lateral border of the dorsum sellae. It should be noted that the upper surface of the dorsum sellae frequently carries indentations that relate especially to the course of the posterior communicating artery.

Tentorial Notch
(Fig. SA 57)

The tentorium cerebelli, like the falx cerebri and the falx cerebelli, constitutes part of the internal skeleton of the skull (see Lang 1985 for further details). Data on the relative positions of the tentorial notch and midbrain were published earlier (Lang 1983, 1985). The falx and tentorium are composed of collagen fibers which limit the mobility of the structures they enclose and support. Width and length measurements of the tentorial notch were performed in our material with the remaining parts of the skull and dura left intact (Horn 1978). The basal width of the tentorial notch was found to be 30.25 (25–36) mm. We performed a second width measurement at the level of the inferior colliculi of the midbrain, finding the tentorial notch (in the taut condition) to be 25.6 (19–33) mm wide in this area. The term "Meynert's axis" has long been used to denote the axis of the midbrain and lower portions of the brain stem (Lang 1985). The axis of the diencephalon extending forward from the midbrain axis is known as "Forell's axis". It is believed that the angulation produced by the narrow but relatively high tentorial notch allows the midbrain to move downward and backward in response to minor frontal and occipital trauma without causing damage to adjacent structures. By contrast, the space available for lateral midbrain displacements is only 1–1.5 mm wide alongside the anterior portions of the midbrain (Lang 1985). The length of the tentorial notch (measured from the dorsum sellae) is 47.05 (38–58) mm. By gender, the mean length of the notch was 46.58 mm in men and 47.95 mm in women.

Arachnoid

The anatomy of the subarachnoid spaces in corrosion preparations was detailed in an earlier publication (Lang 1973), where it was emphasized that all these spaces communicate with one another but are permeated by connective-tissue strands of varying density (arachnoid trabeculae). Especially after aneurysmatic hemorrhage,

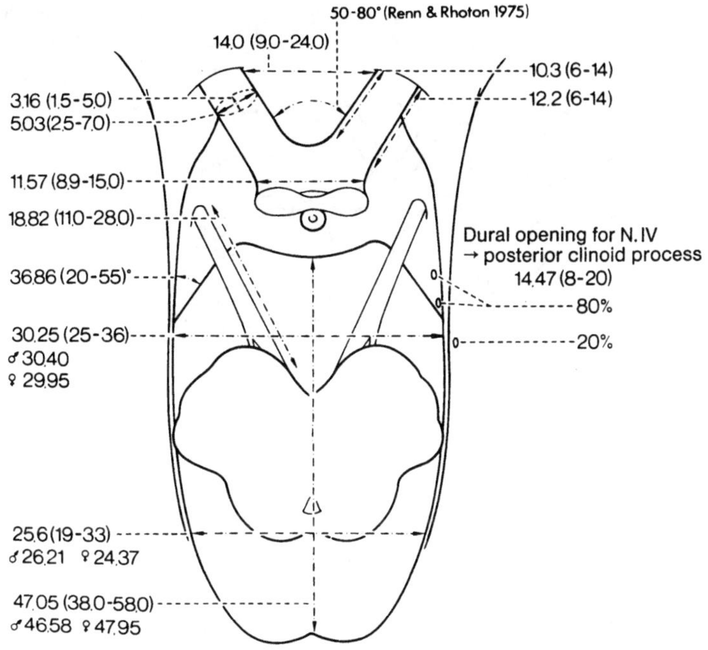

Fig. SA 57. Width of the tentorial notch at different levels, distance between the dorsum sellae and uppermost part, length of the oculomotor nerve, angle between the petroclinoid folds, cross-sectional dimensions of the intracranial part of the optic nerve, distance between the optic canals, width of the chiasm, and length of the medial and lateral borders of the optic nerve. The dural opening for the trochlear nerve and the angle between the optic nerves are also shown (Renn and Rhoton 1975). Mean and extreme values are stated in mm, and some sex differences are noted (from Lang 1985)

the passageways that link the different parts of the subarachnoid cisterns can become obstructed by blood clots. Yasargil et al. (1976) discussed aspects of the surgical anatomy of these cisterns. They applied the term "carotid cistern" to the space whose lateral wall is deep to the internal carotid artery and to the area of origin of the anterior choroid artery and posterior communicating artery and their branches. We refer to this space as the anteroinferior extension of the ambient cistern. The lateral arachnoid covering of the carotid cistern may be opened to expose the branches of the anterior choroid artery and posterior communicating artery which we call the inferior diencephalic branches. Especially the anterior branches of these vessels are often fused with the arachnoid. Figures SA 58 and SA 59 illustrate the course of these important arterial branches to the diencephalon. Posteriorly, the peripeduncular part of the ambient cistern contains a CSF layer only 1–1.5 mm thick which cushions the tentorial notch at its medial border. The trochlear nerve fuses with the lateral wall of the inferior portions of the arachnoid of the ambient cistern. The nerve can be identified and protected during surgery by displacing the cistern wall. Opening the ambient cistern exposes the arteries and veins supplying the mesencephalon. Figure SA 60 illustrates the most frequent arrangement of the arteries of the mesencephalon and their branches; Fig. SA 61 shows the most common arrangement of the superficial veins. Especially in mass effects caused by supra- or infratentorial neoplasms or more acutely by intracranial hemorrhages (subarachnoid, epidural, etc.), the close proximity of the free border of the tentorium to the mesencephalon and diencephalon can cause direct or indirect damage to the fiber tracts and nuclei by compromising their blood supply. Thus the location of the fiber tracts and nuclei in the mesencephalon is of practical im-

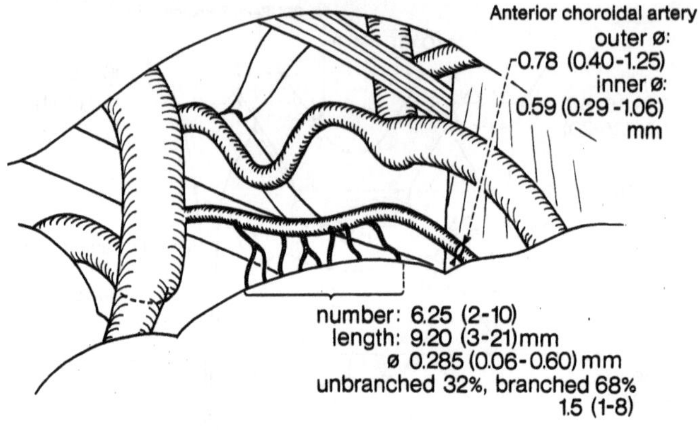

Fig. SA 58. Anterior choroidal artery, diameter and branches to the diencephalon (Lang 1988)

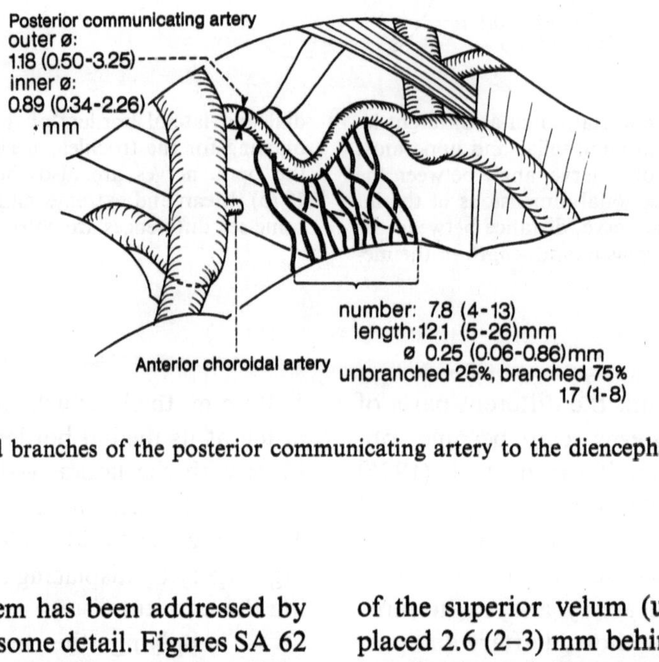

Fig. SA 59. Diameter and branches of the posterior communicating artery to the diencephalon. Mean values (extremals) (from Lang 1988)

portance. This problem has been addressed by Schürmann (1985) in some detail. Figures SA 62 and SA 63 show the major fiber systems of the anterior and posterior portions of the mesencephalon.

The nucleus of the trochlear nerve lies below the floor of the mesencephalic aqueduct at the level of the inferior colliculus. After leaving the nucleus, the fibers of the trochlear nerve first run downward and laterally through the tegmentum and then turn backward around the central gray matter to the upper part of the anterior medullary velum. There they decussate with the contralateral fibers in the limen of the superior medullary velum. This is a thicker zone of the superior velum (up to 1.5 mm) that is placed 2.6 (2–3) mm behind the inferior colliculus (Lang and Deymann-Bühler 1984). As a rule, more than one fiber bundle is seen at the exit zone of the fourth cranial nerve (Lang 1979, 1981, 1983). Their central glial segments are 0.3 (0–1.0) mm long (Lang 1982). The fibers in the first part of the peripheral segment of the nerves are bundled into one trunk, and usually that part of the nerve is surrounded by one of the vermal branches of the superior cerebral artery. Anastomoses between the superior cerebellar artery and the tectal artery also occur in that area. These twigs have a diameter of 0.2 mm or less.

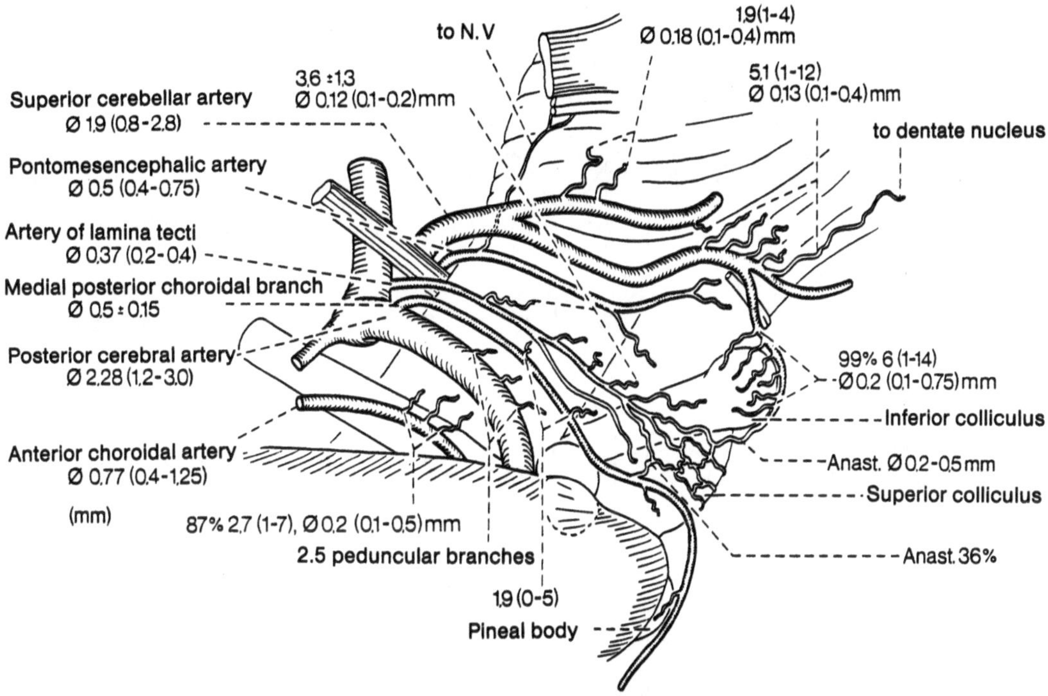

Fig. SA 60. Mesencephalon and its arteries viewed from the right side (parietal region is at the bottom of the picture). The superficial blood supply is derived from the anterior choroidal, posterior cerebellar, medial posterior choroidal, laminae tecti (quadrigemina), pontomesencephalic, and superior cerebellar arteries. The figure indicates the diameters of these vessels, the number of their branches to the mesencephalon, and consistent and less common anastomoses. Mean and extreme values are expressed in mm (from Lang 1985)

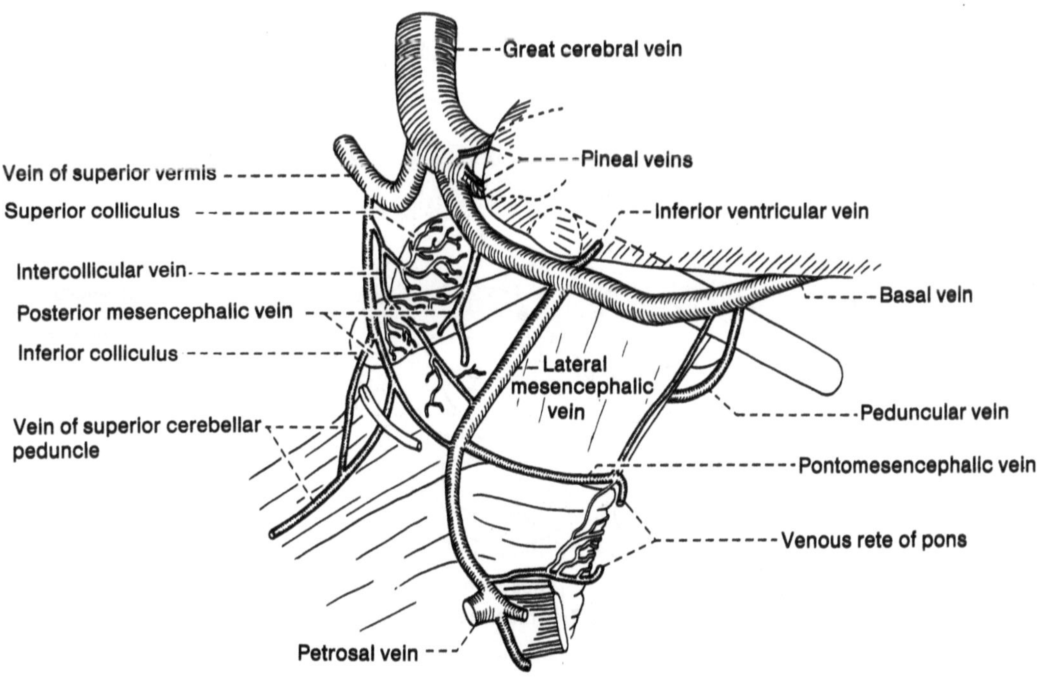

Fig. SA 61. Superficial veins of the mesencephalon, viewed from the right side

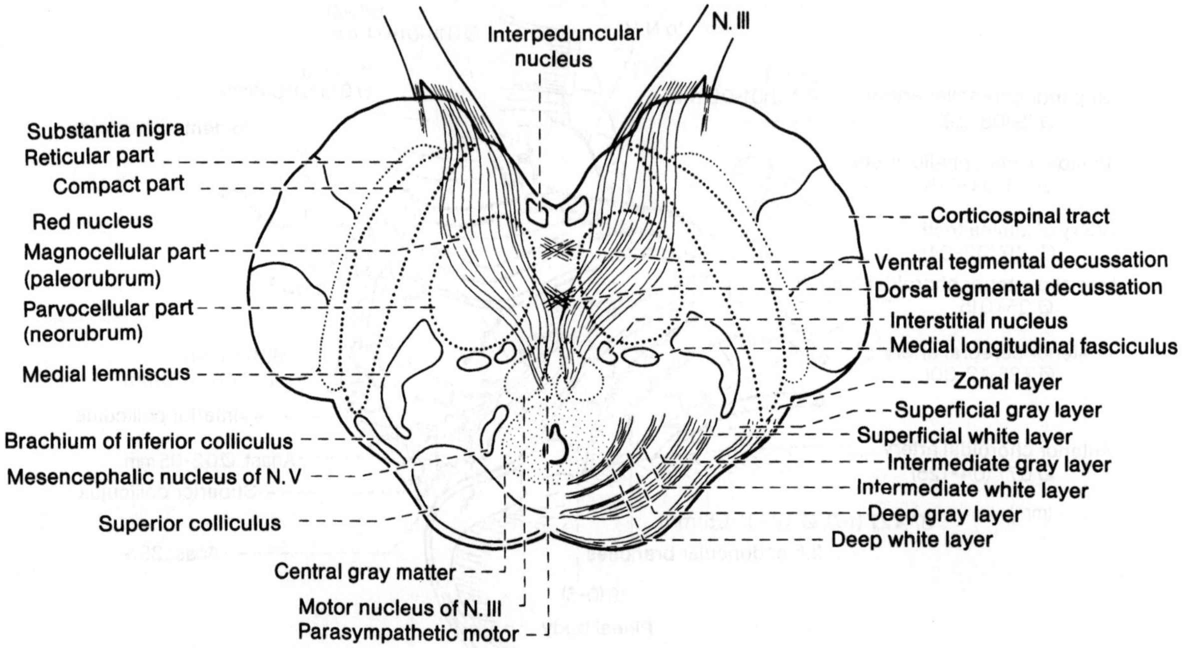

Fig. SA 62. Fiber systems and some nuclei in the superficial part of the mesencephalon (Lang 1985)

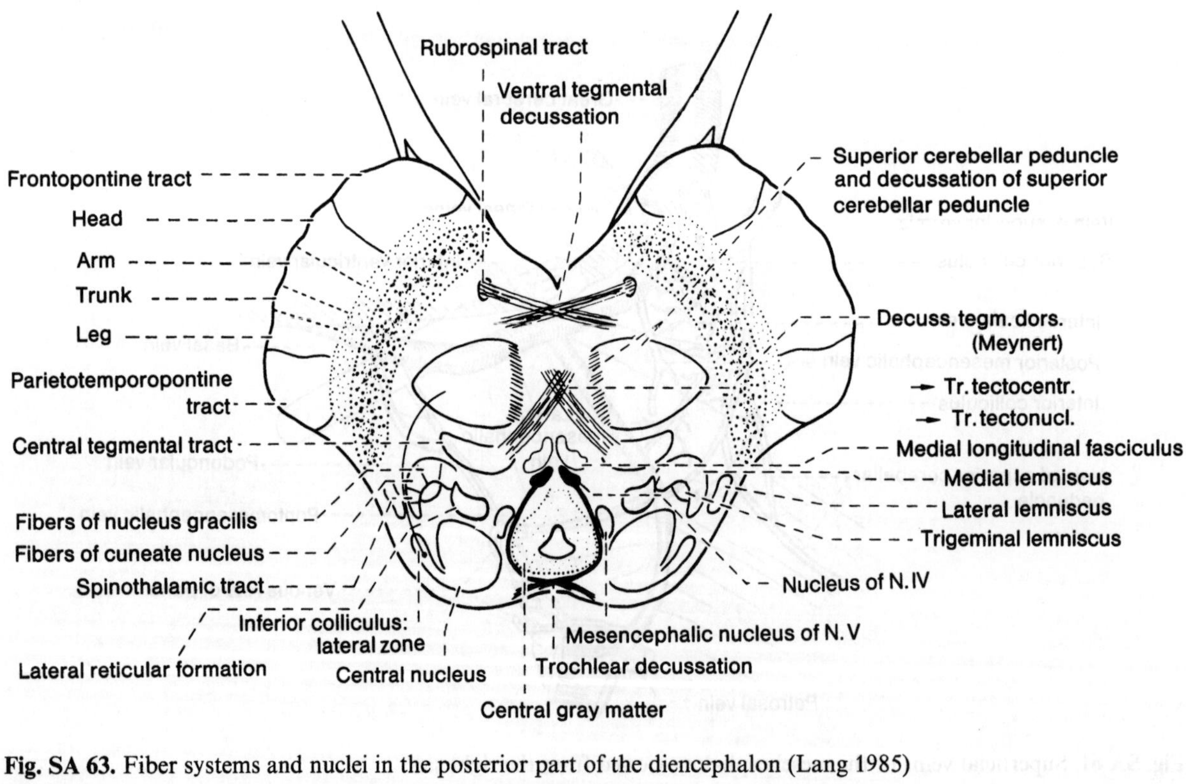

Fig. SA 63. Fiber systems and nuclei in the posterior part of the diencephalon (Lang 1985)

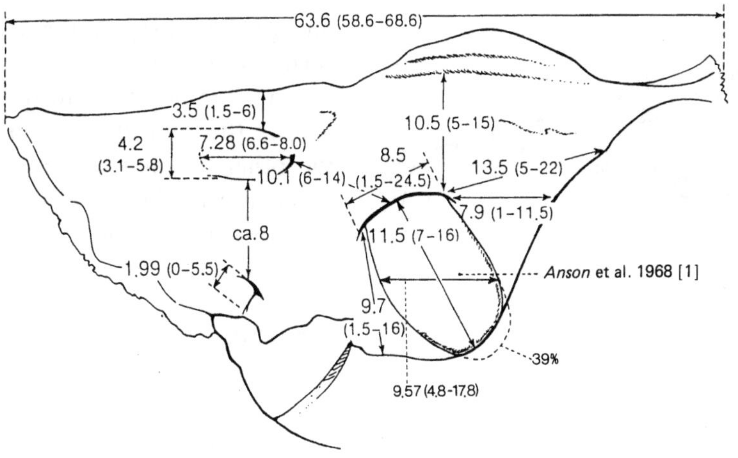

Fig. SA 64. Posterior surface of the right petrous bone. Measurements of dimensions and distances of the internal porus acusticus, the janua arcuata, and the endolymphatic rim and sac. Mean (and extreme) values in mm. The length of the sac is from Anson et al. 1968 (Lang 1984)

The trochlear nerve takes a variable course in the lateral wall of the cavernous sinus. In about 54% of cases the nerve runs closely adjacent to the ophthalmic nerve in its posterior portions. In about 31% it runs forward on the deep aspect of the oculomotor nerve, and in 8.1% it courses between the oculomotor and ophthalmic nerves. In another 7% the trochlear nerve runs first on the deep surface of the oculomotor nerve before passing to and accompanying the ophthalmic nerve farther distally (see Lang and Reiter 1985 for further details).

Cerebellopontine Angle

The cerebellopontine angle (CPA, acousticocerebellar recess, pontomedullocerebellar space, etc.) is bounded anteriorly by the dura of the posterior cranial fossa covering the back surface of the petrosal bone and clivus, and posteriorly by the pons and middle cerebellar peduncle above and by the digastric lobe and flocculus below. Rostrally the sixth, seventh, and eighth cranial nerves and the nervus intermedius exit or enter the brain stem in this region, and more caudally the ninth, tenth, and eleventh cranial nerves. Structures of surgical importance in the CPA region are the flocculus of the cerebellum and the lateral aperture of the fourth ventricle.

In a broader sense the CPA region may be considered to include the portion of the trigeminal nerve which traverses the posterior cranial fossa.

The structures on the posterior surface of the petrous bone are important landmarks for all operations in the CPA region. Figure SA 64 shows the values that we measured for the length of the petrous bone, the distance from the internal porus to the superior margin of the petrous bone, the width and height of the internal acoustic porus, the distance from the porus to the janua arcuata (below which the cochlear duct terminates), the distance from the rima of the endolymphatic sac to various points, the width of the sac, etc. Anson et al. (1968), among others, also determined the length of the endolymphatic sac in the posterior fossa. Lang and Hack (1985) showed that the endolymphatic sac is in contact with the sinus in 61% of cases and overlaps it in 39%. Figure SA 65 shows the entry and exit sites of the lower cranial nerves at the brainstem, and Fig. SA 66 shows the relative spacings of the dural openings for those nerves. The intracisternal lengths of the cranial nerves are shown in Figs. SA 65 and SA 70, which also indicate the length of their central segments (Lang 1982). The central segments of the cranial nerves are parts of the brain. Their axons receive their myelin sheaths not from

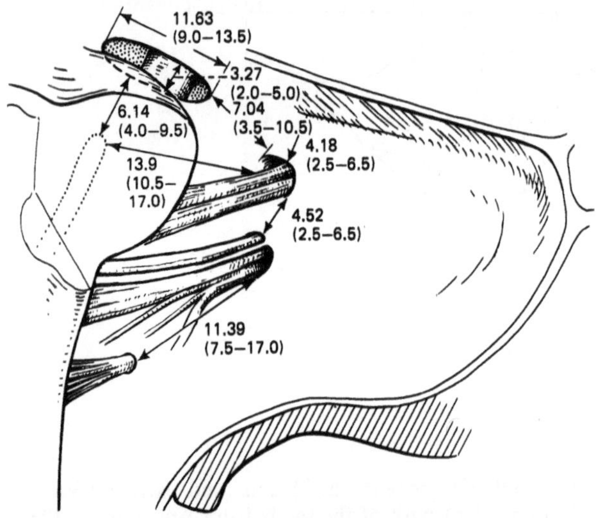

Fig. SA 65. Length of cranial nerves. *Left side*: length of the central parts (*black*). *Right side*: intracisternal length between exit and entry zones of the nerves and dural openings. Mean (and extreme) values in mm

Schwann cells but from oligodendrocytes. In the case of the vestibulocochlear nerve, for example, the junction between the central and peripheral segments lies close to the internal porus acusticus or occasionally within the internal acoustic meatus or posterior fossa. We found the length of the central vestibulocochlear nerve segment to be 10 (6–15) mm. The nerves were stretched out for these measurements, avoiding the slight shrinkage effects that occur with histologic processing. We pointed out in 1982 that pia mater invests the central portions of the eighth (and the other) cranial nerves and usually contains pigment cells. These cells are visible through the operating microscope.

Abducent Nerve

(Figs. SA 67–SA 69)

The nucleus of the abducent nerve lies directly below the facial colliculus on the floor of the rhomboid fossa. It receives fibers from the corticonuclear tract of the contralateral hemisphere, the medial longitudinal fasciculus, the tectobulbar tract, and the reticular formation. Its efferent axons descend ventrally through the pons and surface at the caudal border of the pons, just above the pyramid of the medulla. Occasionally the entire nerve emerges up to 8 mm above the bulbopontine sulcus, or two or three bundles of nerve fibers may be encountered at the exit zone. The medial border of the nerve(s) is 3.93 (2.0–6.5) mm from the midline. In our material we most often found two abducent fiber bundles emerging from the brainstem and uniting shortly thereafter. We found the sixth

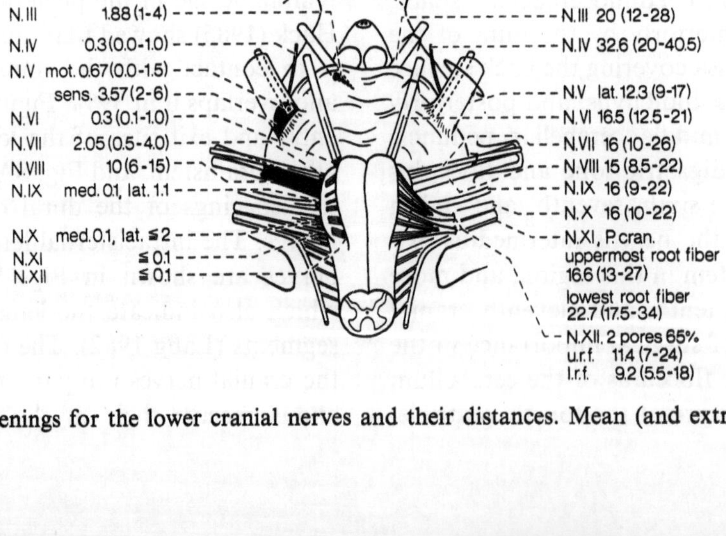

Fig. SA 66. Dural openings for the lower cranial nerves and their distances. Mean (and extreme) values in mm

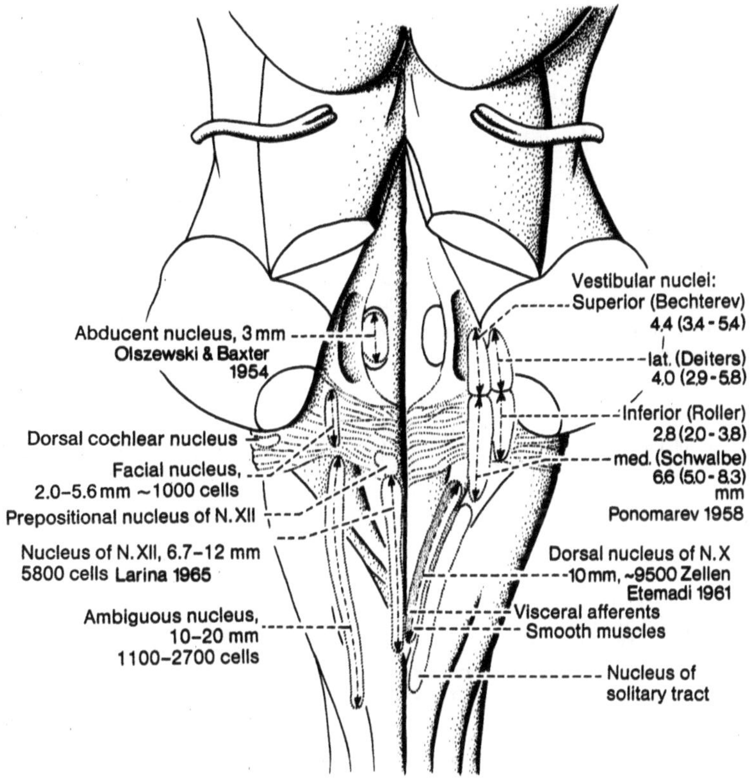

Fig. SA 67. Nuclei below the floor of the rhomboid fossa, location and measurements of different authors

cranial nerve to be composed of 3700 (1946–8136) myelinated fibers having diameters of 4.9 μm or more. The central segment of the abducent nerve in our material is only 0.3 (0.1–1.0) mm long. Nathan et al. (1974) found two nerve fiber bundles in the posterior cranial fossa in 7.5% of cases. The course of the abducent nerve(s) to the anterior inferior cerebellar artery is variable. The nerves run on the dorsal surface of the artery in 79% of cases, below it in 16%, and in 5% the vessel runs between two flanking abducent nerve bundles (Brunner 1978). The abducent nerve segment within the posterior fossa is 15.9 (11–22) mm long. It traverses a slitlike opening in the dura mater of the clivus. Duplicated nerves may pierce the dura at sites separated by as much as 4.5 mm. The dural pore for the sixth cranial nerve lies 6.14 (4.0–9.5) mm below the inferior border of the trigeminal pore and 13.9 (10.5–17.0) mm medial to the medial rim of the internal porus acusticus.

Having pierced the dura, the nerve, enclosed in an arachnoid sheath and a prolongation of dura, runs along the medial border of the inferior petrosal sinus and then through Dorello's canal toward the apex of the petrous bone. Next it traverses the cavernous sinus, passing around the lateral side of the internal carotid artery.

Facial Nerve (Fig. SA 68)

The nucleus of the facial nerve lies 4–5 mm below the anterior floor of the rhomboid fossa and medial to the medial vestibular nucleus. Vraa-Jensen (1942) states the dimensions of the nucleus to be 3–3.5 mm long by 2.5–3 mm wide. Approximately 1 mm high, the nucleus lies in the lateral reticular formation with its greater portion in the dorsal part of the pons and its lesser portion in the medulla oblongata. It is known that the upper part of the nucleus, which

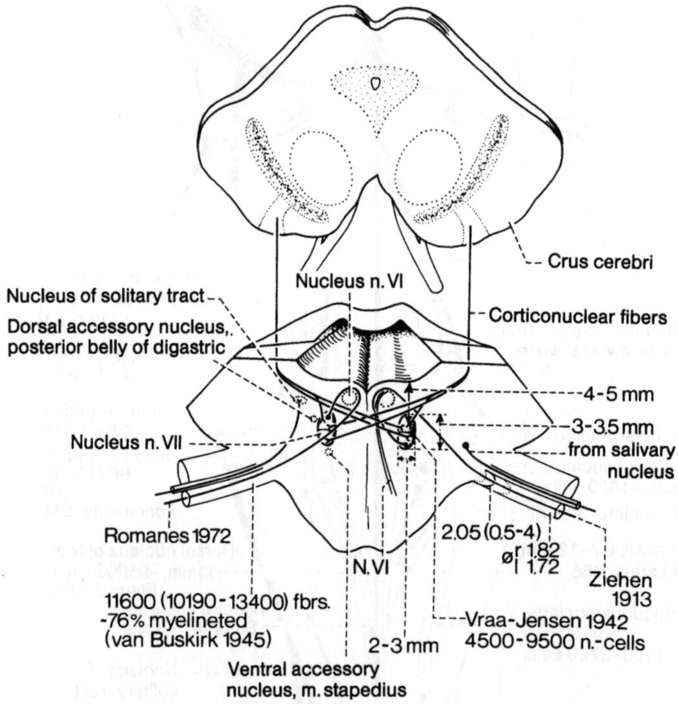

Fig. SA 68. Internal genu of the facial nerve fibers in their course to the abducent nucleus. The fibers encircle the medial side of the abducent nucleus in Ziehen's (1913) and our specimens, and the lateral side in the material of Romanes (1972). The corticonuclear fibers pass to the rostral facial nucleus from both cerebral hemispheres and to the caudal facial nucleus from the contralateral side only. Length measurements and fiber counts are from Vraa-Jensen (1942), van Buskirk (1945), and others

supplies the muscles of the forehead, receives fibers from both cerebral hemispheres, while the lower part, supplying the muscles of the lower part of the face, receives fibers only from the contralateral hemisphere (helpful in differentiating central from peripheral facial nerve paralysis).

The axons of the facial nucleus run upward and dorsally to the medial surface of the abducent nucleus, wind around the dorsal side of the nucleus, and pass downward and laterally to the nerve exit zones. Its loop around the abducent nucleus is called the internal genu of the facial nerve. The intracerebral length of the facial nerve in our material was approximately 16 mm. The exit zone of the nerve is placed 11.8 (9.5–14.5) mm from the midline. The seventh cranial nerve has an oval cross-section with a mean maximum diameter of 1.82 mm on the right side and 1.72 mm on the left side. Van Buskirk (1945) states that the nerve contains 11,600 fibers, 76% of which are myelinated and 24% nonmyelinated. The central segment of the facial nerve was 2.05 (0.5–4.0) mm long in our material (see Fig. SA 70). The central segment of the seventh cranial nerve, like that of the fifth and eighth nerves, is susceptible to irritation by pressure from adjacent arteries, veins, and tumors, resulting in hemifacial spasm. Structures running in proximity to the central segment of the seventh nerve are the anterior inferior cerebellar artery, the vertebral artery, and possibly the posterior inferior cerebellar artery. We determined that the facial nerve was 15.8 (9–26) mm long between its exit zone from the brain and the porus acusticus. Usually the facial nerve runs on the medial aspect of the vestibulocochlear nerve. In about 65% of our

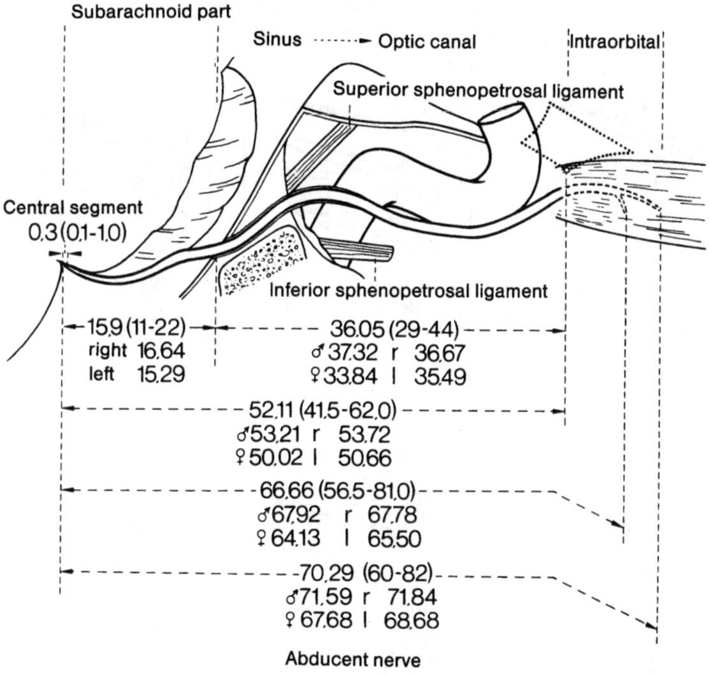

Fig. SA 69. Segments of the abducent nerve viewed from the right side. The distance between the exit zone from the brain and site of passage through the dura (mean value 15.9 mm) is indicated. The segment in the inferior petrosal sinus and in the cavernous sinus extending to the lower border of the orbital opening of the optic canal has a mean length of 36.05 mm. The mean distance between the exit from the brain and this point is 52.11 mm. The most posterior nerve branch enters the lateral rectus muscle 66.66 mm from the nerve exit site, the most anterior branch 70.29 mm. Mean (and extreme) values are stated in mm. Right-left differences and sex differences are indicated (after Lang and Reiter 1983)

material we observed looping of the anterior or posterior inferior cerebellar artery adjacent to the facial nerve, nervus intermedius, and vestibulocochlear nerve in the area of the porus acusticus. Sunderland (1945) and Mazzoni (1969) made similar observations (see Fig. SA 71).

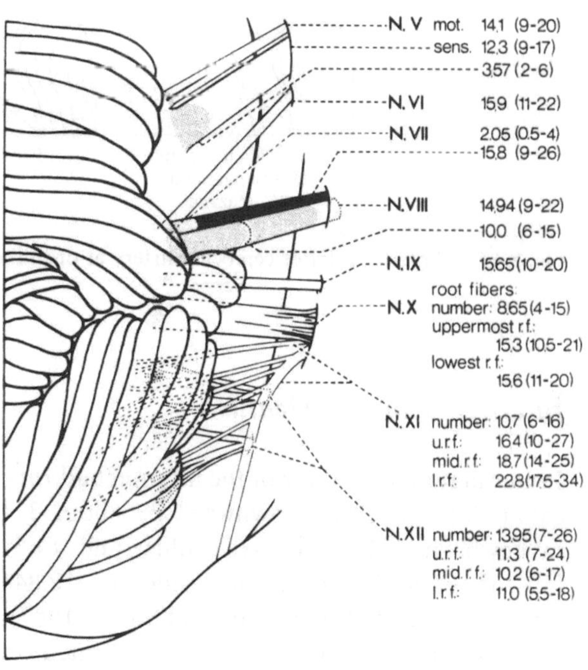

Fig. SA 70. Length of the lower cranial nerves in the posterior fossa. Mean (and extreme) values in mm. Also indicated are the lengths of the main central segments of these nerves and the number and length of the root fibers of the tenth, eleventh, and twelfth nerves (Lang and Reiter 1984)

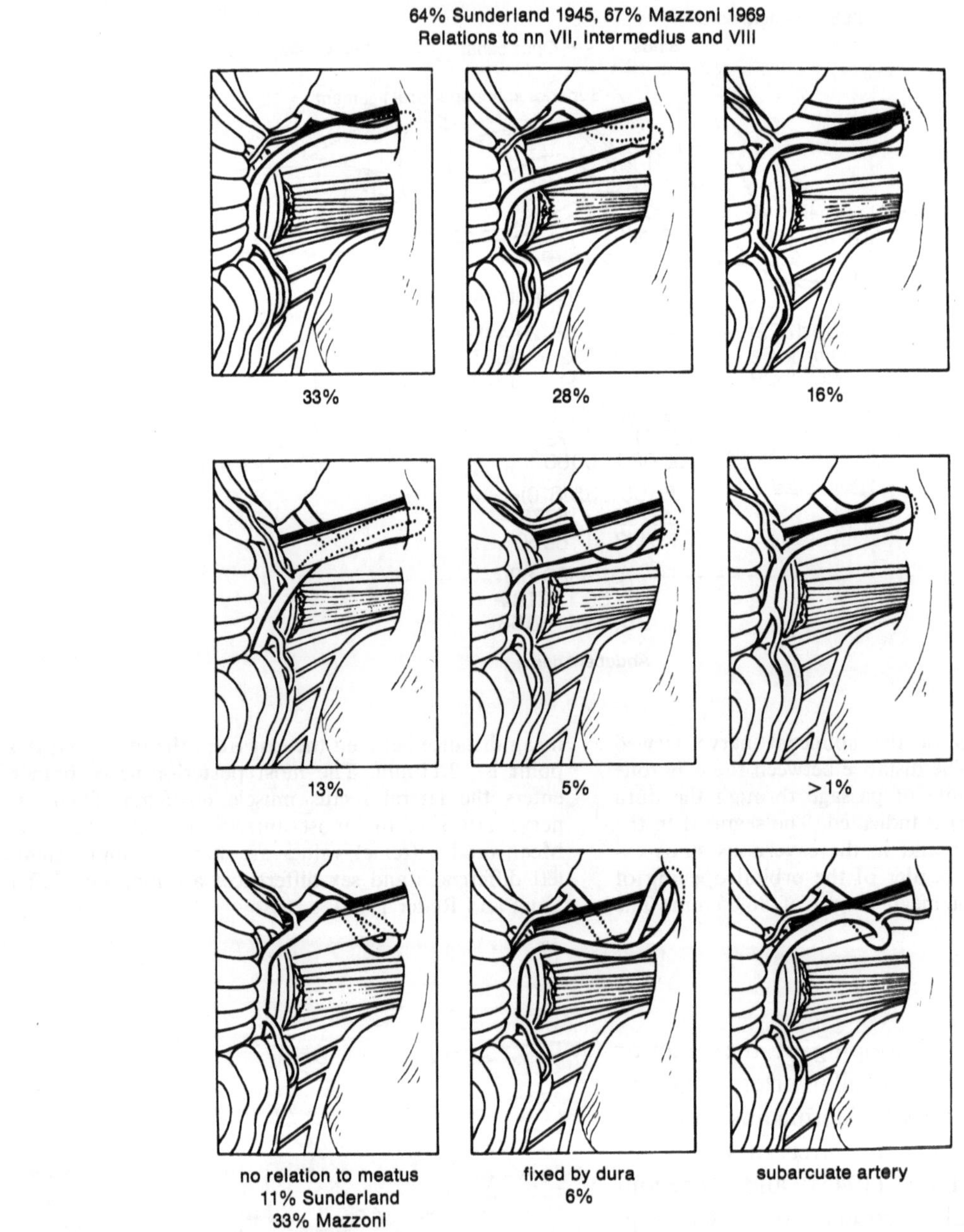

Fig. SA 71. Anterior inferior cerebellar artery at or in the meatus

Internal Acoustic Meatus

In our material the floor of the internal auditory canal slopes laterally downward by about 37° in newborns, 21° in one-year-olds, and 14.3° (5°–35°) in adults on the right side and 12.84° (4°–29°) on the left side (Lang and Stöber 1987). In the 41 petrous bones that were sectioned on the coronal plane, the length of the internal acoustic meatus was 12.33 (5.8–18.2) mm. It measured 4.37 (1.5–7.5) mm high at the porus, 4.37 (2.3–6.1) mm at its midportion, and 3.68 mm in the area of the transverse crest. It should be noted that the length of the canal was measured along its upper aspect as far as the base of the transverse crest. The floor of

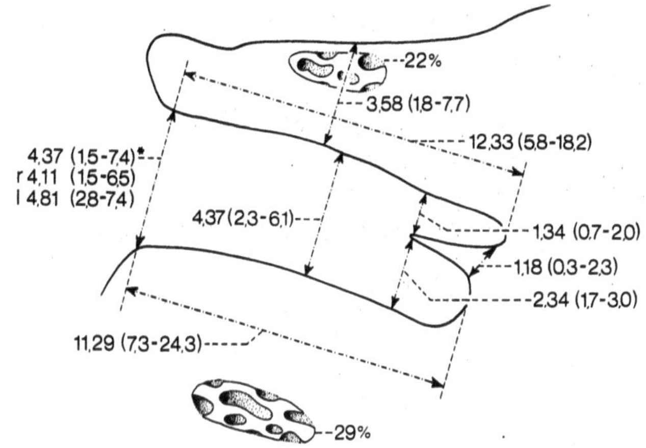

Fig. SA 72. Dimensions of the internal acoustic meatus in coronal section. The development of the suprameatal and inframeatal mastoid cells is indicated. Mean (and extreme) values are stated in mm (Lang and Hack 1985)

the canal is slightly shorter on average. We found air cells above the internal acoustic meatus in about 22% of cases and below it in 29%. Mastoid cells were present in the lateral lip of the porus acusticus in 17% (Lang and Hack 1985; see Fig. SA 72). In the neurosurgical approach to the internal acoustic meatus, the proximity of structures in the peri- and endolymphatic system is a major concern. Thus, for example, the posterior limb of the anterior semicircular canal or the common crus may be placed as little as 0.9 mm from the posterior surface of the petrous bone and 5.3 mm lateral to the lip of the porus. The endolymphatic sac may be placed 8.5 mm lateral to the lip of the porus (Lang and Hack 1985). When the internal acoustic meatus is approached from the floor of the middle fossa, it is useful to know the height of the roof of the internal meatus. This is equal to 3.58 (1.8–7.7) mm in our material (Lang and Stöber 1987). The labyrinthine part of the facial nerve is also exposed in this approach. It should be noted that the meatal foramen of the facial canal (opening of the Fallopian canal on the fundus of the internal acoustic meatus) is 1.19 (0.6–1.99) mm wide in our material. The opening is larger on the right side than on the left and tends to be larger in men than in women. In 15% of cases the geniculate ganglion lacks a bony coverage.

Vestibulocochlear Nerve

Current anatomic nomenclature (*Nomina Anatomica* 1983) recognizes both a vestibular root and a cochlear root for the eighth cranial nerve. The vestibular part of the eighth nerve is known also as the vestibular nerve and is subdivided into a superior (rostral) part and an inferior (caudal) part. The superior part receives fibers from the lateral and anterior ampullary nerves and also from the utricle. The portion of the nerve that conducts fibers from these endolymphatic systems is called the utriculoampullary nerve. The inferior part transmits fibers from the posterior ampullary nerve and saccular nerve. In the fundal region of the acoustic meatus, the fibers pass to the vestibular ganglion. Naufal and Schuknecht (1972) reported that this ganglion contains an average of 18,440 bipolar ganglion cells. Bergström (1973) counted 11,800 fibers in the superior vestibular part. In the inferior vestibular part, some 2500 fibers pass from the posterior ampulla while other fibers pass from the cochleosaccular nerve, the vestibulocochlear nerve, and from the saccule. The inferior vestibular part contains roughly 6500 fibers. The cochlear part contains some 30,000 fibers, whose ganglia are lodged in the cochlear (spiral)

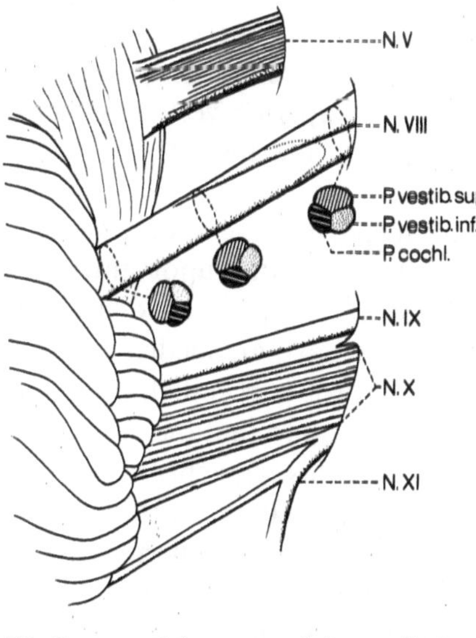

Fig. SA 73. Course of the parts of the vestibulocochlear nerve in the posterior fossa and near the brain stem (after division of the nerve parts between the fundus of the meatus and the brain stem) (Lang 1988)

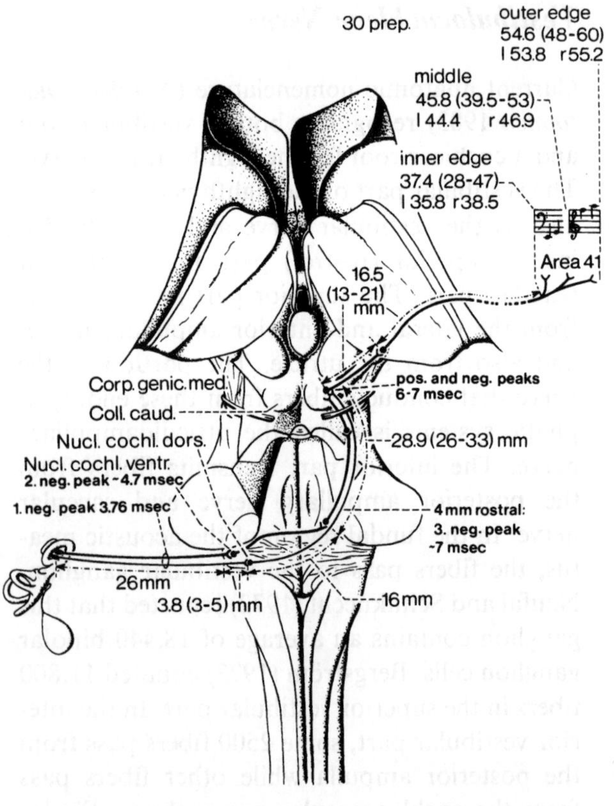

Fig. SA 74. Measurements of the principal pathways of the cochlear part of the eighth nerve, and the electrophysiologic data of Möller and Jannetta (1982, 1983)

ganglion in the modiolus of the cochlea. Approximately 200 efferent fibers have been identified in the vestibular nerve. Within the internal acoustic meatus the cochlear root runs anteromedially, the superior vestibular root laterally and superiorly, and the inferior vestibular part laterally and inferiorly. The fiber bundles of the vestibulocochlear nerve undergo rotation in the posterior fossa, so that upon entering the brain the cochlear part is positioned laterally with the inferior vestibular part medial to it and the superior vestibular part still farther medially. It is not uncommon to find the nervus intermedius emerging with this segment from the brain.

Compression by adjacent arteries, veins, or tumors can produce a hyperreactive vestibulocochlear neuropathy characterized by tinnitus, hyperacusis, diplacusis, vertigo, and hearing loss. These disturbances are caused most frequently by the anterior inferior cerebellar artery; the second most frequent offender is the posterior inferior cerebellar artery. Vestibular nerve lesions are characterized by vertigo, cochlear nerve lesions by tinnitus.

The fibers of the cochlear part of the eighth nerve present a spiral arrangement in the internal acoustic meatus, similar to that seen in the modiolus of the cochlea. The spiral turns are directed counterclockwise on the left side and clockwise on the right side. After entering the brain, the cochlear part runs lateral to the fibers of the inferior cerebellar peduncle to reach the cochlear nuclei (see Lang 1985 for further details).

The fibers of the vestibular nerve curve around the medial aspect of the inferior cerebellar peduncle as they pass to the vestibular nuclei. According to Ponomarev (1958) the superior vestibular nucleus is 4.4 (3.4–5.4) mm long, the medial nucleus 6.6 (5.0–8.3) mm, the lateral nucleus 4.0 (2.9–5.8) mm, and the inferior nucleus 2.8 (2.0–3.8) mm.

The vestibulocochlear nerve presents an oval cross-section near its site of entry into the brain. The longitudinal diameter of this oval measures 3.05 (2.0–5.0) mm in our material, the transverse diameter 1.3 (1.0–2.5) mm. The nerve entry zone is 15 (13–17.5) mm from the midline and 1.36 (0.5–2.0) mm lateral to the exit zone of the facial nerve.

The nervus intermedius usually emerges from the brain close to or jointly with the superior part of the vestibular nerve. Less frequently it emerges between the seventh and eighth cranial nerves. Most of its fibers are 2–4 μm thick, with values ranging from 1.5 to 10 μm.

Glossopharyngeal Nerve
(Figs. SA 44, SA 64, SA 70)

The ninth cranial nerve is the nerve of the third branchial arch. Its fibers arise from and terminate at the same nuclei as those of the tenth nerve. The nucleus ambiguus is a group of large motor nerve cells in the anterior part for the ninth nerve. This nucleus is 10–20 mm long, 3 mm in diameter, and lies 7 mm below the floor of the rhomboid fossa, caudal to the area of the medullary stria. The medial and inferior vestibular nuclei, the nucleus of the solitary tract, and the lateral reticular formation lie dorsal to the nucleus ambiguus, 4 mm below the floor of the rhomboid fossa (3 mm below it at a more caudal level). Farther caudally the nucleus is in close proximity to the spinal tract nucleus of the fifth nerve and to the cuneate nucleus.

Fibers from rostral portions of the nucleus ambiguus supply the muscles of the pharynx.

Parasympathetic secretory fibers arise from the dorsal nucleus of the vagus, which is about 10 mm long and is situated below the ala cineria (trigone). Its caudal part belongs to the vagus nerve. This nucleus has been called the inferior salivatory nucleus by some authors.

The solitary nucleus is the area of termination of the gustatory fibers that course in the ninth cranial nerve (posterior third of tongue).

The sensory fibers of the glossopharyngeal nerve pass to the spinal nucleus of the trigeminal nerve (see Lang 1981 for details).

The fibers of the ninth cranial nerve enter and exit the retro-olivary area 3.2 (1.5–5) mm lateral to the lateral border of the olive and 1.8 (1–3) mm caudal to the bulbopontine sulcus. The motor fibers emerge from the brain at the medial border of the nerve fiber bundle, the sensory fibers at the lateral border. The mean length of the central segment of the motor fibers is only 0.1 mm, that of the sensory fibers 1.1 mm. Usually two closely adjacent fiber bundles traverse the posterior cranial fossa to the dural opening for the ninth nerve. These fiber bundles are 15.65 (10–20) mm in length. The dural opening for the ninth cranial nerve is represented by a small dural pit adjoining the superior ganglion of the ninth nerve. The upper surface of the ganglion is in contact with cerebrospinal fluid and with the outermost end of the perilymphatic duct (see Fig. 31 in Lang 1981). Duplication of the superior ganglion is occasionally observed. The ganglion contains pseudounipolar somatosensory ganglion cells.

Glossopharyngeal Neuralgia

There is no doubt that the ninth cranial nerve, in its intracisternal course, frequently makes contact with the posterior inferior cerebellar artery and less frequently with the anterior inferior cerebellar artery. If these vessels form loops that encroach upon the central segment of the ninth cranial nerve, a significant potential exists for glossopharyngeal neuralgia. This type of disorder has also been described in connection with an unusually long styloid process: pain in the tonsillar region and surrounding structures, in the pharynx, and in the middle ear.

The inferior ganglion of the glossopharyngeal nerve lies in the area of the petrosal fossula (between the jugular fossa and the external opening of the carotid canal). It is usually ovoid in shape, measuring 4.4 (2.1–12) mm long and 2.24 (1.71–3.05) mm wide. Its cross-sectional area is 2.22 (0.88–4.08) mm^2. This ganglion contains the perikarya for sensory and gustatory fibers.

The tympanic nerve generally arises just distal to the inferior ganglion of the glossopharyngeal. The thickness of the nerve 2 mm past its origin was measured in 14 specimens and was found to be 0.33 (0.12–0.91) mm (Vogel 1986). The 1- to 2-mm-long infrapetrous part has connections with vagus nerve fibers in 35% of cases and invariably communicates with facial nerve fibers. After entering the bony canal (in company with a twig from the ascending pharyngeal artery, which may run closely adjacent), the nerve traverses the tympanic canaliculus and runs to the promontory of the labyrinthine wall. This part of the nerve contains two to four intumescences that are thought to be chemoreceptors. Richly vascularized chemodectomas or glomus tumors can arise from these sites and spread along the veins (see Fig. 5 in Lang 1981). The original vessel of these intumescences is the ascending pharyngeal artery with its branches. We additionally found collections of nerve cells in the course of the tympanic nerve. Branches of the tympanic nerve supply the mucosa of the tympanic cavity and mastoid cells as well as the auditory tube. The most superior branch passes upward and forward from the tympanic cavity, unites with branches of the facial nerve, and becomes the lesser petrosal nerve, which supplies the parotid gland after pursuing a complicated course.

Glossopharyngeal Nerve – Its Course in the Parapharyngeal Space

The portion of the ninth nerve in the parapharyngeal space is 1.0 (0.4–1.9) mm wide and 0.9 (0.2–1.0) mm thick in our material (Vogel 1986). The nerve runs lateral to the internal carotid artery and gives off its extracranial branches in an irregular pattern. A thin branch unites with the auricular branch of the vagus nerve, and the adjacent, more distal branch unites with the facial nerve (digastric branch). The next branch given off is the carotid sinus branch, followed most frequently by the pharyngeal rami to the pharyngeal plexus and then the lingual pharyngeal branches. Distal to these, branches to the middle constrictor muscle of the pharynx are observed. Next small branches are given off to its guide muscle, the stylopharyngeus; the final branches of the ninth nerve are lingual. Like Henle (1879), we apply the term "lingual pharyngeal branches" to the glossopharyngeal branches which do not unite with the pharyngeal plexus, but ramify in the mucosa of the pharynx. The branches running on the outer surface of the palatine tonsil form a network called the tonsillar plexus, which supplies the mucosa of the palatine tonsil as well as that of the isthmus faucium and adjacent parts of the soft palate.

Vagus Nerve

(Figs. SA 46, SA 70)

The dorsal nucleus of the vagus nerve is approximately 10 mm long and contains roughly 9500 cells (general visceral efferent and afferent columns) (Etemadi 1961). The upper end of this nucleus is below the vagal trigone, the lower end below the nucleus gracilis. The nucleus ambiguus has connections with corticonuclear fibers from both hemispheres (see Glossopharyngeal Nerve for information on the fibers to the solitary tract nucleus and spinal trigeminal nucleus). The fibers for the voluntary muscles form an internal genu inside the brain (the rest pursuing a straight course to their nuclei). In our material (Lang and Reiter 1985) we counted 8.65 (4.0–15) root fibers of the tenth nerve in the retro-olivary fossa. The uppermost fiber bundle of the tenth nerve has a length of 15.33 (10.5–21.0) mm, the lowermost a length of 15.6 (11.0–20.0) mm between the brainstem and the superior vagal ganglion. The exit (and entry) zone of the upper fiber bundles of the tenth nerve is located 2.70 (1.5–4.0) mm lateral to the lateral border of the olive. Tarlov, in his study of vagus nerve fibers, found that the medial bundles are thinner and contain motor fibers, while the lateral bundles are thicker and contain sensory fibers. The medial ones have a short central segment (0.1 mm). The lateral fibers at the entry zone of the vagus nerve are up to 2 mm long in our material (Lang 1982). Jannetta et al. (1985) observed that pressure on the nerve from arteries or tumors, especially upon the left vagus nerve or adjacent medulla, can have causal significance in essential hypertension. As with the glossopharyngeal nerve, the site of entry of the vagus nerve into the dura mater is marked by a small pit upon which lies the superior vagal ganglion. This site is located 1–3 mm below and behind the analogous site for the superior ganglion of the ninth nerve; both are separated by a dural fold. Like the superior glossopharyngeal ganglion, the superior vagal ganglion is bathed from above by cerebrospinal fluid. It is a spinal ganglion which contains pseudounipolar ganglion cells for the auricular, meningeal, and pharyngeal branches and in some cases for the recurrent laryngeal nerve.

The meningeal branch of the vagus nerve aids in supplying the dura mater of the posterior cranial fossa (see Lang 1985 for details).

The auricular branch of the vagus nerve has major surgical importance due to the possible occurrence of glomus organs in its course. The thin branch arises either from the superior vagal ganglion or just below it and runs laterally along the anterior wall (or occasionally the superior wall) of the jugular fossa. Grooves are frequently found in this area, and small, partially dehiscent canals may be seen. Even this part of the nerve may contain richly vascularized intumescences in its course (see Fig. 5 in Lang 1981). In the area of the lateral wall of the jugular fossa, the nerve and its accompanying vessels enter the mastoid canaliculus, which generally extends for 6 (4–9) mm to the mastoid portion of the Fallopian canal. This part of the nerve establishes connections with the seventh cranial nerve. Then the nerve usually passes behind the facial nerve, or rarely in front of it, through the rest of the canal to the tympanomastoid suture. This nerve segment, too, may contain intumescences. After emerging from the skull, the thin nerve supplies part of the posterior surface of the auricle and the outer surface of the tympanic membrane. Anastomoses between the posterior auricular nerve and facial nerve were invariably present in our material. This part of the vagus nerve is a site of predilection for the development of glomus jugulare tumors.

Accessory Nerve

(Figs. SA 48, SA 70)

The spinal nucleus of the accessory nerve lies in the spinal cord and extends from C_1 to C_5. Its cranial fibers are efferent neurons of the nucleus ambiguus. In our material we found 10.66 (6–16) fiber bundles within the posterior fossa. We estimated a length of 16.42 (10.0–27.0) mm for the uppermost fiber bundles and 22.81 (17.5–34.0) mm for the lowest fiber bundles of the cranial part. The axons of this cranial part (internal ramus of the eleventh nerve) unite with the vagus nerve at various levels below the superior ganglion of the tenth nerve. The cranial fibers are connected by one or two filaments with the superior vagal ganglion. *Gray's Anatomy* states that these are probably the source of the motor fibers which run in the vagus nerve to supply the muscles of the soft palate (except for the tensor veli palatini) and are also distributed with the superior and recurrent laryngeal nerves and possibly also with the cardiac nerves. The roots that form the spinal part of the accessory nerve are described in Lang (1981). These parts of the nerve supply the sternocleidomastoid and trapezius muscles (along with fibers from C2 and C3). In our material the extracranial part of the accessory nerve ran anterior to the internal jugular vein in about 83% of cases, posterior to the vein in 15%, and passed through the vein (or between the inferior petrosal sinus and the vein) in 2%.

Hypoglossal Nerve

(Figs. SA 46, SA 65, SA 66, SA 70)

The hypoglossal nucleus is from 6.7 to 12 mm long (Larina 1965). Its uppermost part lies below the hypoglossal trigone, the lower part in the ventral portion of the central gray matter, close to the median plane. The efferent fibers of the nucleus pass ventrally through the medulla oblongata and emerge from the medulla between the pyramid and olive. We counted 13.95 (7–26) root fiber bundles, which usually are collected into two larger bundles. The course in the posterior cranial fossa of the uppermost root fiber is 11.3 (7–24) mm long, the lower one 11.0 (5.5–18.0) mm. In 65% of cases we found two dural pores for the twelfth nerve (especially on the left side) spaced 4.16 (0.5–9) mm apart. The distance from the lower pore to the vertebral artery in our material was 8.71 (7–15) mm; the distance from the upper pore to the lower rim of the pore for the eleventh nerve, 11.39 (7.5–17.0) mm. The central segment of the twelfth nerve fibers is shorter than 1 mm (like other motor nerve fibers). Inside the hypoglossal canal the fiber bundles unite with each other before the nerve leaves the canal. The nerve fibers are enclosed in an arachnoid sheath and a prolongation of dura and are surrounded by the hypoglossal venous plexus. In most cases one of the meningeal arteries of the posterior fossa traverses the hypoglossal canal. Outside the skull the nerve cross-section measured 1.53 (0.68–2.44) mm by 0.99 (0.46–2.13) mm. Generally the nerve anastomoses with the ninth cranial nerve, with the ventral bundle between the first and second cervical nerves, with the inferior vagal ganglion, and in most cases with the superior ganglion of the sympathetic nerve. In rare cases we found fiber bundles of the twelfth nerve coursing anterior to the vertebral artery in the posterior fossa (Lang 1981) or fibers passing through a hole in the vertebral artery (Lang 1979, Fig. 162).

Anatomy of the Clivus

Various surgical approaches are available for operations in the region of the clivus (e.g., for chordomas or chondromas): subtemporal transtentorial, transcervical, subglossal, and rhinoseptal. Hakuba (1985) reported on the transoral approach to this region. Calcaterra et al. (1973) emphasized that tumors of the nasopharynx (and maxillary sinus, ethmoid cells, palate and facial region) can grow through the foramina of the skull base. They found that these lesions can spread by the perineural route without seeding metastases to regional lymph nodes or other organs. Gabrielsen and Pingman (1964) noted that the skull base tumors known as "chondromas" in the German literature are equivalent to the "osteochondromas" of English and American authors. These tumors arise from cartilage remains of the primordial skull base and initially grow extradurally, although they can penetrate the dura. Their most common sites of occurrence are parasellar, and occasional lesions are found in the middle fossa, posterior fossa, the CPA region, about the petrous apex, and rarely in the area of the petrooccipital suture. Figure SA 75 shows how the position of the notochord changes at the craniocervical junction and in the clivus region during development and indicates the directions in which chordomas (derived from the notochord) may spread (see Lang 1986 for details). Luschka (1856) was probably the first to describe such tumors, which Müller (1858) then related to the notochord. The routes by which chordomas can spread to the posterior fossa, nasopharynx, sphenoid sinus, and the pituitary region of the middle fossa are indicated in the figure. Evidently the course of the notochord is variable in the area of its rostral end. Some researchers describe it as terminating in the area of the dorsum sellae, others at the posterior wall of the pituitary fossa (on which a "sellar spine" is occasionally seen). It appears that we were the first to describe a sellar spine, which we observed in a 23-year-old male (Lang 1977). Since then there have been numerous descriptions of a spiny process projecting into the hypophysis (e.g., Dietemann et al. 1981).

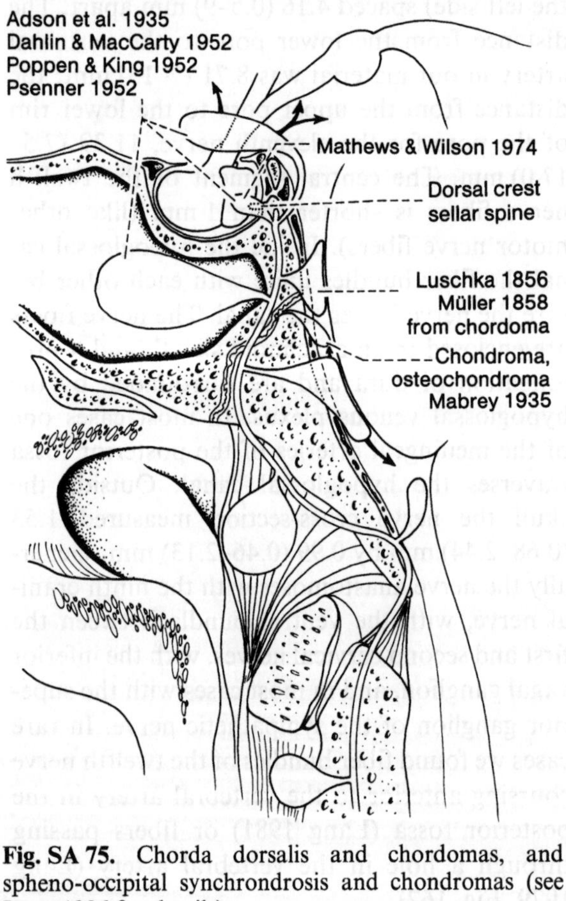

Fig. SA 75. Chorda dorsalis and chordomas, and spheno-occipital synchrondrosis and chondromas (see Lang 1986 for details)

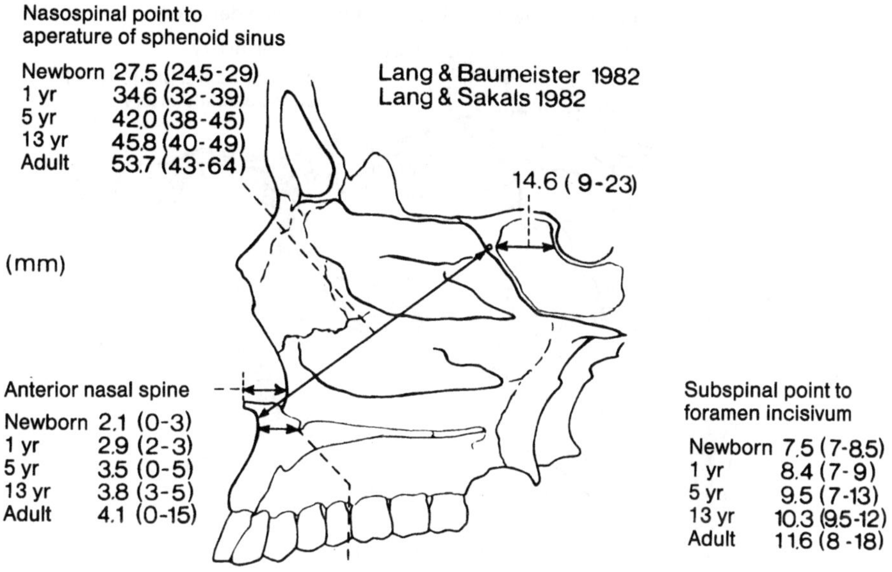

Fig. SA 76. Distances between the subspinal point and the aperture of the sphenoid sinus, and distances from the sinus aperture to the pituitary fossa. Measurements of the position of the foramen incisivum are also given in mm (extremals) (Lang and Baumeister 1982)

Extracranial Surgical Approaches

The *transsphenoidal approach* is made transnasally through the piriform aperture, whose dimensions vary during postnatal growth and in adults (Lang and Baumeister 1982). The distance between the subspinal zone (area below the anterior nasal spine) and the aperture of the sphenoid sinus is 53.7 (43–64) mm in our adult material (see Fig. SA 76, from Lang and Baumeister 1982 and Lang and Sakals 1982).
The pattern of the arterial supply to the nasal septum is shown in Fig. SA 77. In 70% of our material the ostium of the sphenoid sinus was less than 3.5 mm in diameter (Lang and Sakals 1982). In 15% the opening was pinhead-sized, and in 28% the opening was elliptical, usually with its major axis directed vertically. The ostium tends to occur in the upper half of the sphenoid sinus, with other sites being less frequent (see Fig. SA 78). The dimensions of the sinus are variable, and we reported on these in some detail in our 1983, 1985 and 1988 publications. It is important to note that the main septum within the sphenoid sinus is often directed obliquely, and that it is accompanied by additional septa that are oriented transversely and obliquely (see Fig. SA 79). The distance from the ostium of the sphenoid sinus to the sellar floor is 17.1 (12–23) mm in the material of Fujii et al. (1980) and 14.6 (9–23) mm in our material. Removing the sinus mucosa gives access to the anterior clivus region. It was common in our material to find rarefaction of the posterosuperior portions of the clivus (dorsum sellae) with arteries and veins from the pituitary fossa coursing directly on the posterior surface of the clivus below the dura mater of the clivus. Figure SA 80 indicates the thickness of the clivus 8 mm and 11 mm anterior to the basion as well as the cortical thickness of the clivus.

Transoral-Transpalatine Approach
(Fig. SA 81)

In this approach an effort is made to spare the vessels and nerves of the hard and soft palate if at all possible. An important neurovascular foramen in this region is the greater palatine foramen, which in our adult material lies 29.21 (21–40) mm behind the medial alveolar border

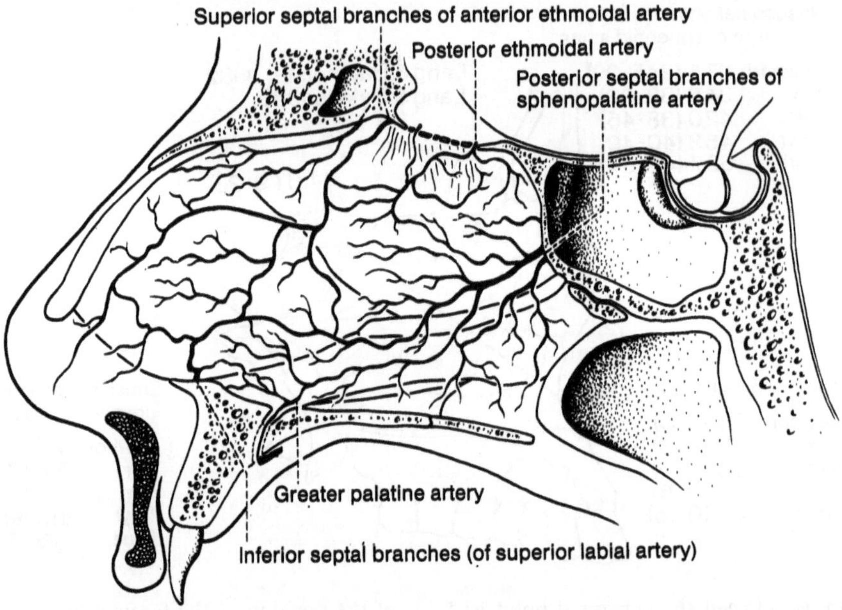

Fig. SA 77. Arteries of the nasal septum (dissection from the medial side after removal of skeletal parts)

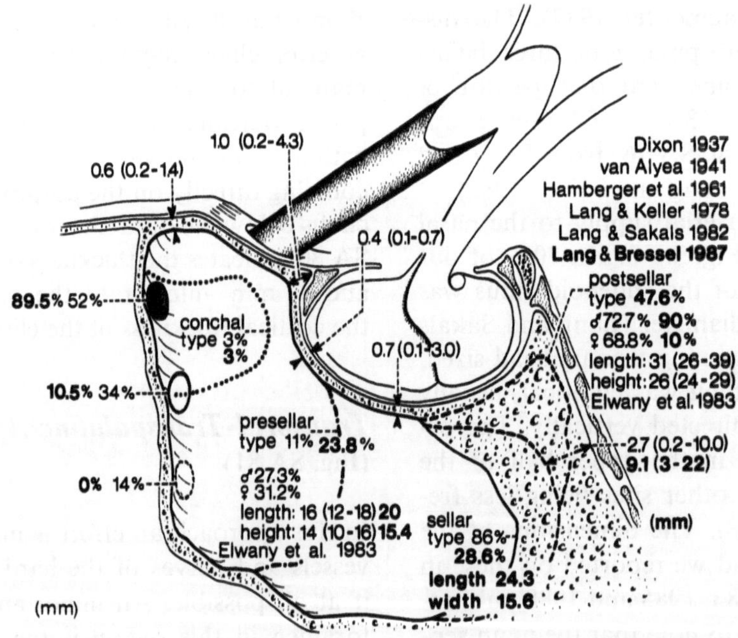

Fig. SA 78. Position of the aperture of the sphenoid sinus, shapes of the sphenoid sinus, and measurements from various authors (Lang 1988)

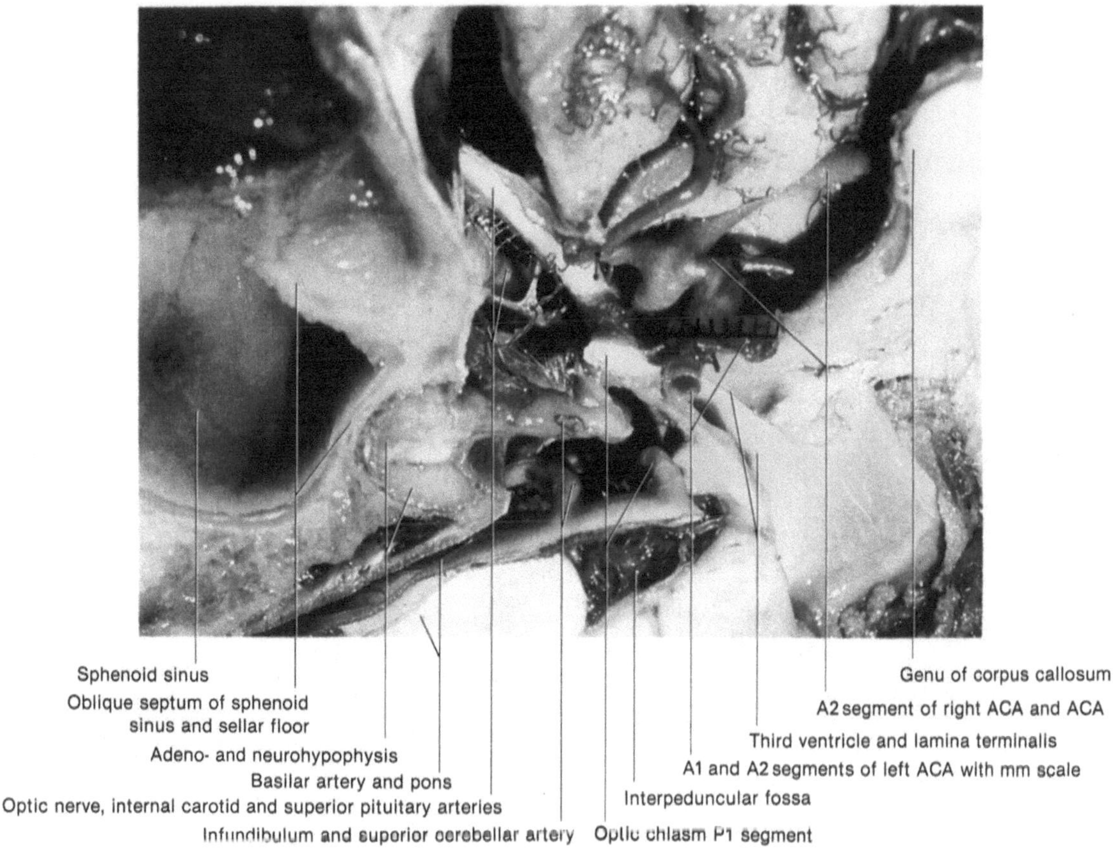

Fig. SA 79. Midsagittal section through the head, viewed from the left front

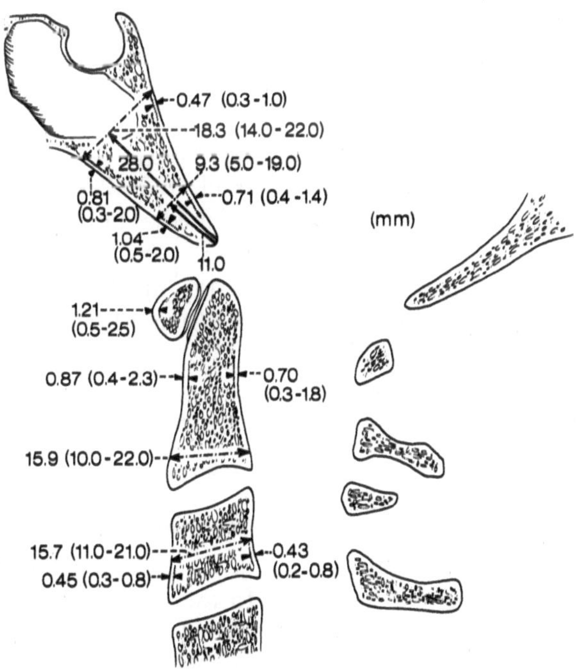

Fig. SA 80. Thickness of the clivus and the upper three vertebrae in different areas. Cortical thicknesses are also shown (after Issing 1985)

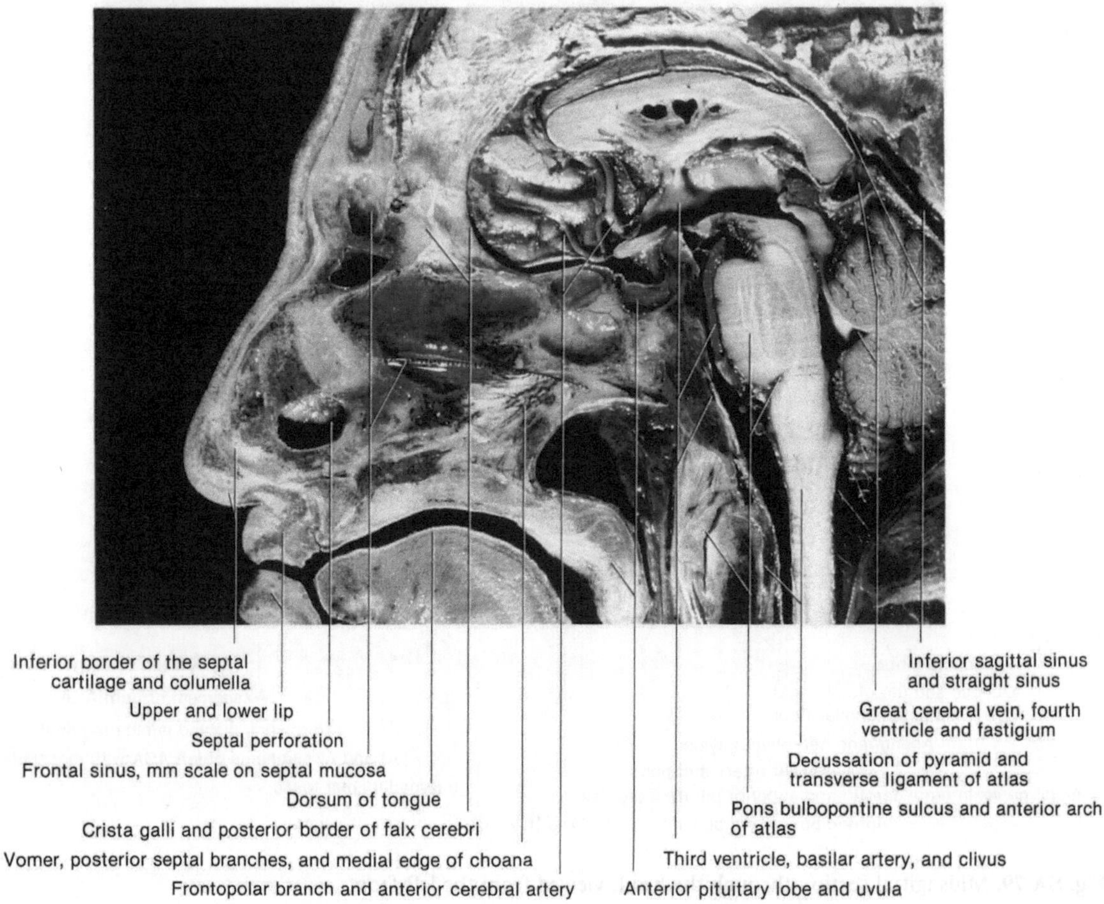

Fig. SA 81. Midsagittal section in a specimen with a perforated septum

of the canine tooth (Lang and Baumeister 1984). This opening has a longitudinal diameter of 5 (3–8) mm in adults and a short diameter of 3.26 (2–6) mm. It transmits the emerging greater palatine artery and greater palatine nerve, which run forward and medially close to the bony palate. The terminal branch of the artery traverses the foramen incisivum and the incisive canal to the anteroinferior part of the nasal septum, where it anastomoses with posterior septal branches from the sphenopalatine artery (see Lang and Baumeister 1984 for further details). Another important structure in this region is the pterygoid hamulus, around which passes the tendon of the tensor veli palatini muscle. The two hamuli are spaced 28.86 (20–34) mm apart in our adult material. It is important to note that the clivus is 22.5 (13–18) mm wide in its anterior portions at the undersurface of the skull, and 42.7 (33–52) mm wide posteriorly at the medial border of the jugular foramen (Issing 1985). The narrow anterior zone is about 11 (8–18) mm long, the wider posterior zone 14.3 (8–20) mm long.

Occipital Condyles
(Fig. SA 82)

The long axes of the occipital condyles converge in an anteromedial direction. The mean angle to the median plane in our material was 25.2° (14°–42°) on the right side and 26.3° (14°–47°) on the left. Ingelmark (1947) determined mean values of 28° in adults and 35.5° in newborns. In our material the articular surfaces of the con-

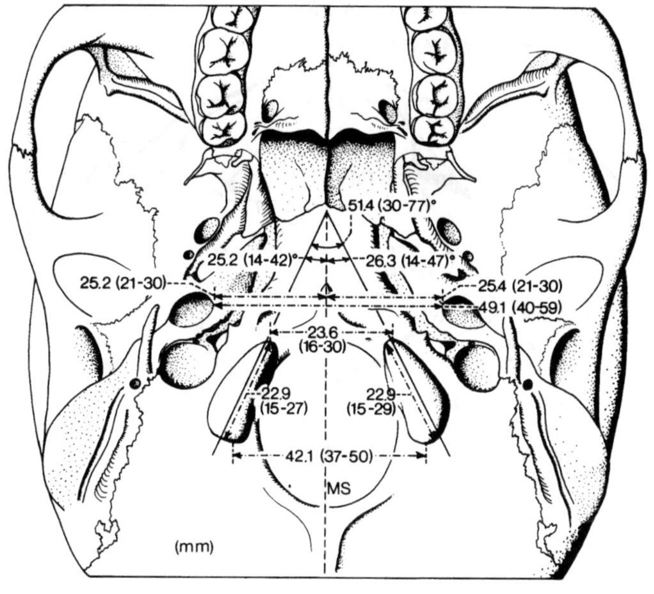

Fig. SA 82. Distances between the anterior and posterior ends of the occipital condyles, their lengths, the sagittal condylar angle, and the angle formed by the long axis of the right and left occipital condyles with the midsagittal plane. The length of the occipital condyles and the paramedian distances of the external openings of the carotid canals and their spacing are shown. Mean and extreme values are stated in mm (from Lang 1986)

dyles are separated by a distance of 23.6 (16–30) mm anteriorly and 42.1 (37–50) mm posteriorly. Issing measured 22.9 (15–29) mm for the length of the articular surface. Bernhard (1976) measured an articular surface area of approximately 1.12 cm^2.

The surface of the condyle presents an oblong oval or bean shape. Not infrequently, we noted a division of the surface into anterior and posterior parts with a ridge between the two articular surfaces. Very rarely the articular surface may present two furrows (Schwegel, quoted in Henle 1871). The ratio of length to width is 2:1. The anterior border is sharp and projects downward along the body of the condyle. The posterior border is usually continuous with the retrocondylar fossa. Strecker (1887), Misch (1905), and Bernhard (1976) describe a variety of condyle shapes, including bean-shaped, prismatic types, flattened types, convex types, flattened convex types, flat types, short and broad, flat and long, small and convex. Right-left differences are often noted in the condyle shapes, even in fetuses (Sergi 1909, 1919). Bernhard (1976) reported a mean value of 11.9 mm for the height of the condyles.

The lateral border of the articular surfaces of the occipital condyles is more elevated than the medial one. Knese (1949/1950) estimated the frontal angle between the two axes to be 124° in men and 127° in women. Low condyles are associated with larger angles (up to 152° in hypoplastic condyles).

In our material the transverse axis of rotation of the major part of the articular surface was 20.53 (11.0–27.0) mm posterior to the basion and 9.57 (6.4–13.3) mm below the FHP (see Fuchs 1980, Fig. 20).

The os odontoideum (ossiculum Bergmann) is an isolated bone situated between the dens axis and occiput. Keller and Neiss (1962) noted an abnormal mobility at the atlantocervical junction caused by separation of the os odontoideum. (See Wackenheim 1974 for more details.)

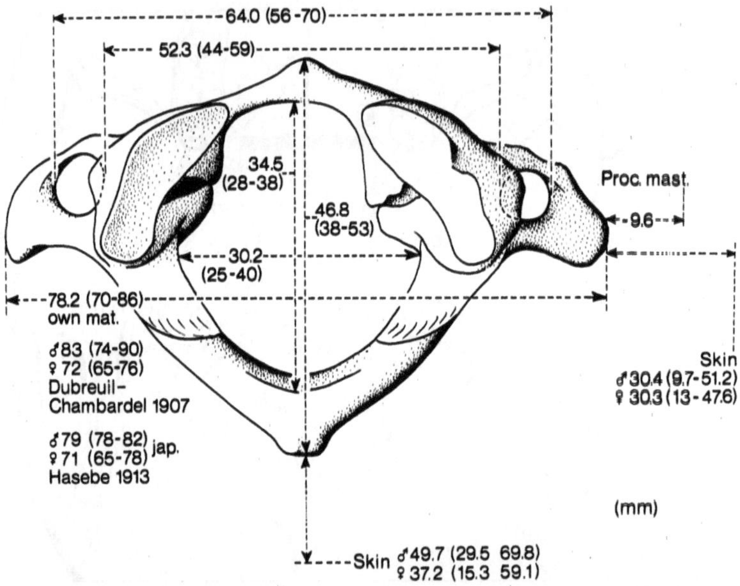

Fig. SA 83. Maximum width of the atlas, distances between the lateral and the medial borders of the transverse foramina, overall length of the atlas, length and width of the space for the dens of the axis and spinal cord. The distances from the lateral border of the atlas to the tip of the mastoid process and to the lateral and dorsal skin are shown. Mean (and extreme) values are stated in mm, and some sex differences are noted (from Lang 1986)

Atlas in Adults (Fig. SA 83)

The anterior arch of the atlas carries the anterior tubercle on its ventral aspect. The posterior surface of the anterior arch is covered with cartilage and articulates with the dens of the axis. The larger posterior arch forms about three-fifths of a complete bony ring. It usually carries a posterior tubercle on its dorsal surface. The anterior and posterior arches converge at the articular parts of the atlas and its lateral masses. The superior articular fovea is covered with cartilage where it articulates with the occipital condyle. The long axis of the two oval or kidney-shaped superior articular facets (which are divisible into anterior and posterior parts) converge in an anteromedial direction (like those of the occipital condyles). Immediately behind the superior articular fovea is a transverse groove for the vertebral artery, its accompanying veins, and the first cervical nerve. The articular process usually overhangs this groove anteriorly. Often there is a bony bridge over the course of the vertebral artery (7% bilateral and 14% unilateral). Even more frequent are incomplete bridges formed by anterior and posterior bony spurs (posterior and lateral ponticuli). Medial to the articular surface is a rough bony part with nutrient foramina to which the transverse ligament of the atlas is attached. The maximum width of the atlas (in the area of the lateral masses) was found to be 83 (74–90) mm in European men and 72 (65–76) mm in European women. Smaller values were found in Japanese (Tsusaki 1924; Dubreuil-Chambardel 1907). Hasebe (1913) found a mean value of 80.9 (73–85) mm in adult Europeans.

The transverse foramen for the vertebral artery and accompanying veins lies between the superior articular fovea and the lateral mass of the atlas.

Axis (Fig. SA 84)

Our measurements of the superior surface of the axis and vertebral canal are shown in Fig. SA 84. The sagittal diameter of the vertebral

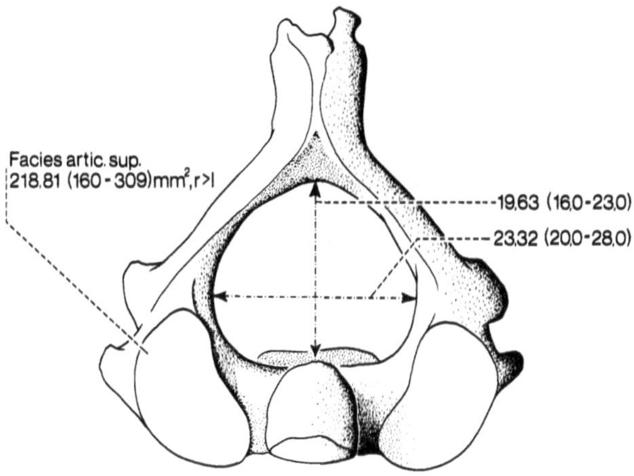

Fig. SA 84. Axis from above. Length and width of the vertebral canal in mm (mean and extreme values) and in the area of the superior articular facet, after Sturm (1981) and Lang (1986)

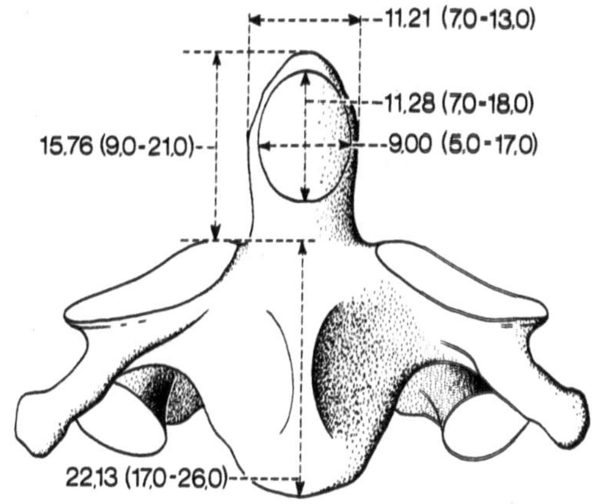

Fig. SA 85. Axis from the front. Measurements of the height of the body and dens of the axis, the width of the dens and the articular surface on the anterior side of the dens. Mean and extreme values are stated in mm (Lang 1986)

canal in our material is larger than the mean diameter of 15.7 mm measured in Japanese men and 15.4 mm in Japanese women (Tsusaki 1924). The mean transverse diameter in our material also was greater than in Japanese men (21.9 mm) and Japanese women (21.6 mm) (Hasebe 1913). The superior articular surface was kidney-shaped in about 38% of our material, presenting in other cases a rounded, elliptical, or other shape (Sturm 1981). The superior articular facets of the axis converge anteriorly at an angle of 134.7° (124°–141°). Frizzi (1915) found the mean length of the facets to be 18.5 (16.4–20.4) mm with a mean width of 16.3 mm on the right side and 16.6 (14.8–17.9) mm on the left side. The cartilage thickness ranges from 0.5 to 1.9 mm (Koebke and Brade 1982).

Anterior Surface of the Axis
(Fig. SA 85)

The body of the axis measured 22.13 (17–26) mm high in our material. Hasebe (1913) found mean values of 19.3 mm in Japanese men and 17.3 mm in Japanese women. The dens in our material has a mean height of 15.7 mm, as compared with 17.9 mm measured by Hasebe for Japanese men and 16.5 mm for Japanese women. It is possible that different methods were used to measure the body and dens. The transverse diameter of the dens in our material is greater than that measured in Japanese. We found a mean diameter of 11.21 mm, as opposed to 10.5 mm and 9.8 mm measured by Hasebe for Japanese men and women. The anterior articular surface of the dens in our material is slightly larger than in Japanese (Tsusaki 1924). The maximum width of the axis as measured by Dwight (1887) was 55–58 mm in Europeans. Hasebe determined values of 57 mm in men and 50.4 mm in women. Helms (1963) measured the radiographic angle between the axes of the dens and the lower surface of the body of the axis, finding values from 42° to 88° (88° is almost straight).

Occasionally the dens is inclined forward or laterally ("scoliosis of the dens"). Helms found angles ranging from +10° (inclined to the right) to −6° (inclined to the left). Krmpotić-Nemanić and Keros (1973) measured the angulation of the dens relative to a horizontal line through the center of the lower surface of the axis. The vertical was established through the center of the lower part of the body of the axis. In 78% of cases the dens was oriented so that it was coaxial with the body of the axis. A less pronounced lordosis was found with a posterior

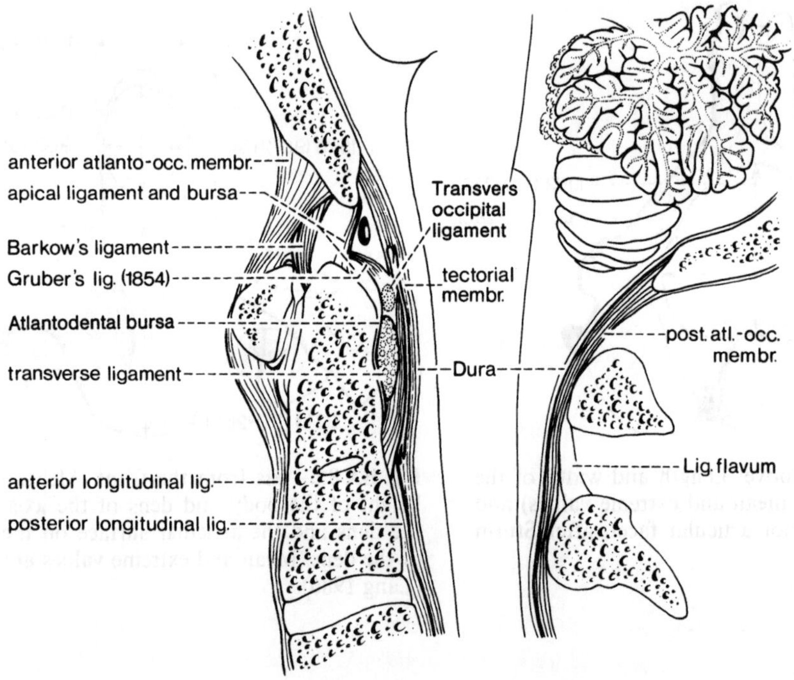

Fig. SA 86. Ligamentous structures between the upper part of the spinal column and the occiput, seen in midsagittal section. The anterior atlantodental articulation and the posterior atlantodental bursa are also shown. Frequently a subdental synchondrosis, pictured here, persists in the axis until about 20 years of age; remains are often seen in older people (Lang 1986)

inclination up to 11°. The dens also may show up to 14° of kyphotic angulation, especially in persons with pronounced lordosis of the cervical spine.

Atlantodental Joint

(Fig. SA 86)

The anterior and medial parts of the capsule of the atlantodental joint are thinner than the posterior and lateral parts. The cavity of this joint sometimes communicates with that between the dens and the transverse ligament of the atlas (Cave 1933, 1934). The latter is termed the "atlantodental bursa" in the *Nomina Anatomica*. The articulating dorsal part of the dens is smooth and is covered by a soft layer of connective tissue with chondrocytes. It is about 0.5 mm thick and articulates with the cartilage-covered anterior surface of the transverse ligament of the atlas. Several recesses in the joint cavity have been described. Koebke (1979) claims that the anterior articular surface of the dens always has an upright oval shape. The posterior articular surface is a transverse oval in 70% of specimens and circular in the rest. It is covered by fibrocartilage. In older persons, degenerative changes are frequently seen on the anterior articular surface of the dens and its facet on the atlas.

Transverse Ligament of the Atlas

(Fig. SA 87)

The medial surfaces of the lateral masses of the atlas usually present several tubercles of attachment for the transverse ligament. The parallel fibers form rounded bands near their sites of attachment, the ligament widening out over the posterior surface of the dens. The ligament is approximately 10 mm wide and 2 mm thick at its midportion. Its upper border is sharp-edged,

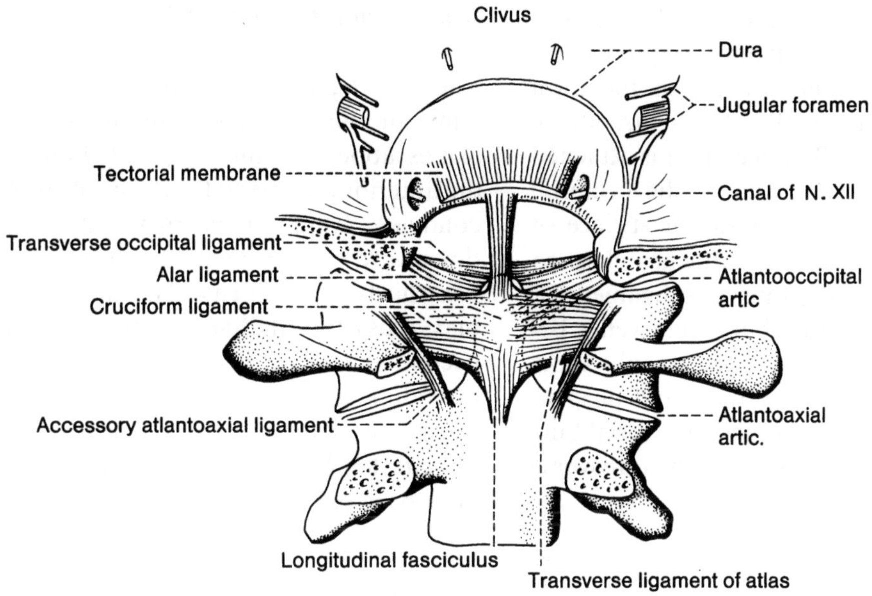

Fig. SA 87. Ligaments of the atlantodental articulation, posterior aspect. Besides the alar ligament, the cruciform ligament and the transverse occipital ligament are also shown. An accessory atlantoaxial ligament is frequently present. The tectorial membrane and dura mater are detached, and the posterior aspect of the lateral atlantoaxial articulation has been dissected free (Lang 1986)

the lower border rounded. It is composed of bundles of collagen fibers which cross one another at acute angles, allowing the ligament to stretch slightly when the cervical spine and head are flexed forward (Stofft 1968). Macalister (quoted in Warwick and Williams 1973) states that a force of 130 kg is needed to rupture this powerful ligament.

Cruciform Ligament of the Atlas
(Fig. SA 87)

The transverse ligament forms the major portion of the cruciform ligament, which is completed by a longitudinal portion. The superior longitudinal band of the ligament is always present. It is enclosed by loose connective tissue and merges with the anterior atlanto-occipital membrane. The inferior longitudinal band attaches to the posterior surface of the body of the axis but is not always present.

Apical Ligament of the Dens
(Fig. SA 86)

The apical ligament, 2–5 mm wide and 2–12 mm long, is without functional significance. It is thought to be a vestige of the notochord. In our experience it is not unusual to find bony deposits in the area of the ligament. We have also drawn attention to a process of the dens which articulates with the basion.

Tectorial Membrane
(Fig. SA 86)

Immediately below the anterior dura, the dens of the axis and the cruciform ligament are covered from behind by a broad and fairly strong ligament called the tectorial membrane. It may be regarded as an upward prolongation of the posterior longitudinal ligament of the spine (Warwick and Williams 1973). This flat ligament consists of two layers. The lateral part joins the capsule of the atlanto-occipital joint. The dorsal part is continuous with the dura mater in the vicinity of the clivus, just above the foramen magnum. The deep part is attached superiorly to the basilar part of the occipital bone and inferiorly to the posterior surface of the body of the axis. It also attaches close to the cruciform ligament (transverse ligament of the atlas). In some cases a bursa intervenes between the two, but usually there is only some loose connective tissue superficial and deep to the transverse ligament. A cruciatotectorial bursa also may be present adjacent to the transverse ligament of the atlas.

Anterior and Posterior Longitudinal Ligaments

Hayashi et al. (1977) examined the spinal columns of 62 adults and 8 fetuses, observing that the anterior longitudinal ligament passes around the lateral surfaces of the vertebral bodies, deep to the long muscle of the neck. The anterior and posterior longitudinal ligaments unite in the vicinity of the intervertebral foramina. The posterior longitudinal ligament lies against the posterior surfaces of the vertebral bodies and is composed of two layers. The deep layer supplies fibers to the annulus fibrosus. The superficial layer is loosely attached to the deep layer medially. Laterally it is entirely separate from it and extends outward to form a connective-tissue membrane that covers the dura mater, the nerve roots, and the vertebral artery. This part may be relatively thick, but elsewhere some parts may be thin or incompletely formed, especially posteriorly. The parts around the nerve roots and vertebral artery usually are easily identified.

Alar Ligament (Fig. SA 87)

The alar ligaments are rounded cords about 8 mm in diameter. They are attached to tuberosities about 10 mm long and 4 mm wide on the anterior and medial surfaces of the occipital condyles, from which they extend medially downward to the lateral surface of the upper two-thirds of the dens. The uppermost fibers may cross the midline to form the transverse occipital ligament. This ligament has a deep part extending to the lateral and posterior border of the dens and a superficial part that is attached in part to the apex of the dens. Other fibers have been seen running to the opposite side.

Vertebral Artery, Transverse Part (Fig. SA 88)

In some 90% of cases the vertebral artery runs upward from C6 within the transverse foramina. These foramina have an anteroposterior diameter of 6.5–7.5 mm on the left side and about 7 mm on the right (Argenson et al. 1980). The foramina and the interspaces between adjacent foramina are traversed by the vertebral venous plexus and by a sympathetic nerve plexus surrounding the artery. This plexus has connections with the vertebral nerve, which usually originates from the stellate ganglion and less frequently from the inferior or superior cervical ganglion. The vertebral nerve was first described by Hirschfeld (1876) and later by Francois Franck (1878, 1899). Van den Broek (1908) and Kunert (1961) drew special attention to this plexus. The plexus is surgically important because of its connections with the cervical ganglia of the sympathetic chain, its connections with cervical nerves, and the much discussed role of these nerves in the pathogenesis of equilibrium disorders, hearing loss, and pain. Besides the vertebral artery and its branches, the vertebral nerve assists the cervical nerves in supplying the joints and ligaments of the vertebral column and the dura mater. Lesions of the vertebral nerve can be caused by arteriosclerotic changes, spinal deformities, lordosis, and lead to vegetative angiospasms (see Lang 1983 for more details).

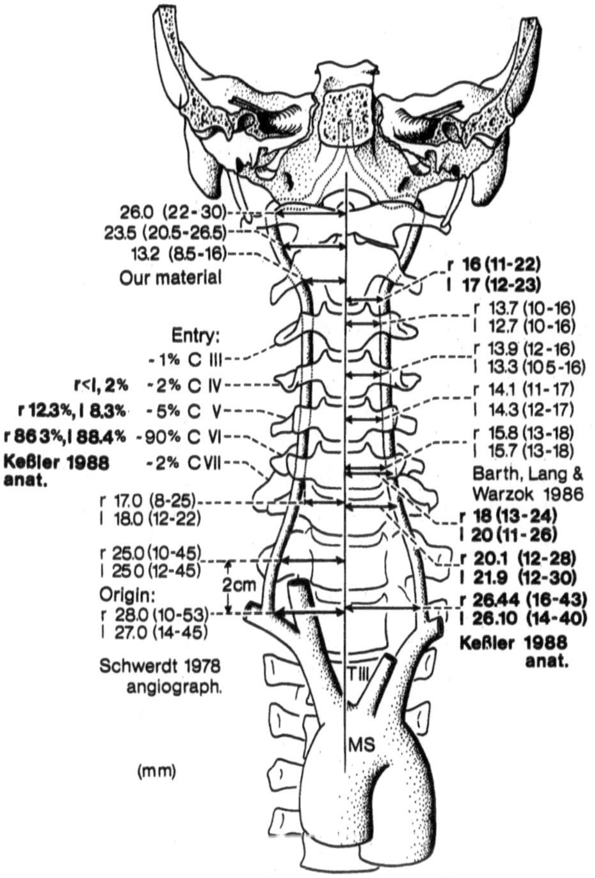

Fig. SA 88. Vertebral artery, distances of its segments from the midline. Schwerdt (1978), Barth et al. (1986) and we ourselves measured the distances from the medial border of the vertebral artery; Kessler measured from the center of the artery in our material. The sites of entry of the vertebral artery into the cervical vertebrae are indicated. These distances are important in all operative approaches to the cervical spine

Vertebral Artery, Axoatlantic Part

(Fig. SA 88)

The axoatlantic part of the vertebral artery is the segment running between the axis and the atlas. It is specially constructed to allow about a 35° freedom of rotation of the head and atlas. Most notably, in its adventitia we found many elastic fibers, and with advancing age the vertebral artery tends to form loops between the axis and atlas. Both lateral and posterior looping of the artery were observed in our material.

Atlantic Part

In our material the medial border of the transverse foramen of the atlas lies 26 (22–30) mm from the midline – farther laterally than the transverse foramen of the axis. In addition, the inferior border of this foramen is placed farther medially than its superior border. At the upper surface of the atlas the vertebral artery curves or angles backward to its sulcus on the atlas. It does not contact this sulcus directly, but generally is separated from it by a venous plexus. The suboccipital nerve also runs dorsally below the artery. This segment of the vertebral artery often gives off muscular branches that anastomose with branches of the occipital artery and deep cervical artery and less frequently with the ascending cervical artery.

Vertebral Artery, Entry into the Subarachnoid Space

Before entering the subarachnoid space along with branches of the vertebral nerve, the vertebral artery pierces the posterior atlanto-occipital membrane and the dura mater. Below the artery are the short root sleeves of the ventral (and often the dorsal) roots of C1. Within the subarachnoid space the vertebral artery takes either a straight or (especially in older persons) a curved path to the contralateral homonymous artery. As it does so, the artery curves around first the lateral and then the anterior aspect of the spinal cord and medulla. In two-thirds of our specimens the artery unites with the opposite artery at the lower end of the pons to form the basilar artery. The intracisternal length of the vertebral artery measured 25.4 (19–35) mm in our adult material.

Arterial Supply of the CNS at the Craniocervical Junction

(Fig. SA 89)

Radicular Arteries

Unlike other workers (Noeske 1958; Piscol 1972), we found a number of specimens in which arteries accompanied the ventral and dorsal roots of C_1 to the spinal cord and brainstem. The diameters of the vessels at C_2, for example, averaged 400 µm on the right side and 300 µm on the left side; the diameters at C_1 averaged 800 µm on the right side and 700 µm on the left. The ventral radicular arteries usually form anastomoses with the anterior spinal artery and adjacent arteries of the spinal cord and medulla oblongata.

Anterior Spinal Artery

(Fig. SA 89)

Following up on the work of Stopford (1915, 1916), Wollschlaeger and Wollschlaeger (1967) and others, the anterior spinal artery was investigated in our material (Brunner 1978). This vessel arises 5.8 (1–13) mm proximal to the union of the two vertebral arteries. It unites with the opposite anterior spinal artery after a course of 13.9 (5–38) mm caudal to the pontomedullary junction. The anterior spinal artery has an outer diameter of 0.75 (0.245–0.9) mm and in 10% of cases is absent on one side. In about 13% both anterior spinal arteries run downward for some distance before uniting with each other. An accessory anterior spinal artery is present in 38% of cases. This vessel arises distal to the main artery and sends branches to the pyramids, the anterior median fissure, and the pontomedullary sulcus. Branches from the anterior spinal artery proper to the pyramids were seen in 55% of cases.

Posterior Inferior Cerebellar Artery

(Fig. SA 89)

The posterior inferior cerebellar artery (PICA) arose from the vertebral artery in 79% of the material of Adachi (1928) and in about 90% of our earlier material (Lang and Kollmannsberger 1961; Lang and Müller 1975). Various authors report the PICA arising from the basilar artery in 6%–10% of their material. Extradural origins of the PICA are not unusual (Lang 1985). Bilateral absence of the PICA was confirmed in slightly more than 4% of the material of Adachi (1928) and in 2% of the material of Lang and Kollmannsberger (1961). Brunner (1978) noted unilateral absence in 7.3% and bilateral absence in 3.6%. In these cases the area normally supplied by the PICA receives blood from a strongly developed anterior inferior cerebellar artery. In 0.9% of our material the PICA was duplicated on one side. When the vessel arose from the vertebral artery, it sprang from its proximal third in 50%, middle third in 27.6%, and distal (cranial) third in 15.3%. Figure SA 89 illustrates the vertebral arteries, posterior inferior cerebellar arteries, basilar artery, superior cerebellar arteries, posterior cerebellar arteries, in addition to smaller vessels including the anterior inferior cerebellar artery and the branches to the pons.

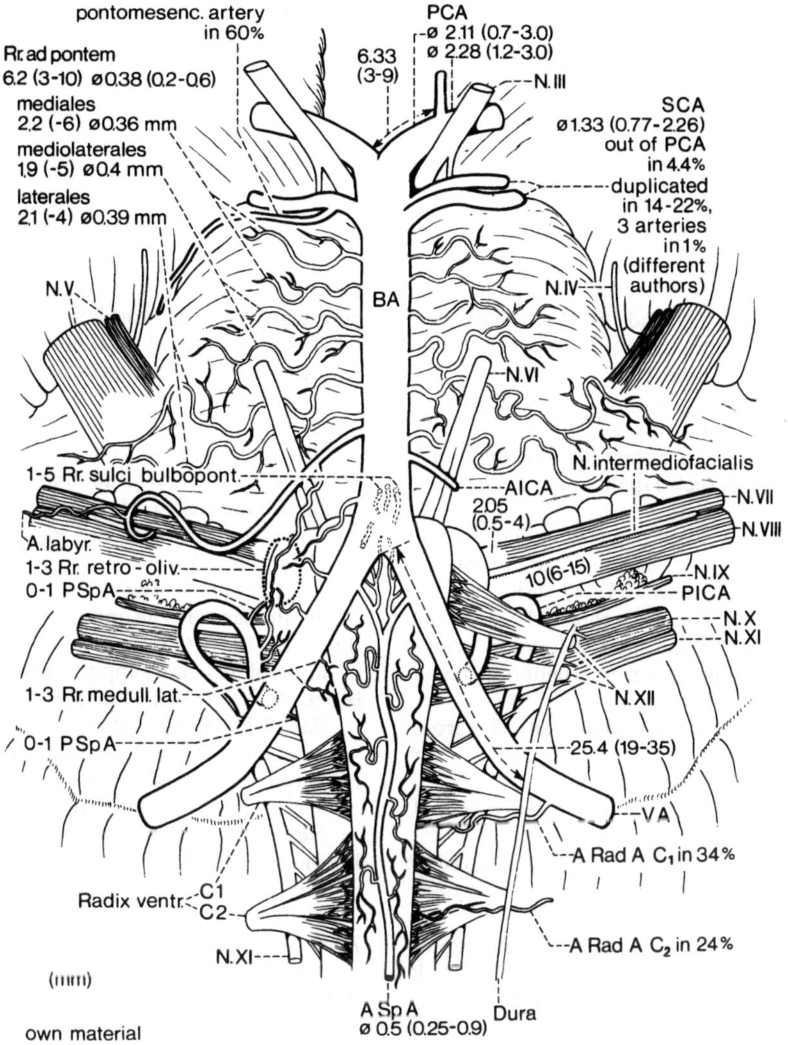

Fig. SA 89. Vertebral and basilar arteries, their lengths and branches in the area of the craniocervical junction and posterior cranial fossa, anteroinferior aspect. The lengths of the central segments of the seventh and eighth nerves and the multiple origins of the superior cerebellar artery are shown (from Lang in press)

References

Adachi B (1904a) Die Orbita und die Hauptmaße des Schädels der Japaner und die Methode der Orbitalmessung. Z Morphol Anthropol 7:379–480

Adachi B (1904b) Topographische Lage des Augapfels der Japaner. Z Morphol Anthropol 7:481–501

Adachi B (1928) Das Arteriensystem der Japaner, vol I u. II. Verlag der Kaiserlich-Japanischen Universität, Kyoto

Adson AW, Kernohan JW, Woltman HW (1935) Cranial and cervical chordomas: clinical and histologic study. Arch Neurol Psychiatry 33:247–261

Anderson RD, Liebeskind A, Schechter M, Zingesser L (1972) Aneurysms of the internal carotid artery in the carotid canal of the petrous temporal bone. Radiology 102:639–642

Anson BJ, Warpeha RL, Rensink MJ (1968) The gross and macroscopic anatomy of the labyrinths. Ann Otol Rhinol Laryngol 77/4:1–25

Arey LB (1950) The craniopharyngeal canal reviewed and reinterpreted. Anat Rec 106:1–16

Argenson C, Francke JP, Sylla S, Dintimille H, Papasian S, di Marino V (1980) The vertebral arteries (segments V1 and V2). Anat Clin 2:29–41

Arnold G, Huhn P, Clahsen H (1980) Zur topographischen Anatomie der V. jugularis interna im Hinblick auf verschiedene Punktionsverfahren und Komplikationen beim zentralen Venenkatheter. Verh Anat Ges 74:809–811

Austin JH, Stears JC (1971) Familial hypoplasia of both internal carotid arteries. Arch Neurol 24:1–10

Barth H, Lang G, Warzok R (1986) Untersuchungen zur klinisch-topographischen Anatomie der Regio intervertebralis lateralis im Bereich des 3. bis 7. Halswirbelkörpers. Anat Anz 162:175–193

Bast R (1982) A. alveolaris inferior, Verlauf und Verzweigungstypen. Dissertation, University of Würzburg

Batujeff N (1889) Eine seltene Arterienanomalie (Ursprung der A. basilaris aus der A. carotis interna). Anat Anz 4:282–285

Baumel JJ, Vanderheiden JP, McElenney JE (1971) The auriculotemporal nerve of man. Am J Anat 130:431–440

Begg AC (1961) Radiographic demonstration of the hypoglossal artery. A rare type of persistent anomalous carotid-basilar anastomosis. Clin Radiol 12:187–189

Bergerhoff W (1960) Die Sella turcica im Röntgenbild. JA Barth, Leipzig

Bergland R, Ray B, Torack R (1968) Anatomical variations in the pituitary gland and adjacent structures in 225 human autopsy cases. J Neurosurg 28:93–99

Bergström B (1973) Morphology of the vestibular nerve. II. The number of myelinated vestibular nerve fibers in man at various ages. Acta Otolaryngol (Stockh) 76:173–179

Berke RN (1954) A modified Krönlein operation. Arch Ophthalmol 51:609–632

Bernhard W (1976) Kraniometrische Untersuchungen zur funktionellen Morphologie des oberen Kopfgelenkes beim Menschen. Gegenbaurs Morphol Jahrb 122/4:497–534

Boyd GI (1930/31) The emissary foramina of the cranium in man and the anthropoids. J Anat 65:108–121

Boyd JD (1937) Observations on the human carotid sinus and its nerve supply. Anat Anz 84:386–399

Broek AJP van den (1908) Untersuchungen über den Bau des sympathischen Nervensystems der Säugetiere. Gegenbaurs Morphol Jahrb 37:202–288

Bruneton JN, Drouillard JP, Sabatier JC, Elie GP, Tavernier JF (1949) Normal variants of the sella turcica. Neuroradiology 131:99–110

Brunner FX (1978) Über die Arterien des Hirnstammes, Vorkommen, Zahl, Durchmesser und Variationen. Dissertation, University of Würzburg

Bucy PC (1936) Carotid sinus nerve in man. Arch Intern Med 58:418–432

Bulatnikow TJ (1915) Regio latero-pharyngea. Topographie ihrer Arterien im Zusammenhang mit der Frage über gefährliche Blutungen bei operativen Eingriffen in der Regio tonsillaris. Arch Laryngol Rhinol 29:225–281

Burns A (1811) Observations on the surgical anatomy of the head and neck. Edinbourg

Cairney J (1924) Tortuosity of the cervical segment of the internal carotid artery J Anat 59:87–96

Calcaterra TC, Cherney EF, Hanafee WF (1973) Normal variations in size and neoplastic changes of skull foramina. Laryngoscope 83:1385–1397

Calverley JR, Millikan CH (1961) Complications of carotid manipulation. Neurology (Minneap) 11:185–189

Carpue C (1816) An account of two successful operations restoring a lost nose from the integuments of the forehead in the case of two officers of his Majesty's army. Longman, London

Casberg MA (1950) The clinical significance of the cervical fascial planes. Surg Clin North Am 30:1415–1434

Cave JE (1933/34) On the occipito-atlanto-axial articulations. J Anat 68:416–428

Coller FA, Yglesias L (1935) Infections of the lip and face. Surg Gynecol Obstet 60:277–290

Conley JJ (1956) The surgical approach to the pterygoid area. Am Surg 144:39–43

Converse JM (1942) New forehead flap for nasal reconstruction. Proc R Soc Med 35:811–812
Converse JM, Coccaro PJ, Becker M, Wood-Smith D (1973) On hemifacial microsomia. Plast Reconstr Surg 51:268–279
Cornell SH (1969) Jugular venography. Am J Roentgenol 106:303–307
Costen JB (1934) A syndrome of ear and sinus symptoms dependent upon disturbed function of the temporomandibular joint. Ann Otol Rhinol Laryngol 43:1–15
Czerwinski F (1981) Variability of the course of external carotid artery and its rami in man in the light of anatomical and radiological studies. Folia Morphol (Warsz) XL:449–453
Dahlin DC, MacCarty CS (1952) Chordoma. A study of fifty-nine cases. Cancer 5:1170–1178
Dausacker J (1974) Praktisch anatomische Befunde an der mittleren und hinteren Schädelgrube. Dissertation, University of Würzburg
De Castro Correia P, Zani R (1973) Surgical anatomy of the facial nerve as related to ancillary operations in rhytidoplasty. Plast Reconstr Surg 52:549–552
Delens E (1870) (cited in Hamby 1952)
Denecke HJ (1961) Zur präparatorischen und reparatorischen Chirurgie des N. facialis. Z Laryngol Rhinol Otol 40/5:380–383
Denecke HJ (1966) Zur Chirurgie ausgedehnter Glomustumoren im Bereich des Foramen jugulare. Arch Klin Exp Ohr Nasen Kehlkopfheilkd 187:656
Dietemann JL, Lang J, Francke JP, Clarisse J, Bonneville JF, Wackenheim A (1981) Anatomy and radiology of the sellar spine. Neuroradiology 21:5–7
Dittel L (1857) Die Topographie der Halsfascien. Vienna
Dixon FW (1937) A comparative study of the sphenoid sinus (a study of 1600 skulls). Ann Otol Rhinol Laryngol 46:687–698
Dubreuil-Chambardel L (1907) Variationes sexuelles de l'atlas. Bull Soc Antropol Paris s 5: T 8 (after Tsusaki T 1924)
Dwight T (1887) Account of two spines with cervical ribs, one of which has a vertebra suppressed, and absence of the anterior arch of the atlas. J Anat Physiol 21:539–550
Edington GH (1901) Tortuosity of both internal carotid arteries. Med J (Lond) 2:1526–1527
Eisler P (1912) Die Muskeln des Stammes. In: Bardelebens Handbuch des Menschen, vol 2. Fischer, Jena
Elwany S, Yacout YM, Talaat M, Gunied A, El-Nahass M, Talaat M (1983) Surgical anatomy of the sphenoid sinus. J Laryngol Otol 97:227–241
Engel A (1975) Ursprungs- und Verlaufsvariationen der ersten Ophthalmica-Strecke. Dissertation, University of Würzburg
Engström H, Rexed B (1940) Über die Kaliberverhältnisse der Nervenfasern im N. stato-acusticus des Menschen. Z Mikrosk Anat Forsch 47:448–455
Ernst T, Inke G (1962) Variationen der sensiblen Hauptäste des N. mandibularis beim Menschen. Z Anat Entwicklungsgesch 123:126–136
Etemadi AA (1961) The dorsal motor nucleus of the vagus. Acta Anat (Basel) 47:328–332
Fichtl H (1989) Scientific researchments at the Department of Anatomy, University of Würzburg
Fink J (1978) Untersuchungen im Bereich der Fissura sphenomaxillaris, des Canalis palatinus major und des harten Gaumens. Dissertation, University of Würzburg
Fisher AGT (1915) Sigmoid tortuosity of the internal carotid artery and its relation to tonsil and pharynx. Lancet 2:128 (after Weibel and Fields 1965)
Fluur E (1964) Parapharyngeal tumors. Arch Otolaryngol 80:557–565
Franck F (1899) Anatomie du nerf vertébral chez l'homme et les mammiferes. J Physiol de Pathol Géné I (after Broek AJP van den 1908)
Francke JP, Macke J, Clarisse J, Libersa JC, Dobbelaero P (1982) The internal carotid arteries. Anat Clin 3:243–261
Franke H (1963) Über das Karotissinus-Syndrom und den sogenannten hyperaktiven Karotissinus-Reflex. Schattauer, Stuttgart
Freckmann N (1981) In: Samii M, Jannetta PJ (eds) The cranial nerves. Anatomy, pathology, pathophysiology, diagnosis, treatment. Springer, Berlin Heidelberg New York
Frizzi E (1915) Über die Wirbelsäule der Baining (Neu-Pommern). Z Morphol Anthropol 17
Fuchs E (1980) Untersuchung über die Gelenkflächen der Articulatio atlanto occipitalis. Dissertation, University of Würzburg
Fujii K, Lenkey C, Rhoton AL (1980a) Microsurgical anatomy of the choroidal arteries: lateral and third ventricles. J Neurosurg 52:165–188
Fujii K, Lenkey C, Rhoton Al (1980b) Microsurgical anatomy of the choroidal arteries. Fourth ventricle and cerebellopontine angles. J Neurosurg 52:504–524
Gabrielsen TO, Bookstein JJ (1968) Jugular venography by catheter approach from the arm. Radiology 91:378–379
Gabrielsen TO, Kingman AF (1964) Osteocartilaginous tumors of the base of the skull. Am J Roentgenol Radium Ther Nucl Med 91/4:1016–1023
Garretson HD, Elvidge AR (1963) Glossopharyngeal neuralgia with asystole and seizures. Arch Neurol 8:26–31
Gaughran GRL (1957) Fasciae of the masticator space. Anat Rec 129:383–400
Gerlach J, Jensen H-P, Spuler H, Viehweger G (1962) Die Persistenz der Arteria primitiva hypoglossica. Arch Psychiatry Ges Neurol 203:164–172
Gillies HD (1935) The development and scope of plastic surgery. Northwest Univ Med School Bull 35:1
Gisselsson L (1947) Intranasal forms of encephalomeningocele. Acta Otolaryngol (Stockh) 35:519–531
Griffin CJ (1962) Glomus tumor in the bilaminar zone of the human temporomandibular meniscus. Aust Dent 7:377–380
Grodinsky M, Holyoke EA (1938) The fasciae and fascial space of the head, neck and adjacent regions. Am J Anat 63:367–408
Gross SW, Holzman A (1954) Aneurysm of common carotid artery in the neck. J Neurosurg 11:209–213

Grote G (1901) Die Varietäten der Arteria temporalis superficialis. Z Morphol u Anthropol III:1–20

Gudmundsson K, Rhoton AL Jr, Rushton JG (1971) Detailed anatomy of the intracranial portion of the trigeminal nerve. J Neurosurg 35:592–600

Guerrier Y, Bolönyi F (1948) L'innervation de l'articulation temporo-maxillaire. Ann Otolaryngol 65:109–111

Guild SR (1941) A hitherto unrecognized structure, the glomus jugularis, in man. Anat Rec 79:29

Hakuba A (1985) Transoral approach for atlantoaxial dislocation. Neurosurgeons (proceeding of the 4th annual meeting of the Japan congress of neurological surgery) 4:231–236

Hall C (1934) The parapharyngeal space: an anatomical and clinical study. Ann Otol Rhinol Laryngol 43:793–812

Hamberger CA, Hammer G, Norlen G, et al. (1961) Transantrosphenoidal hypophysectomy. Arch Otolaryngol 74:2–8

Hamby WB (1952) Intracranial aneurysma. Thomas, Springfield

Hansson T, Nordström B (1977) Thickness of the soft tissue layers and articular disk in temporomandibular joints with deviations in form. Acta Odontol Scand 35:281–288

Hardy J (1969) Transsphenoidal microsurgery of the normal and pathological pituitary. Clin Neurosurg 16:185–217

Harris FS, Rhoton AL Jr (1976) Anatomy of the cavernous sinus. A microsurgical study. J Neurosurg 45:169–180

Harris W (1926) Neuritis and neuralgia. Oxford University Press, New York

Hasebe K (1913) Die Wirbelsäule der Japaner. Morphol Anthropol 15 (after Tsusaki 1924)

Hassler O (1961) Morphological studies on the large cerebral arteries. With reference to the aetiology of subarachnoid haemorrhage. Appelberg, Uppsala

Hayashi K, Yabuki T, Kurokawa T, Seki H, Hogaki M, Minoura S (1977) The anterior and the posterior longitudinal ligaments of the lower cervical spine. J Anat 124/3:633–636

Hayreh SS, Dass R (1962a) The ophthalmic artery. I. Origin and intra-cranial and intracanalicular course. Br J Ophthalmol 46:65–98

Hayreh SS, Dass R (1962b) The ophthalmic artery. II. Intra-orbital course. Br J Ophthalmol 46:165–185

Helms J (1963) Über den Winkel zwischen Dens und Epistropheus. Dissertation, University of Munich

Henle J (1871) Handbuch der systematischen Anatomie des Menschen, 3rd edn. Vieweg, Braunschweig

Henschen F (1961) Zur Histologie und Pathogenese der Kleinhirnbrückenwinkeltumoren. Arch Psychiatr Nervenkrankh 56:20–122

Hirschfeld L (1866) Névrologie et esthésiologie, 2nd édn. Paris

Hochstetter F (1940) Über die Taenia interclinoidea, die Commissura alicochlearis und die Cartilago supracochlearis des menschlichen Primordialkraniums. Morphol Jahrb 84:220–243

Hoffman HH, Schnitzelein HN (1961) The numbers of nerve fibers in the vagus nerve of man. Anat Rec 139:429–434

Hoffmann H (1973) Der supra- und intradiscoidale Gelenkspalt des menschlichen Kiefergelenks. Dissertation, University of Würzburg

Hogg SP, Kratz RC (1958) Surgical exposure of the facial nerve. Arch Otolaryngol 67:560–561

Horn W (1978) Variationen am Sinus cavernosus und benachbarter Regionen. Dissertation, University of Würzburg

Hyrtl J (1853) Handbuch der topographischen Anatomie, vol 1. Braumüller, Vienna, p 192

Hyrtl J (1859) Lehrbuch der Anatomie des Menschen, mit Rücksicht auf physiologische Begründung und praktische Anwendung, 6th edn. Braumüller, Vienna

Hyrtl J (1862) Der Sinus ophthalmo-petrosus. Wien Med Wochenschr 19:291–292

Hyrtl J (1885) Lehrbuch der Anatomie des Menschen mit Rücksicht auf physiologische Begründung und praktische Anwendung, 18th edn. Braumüller, Vienna

Ingelmark BE (1947) Über das craniovertebrale Grenzgebiet beim Menschen. Acta Anat [Suppl] (Basel) 6:1–116

Issing P (1985) Scientific researchments at the Department of Anatomy, University of Würzburg

Jackson FE (1964) Syncope associated with persistent hypoglossal artery. Case report. J Neurosurg 21:139–141

Jacod M (1921) Sur la propagation intracranienne des sarcomes du carrefour pétro-sphénoïdal: paralysie des 2°, 3°, 4°, 5°, et 6° paires crâniennes. Rev Neurol (Paris) 38:33–38

Jannetta PJ (1977) Observations on the etiology of trigeminal neuralgia, hemifacial spasm, acoustic nerve dysfunction, and glossopharyngeal neuralgia. Definitive microsurgical treatment and results in 117 patients. Neurochirurgia (Stuttg) 20:145–154

Jannetta PJ, Dujovny M, Gendell HM, Segal R, Wolfson S (1981) Neurovascular compression of the left hind brain and the vagus nerve in neurogenic "essential" hypertension. In: Dietz H, Metzel E, Langmaid C (eds) Neurological surgery. Abstracts of the 7th international congress of neurological surgery, Munich, July 12–18, 1981. Supplement to Neurochirurgia. Thieme, Stuttgart

Jannetta PJ, Segal R, Wolfson SK (1985) Neurogenic hypertension: Etiology and surgical treatment. Ann Surg 201:391–398

Jazuta KZ (1928) Zur topographischen Anatomie der Carotidenarterien. Anat Anz 59:148–153

Joessel (1878) Neue Anomalien der Carotis externa und der Maxillaris interna. Arch Anat Physiol 433–437

Juvara E (1870) Anatomie de la région ptérygomaxillaire. Thesis, University of Paris

Kagerbauer Ch (1985) Scientific researchments at the Department of Anatomy, University of Würzburg

Kantor H (1905) Tiefe Teilung der Arteria carotis communis. Anat Anz 26:492–496

Karma P, Räsänen O, Kärjä J (1977) Nasal gliomas: a review and report of two cases. Laryngoscope 87:1169–1179

Keen WW, Funke J (1906) Tumors of the carotid gland JAMA 47:469–479, 566–570

Keller HL, Neiss A (1962) Abnorme Beweglichkeit der Occipito-Zervikalgegend beim Os odontoideum. Acta Radiol 57:145–155

Kelly AB (1925) Tortuosity of the internal carotid in relation to the pharynx. J Laryngol 40:15

Keros P (1962) Über die praktische Bedeutung der Niveauunterschiede der Lamina cribrosa des Ethmoids. Z Laryngol Rhinol 11:808

Kessler (1989) – Scientific researchments at the Department of Anatomy, University of Würzburg

Kitamura H (1974) Development of temporomandibular joint innervation. Bull Tokyo Med Dent Univ 21:83–85

Knese H (1949/50) Kopfgelenk, Kopfhaltung und Kopfbewegung des Menschen. Z Anat Entwicklungsgesch 114:67–107

Koos WT, Spetzler RF, Pendl G, Perneczky A, Lang J (1985) Color atlas of microneurosurgery. Thieme, Stuttgart

Koebke J (1979) Morphological and functional studies on the odontoid process of the human axis. Anat Embryol (Berl) 155:197–208

Koebke J, Brade H (1982) Morphological and functional studies on the lateral joints of the first and second cervical vertebrae in man. Anat Embryol (Berl) 164:265–275

Krauss J (1987) Messungen zur cranio-cerebralen Topographie. Dissertation, University of Würzburg

Križan Z (1956) Beitrag zur Kenntnis des dritten Trigeminusastes. Pract Oto Rhinolaryngol 18:144

Križan Z (1960a) Über die fraglichen Korrelationen und über die Entwicklung einiger Typen der A. maxillaris. Acta Anat (Basel) 42:71–87

Križan Z (1960b) Beiträge zur deskriptiven und topographischen Anatomie der A. maxillaris. Acta Anat (Basel) 41:319–333

Krmpotić-Nemanić J, Keros P (1973) Funktionale Bedeutung der Adaption des Dens axis beim Menschen. Verh Anat Ges 67:393–397

Krönlein RU (1889) Zur Pathologie und operativen Behandlung der Dermoidcysten der Orbita. Klin Chir 4:149–163

Kunert W (1961) Arteria vertebralis und Halswirbelsäule. Experimentelle und klinische Untersuchungen über die Strömungsverhältnisse in den Vertebralarterien. In: Junghanns H (ed) Die Wirbelsäule in Forschung und Praxis, vol 20. Hippokrates, Stuttgart

Lang J (1973) Vaskularisation der Dura mater cerebri. II. Vaskularisierte Durazotten am Eingang in den Canalis opticus. Z Anat Entwicklungsgesch 141:223–236

Lang J (1974) Eintritt und Verlauf der Hirnnerven (III, IV, VI) "im" Sinus cavernosus. Z Anat Entwicklungsgesch 145:87–99

Lang J (1975) Über die Vascularisation der Periorbita. Gegenbaurs Morphol Jahrb 121:174–191

Lang J (1977) Structure and postnatal organization of heretofore uninvestigated and infrequent ossification of the sella turcica region. Acta Anat (Basel) 99:121–139

Lang J (1979) Gehirn- und Augenschädel. In: Lanz T von, Wachsmuth W (eds) Praktische Anatomie. Ein Lehr- und Hilfsbuch der anatomischen Grundlagen ärztlichen Handelns, vol 1/B. Springer, Berlin Heidelberg New York

Lang J (1981) Klinische Anatomie des Kopfes: Neurokranium, Orbita, kraniozervikaler Übergang. Springer, Berlin Heidelberg New York

Lang J (1982) Neue Ergebnisse zur Anatomie der Orbita. Fortschr Ophthalmol 79:3–10

Lang J (1983) Clinical anatomy of the head. Neurocranium-orbit-craniocervical regions. Springer, Berlin Heidelberg New York

Lang J (1984) Clinical anatomy of the cerebellopontine angle and internal acoustic meatus. Adv Otorhinolaryngol 34:8–24

Lang J (1985a) Circulus arteriosus cerebri, Variationen und Anomalien sowie seine Rami centrales. In: Voth D, Glees P (eds) Der zerebrale Angiospasmus. Experimentelle und klinische Grundlagen, Fortschritte der Diagnostik und Therapie. De Gruyter, Berlin, pp 3–18

Lang J (1985b) Übergeordnete Systeme. In: Lanz T von, Wachsmuth W (eds) Praktische Anatomie. Ein Lehr- und Hilfsbuch der anatomischen Grundlagen ärztlichen Handelns, vol 1/A. Springer, Berlin Heidelberg New York

Lang J (1985c) Anatomie der tiefliegenden Hirnstrukturen, insbesondere des Mittelhirns. In: Schürmann K (ed) Der zerebrale Notfall. Ein interdisziplinäres Problem. Urban und Schwarzenberg, Munich, pp 1–30

Lang J (1986) Topographical anatomy of the skull base and adjacent tissues. In: Scheunemann H, Schürmann K, Helms J (eds) Tumors of the skull base. Extra- and intracranial surgery of skull base tumors. De Gruyter, Berlin

Lang J (1987) Inferior skull base anatomy. In: Sekhar LN, Schramm VL Jr (eds) Tumors of the cranial base: diagnosis and treatment. Futura, Mount Kisco NY

Lang J (1988) Cerebellopontine angle and temporal bone. Second Microneurosurgical Anatomy Seminar: Surgical anatomy for microneurosurgery. 27 March 1988 (suppl) pp 37–47

Lang J (1988) Klinische Anatomie der Nase, Nasenhöhle und Nebenhöhlen. Grundlagen für Diagnostik und Operation. Thieme, Stuttgart

Lang J, Baldauf R (1983) Beitrag zur Gefäßversorgung des Rückenmarks. Gegenbaurs Morphol Jahrb 129:57–95

Lang J, Baumeister R (1982) Über das postnatale Wachstum der Nasenhöhle. Gegenbaurs Morphol Jahrb 128:354–393

Lang J, Baumeister R (1984) Postnatale Entwicklung der Gaumenbreite und -höhe und die Foramina palatina. Anat Anz 155:151–167

Lang J, Brückner B (1981) Über dicke und dünne Zonen des Neurocranium, Impressiones gyrorum und Foramina parietalia bei Kindern und Erwachsenen. Anat Anz 149:11–50

Lang J, Brunner FX (1978) Rami diencephalici inferiores anteriores, inferiores, inferiores posteriores and inferiores laterales posteriores – Anzahl, Durchmesser, Ursprungs- und Verlaufsvariationen. Verh Anat Ges 72:429–431

Lang J, Deymann-Bühler B (1984) Über die Größe bestimmter Mittelhirnstrukturen (Messungen an der Außenseite). J Hirnforsch 25:375–384

Lang J, Götzfried HP (1982) Über praktisch-ärztlich wichtige Maße an der Fossa cranialis media. Anat Anz 151:433–453

Lang J, Hack C (1985) Über Lage und Lagevariationen der Kanalsysteme im Os temporale. Teil I. Kanäle der Pars petrosa zwischen Margo superior und Meatus acusticus internus. HNO 33:176–179

Lang J, Hack C (1985) Über Lage und Lagevariationen der Kanalsysteme im Os temporale. Teil II. Kanäle der Pars petrosa zwischen Meatus acusticus internus und Facies inferior partis petrosae. HNO 33:279–284

Lang J, Haas R (1979) Neue Befunde zur Bodenregion der Fossa cranialis anterior. Verh Anat Ges 73:77–86

Lang J, Heilek E (1984) Anatomisch-klinische Befunde zur A. pharyngea ascendens. Anat Anz 156:177–207

Lang J, Hetterich A (1983) Beitrag zur postnatalen Entwicklung des Processus pterygoideus. Anat Anz 154:1–32

Lang J, Issing P (in press) Über Messungen am Clivus, den Foramina an der Basis cranii externa und den oberen drei Halswirbeln. Anat Anz (to be published)

Lang J, Kageyama I (1989) The anatomy of the ophthalmic artery and its branches. 83rd Meeting of the Anatomische Gesellschaft in Zürich, 20–23 March 1988. Verh Anat Ges

Lang J, Keller H (1978) Über die hintere Pfortenregion der Fossa pterygopalatina und die Lage des Ganglion pterygopalatinum. Gegenbaurs Morphol Jahrb 124:207–214

Lang J, Kollmannsberger A (1961) Beitrag zur Anatomie der Kleinhirnarterien. Gegenbaurs Morphol Jahrb 102:170–179

Lang J, Müller J (1975) Über bisher unbekannte topographische Beziehungen von Kleinhirnarterien. Verh Anat Ges 69:823–828

Lang J, Müller J (1977) Weitere Befunde über Kleinhirnarterien. Verh Anat Ges 71:713–717

Lang J, Niederfeilner J (1975) Über Fovea und Tuberculum articulare des Kiefergelenks. Verh Anat Ges 69:815–822

Lang J, Öder M (1984) Über die Biomorphose der Mandibula. Gegenbaurs Morphol Jahr 139:185–234

Lang J, Oehmann G (1976) Formentwicklung des Canalis opticus, seine Maße und Einstellung zu den Schädelebenen. Verh Anat Ges 70:567–574

Lang J, Papke J (1984) Über die klinische Anatomie des Paries inferior orbitae und dessen Nachbarstrukturen. Gegenbaurs Morphol Jahrb 130:1–47

Lang J, Reiter U (1984) Über den Verlauf der Hirnnerven in der Seitenwand des Sinus cavernosus. Neurochirurgia (Stuttg) 27:93–97

Lang J, Reiter U (1985) Über den Verlauf des N. abducens vor der Austrittszone aus dem zentralnervösen Organ bis zum M. rectus lateralis. Neurochirurgia (Stuttg) 28:1–5

Lang J, Reiter W (1983) Über den intraorbitalen Verlauf des n. abducens. Morphol Med 3:173–178

Lang J, Reiter W (1987) Über die dem Orbitadach und -rand angelagerten Strecken des N. ophthalmicus und seiner Äste. Neurochirurgia (Stuttg) 30:129–134

Lang J, Ricker K (1970) Bau und Funktion des subgaleotischen Verschiebegewebes. Z Anat Entwicklungsgesch 132:272–281

Lang J, Roth C (1984) Über die Fläche des Bodens der vorderen Schädelgrube und des Augenhöhlendachs sowie einige Winkel und Maße der Orbita. Anat Anz 156:1–19

Lang J, Sakals E (1981) Über die Höhe der Cavitas nasi, die Länge ihres Bodens und Maße sowie Anordnung der Conchae nasales und der Apertura sinus sphenoidalis. Anat Anz 149:297–318

Lang J, Sakals E (1982) Über den Recessus spheno-ethmoidalis, die Apertura nasalis des Ductus nasolacrimalis und den Hiatus semilunaris. Anat Anz 152:393–412

Lang J, Schäfer K (1976) Über Ursprung und Versorgungsgebiete der intracavernösen Stecke der A. carotis interna. Gegenbaurs Morphol Jahrb 122:182–202

Lang J, Schäfer W (1977) Fossa cranii, praktisch-anatomisch. Verh Anat Ges 71:1273–1278

Lang J, Schäfer K (1979) Arteriae ethmoidales: Ursprung, Verlauf, Versorgungsgebiete und Anastomosen. Acta Anat (Basel) 104:183–197

Lang J, Schlehahn F (1978) Foramina ethmoidalia und Canales ethmoidales. Verh Anat Ges 72:433–435

Lang J, Schlehahn F (1981) Über die postnatale Entwicklung der Fissura orbitalis. Gegenbaurs Morphol Jahrb 127:849–859

Lang J, Schreiber T (1983) Über Form und Lage des Foramen jugulare (Fossa jugularis), des Canalis caroticus und des Foramen stylomastoideum sowie deren postnatale Lageveränderungen. HNO 31:80–87

Lang J, Schulz F (1985) Über die Variabilität der Nasenarterien. Gegenbaurs Morphol Jahrb 131:551–566

Lang J, Strobel FJ (1978) Über den Einbau des Ganglion trigeminale. Verh Anat Ges 72:437–439

Lang J, Stöber G (1987) Über Lage und Lagevariationen der Kanalsysteme des Os temporale und Frontalschnitten. Gegenbaurs Morphol Jahrb 133:249–289

Lang J, Tisch-Rottensteiner K (1976) Lage und Form der Foramina der Fossa cranii media. Verh Anat Ges 70:557–565

Lang J, Tisch-Rottensteiner KF (1977) Über Formavarianten der Sella turcica. Verh Anat Ges 71:1279–1282

Lang J, Urban A (1977) Verlaufsvariationen der Pars pterygopalatina a. maxillaris. Verh Anat Ges 71:731–734

Lang J, Weigel M (1983) Nerve vessel relations in jugular foramen region. Anat Clin 5:1–16

Lang J, Schlehahn F, Jensen HP, Lemke J, Klinge H, Muhtaroglu U (1976) Cranio-cerebral topography as a basis for interpreting computed tomograms. In: Lanksch W, Kazner E, Grumme T, et al. (eds) Cranial computerized tomography. Springer, Berlin Heidelberg New York

Lang J, Horn T, von den Eichen U (1980) Über die äußeren Augenmuskeln und ihre Ansatzzonen. Gegenbaurs Morphol Jahrb 126:817–840

Lang J, Stefanec P, Breitenbach W (1983) Über Form und Maße des Ventriculus tertius, von Sehbahnteilen des N. oculomotorius. Neuchirurgia (Stuttg) 26:1–5

Lang J, Maier R, Schafhauser O (1984) Über die postnatale Vergrößeruing der Foramina rotundum, ovale et spinosum und deren Lageveränderungen. Anat Anz 156:351–387

Lanz T von, Wachsmuth W (1955) Praktische Anatomie. Ein Lehr- und Hilfsbuch der anatomischen Grundlagen ärztlichen Handelns. Hals, vol 1/2. Springer, Berlin Heidelberg New York

Larina VN (1965) Der Nucleus n. hypoglossi des Menschen, Topographie, makro- und mikroskopische Beschreibung, Zahl der Ganglienzellen (in Russian). Arkh Anat 48:77–82

Larsell O (1951) Anatomy of the nervous system, 2nd edn. Appleton-Century-Crofts, New York

Lasjaunias P, Moret J (1976) The ascending pharyngeal artery: normal and pathological radioanatomy. Neuroradiology 11:77–82

Lauber H (1901) Über einige Varietäten im Verlaufe der Arteria maxillaris interna. Anat Anz 19:444–448

Lazorthes G, Daraux H, Gaubert J (1961) Etude de la vascularisation artérielle des formations optiques nerf, chiasma et baudelettes. Bull Soc Ophthalmol Fr 74:276

Lazorthes G, Gouaze A, Zadeh JO, Santini JJ, Lazorthes Y, Burdin P (1971) Arterial vascularisation of the spinal cord. J Neurosurg 35:253–262

Lhermitte F, Gautier J-C, Poirier J, Tyrer JH (1968) Hypoplysia of the carotid artery. Neurology (Minneap) 18:439–446

Lie TA (1968) Congenital anomalies of the carotid arteries including the carotid-basilar and carotid-vertebral anastomoses; an angiographic study and a review of the literature. Excerpta Medica, Amsterdam

Lippert H, Pabst R (1985) Arterial variations in man. Classifications and frequency. Bergmann, Munich

Löwy R (1910) Über das topographische Verhalten des nervus hypoglossus zur Vena jugularis interna. Anat Anz 37:10–12

Lowman RM, Robinson F, McAllister WB (1966) The craniopharyngeus canal. Acta Radiol (Stockh) 5:41

Lubosch W (1906) Über Variationen am Tuberculum articulare des Kiefergelenks des Menschen und ihre morphologische Bedeutung. Gegenbaurs Morphol Jahrb 35:322–353

Luschka H von (1856) Die sensitiven Zweige des Zungenfleischnerven des Menschen. Müllers Arch 62–82

Luschka H von (1861) Die Venen des menschlichen Halses. Denkschr Koenigl Akad Wissensch [Math Naturw Cl] 20:199–226

Luschka H von (1862) Die Anatomie des menschlichen Halses, vol 1. Laupp'sche Buchhandlung, Tübingen

Mabrey RE (1935) Chordoma. A study of 150 cases. Am J Cancer 25:501–517

Manelfe C, Starling-Jardim D, Touibi S, Bonafè A, David J (1978) Transsphenoidal encephalocele associated with agenesis of corpus callosum: value of metrizamide computed cisternography. J Comput Assist Tomogr 2:356–361

Mangold U, Lierse W, Pfeifer G (1980) Die Arterien der Stirn als Grundlage des Nasenersatzes mit Stirnlappen. Acta Anat (Basel) 107:18–25

Maniscalco JE, Habal MB (1978) Microanatomy of the optic canal. J Neurosurg 48:402–406

Mathews W, Wilson CB (1974) Ectopic intrasellar chordoma. J Neurosurg 39:260–263

Matsuda I (1977) Bilateral anomalous occipital artery of internal carotid origin: case report. Arch Jpn Chir 46:57–61

Mazzoni A (1969) Internal auditory canal arterial relations at the porus acusticus. Ann Otol Rhinol Laryngol 78/4:797–814

McLachlan MSF, Williams ED, Fortt RW, et al. (1968a) Estimation of pituitary gland dimensions from radiographs of the sella turcica. A post-mortem study. Br J Radiol 41:323–331

McLachlan MSF, Williams ED, Doyle FH (1968b) Applied anatomy of the pituitary gland and fossa. Br J Radiol 41:782–788

McMurtry JG, Melvin DY (1966) Extracranial carotid artery occlusion by an anomalous digastric muscle. J Neurosurg 24:108–110

Merkel F (1892) Über die Halsfascie. Anatomische Hefte, vol 1. Bergmann, Wiesbaden, pp 77–111

Meuer H-W (1983) Anatomische Befunde zu den Aa. thyreoideae. Dissertation, University of Würzburg

Miehlke A (1973) Surgery of the facial nerve, 2nd edn. Saunders, Philadelphia

Miles AEW (1950) Chondrosarcoma of the maxilla. Br Dent J 88:257–269

Milosslawski M (1903) Die Sinus frontales. Dissertation, Moscow

Misch M (1905) Beiträge zur Kenntnis der Gelenkfortsätze des menschlichen Hinterhauptes und der Varietäten in ihrem Bereich. Günther, Berlin

Mitterwallner F von (1955) Variationsstatistische Untersuchungen an den Hirngefäßen. Acta Anat 24:51–88

Moffett BC (1957) The prenatal development of the human temporomandibular joint. Contrib Embryol 243:19–28

Moffett BC (1964) The development of discs and fibrous articular tissue in the temporomandibular and clavicular joints. Anat Rec 148:313

Møller AR, Jannetta PJ (1982) Auditory evoked potentials recorded intracranially from the brain stem in man. Exp Neurol 78:144–157

Møller AR, Jannetta PJ (1983a) Monitoring auditory functions during cranial nerve microvascular decompression operations by direct recording from the eighth nerve. J Neurosurg 59:493–499

Morris ED, Moffat DB (1956) Abnormal origin of the basilar artery from the cervical part of the internal carotid and its embryological significance. Anat Rec 125:701–711

Müller F (1952) Die Bedeutung der Sellabrücke für das Auge. Klin Monatsbl Augenheilkd 120:298–302

Müller G (1985) Zur Verankerung der Venae ophthalmicae. Verh Anat Ges 79:473–475

Müller H (1858) Über das Vorkommen von Resten der Chorda dorsalis bei Menschen nach der Geburt und über die Verhältnisse zu den Gallertgeschwülsten am Clivus. Z Rat Med 2:202–229
Müller T (1985) Über die Verbreitung des N. glossopharyngeus im Bereich des Gaumens und die Anastomosen des N. hypoglossus im Spatium parapharyngeum. Dissertation, University of Würzburg
Müsebeck K, Karst H (1967) Zur familiären Häufung medianer Dermoidfisteln der Nase. HNO 15:326–328
Mulligan RM (1950) Chemodectoma in the dog (abstract). Am J Pathol 26:680
Nathan H, Quaknine G, Kosary IZ (1974) The abducens nerve. J Neurosurg 41:561–566
Naufal PM, Schuknecht HF (1972) Vestibular, facial and oculomotor neuropathy in diabetes mellitus. Arch Otolaryngol 96:468 (after Bergström 1973)
Navarro JAC, Filho JLT, Zorzetto NL (1982) Anatomy of the maxillary artery into the pterygomaxillopalatine fossa. Anat Anz 152:413–433
Neiß A (1956) Die Sellabrücke, eine Erscheinungsform des Foramen caroticoclinoideum. Fortschr Geb Rontgenstr Nuklearmed 84:70–72
Noeske K (1958) Über die arterielle Versorgung des menschlichen Rückenmarks. Gegenbaurs Morphol Jahrb 99:455–497
Nomina Anatomica (1983) 5th edn, approved by the 11th international congress of anatomists at Mexico City, 1980. Williams and Wilkins, Baltimore
Oberbeckmann J, Lautenbach E (1979a) Nervenfasern am tierischen und menschlichen Kiefergelenk, part I. ZWR 88:511–516
Oberbeckmann J, Lautenbach E (1979b) Nervenfasern am tierischen und menschlichen Kiefergelenk, part II. ZWR 88:552–557
Oertel O (1922) Über die Persistenz embryonaler Verbindungen zwischen der A. carotis interna und der A. vertebralis. Verh Anat Ges 31:281–295
Oliveira Y de (1979) Le processus rétro-articulaire ou tubercule rétro-mandibulaire du squelette crânien chez l'homme. Acta Anat (Basel) 104:211–219
Overton SB, Ritter FN (1973) A high-placed jugular bulb in the middle ear. A clinical and temporal bone study. Laryngoscope 83:1986–1991
Pahnke J, Lüdinghausen M von (1989) Topographische Anatomie der Tuba auditiva und ihre Darstellung in CAD-Technik. Verh Anat Ges (in press)
Parkinson D (1965) A surgical approach to the cavernous portion of the carotid artery. J Neurosurg 23:474–483
Parry CH (1799) An inquiry into the symptoms and causes of the syncope anginosa, commonly called angina pectoris. Cruttwell, Bath
Pasternack JG, Lillie R, Jones RA (1933) Metastasizing chondrosarcoma of the coronoid process in the mandible. Arch Pathol 15:649–654
Paullus WS, Pait TG, Rhoton AL Jr (1977) Microsurgical exposure of the petrous portion of the carotid artery. J Neurosurg 47:713–726
Perlmutter D, Rhoton AL Jr (1976) Microsurgical anatomy of the anterior cerebral–anterior communicating–recurrent artery complex. J Neurosurg 45:259–272
Perović D (1958) Über eine eigenartige normale Bildung am menschlichen Vomer sowie über die wahre Umrandung der Choanen. Jugoslavenska Akademija Znanosti i Umjetnosti, Zagreb (Rad knj 316:5–58)
Pfeifer G (1974) Systematik und Morphologie der kraniofazialen Anomalien. Orthop Chir Kiefer Gesichtsbereich XVIII:1–14
Pfeifer G (1978) Wiederherstellung der Nasenform bei partiellen und totalen Defekten. In: Schuchardt K, Schilli W (eds) Fortschritte der Kiefer- und Gesichtschirurgie. Thieme, Stuttgart
Piscol K (1972) Die Blutversorgung des Rückenmarkes und ihre klinische Relevanz. Springer, Berlin Heidelberg New York (Schriftenr Neurol 8)
Platzer W (1957) Zur Anatomie der "Sellabrücke" und ihrer Beziehung zur A. carotis interna. Fortschr Geb Röntgenstr Nuklearmed 87/5:613–616
Poisel S, Golth D (1974) Zur Variabilität der großen Arterien im Trigonum caroticum. Wien Med Wochenschr 15:Apr 13
Pollock JA, Newton TH (1971) Encephalocele and cranium bifidum. In: Newton TH, Potts DG (eds) Radiology of the skull and brain. Mosby, St Louis, pp 634–647
Ponomarev VS (1958) Density of cells in the vestibular nuclei in man. Vopr Neirokhir (Moskva) 22:24–27
Poppen JL, King AB (1952) Chordoma: Experience with thirteen cases. J Neurosurg 9:139–163
Poulsen K (1886) Über die Fascien und die interfascialen Räume des Halses. Z Chir 23:223–272
Psenner L (1952) Beitrag zur Klinik und zur Röntgendiagnostik des Chordoms der Schädelbasis. ROFO 77/4:425–433
Quain R (1844) The anatomy of the arteries of the human body and its application to pathology and operative surgery, with a series of lithographic drawings. Taylor and Walton, London
Reinbach W (1963a) Das Cranium eines menschlichen Embryos von 93 mm Sch.-St. Länge (Zur Morphologie des Cranium älterer menschlicher Feten I). Z Anat Entwicklungsgesch 124:1–50
Reinbach W (1963b) Die Lamina alaris (Voit) am Occipitalpfeiler des Säugercraniums sowie eine weitere lamellenförmige Bildung in dieser Region bei *Zaedyus minutus* (Ameghino). Z Anat Entwicklungsgesch 124:51–56
Rektoržik E (1858) Über das Vorkommen eines Sinus venosus im Canalis caroticus des Menschen. Sitzungsber Math Naturwiss Cl Koenigl Akad Wiss 33:466–470
Renn WH, Rhoton AL Jr (1975) Microsurgical anatomy of the sellar region. J Neurosurg 43:288–298
Romanes G-J (1972) Cunningham's text book of anatomy. 2nd edn. Oxford University Press, London
Rosenwasser H (1945) Carotid body tumor of the middle ear and mastoid. Arch Otolaryngol 41:64–67
Rowlands RP, Swan RHJ (1902) Tortuosity of both internal carotid arteries. Br Med J i:76
Samii M, Jannetta PJ (1981) The cranial nerves. Anatomy – pathology – pathophysiology – diagnosis – treatment. Springer, Berlin Heidelberg New York

Schiller A (1978) Caput mandibulae: Einstellung, Form und Knorpelfläche. Dissertation, University of Würzburg

Schmidt H-M (1974) Über Maße und Niveaudifferenzen der Medianstrukturen der vorderen Schädelgrube des Menschen. Gegenbaurs Morphol Jahrb 120:538–559

Schmidt H-M (1976) Gelenkflächenform und Spaltlinienbild der Trochlea tali. Verh Anat Ges 70:621–626

Schmidt MB (1900) Über seltene Spaltbildungen im Bereiche des mittleren Stirnfortsatzes. Arch Pathol Anat 162:340 (after Zook et al. 1984)

Schröder F (1967) Bildung von Gesichtshautlappen unter besonderer Berücksichtigung der Gefäßversorgung nach Entfernung von Gesichtstumoren. Chir Plast Rekonstr 3:184–197

Schürmann K (1985) Der cerebrale Notfall. Ein interdisziplinäres Problem. Urban und Schwarzenberg, Munich

Schubert M (1976) Praktisch-anatomische Befunde in der Fossa cranii posterior. Dissertation, University of Würzburg

Schumacher GH (1961) Die Kiefermuskeln des Menschen als funktionelles System. Wissensch Z Universität Rostock vol 10, mathematical-natural sciences series issue 1

Schumacher GH (1976) Über einige Aspekte der experimentellen Teratologie. Anat Anz 140:337–344

Schumacher GH, Lau H, Freund E, Schultz M, Himstedt HW, Menning A (1976) Zur Topographie der muskulären Nervenausbreitungen. 9. Kaumuskeln, M. pterygoideus lateralis und medialis, verschiedene Kautypenvertreter. Anat Anz 139:71–87

Schwalbe G (1901a) Über die Fontanella metopica (media-frontalis) und ihre Bildungen. Z Morphol Anthropol 3:93–129

Schwalbe G (1901b) Über den supranasalen Theil der Stirnnaht. Z Morphol Anthropol 3:208–220

Schweizer O, Leak GH (1952) A study of spinal fluid pressures in operations requiring removal of both internal jugular veins. Ann Surg 136:948

Schwerdt K (1978) Form- und Lagevariationen der extracraniellen Arteria vertebralis im Angiogramm. Dissertation, University of Würzburg

Sergi G (1909/10) Sull'arimmetria dei condili occipitali nell'uomo. Atti Soc Ron Antropol 15:173

Shah AC, Srivastava HC (1965) Bifurcation of the common carotid artery. Indian J Surg 27:662–664

Shealy CN, Jackson CCR, Pearson O, Kaufmann B (1968) Submucosal infranasal transsphenoidal hypophysectomy. Bull Los Angeles Neurol Soc 33:185

Singer E (1935) Fasciae of the human body and their relation to the organs they envelop. Williams and Wilkins, Baltimore

Sjöqvist O (1938) Studies on pain conduction in the trigeminal nerve. Acta Psychiatr (Copenh) 17:1–139

Skopakoff C (1968) Über die Variabilität im Verlauf der A. maxillaris. Anat Anz 123:534–546

Smith CG (1941) Incidence of atrophy of the olfactory nerves in man. Arch Otolaryngol 34:533–539

Smith D, Larsen JL (1979) On the symmetry and asymmetry of the bifurcation of the common carotid artery. Neuroradiology 17:245–247

Smith GM (1902) Tortuosity of internal carotid artery. Br Med J 1:1602

Smith KR, Nelson JS, Dooley JM (1968) Bilateral "hypoplasia" of the internal carotid arteries. Neurology (Minneap) 18:1149–1156

Sömmerring ST von (1791) Vom Baue des menschlichen Körpers. Erster Theil: Knochenlehre. Varrentrapp u Wenner, Frankfurt a.M.

Sömmerring ST von (1792a) Über den natürlichen Unterschied der Gesichtszüge in Menschen. Vossische Buchhandlung, Berlin

Sömmerring ST von (1792b) Vom Bau des menschlichen Körpers. Teil 4. Gefäßlehre. Varrentrapp und Wenner, Frankfurt/M

Sömmerring ST von (1796) De corporis humani Fabrica. Lat. donata, ab ipso auctore aucta et em. T. 1–5. Traiecti a.M. Varrentrappius et Wennerus 1794–1800. 4 Bde. T 3 De musculis tendinibus et bursis mucosis. 1796

Soemmerring ST von (1806) Abbildungen der menschlichen Organe des Geschmackes und der Stimme. Varrentrapp u. Wenner, Frankfurt a.M.

Soemmerring ST von (1841) Hirn- und Nervenlehre. Umgearbeitet von G. Valentin. Voß, Leipzig

Spallone A, Cantore G (1981) The role of extracranial carotid abnormalities in the genesis of cerebral aneurysms. J Neurosurg 55:693–700

Stock AL, Collins HP, Davidson TM (1980) Anatomy of the superficial temporal artery. Head Neck Surg 2:466–469

Stofft E (1968) Das Ligamentum transversum atlantis als funktionellstrukturierter Dens-Halteapparat. Anat Anz 123:157–168

Stopford JSB (1916) The arteries of the pons and medulla oblongata. J Anat Physiol 50:131–164

Strand SO (1958) Primary tumors of the infra-temporal and pterygopalatine fossae. Arch Otolaryngol 68:437–450

Strecker C (1887) Über die Condylen des Hinterhauptes. Arch Anat Entwicklungsgesch [Anat Abt] 301

Sturm R (1981) Gelenkspalt und Gelenkkapsel der Articulatio atlantoaxialis lateralis. Dissertation, University of Würzburg

Sunderland S (1945) Arterial relations of the internal auditory meatus. Brain 68:23–27

Tabb HG, Tannehill JF (1973) The tympanomastoid fissure: a reliable approach to the facial nerve in parotid surgery. South Med J 66/11:1273–1276

Tabb HG, Scalco AN, Fraser SF (1970) Exposure of the facial nerve in parotid surgery. Laryngoscope 80:559–567

Tanaka T (1932a) Ganglion sphenopalatinum des Menschen. Arbeiten aus der 3. Abteilung des Anat. Inst. der Kaiserl. Univ. Kyoto 3:91–115

Tanaka T (1932b) Ganglion oticum. Arb. 3. Abt. Anat. Inst. Kyoto, (A) 3:41–49

Tarlov IM (1937a) Structure of the nerve root. I. Nature of the junction between the central and the peripheral nervous system. Arch Neurol Psychiatry 37:555–583

Tarlov IM (1937b) Structure of the nerve root. II. Differentiation of sensory from motor roots; observations on identification of function in roots of mixed cranial nerves. Arch Neurol Psychiatry 37:1338–1355

Taveras JM, Wood EH (1964) Diagnostic neuroradiology. Williams and Wilkins, Baltimore

Tessier P (1976) Anatomical classification of facial, cranio-facial and laterofacial clefts. J Maxillofac Surg 4:69–92

Teufel J (1964) Einbau der Arteria carotis interna in den Canalis caroticus unter Berücksichtigung des transbasalen Venenabflusses. Gegenbaurs Morphol Jahrb 106/2:188–274

Tharp B, Heyman A, Pfeiffer J, et al. (1965) Cerebral ischemia: result of hypoplasia of internal carotid artery. Arch Neurol 12:160–164

Thilander B (1962) Innervation of the temporomandibular disc in man. Acta Odontol Scand 22:151–156

Thorsteinsdottir K (1982) Über Faserzahlen des N. oculomotorius, N. trochlearis, N. abducens, N. ophthalmicus, N. maxillaris und N. mandibularis sowie die Faszikelzahl des N. maxillaris. Dissertation, University of Würzburg

Todman RC (1960) Fatal case of spontaneous hemorrhage from internal carotid artery resulting from retropharyngeal infection. J Laryngol 74:493–496

Trotter W (1911) On certain clinically obscure tumors infiltrating the naso-pharyngeal wall. Trans Med Soc Lond 34:372–378

Tsusaki T (1924) Über den Atlas und Epistropheus bei den eingeborenen Formosanern. Folia Anat Jpn 11:221–246

Turvey TA, Fonseca RJ, Hill C (1980) The anatomy of the internal maxillary artery in the pterygopalatine fossa: its relationship to maxillary surgery. J Oral Surg 38:92–95

Urban A (1974) Topographie der Pars pterygopalatina der A. maxillaris aus frontaler Sicht. Dissertation, University of Würzburg

Van Alyea OE (1941) Sphenoid sinus. Anatomic study, with consideration of the clinical significance of the structural characteristics of the sphenoid sinus. Arch Otolaryngol 34:225–253

Van Buskirk A (1945) The seventh nerve complex. J Comp Neurol 82:303–333

Velpeau A (1830) A treatise on surgical anatomy or the anatomy of the regions, vol 1. Wood, New York

Vogler C (1936) Beitrag zu den Lagebeziehungen der tiefen Gesichtsschlagader. Dissertation, Munich

Vraa-Jensen G (1942) The motor nucleus of the facial nerve. Munksgaard, Copenhagen

Wackenheim A (1974) Roentgen diagnosis of the craniovertebral region. Springer, Berlin Heidelberg New York

Walker E, Moore WW, Simpson JR (1952) Intranasal encephalocele. Arch Otolaryngol 55:182–187

Warwick R, Williams PL (1973) Gray's anatomy, 35th edn. Longman, London

Weaver kDF, Young DJ (1964) Retropharyngeal hemorrhage from the carotid arteries. Ann Otol Rhinol Laryngol 73:541–554

Weber-Liel FE (1873) Über das Wesen und die Heilbarkeit der häufigsten Form progressiver Schwerhörigkeit. Hirschwald, Berlin, pp 1–205

Weber-Liel FE (1897) Experimenteller Nachweis einer freien Kommunication der endolymphatischen Räume des menschlichen Ohrlabyrinths mit extracraniellen Räumen. Arch Pathol Anat Physiol Klin Med 77/7:207–226

Weibel J, Fields WS (1965a) Tortuosity, coiling, and kinking of the internal carotid artery. I. Etiology and radiographic anatomy. Neurology (Minneap) 15:7–18

Weibel J, Fields WS (1965b) Tortuosity, coiling, and kinking of the internal carotid artery. II. Relationship of morphological variation to cerebrovascular insufficiency. Neurology (Minneap) 15:462–468

Weisenburg TH (1910) Cerebello-pontile tumor diagnose for six years as tic douloureux. JAMA LIV:1600–1604

Whitaker SR, Sprinkle PM, Chou SM (1981) Nasal glioma. Arch Otolaryngol 107:550–554

Williamson WP, Barelli PA (1951) Intranasal encephalocele. J Neurosurg 8:231–235

Wishart ES (1923) Retropharyngeal abscess and erosion of internal carotid artery: with pathological specimen. Can Med Assoc J 13:635

Wollschlaeger G, Wollschlaeger PB, Lucas FV, Lopez VF (1967) Experience and result with postmortem cerebral angiography performed as routine procedure of the autopsy. Am J Roentgenol 101:68–87

Wullstein HL (1985) Diskussion in La Napoule

Yasargil MG, Kasdaglis K, Jain KK, Weber H-P (1976) Anatomical observations of the subarachnoidal cisterns of the brain during surgery. J Neurosurg 44:298–302

Yasargil MG, Smith RD, Young PH, Teddy PJ (1984) Microsurgical anatomy of the basal cisterns and vessels of the brain, diagnostic studies, general operative techniques and pathological considerations of the intracranial aneurysms. Thieme, Stuttgart

Young RF, Stevens R (1979) Unmyelinated axons in the trigeminal motor root of human and cat. J Comp Neurol 183:205–214

Zehm S (1966) Die Topographie des retromaxillären Raumes in chirurgischer Sicht. Habilitationsschrift, University of Würzburg

Zenker W (1955) Das "Spatium buccotemporale" und die anderen Fascienräume der tiefen seitlichen Gesichtsregion. Z Anat Entwicklungsgesch 118:371–390

Zenker W, Zenker A (1955) Die Tätigkeit der Kiefermuskeln und ihre elektromyographische Analyse. Z Anat Entwicklungsgesch 119:174–200

Ziehen T (1913) Das Gehirn. II. Mikroskopische Anatomie, Aufgaben und Methoden. Anatomie des Centralnervensystems 1. Teil. Fischer, Jena

Zook EG, Nickey WM, Pribaz JJ (1984) Heterotropic brain tissue in the scalp. Plast Reconstr Surg 73:660–663

Surgery of the Anterior Skull Base (AS)

Surgery of Malformations of the Anterior Skull Base

Introductory Remarks. In discussing the surgical treatment of malformations of the anterior skull base, we must recognize two major groups:

1) Closure defects of the skull and brain–the fistulas, cysts, and celes (frontobasal dysraphic anomalies).
2) The various types of craniofacial synostosis and dysostosis.

Closure defects of the skull and frontobasal dysraphic anomalies are classified either by the site of the herniation (Table 1) or by its contents (Table 2, E. Meyer 1968). The simplest cleft malformation in the frontobasal region is the dermal sinus, which may be accompanied by dermoid cysts. This class includes a large portion of the congenital *nasal fistulas* and *dermoid cysts* of the nose, which are infrequently seen by the ear, nose and throat surgeon (Fig. AS 1a-c). Lannelongue (1891) quotes Cruvelhier, who in 1817 described a patient with a hairy depression on the dorsum of the nose. According to Denecke and Meyer (1964), the first case of a nasal dermoid cyst was published in Germany by Bramann (1890) and in the U.S. by Birkett (1901) (see references in Stupka 1938, Sessions 1982). These fistulas may extend from the skin to the cranial bone (Fig. AS 1a), to the dura through an opening in the cranium (Fig. AS 1b), or even into the intracranial subarachnoid space (Fig. AS 1c). The external opening in the skin may be inconspicuous and masked by a pigmented spot, so the condition may go undiagnosed until a subcutaneous fistulitis supervenes, possibly accompanied by intracranial complications. The fistulous opening is most commonly located on the nasal dorsum (Draf and Nagel 1971). Dermoid cysts may form along the course of the fistula, occurring anterior to the frontal bone, epidurally, or subdurally. With a subdural epidermoid cyst, a supervening inflammatory complication can produce symptoms of meningitis, brain abscess, or brain tumor; the possibility of such an anomaly should be considered whenever unexplained meningitis appears.

Table 1. Classification of frontobasal dysraphic anomalies by site of occurrence

1. Nasal fistulas
2. Nasal fistulas with cysts
3. Encephaloceles
   3.1 Frontoethmoidal
      a) Nasofrontal
      b) Nasoethmoidal
      c) Naso-orbital
   3.2 Spheno-orbital
   3.3 Sphenomaxillary
   3.4 Nasopharyngeal
      a) Transethmoidal
      b) Sphenoethmoidal
      c) Sphenopharyngeal

Table 2. Classification of frontobasal dysraphic anomalies by the contents of the sac

1. Dermal sinus
2. Dermal sinus with dermal cyst
3. Encephaloceles
   3.1 Meningocele
   3.2 Meningoencephalocele
   3.3 Encephalocystocele
   3.4 Encephalocystomeningocele

Occasionally epithelial cells can be demonstrated in the cerebrospinal fluid. With meningitis, staphylococci can be recovered from the fluid. Because the bony defect may be quite small, it is not always visible on roentgenograms. Differential diagnosis is not difficult in the presence of a fistula. If meningitis is present, its diverse etiologies must be considered.

Although these lesions may appear to be minor in the absence of complications, their early, complete removal is necessary to prevent progressive damage to the dorsal nasal skin from recurrent fistulization and to avoid intracranial complications.

Encephaloceles (Fig. AS 2a-d) result from congenital openings in the midline region of the skull, often at the junction of the chondro- and desmocranium, which permit meninges, brain substance, or both to herniate from the cranial cavity (Gerlach et al. 1967). Data on the prevalence of encephaloceles range from 1 in 2500 to 1 in 25,000 normal births. Their association with other closure disorders (e.g., of the spine) is less common.

A meningocele is a cerebrospinal fluid-filled hernial sac that is lined and covered by meninges. A sac that additionally contains brain tissue or other glial matter is referred to as a *meningoencephalocele*. An encephalocystocele is formed by the herniation of brain and fluid-filled portions of the ventricles through the osseous defect.

The severest grade of herniation is the *encephalocystomeningocele*, in which portions of the brain and ventricles are accompanied by a large collection of cerebrospinal fluid in the meningeal space (Fig. AS 3).

The great majority of cephaloceles are located along the sagittal line.

Encephaloceles of the anterior skull base include:

1) *Frontoethmoidal encephaloceles* (Fig. AS 2a-b), which comprise nasofrontal, nasoethmoidal, and naso-orbital forms. Their common internal hernial opening is located adjacent or anterior to the ethmoid bone, in proximity to the cecal foramen. The sac may project through the nasal root (nasofrontal encephalocele) or laterally between the frontal and nasal bones (nasoethmoidal encephalocele).

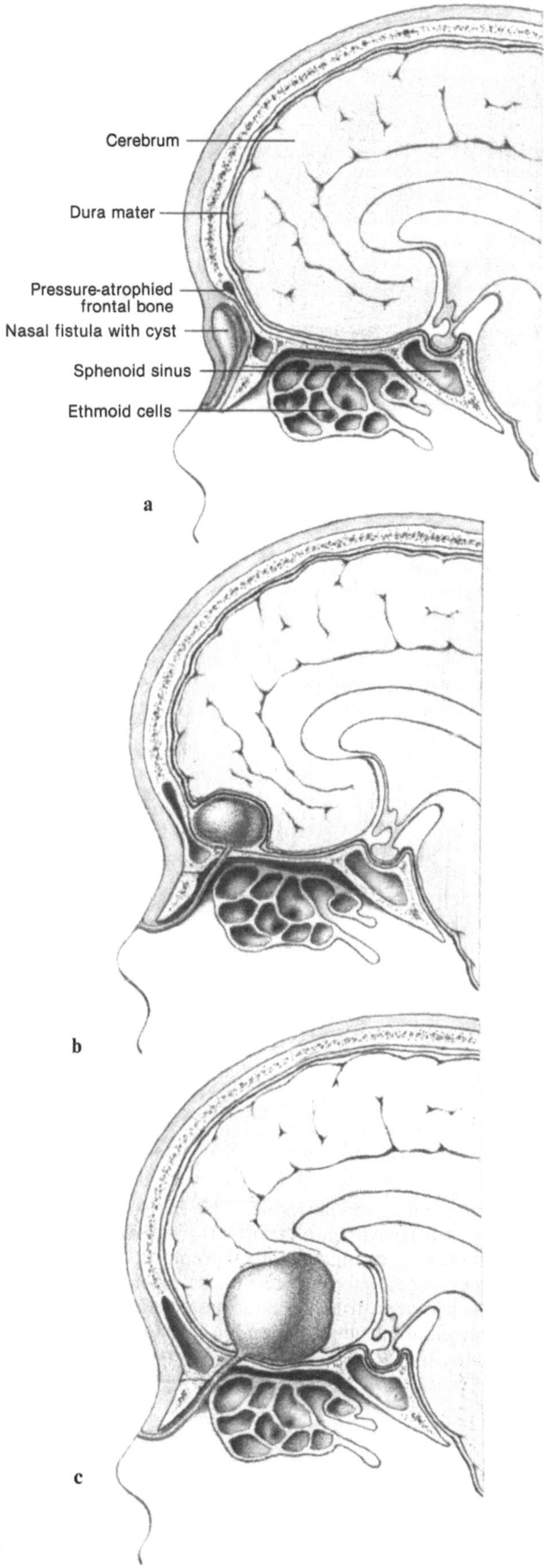

Fig. AS 1 a–c. Nasal fistulas and cysts.
a Nasal fistula with cyst anterior to the frontal bone, which has been thinned by pressure atrophy.
b Nasal fistula extending through the skull base into the cranial cavity, where it communicates with an extradural cyst.
c Nasal fistula with an associated intracerebral cyst

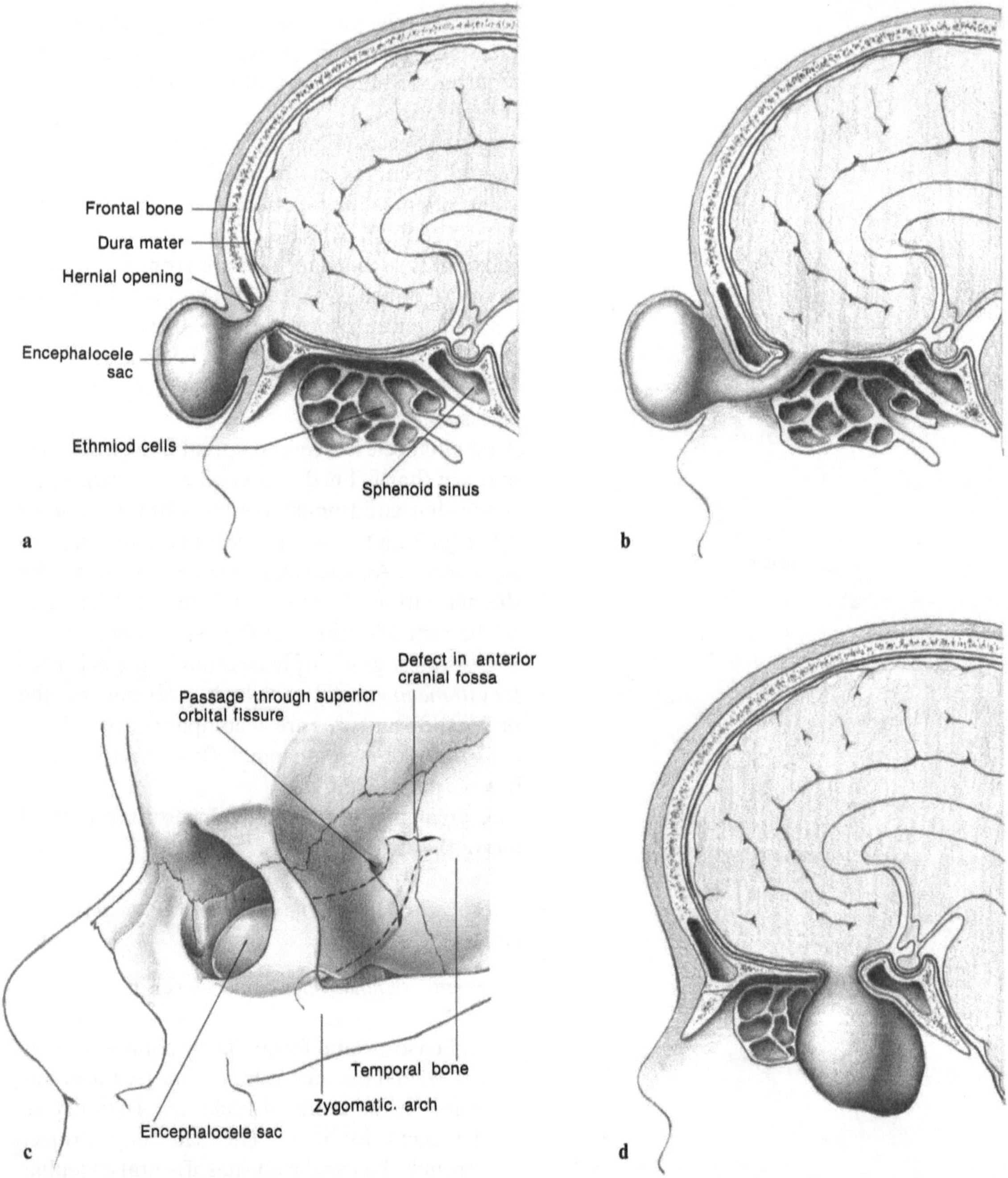

Fig. AS 2a–d. Encephaloceles of the anterior skull base. **a, b** Frontoethmoidal encephaloceles.
a Nasofrontal encephalocele. The hernial opening is located on the midline over the root of the nose.
b Nasoethmoidal encephalocele. The hernial opening is situated more laterally between the frontal and nasal bones.
c Spheno-orbital encephalocele. The hernia projects from the cranial cavity into the orbit through the superior orbital fissure, causing unilateral proptosis.
d Nasopharyngeal encephalocele of the sphenoethmoid type. The hernia protrudes into the nasal cavity or pharynx through an opening between the sphenoid and ethmoid bones

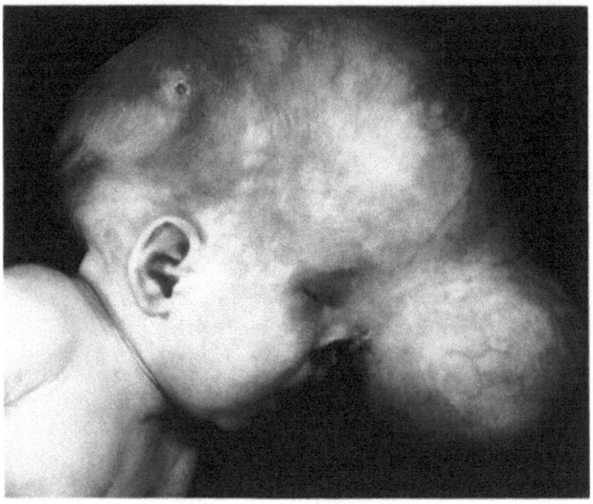

Fig. AS 3. Massive encephalocystomeningocele in an infant with cleft palate

In the naso-orbital form, the herniation occurs in the anterior portion of the medial orbital wall.

2) *Spheno-orbital encephaloceles* (Fig. AS 2c), which project into the orbit through the superior orbital fissure and produce a unilateral proptosis (Bushe and Glees 1968).
3) *Sphenomaxillary encephaloceles*. These are extremely rare and pass through the orbital cavity into the "sphenomaxillary fossa" situated in the posterior nasal region between the anterior wall of the sphenoid sinus and the posterior wall of the maxillary sinus.
4) *Nasopharyngeal encephaloceles*. The transethmoidal form projects into the nasal cavity, the sphenoethmoidal form enters the nasal or pharyngeal space between the sphenoid and ethmoid bones (Fig. AS 2d), and the sphenopharyngeal form protrudes into the pharynx through the sphenoid.

The naso-orbital encephaloceles are manifested *clinically* by a rounded bulge at the inner canthus of the eye. Differentiation is required from traumatic encephalocele, ethmoid-frontal sinus mucocele, and simple atheroma. E. Meyer (1968) states that large naso-orbital encephaloceles cause ocular displacement and can lead to blindness from optic nerve atrophy. The spheno-orbital encephaloceles are more difficult to diagnose. They cause proptosis and decreased ocular motility. Neurinoma, hemangioma, and glioma should be considered in differential diagnosis. A common feature of encephaloceles that enter the nasal and nasopharyngeal space is impairment of nasal respiration; these lesions are easily mistaken clinically for nasal polyps or tonsillar hyperplasia – the latter especially because adenoid vegetations are a frequent cause of impaired nasal respiration in children. Not infrequently, the diagnosis is made only after meningitis develops following an adenotomy or nasal polyp removal. In doubtful cases endoscopy of the nasopharynx will reveal the sacs as smooth, pulsating masses.

The *operative treatment* of nasal fistulas and cysts should be preceded by a selective diagnostic evaluation, even in patients with small fistulas. The workup should include endoscopy, radiographs, and computed tomography (CT) of the anterior skull base. The need for contrast visualization of the fistula is controversial. We do not perform a contrast study preoperatively, nor do we stain the fistula intraoperatively with a dye. Very often the fistulous tracts are occluded by desquamated epithelium, and in these cases contrast visualization would be misleading. If an attempt is made at operation to fill the fistulous tract with methylene blue, again only a portion of the fistula may be visualized because of epithelial occlusion. With forcible injection, dye can easily leak from the fistula and obscure the field.

Technique for the Surgical Removal of Nasal Fistulas, Cysts, and Meningoceles
(Fig. AS 4a-d)

Basically, nasal fistulas and cysts are treated by cutting around the external opening and then following the fistulous tract with the aid of a magnifying loupe or operating microscope to make certain that all epithelium-lined outpouchings are removed.

A probe is inserted into the tract before cutting around the fistulous opening. The outer skin is split on the midline using an irregular incision (with about 5-mm jogs) to obtain a less visible

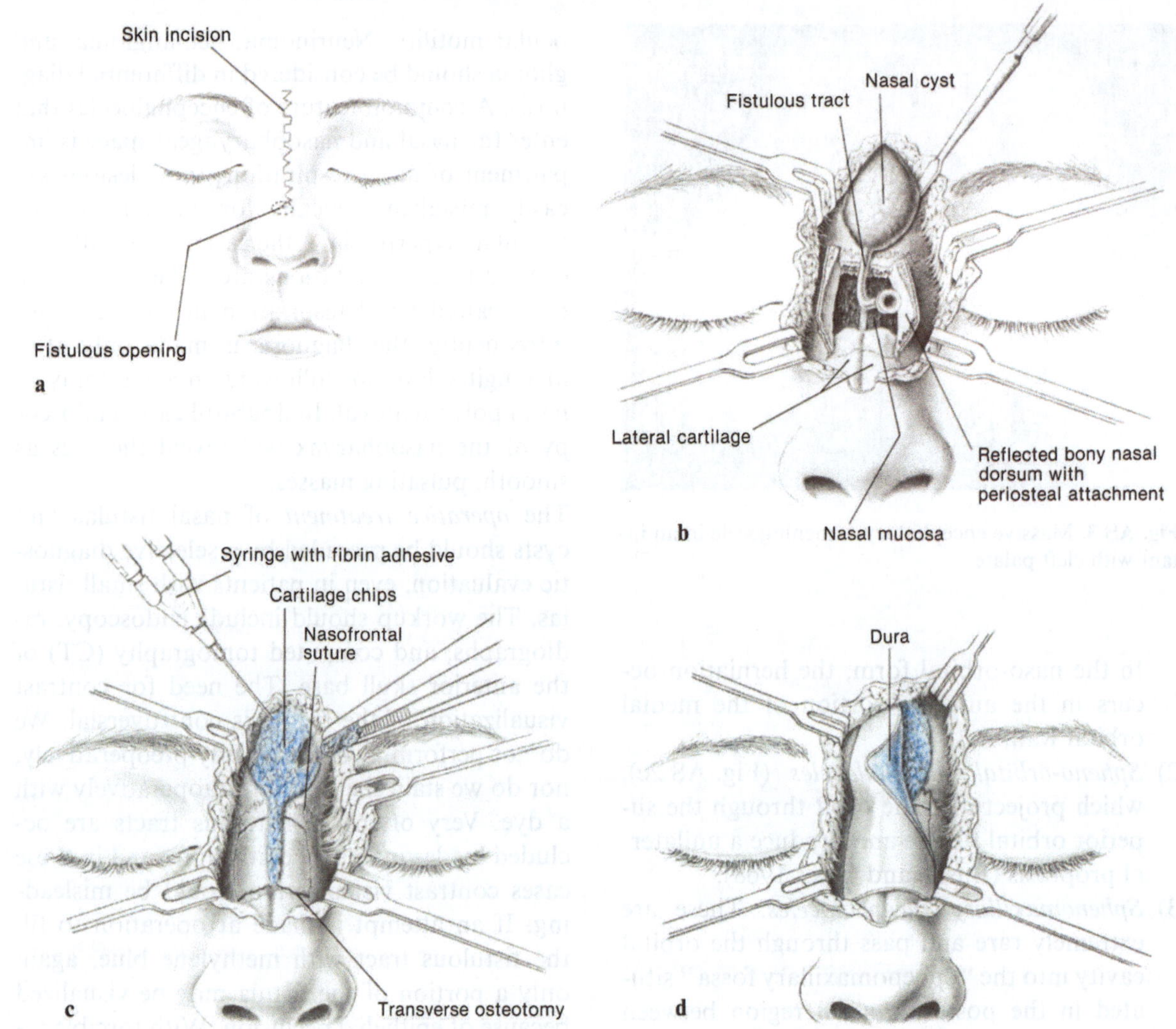

Fig. AS 4a–d. Technique for operative removal of nasal fistulas and cysts.
a The fistulous opening is outlined with a scalpel, and an irregular, "elective-type" skin incision is made on the midline (Borges 1973) to obtain a less obvious scar.
b The nasal mucosa having been stripped at the junction of the cartilaginous and osseous nose, the bony nasal dorsum is mobilized by bilateral median and transverse osteotomies and opened in trap-door fashion on the attached periosteum to expose the fistulous tract.
c The surgical defect is filled with cartilage chips measuring about 3 mm on a side. The chips are bonded together with fibrin adhesive. The nasal dorsal flaps have been swung back into place.
d The glabella and bony nasal dorsum are covered with stored dura to obtain a smooth contour

scar (Borges 1973). If it is found that the fistula passes upward under the bony and cartilaginous framework of the nose, a median osteotomy of the frontal process of the maxillary bone is performed. This can be extended superiorly with a transverse osteotomy. First the nasal mucosa is carefully separated and displaced inferiorly. If necessary, the lateral cartilages may be resected without injury to the nasal mucosa. The bony nasal dorsum is then reflected laterally on both sides, preserving its periosteal attachments, to create sufficient working room and to minimize the removal of dorsal bone. The fistula or cyst is separated from its bed along with the periosteum. A fistula penetrating the floor of the frontal sinus often will extend to the dura of the anterior cranial fossa, from which the epithelium must be dissected under magnifica-

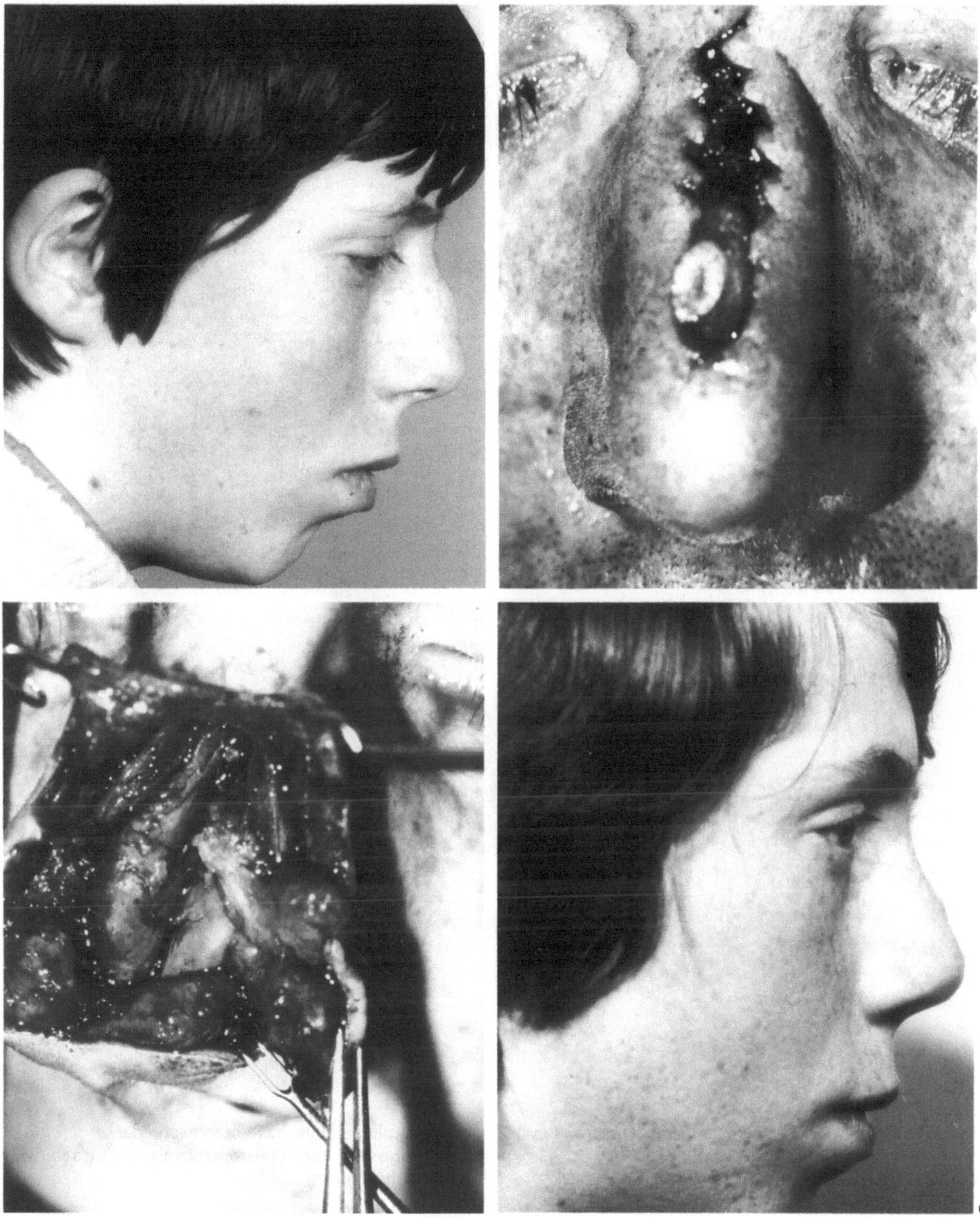

a b c d

Fig. AS 5a–d. Surgical treatment of a dorsal nasal fistula extending to the dura. The patient had had multiple previous operations.
a Fistula-related inflammatory swelling of the nasal dorsum.
b An irregular vertical ("elective") incision is made after cutting around the fistulous opening.
c The fistula, which passes upward between the nasal bones, is exposed by reflecting the periosteally based frontal process of the maxillary bone toward the skull base.
d Appearance of the patient several weeks after surgery

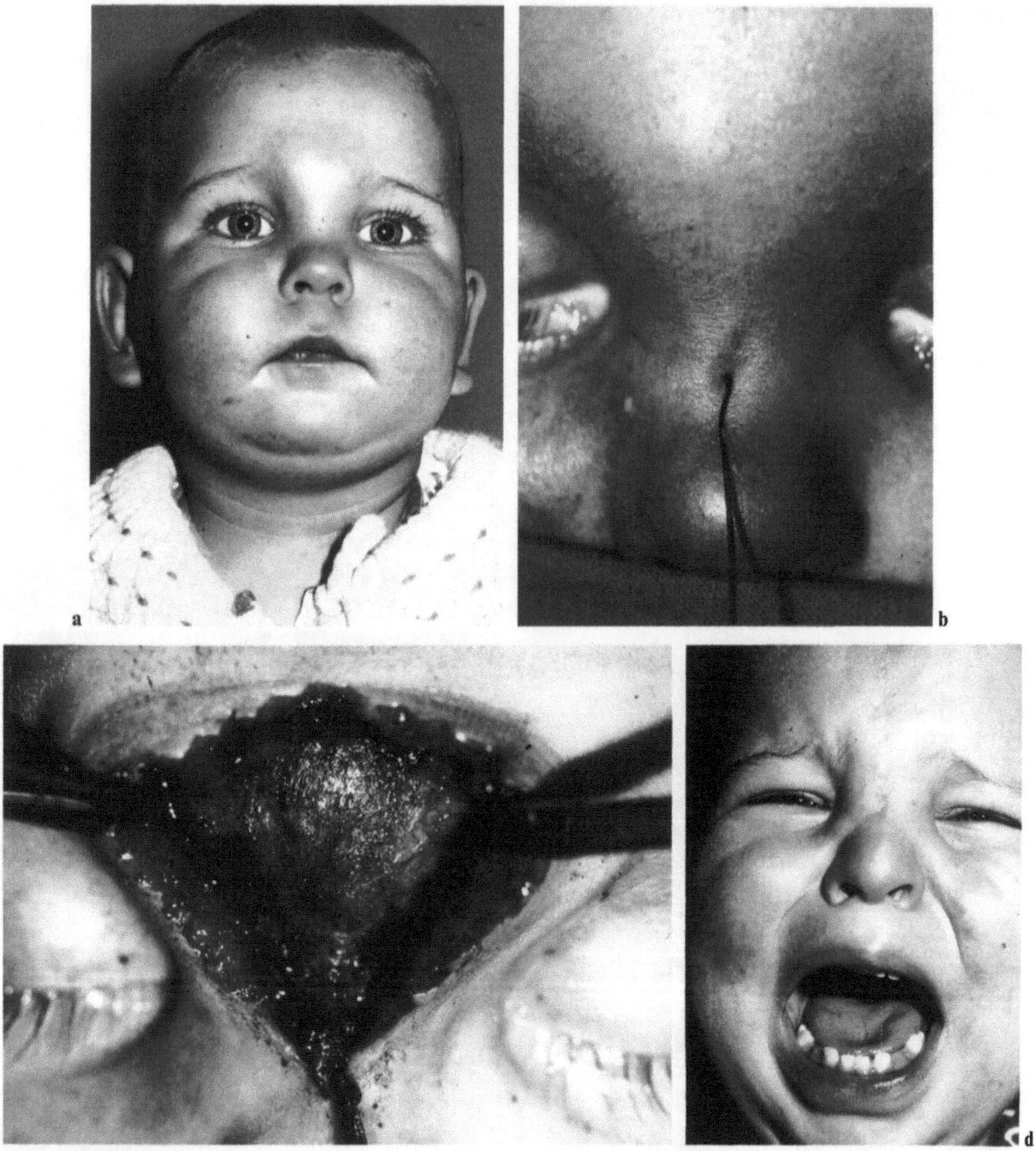

Fig. AS 6a–d. Frontobasal subcutaneous epidermal cyst combined with a fistula.
a, b Preoperative appearance.
c The fistula and cyst have been exposed.
d Appearance 6 weeks postoperatively, with a relatively unobtrusive scar

tion. The lateral bony nasal wall is then swung back into place on its periosteal hinge.
The defect formed by removal of the fistula or cyst can be satisfactorily filled with autogenous cartilage from the nasal septum or ear, or even with banked cartilage if that is the only option (greater risk of infection!). The graft material can be covered with stored dura or fascia to restore an acceptable appearance to the nasal bridge (see illustrative case in Fig. AS 5a-d).

A similar procedure was used to treat a fronto-basal epidermal cyst associated with a dermal sinus and osseous destruction in an 18-month-old boy (Fig. AS 6a-d).

In our experience, the surgeon treating a nasal fistula or cyst must be prepared for the necessity of opening the subarachnoid space and performing a duraplasty, as the lesion may communicate with the intracranial cavity. The same possibility exists in the patient who presents with a rounded, firm or tense swelling on the nasal dorsum, which may be a meningocele (Fig. AS 7). For removal, the overlying skin is incised on the midline, or else the lesion is progressively isolated from the nose after raising a superiorly based skin flap (Fig. AS 8a-b). When the cranial defect has been reached through the bony nasal framework, the hernial sac is removed, and a duraplasty is performed to seal the subarachnoid space (see pp. 131–138).

It is recommended that large encephaloceles, especially those projecting into the nasopharynx, be exposed through a transfrontal intradural approach, reduced into the cranium, and secured with a pericranial flap (Fig. AS 21a-b).

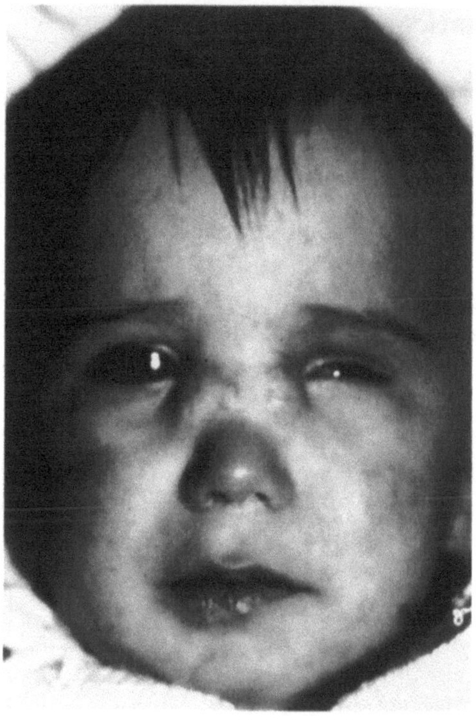

Fig. AS 7. The smooth, rounded, firm swelling over the nasal dorsum was found to be a meningocele at operation. Duraplasty was performed following removal of the sac

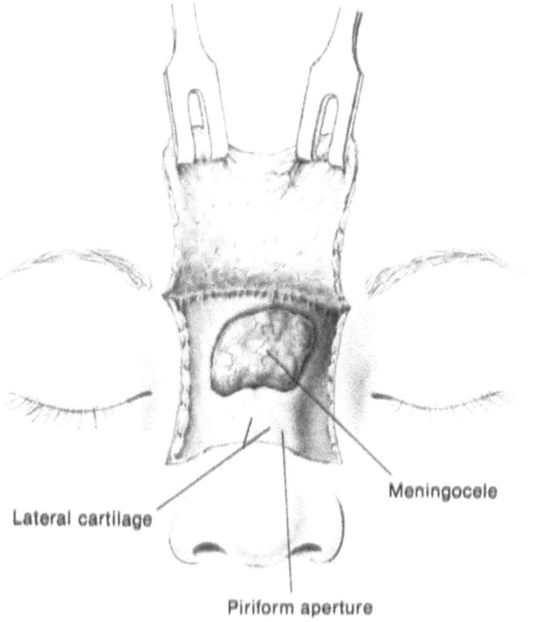

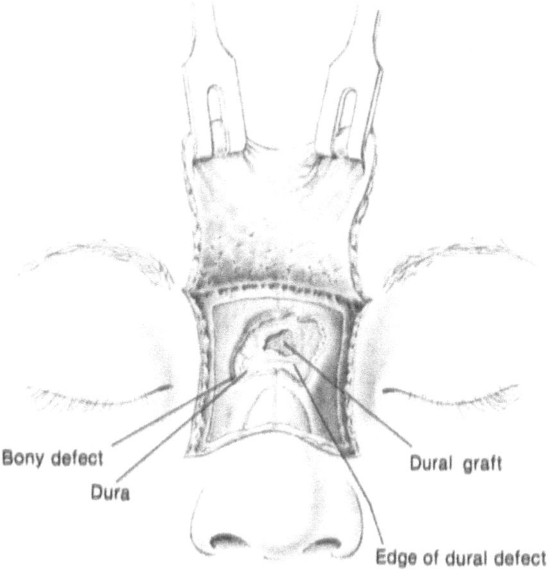

Fig. AS 8a, b. Surgical repair of a meningocele on the nasal dorsum.
a The dorsal skin flap is reflected upward, and the dura is exposed.
b After removal of the sac, the resulting dural defect is closed with stored dura and fibrin adhesive

Remarks on Craniofacial Surgery

In patients with *craniofacial synostoses* and *dysostoses*, extensive osteotomies and skeletal corrections can be a highly effective means of restoring craniofacial morphology and preserving function (Fig. AS 9a-e). Webster and Deming had already published in 1950 on the surgical treatment of the bifid nose. Epochal pioneering work in this field was done by Tessier and coworkers (Tessier 1967, 1971), and various groups of authors in recent years have expanded upon those earlier studies (Converse et al. 1977, David et al. 1982, Mühlbauer and Anderl 1983, Mühling et al. 1984, Munroe and Das 1979, Van der Meulen et al. 1983). These difficult procedures require the combined efforts of an experienced team of plastic surgeons, ophthalmologic surgeons, neurosurgeons, maxillofacial surgeons, and otolaryngologic surgeons, who preferably have been working together for some years.

It would exceed the scope of this monograph to give a detailed account of the treatment of these complex malformations involving the whole skull. One such case is illustrated in Fig. AS 10a-f, which shows the surgical repair of a craniosynostosis with fronto-orbital advancement in a 6-month-old boy.

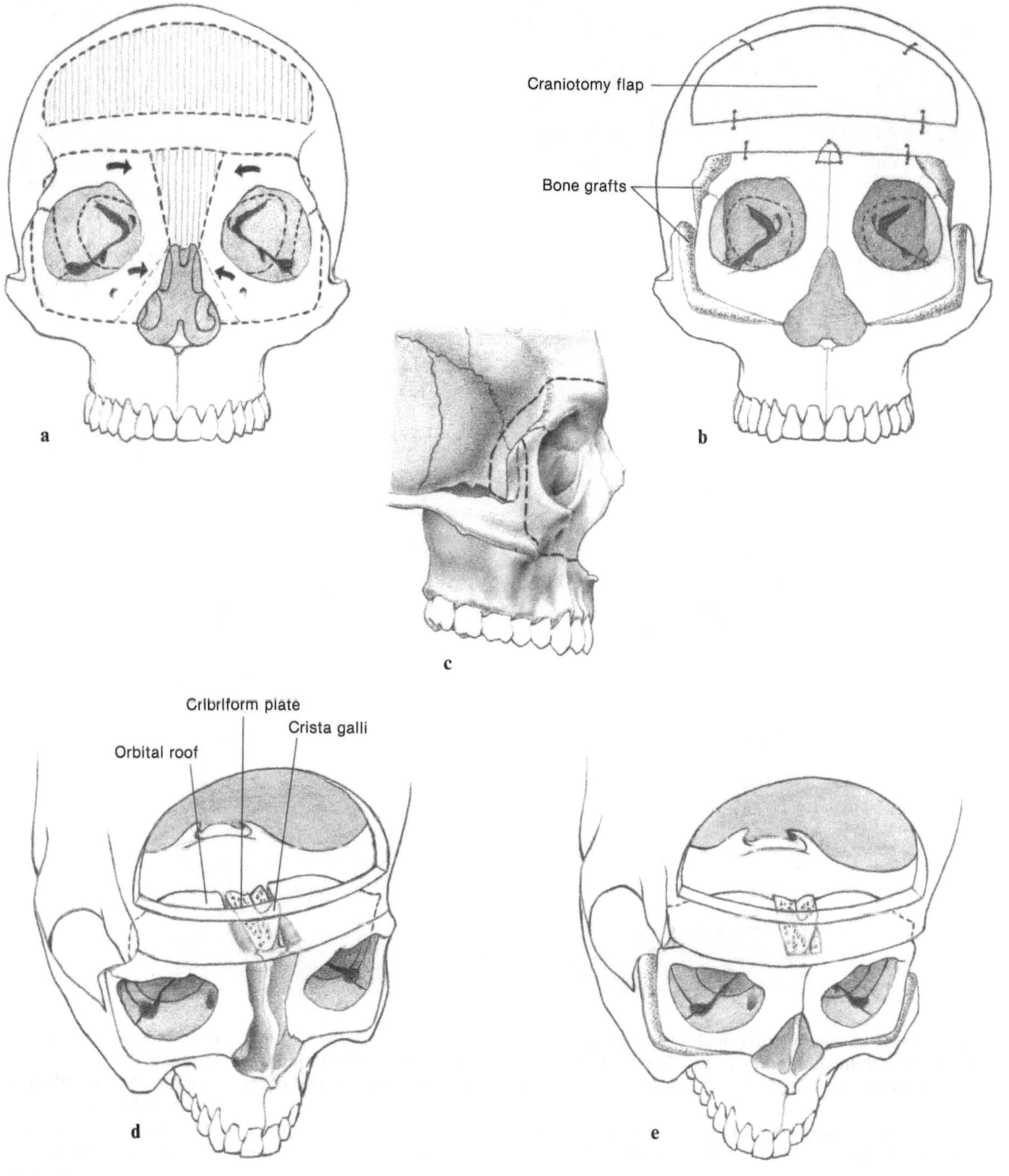

Fig. AS 9a–e. Craniofacial procedure of Tessier and Converse (1971, 1977) with complete mobilization of the lateral orbital wall.
a Osteotomy lines.
b Situation after displacement of the orbital walls and wire fixation.
c The lateral orbital margin is split. The remaining lateral orbital wall is mobilized after performing the osteotomy indicated by the *broken lines*.
d Technique (of Converse) for preserving the cribriform plate.
e Closure of the defect in the anterior cranial floor

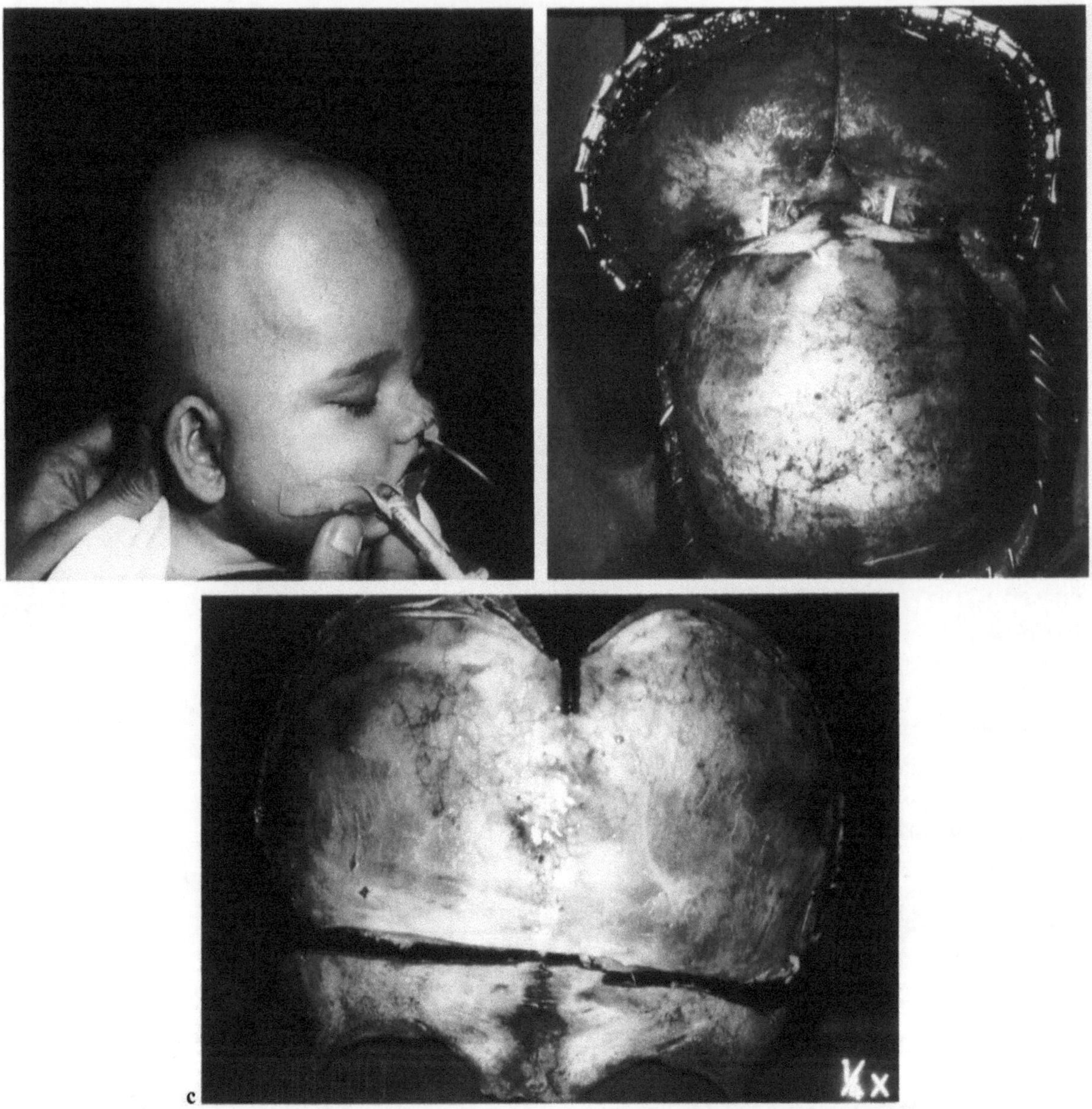

Fig. AS 10a–f. Surgical treatment of craniosynostosis with fronto-orbital advancement in a 6-month-old boy.
a Cranial deformity has resulted from premature fusion of the cranial sutures.
b A bitemporal skin incision is made, and a scalp flap is mobilized. The flap is reflected inferiorly to the nasal root, and the orbital contents are displaced downward on both sides. The supraorbital nerves are marked and preserved.
c The frontal bone and supraorbital ridge are temporarily removed.
d The orbital ridge is reinserted, advancing it about 2 cm anteriorly and rotating it 30° caudally.
e Situation at the end of the procedure, before soft-tissue closure. After replacement of the frontal bone, the posterior cranial vault is opened in tulip-petal fashion by corresponding bone resections. The individual bony plates are attached only at the skull base, thus permitting the brain to expand with future growth. The fronto-orbital advancement also corrects the preexisting fronto-orbital deformity.
f The patient one year postoperatively

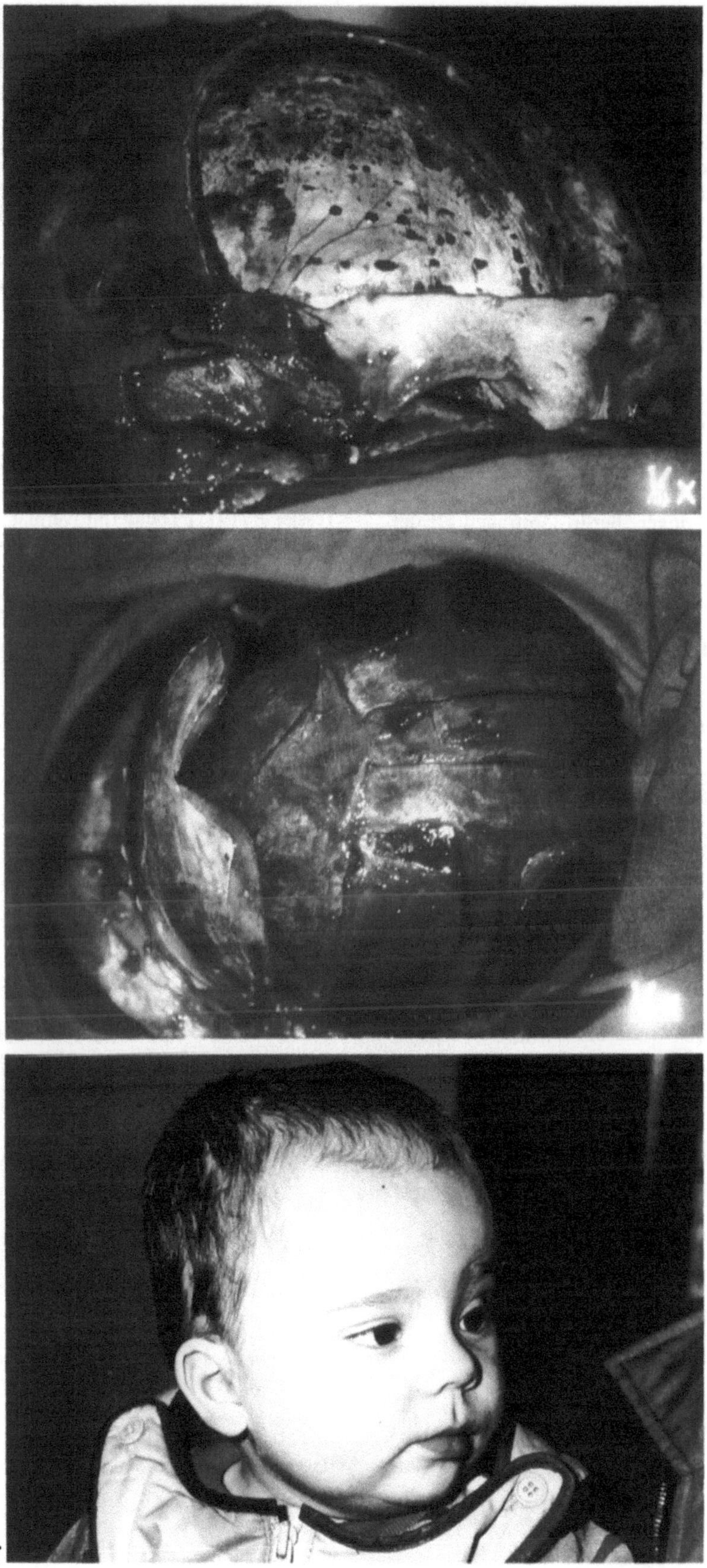

d

e

f

References

Birkett HS (1901) Report of two cases of dermoid cyst of the nose. NY Med J. 73:91

Borges AF (1973) Elective incision and scar revision. Little Brown, Boston

Braman (1890) Über die Dermoide der Nase. Langenbecks Arch Klin Chir 40:101

Bushe KA, Glees P (1968) Chirurgie des Gehirns und Rückenmarks im Kindes- und Jugendalter. Hippokrates, Stuttgart, p 971

Converse JM, McCarthy JG, Wood-Smith D, Coccaro PJ (1977) Principles of craniofacial surgery. In: Reconstructive plastic surgery, Vol 4, p 2427. Saunders, Philadelphia London Toronto

David DJ, Paswillo D, Simpson D (1982) The craniosynostoses. Springer, Berlin Heidelberg New York

Denecke HJ, Meyer R (1964) Plastische Operationen an Kopf und Hals. Springer, Berlin Göttingen Heidelberg New York, pp 302ff

Draf W, Nagel F (1971) Eine Nasenstegfistel als seltene Mißbildung. Diagnostische Möglichkeiten der Tomographie. Mschr Ohr Nas Kehlk Heilkd 105:156

Gerlach G, Jensen HP, Koos W, Krons H (1967) Pädiatrische Neurochirurgie. In: Fehlbildungen des Gehirns. Thieme, Stuttgart, p 239

Lannelongue R, Minard V (1891) Affectiones congenitales. Asselin et Houzeau, Paris

Meyer E (1968) Mißbildungen und angeborene Störungen. In: Bushe KA, Glees P (eds) Chirurgie des Gehirns und Rückenmarks im Kindes- und Jugendalter. Hippokrates, Stuttgart, pp 948–991

Mühlbauer W, Anderl H (1983) Kraniofaziale Fehlbildungen und ihre operative Behandlung. Thieme, Stuttgart New York

Mühling J, Reuther J, Sörensen N (1984) Operative Behandlung kraniofazialer Fehlbildungen. Kinderarzt 15:1022–1023

Munro JR, Das SK (1979) Improving results in orbital hypertelorism correction. Ann Plast Surg 2:499

Sessions RB (1982) Nasal dermal sinuses – New concepts and explanations. Laryngoscope 92. Suppl 29

Stupka W (1938) Die Mißbildungen und Anomalien der Nase und des Nasenrachenraumes. Springer, Vienna

Tessier P (1967) Osteotomies totales de la face. Syndrome de Crouzon, Syndrome D'Apert. Oxycephalis, Scapho cephalis, Turri cephalis. Ann Chiru Plast 12:273

Tessier P (1971) The definitive plastic surgical treatment of the severe facial deformities of craniofacial dysostosis, Crouzon's and Apert's desease. Plast Reconstr Surg 48:419

Van der Meulen JC, Mazda R, Vermey-Keers C, Stricker M, Raphael B (1983) A morphogenetic classification of craniofacial malformations. Plas Reconstr Surg 71:560–572

Webster JP, Deming EG (1950) Surgical treatment of the bifid nose. Plast Reconstr Surg 6:1

Surgery of Traumatic Lesions of the Anterior Skull Base

Introductory Remarks on Diagnosis and Indications for Operation. The interdisciplinary diagnosis of frontobasal injuries should take into account potential lesions of the midfacial region, orbit, paranasal sinuses, and intracranial cavity (Samii and Draf 1978). In the treatment plan that emerges from this evaluation, specific surgical measures are defined, and their sequencing is coordinated among the otorhinolaryngologist, neurosurgeon, and maxillofacial surgeon (and ophthalmologist if required). Many studies have been published offering guidelines on rhinosurgical and neurosurgical treatment methods (Boenninghaus 1960, Dietz 1970, Escher 1960, 1967, 1969, Kley 1967, 1968, Naumann 1974, Probst 1971, Samii and Brihaye 1983, Seiferth 1954, Seiferth and Wustrow 1977, Bock 1983, Voss 1936). The status of oromaxillofacial surgery is summarized by Schuchardt (1966).

Despite basic agreement among the different specialties, there is diversity of opinion concerning the selection of surgical approaches and the timing of intervention.

At the time the patient with a frontobasal injury is admitted, an initial *joint* consultation should be held to decide what special diagnostic investigations are required.

Cerebrospinal fluid leakage from the nose or nasopharynx demands accurate *localization* of the site of the leak and subsequent operative repair, even if the leak stops spontaneously after it is detected. The cicatricial healing of dural tears in areas of the skull base that are in contact with the nose or paranasal sinuses (the "rhinobase", Wullstein 1972) does not adequately seal off the cranial cavity. Because of the normal bacterial flora that colonize the nose and paranasal sinuses, intracranial complications such as meningitis, encephalitis, or brain abscess can develop even years later unless the leak is definitively sealed by appropriate duraplasty.

A cerebrospinal fluid leak may remain clinically undetected for some time before complications arise, and so the examiner should make a specific search for cerebrospinal fluid leaks in patients who present with corresponding injuries. *Provocative measures* include head-down positioning and jugular vein compression. A watery discharge from the nose that does not contain blood can be differentiated from nasal secretion with a *glucose test strip* owing to the high glucose content of cerebrospinal fluid. However, the high sugar content of blood makes this test unreliable in trauma patients who have bleeding. An important diagnostic aid in such cases is the *halo sign*, or a colorless wet circle surrounding a bloody stain on the pillowcase or on a gauze pad held beneath the nose.

Recently, two new more specific and sensitive methods make it possible to identify even small amounts of cerebrospinal fluid. One method is based on measurement of β_2-transferrin, a transferrin variant found only in cerebrospinal fluid (Oberascher 1988), whereas the other one is based on determination of the albumin-prealbumin-ratio (Bohner and Hesse 1989). For the diagnosis of a cerebrospinal fistula β_2-transferrin is a highly sensitive parameter, but its determination by the proposed electrophoretical procedure is time-consuming and needs a lot of methodical experience. The determination of the ratio of the concentrations of albumin and prealbumin by nephelometry is a further possibility to identify pure of almost pure cerebrospinal fluid. This method is fast and easy to perform and therefore more convenient to the clinical routine laboratory.

However, on the basis of the both forementioned methods cerebrospinal fluid can be differentiated unambiguously from other secretions, and false negative results are only caused by high contamination of cerebrospinal fluid with blood or nasal secretion.

In particularly difficult cases, the leak can be localized by injecting dye, usually fluorescein, into the lumbar canal. The stained cerebrospinal fluid is easily detected with a nasal endoscope equipped with a special blue filter (Denecke 1956/1958, Messerklinger 1972). The intrathecal injection of fluorescein should be used with caution in patients who are prone to seizures. Also, one should try to use as small a volume of fluorescein as possible (2 ml of 5% fluorescein), since several occurrences of epileptiform states have been described (Mahaley et al. 1966, Mees and Beyer 1982, Wallace et al. 1972). It is prudent to keep the patient under observation for 4–6 hours following the examination. Messerklinger (1984, personal communication) has the fluorescein solution freshly prepared for each examination and has never experienced a serious incident. This is consistent with our own experience.

Both the *fluorescein test* and modern radioisotope methods of localization using intralumbar injections of iodine 131-albuminyterbium 169 and indium 111 are positive only if cerebrospinal fluid is actively leaking; they are negative if the dural opening is temporarily occluded (Table 3).

Samii and Draf (1978) have also obtained false-positive results in RISA isotope studies.

Radiologic studies are of major importance. While plain films of the skull in the AP, lateral, semiaxial, and basal projections are good for demonstrating the extent of fractures and evaluating for pneumatocele, some cases will require special views such as the tangential projection for a suspected depressed fracture of the frontal sinus, or Rhese views. Brandt (1959) recommends "eyeglass" views for delineating the orbital margins. Grote (1966 a,b) emphasizes the value of stereoradiography as an adjunct to routine films, while Metzger et al. (1965) and Reisner and Gosepath (1973) state that cranial tomography employing a hypocycloidal figure of motion should remain a routine part of the evaluation of facial and anterior skull base injuries.

Table 3. Possible mechanisms for the temporary obturation of a dural tear

1. Clotted blood
2. Lacerated mucosa
3. Prolapsed or edematous brain
4. Orbital tissue

Increasingly, it appears that refined techniques of CT imaging are capable of replacing conventional tomography. Modern CT equipment provides improved resolution of osseous features and can delineate fractures of even very thin bony plates without increasing the radiation exposure (Rettinger and Kalender 1981). This makes it possible to diagnose bony injuries and evaluate the extent of brain trauma in a single investigation, completely eliminating the need for conventional X-ray films in many cases.

The majority of cerebrospinal fluid leaks result from dural injury at the ethmoid roof. Tönnis and Frowein (1952) attribute this to the firm attachment of the dura to the bone and the relative thickness of the skull base in that area, as well as the favorable conditions for drainage. Most leaks occur not in the cribriform plate but in the adjacent ethmoid roof. The second most common cause of cerebrospinal fluid leakage is fracture of the posterior wall of the frontal sinus; relatively few leaks come by way of the sphenoid sinus. The dural defect in sphenoid leaks usually is located in the region of the tuberculum sellae and anterior wall of the sella, rather than on the planum sphenoidale. With extensive comminuted injuries of the anterior skull base, the frontal sinus, ethmoid cells, and sphenoid sinus may all be involved concurrently. Cerebrospinal fluid can also escape through dural openings formed by the avulsion of olfactory nerve fibers and especially by occipital violence with a contre coup injury (Grote 1966 a,b). Cerebrospinal rhinorrhea occasionally results from a defect in the petrous bone in either the middle or posterior cranial fossa. The tympanic membrane must be intact for this paradoxical type of rhinorrhea to occur. In a study by Dietz (1966), conventional tomographic imaging was unable to delineate a frontobasal fracture in approximately 15% of patients. A diagnosis cannot be made in these cases in the absence of a clinically overt cerebrospinal fluid leak. The pneumatocele, which is clearly visible even on plain skull films, is pathognomonic for a dural defect even in the absence of a manifest leak. With CT it is possible to identify very small air bubbles in the intracranial cavity as evidence of a dural injury. Despite technical refinements, there are still a certain percentage of fractures that are not demonstrable on CT scans, even in the presence of frank cerebrospinal fluid leakage.

The *timing of operative treatment* depends on the patient's general condition, the type of injury, and the varying temporal requirements of the specialties involved. Life-threatening bleeding is the only justification for emergency surgery without special preoperative studies. In all other cases a swift but thorough diagnostic evaluation is an absolute prerequisite for adequate surgical planning. It must be considered that once the patient's respiration and cardiovascular status have been stabilized, his general condition may be better a short time after the injury than several days later. This means that the early postinjury period may be favorable for operative procedures that are not too extensive. Operative intervention cannot be delayed for too long in cases where bony skull injury is associated with extensive injury to the facial soft tissues. Nasal fractures, which may be assigned a low priority initially, should be treated in the first five days in order to lessen the psychological impact of disfigurement. Midfacial fractures that involve the masticatory apparatus should be reduced and stabilized within the first 14 to 21 days. Duraplasty, if required, should be performed *after* any forced surgical manipulations of the jaw, which otherwise could disrupt the dural closure. Duraplasty may be deferred for up to 4–6 weeks if necessary while high-dosage antibiotic coverage is maintained. In children, reduction of the facial bones should be accomplished as soon after the injury as possible, as the fragments will become fixed within 3–4 days after the injury (Krausen and Samuel 1979).

We share the opinion of Kley (1974) and Scheunemann (1974) that thorough, primary excavation of the paranasal sinuses is not necessary as long as consistent follow-up of the trauma patient is maintained.

The complete and possibly bilateral debridement of the paranasal sinuses in severe midfacial fractures might further weaken the facial skeleton and compound the difficulty of reconstruction, especially in terms of maxillary suspension. It is our experience, moreover, that initially healthy paranasal sinus mucosa displays a good healing tendency even after severe trauma, and it is not unusual for X-rays to show normal radiolucency by 6–8 weeks postinjury (Fig. AS 24d). If this is not the case, secondary debridement of the injured paranasal sinuses is advised following duraplasty to remove a potential source of intracranial infection. By this time the facial bones will already have consolidated to some degree.

For a systematic discussion of *surgical approaches* and techniques, it is convenient to subdivide the anterior skull base into a medial portion contiguous with the nose and paranasal sinuses (the "rhinobase" of Wullstein 1972) and a lateral portion that includes the orbital roof and lesser wing of the sphenoid.

The *choice of approach* for the surgical closure of a frontobasal dural defect must meet the following criteria:

1) Provide wide exposure of the dural defect.
2) Involve a minimum of surgical stress.
3) Preserve olfactory sensation if possible.

It is possible to preserve olfactory sensation when exposing the anterior skull base transfacially and also in the transfrontal intradural approach by microsurgical dissection of the olfactory nerve. The transfrontal extradural approach to the anterior skull base described by Unterberger (1958) involves division of the olfactory fibers in cases requiring bilateral exposure of the cribriform plate, due to the necessity of elevating the dura. Thus, this technique generally is acceptable only if anosmia is already present as a result of the trauma. The transfrontal extradural exposure of the posterior wall of the frontal sinus and anterolateral skull base allows preservation of the olfactory fibers.

With *circumscribed* bony and dural defects involving the posterior wall of the frontal sinus and areas of the skull base bordering on the sphenoid and ethmoid sinuses, the *rhinosurgical fronto-orbital approach* is preferred and may be combined with appropriate open treatment measures on the paranasal sinuses. It is possible to preserve olfactory sensation in many cases with this approach. The rhinosurgical technique is especially suitable for the repair of cerebrospinal fluid leaks through the sphenoid sinus. The neurosurgical transfrontal intradural approach is less satisfactory in these cases, as it is more difficult and time-consuming and cannot always ensure adequate coverage of the sphenoid sinus posterior wall with a galeal pericranial flap. Moreover, when there is forward displacement of the optic chiasm "chiasma prefix" associated with a fracture of the posterior wall of the sphenoid sinus, vision may be jeopardized in cases where the galeal pericranial flap has to be interposed between the anterior wall of the sella and the optic chiasm.

There are two situations in which the neurosurgical *transfrontal intradural approach* is preferred: 1) When there is cerebrospinal fluid leakage from a comminuted fracture of the anterior skull base. These cases are almost always accompanied by extensive dural tearing and cerebral prolapse. The transfacial, rhinosurgical approach is not appropriate, as extensive debridement of the skull base would be necessary in order to evaluate the dural injury. Aside from the fact that the dural tears in these cases often extend beyond the rhinobase and are inaccessible to rhinosurgery, the approach might compromise the stability of the skull base and complicate subsequent dural repair. 2) With a frontobasal cerebrospinal fluid leak, regardless of its location and extent, accompanied by an enlarging intracranial mass lesion and impending tentorial herniation, *surgical decompression* of the intracranial space must be combined with repair of the dural defect. Early-stage intracranial hemorrhages, contusions, encephalitic foci, and abscesses *not* accompanied by a rise of intracranial pressure are rarely an indication for immediate neurosurgical intervention.

Serial CT observations have shown that these lesions can regress under conservative treatment with corticosteroids and antibiotics, enabling the surgeon to repair the cerebrospinal fluid leak under more favorable conditions at a later time (Fig. AS 11).

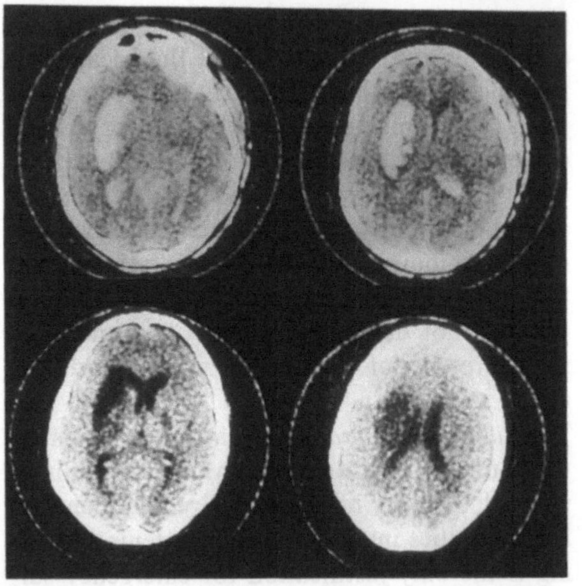

Fig. AS 11. Serial CT observations of a traumatic intracerebral hemorrhage with an intraventricular component (*upper scans*). The hematoma was largely reabsorbed after 3 weeks' conservative therapy (*lower scans*)

The transfrontal extradural approach, as advocated for rhinosurgeons by Unterberger (1958) and for neurosurgeons by Teachenor (1927) and others (see refs. in Dietz 1970), may be acceptable for comminuted fractures of the anterior skull base. Iatrogenic meningeal damage occasionally occurs during elevation of the dura from the olfactory grooves. The transfrontal extradural approach and intradural approach each have their advantages and disadvantages. While the intradural space does not need to be widely opened in the brain-sparing transfrontal extradural approach, the latter gives somewhat poorer exposure of the posterior portions of the anterior skull base (lesser sphenoid wing, planum sphenoidale, optic canal). An advantage of both approaches is that they avoid additional weakening of the cranial base.

Nasal packing, which is necessary in the presence of heavy bleeding, exacerbates the risk of an ascending intracranial complication and should be removed as soon as possible. It is not uncommon for bleeding to arrest spontaneously on completion of the maxillary phase of the operation.

Operative Technique

Principles of Duraplasty in the Region of the Skull Base

The watertight closure of a dural defect in the region of the anterior skull base often cannot be achieved by direct suturing of the dural margins, because the dura is relatively adherent to the bone in that area, and a dural tear is frequently compounded by loss of substance. Suturing of the dura should be combined with plastic repair whenever possible (Kley 1968). Simple closure of a dural defect with tissue adhesive is not sufficient.

Consistently good results are obtained with homologous *lyophilized or solvent-dried cadaver dura* (Burmeister 1962, Crawford 1957, Weickmann and Steinle 1960). This material is available in various sizes and must be softened in physiologic saline or Ringer's solution before use. The relatively stiff material can be made even more supple by placing it in a piece of moisted gauze and rolling it between the fingers. This is particularly useful when the graft has to be tucked into a corner, as in the sphenoid sinus.

An excellent material is *autogenous fascia lata* (Kirschner 1909a, b). A second operation is necessary to obtain the graft, which is taken about a handwidth below the trochanter of the femur through a longitudinal incision on the lateral side of the thigh. After division and retraction of the subcutaneous fat, the fascia lata graft is outlined with a scalpel and removed. Advantages of autogenous fascia lata are its excellent pliancy and favorable healing potential.

Pedicled mucoperiosteal flaps or pure *mucosal flaps* (Berendes 1956, Draf and Samii 1983, Hirsch 1955, Minnigerode 1967, Schreiner and Herrmann 1967) are recommended as adjuncts to duraplasty in difficult areas (see Midline Problem, p. 133) to reinforce the watertight closure. Because of the inflammatory mucosal reaction that accompanies diseases of the nose and paranasal sinuses, mucosal flaps are not suitable by themselves for the repair of dural defects (Boenninghaus 1974, Kley 1968).

The *galeal pericranial flap*, which is obtainable from a coronal incision or an incision beneath the brow, makes an excellent closure material. The inferiorly based galeal pericranial flap (Berendes 1959, Dumas and Laignel-Cavastine 1914, Tönnis and Frowein 1952, etc.) is the material of choice for resurfacing the cranial floor following osteoplastic craniotomy in the transfrontal intra- and extradural approaches. It is less suitable in the fronto-orbital transfacial approach, where other materials such as fascia lata and stored dura are generally used.

Autogenous *fat grafts* attached with fibrin adhesive have proved useful in reinforcing the closure of a cerebrospinal fluid leak with a dural or fascial graft, especially in the sphenoid sinus (Draf 1980). A similar technique is used in the mastoid after operations on the internal auditory canal.

Techniques of Fronto-Orbital Repair of Circumscribed Dural Injuries of the Anterior Skull Base

The technique for repairing circumscribed dural tears from below is dictated by the site of the injury. We have found the preoperative intrathecal injection of 2 ml of 5% freshly prepared fluorescein solution (Messerklinger 1984, personal communication) to be helpful in localizing the leak and assessing the integrity of the repair. The operating microscope is used in this procedure.

Duraplasty in the Region of the Posterior Wall of the Frontal Sinus
(Fig. AS 12a–c)

In circumscribed, caudally situated posterior-wall fractures of the frontal sinus with possible involvement of the ethmoid roof and suspicion of cerebrospinal fluid leakage, the frontal sinus and ethmoid cells are opened through a Jansen-Ritter incision beneath the brow (see Boenninghaus 1974, Theissing and Theissing 1971). The mucosa is stripped from the frontal and

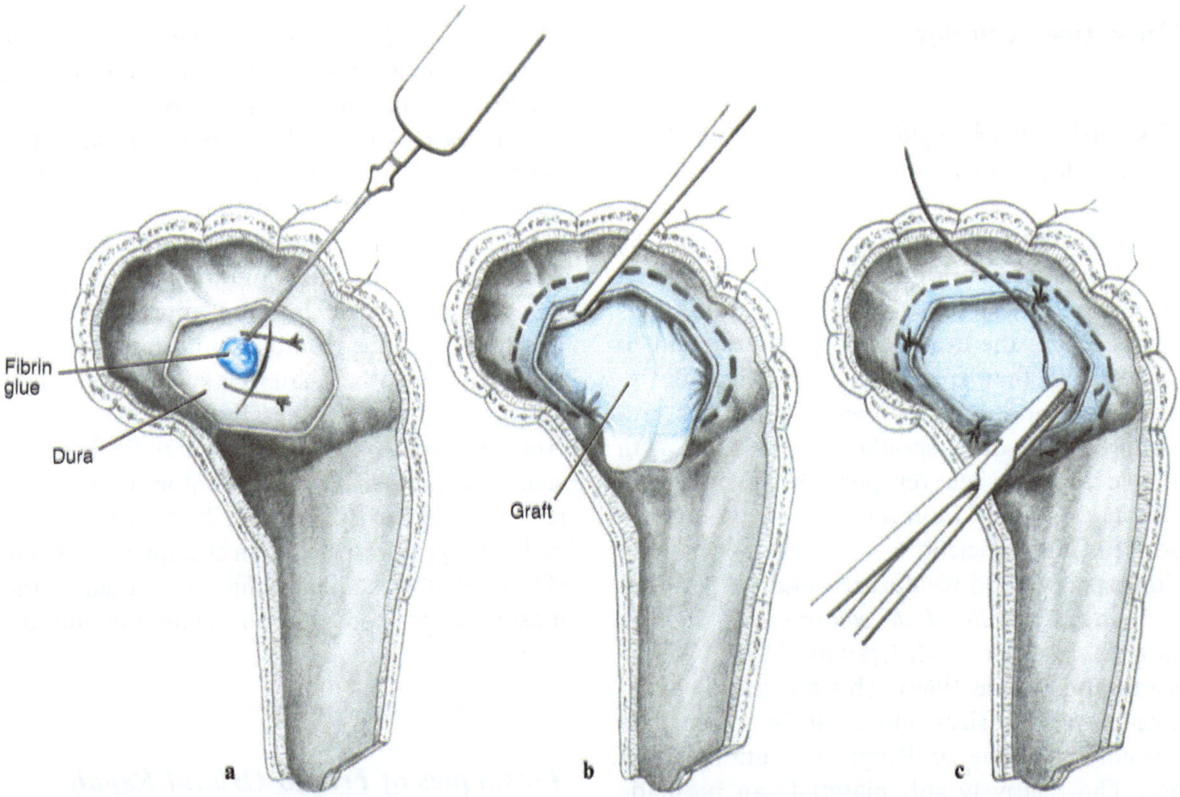

Fig. AS 12a–c. Duraplasty at the posterior wall of the frontal sinus.
a The torn dura is reapproximated with sutures, and fibrin adhesive is applied.
b The dura is covered with a graft tucked between the dura and bone edge (---).
c The graft is additionally secured with sutures placed through drill holes in the bone

ethmoid sinuses, allowing inspection of the posterior wall of the frontal sinus and skull base. The bony defect is enlarged with a diamond burr, punch forceps, and small elevators to give wide exposure of the dural lesion. The operating microscope is used in areas where visualization is difficult. The dura is closed as securely as possible with direct sutures, whereupon the sutures and residual defect are covered with a dural or fascial graft tucked between the bone and dura; additional fixation with fibrin adhesive is recommended. With extensive defects, the duraplasty can be further reinforced with sutures placed through the bony margins. The threads are not tied until all sutures have been placed. It is important that the graft be supported by an intranasal ointment pack, which remains in place for about 14 days until the graft material has become fixed by granulations.

The addition of an antibiotic-containing ointment or Xerform ointment (Osterwald 1977, personal communication) to the packing has several advantages: 1) it helps the packing conform to the graft surface, 2) it prevents adhesion of the packing to the graft, 3) it aids the development of granulations, and 4) it inhibits local infection. Decades of experience have confirmed the value of this type of intranasal packing in transfacial operations on the dura.

Acrylic tissue adhesive was once commonly used, either alone or in conjunction with other materials, but it is a foreign substance that incites an inflammatory response and is resistant to absorption. For this reason, and because of problems relating to the heat of polymerization, this material is now considered to be obsolete. Fibrin adhesive offers a more compatible, biologic means for the joining of tissues.

Duraplasty in the Region of the Ethmoid Roof
(Fig. AS 13a,b)

A similar duraplasty technique is used for circumscribed injuries of the ethmoid roof. The duraplasty in these cases can be additionally covered with a large flap of nasal mucosa (Berendes 1956). Minnigerode (1967) uses a mucoperiosteal flap following complete exenteration of the ethmoid cells. The middle turbinate is deboned to obtain a flap of adequate size. Generally these techniques are most suitable for late operations. They may be unsatisfactory in early operations because of concomitant injuries to the nasal mucosa. The mucoperiosteal flap can be secured with fibrin adhesive.

Duraplasty and the "Midline Problem"

A special problem is posed by unilateral or bilateral circumscribed ethmoid fractures that involve the cribriform plate in the midline region (Draf 1980). The graft can be readily interposed between the dura and bone laterally, but medially this would cause additional trauma to the olfactory fibers. This problem led to the development of several techniques in which the dural graft is applied over the dural defect and adjacent medial bone and is reinforced with a mucoperiosteal flap.
In the modification of Kley (1973), the dural graft is tucked between the dura and bone on the lateral side in standard fashion, and medial-

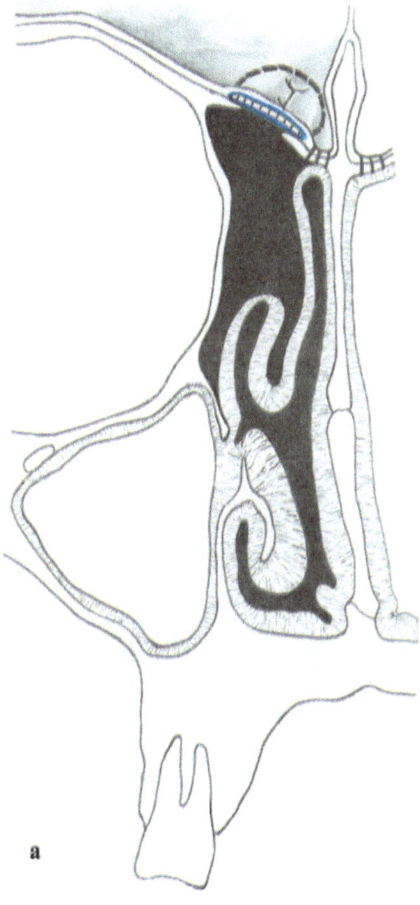

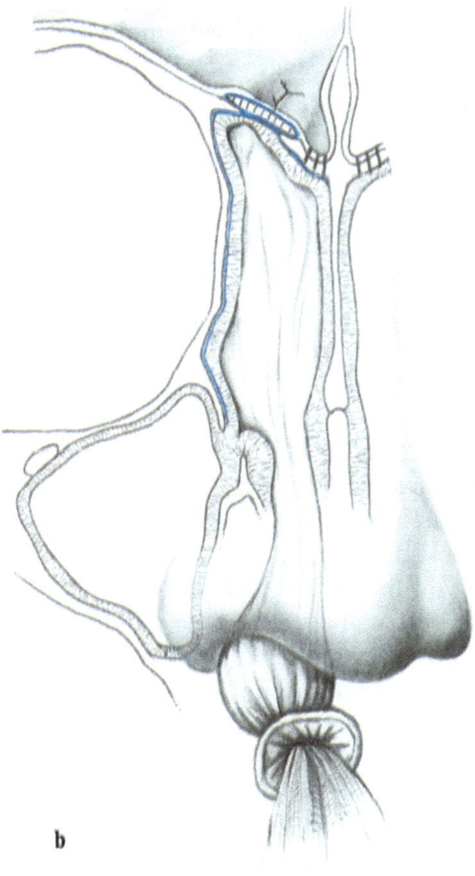

Fig. AS 13a, b. Duraplasty in the area of the ethmoid roof.
a The ethmoid cells are exenterated to expose the area of injury, sparing the lateral nasal mucosa and the mucosa of the middle turbinate. The *broken line* indicates the outline of the graft interposed between the bone and dura. The fibrin adhesive is colored blue.
b The nasal mucosa is attached over the duraplasty with adhesive and supported with packing

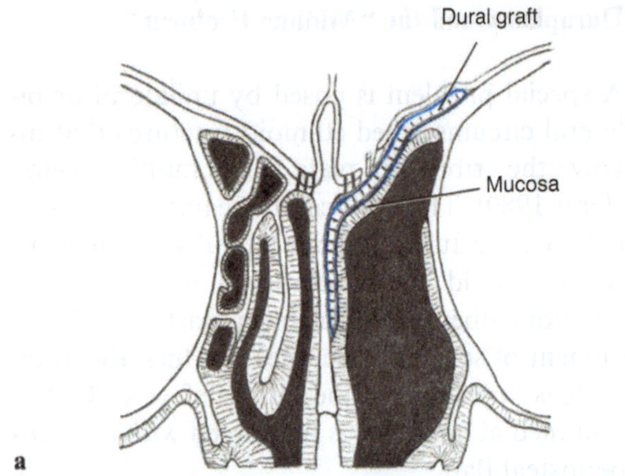

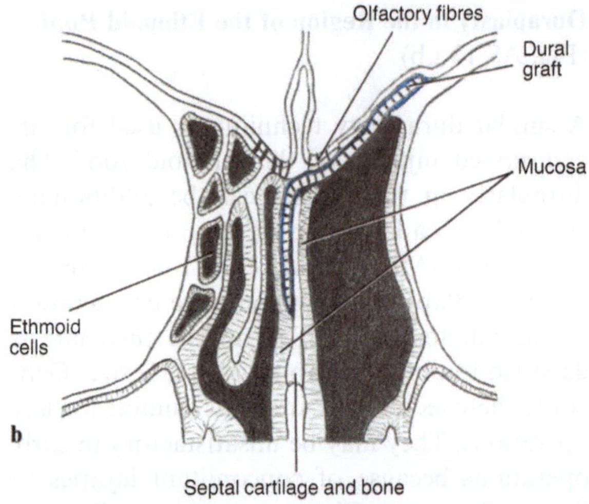

Fig. AS 14a, b. Kley duraplasty (1967) for unilateral fracture of the rhinobase close to the midline.
a After ipsilateral ethmoidectomy and exposure of the fracture, the preserved dural graft is interposed laterally between the bony skull base and dura. The graft is secured medially by fixing it to the perpendicular plate of the septum with fibrin adhesive and covering it with mucosa stripped from the ethmoid roof, cribriform plate, and ipsilateral upper septum.
b Kley's modification of the extradural duraplasty (Draf 1980). The preserved dural graft is tucked beneath the septal mucosa of the opposite side after removing the upper border of the septum. This technique is recommended when the ipsilateral septal mucosa cannot be used

ly a flap of mucoperiosteum is dissected off the bony septum and interposed between the perpendicular plate of the nasal septum and the detached mucosa (Fig. AS 14a). The mucoperiosteal flap is held in place with fibrin adhesive and packing. The graft can be fixed even more securely on the medial side by resecting a narrow strip from the upper edge of the septum, mobilizing the contralateral mucoperiosteum as necessary, and interposing the graft between it and the perpendicular plate on the opposite side (Fig. AS 14b). Bilateral nasal packing is inserted to complete the operation. One disadvantage is the danger of injury to the olfactory fibers when mobilizing the contralateral mucosa.

In a unilateral fracture of the ethmoid roof with extension into the cribriform plate, the extradural duraplasty of Schreiner and Herrmann (1967) is advantageous. After removal of the

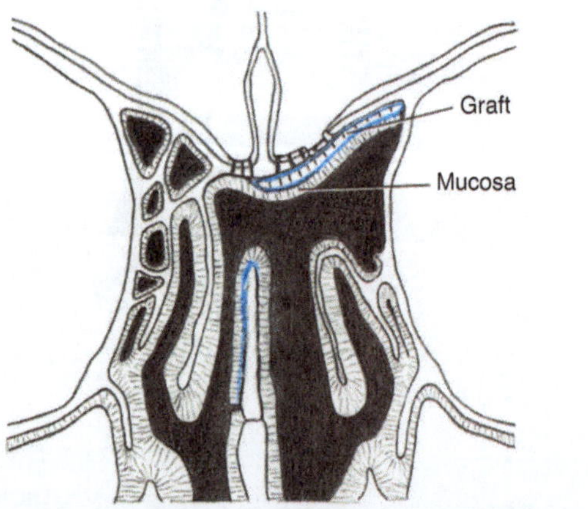

Fig. AS 15. Duraplasty of Schreiner and Herrmann (1967). Preferred dura is applied over the fracture site, and the graft is reinforced with a laterally based flap of septal mucosa from the opposite side. A septal mucosal flap ipsilateral to the side of the injury is swung over the upper border of the septum to give epithelial coverage

superior border of the nasal septum, the septal mucosa on the healthy side is swung across the midline on a lateral pedicle to the side affected by the fracture and attached over the dural graft with adhesive (Fig. AS 15).
With a bilateral ethmoid roof fracture that involves the olfactory groove, a bilateral ethmoidectomy is needed to obtain wide exposure of the whole anterior skull base.
In such cases we exenterate the ethmoid cells bilaterally while preserving the nasal mucosa (Draf and Samii 1983) and create mucosal flaps based on the septum. These may include the covering of the middle turbinate, depending on the flap length required. By dissecting the mucosa from the ethmoid roof and cribriform plate with division of the olfactory fibers, the midportion of the anterior skull base can be widely exposed, and dural injuries can be repaired extradurally with a dural graft (Fig. AS 16a). The mucosal flaps are secured over the duraplasty with fibrin adhesive and supported with packing (Fig. AS 16b).

This technique is most appropriate for late operations. Difficulties may be encountered in fresh injuries with extensive tears of the nasal mucosa, and the transfrontal approach from below may be preferable in some cases.

Duraplasty in the Sphenoid Sinus

Cerebrospinal fluid leaks into the sphenoid sinus are a challenge to diagnosis and treatment. They may be unilateral or bilateral, and they can occur in association with circumscribed fractures of the sphenoid sinus as well as comminuted fractures of the skull base. In the primary rhinosurgical management of a frontobasal head injury, the surgeon, guided by radiologic findings, should explore the entire skull base, including the sphenoid sinus, for the presence of dural defects. Because of the difficulty of visualizing the interior of the recess, even with the binocular operating microscope, it is recommended that an endoscope with angled optics

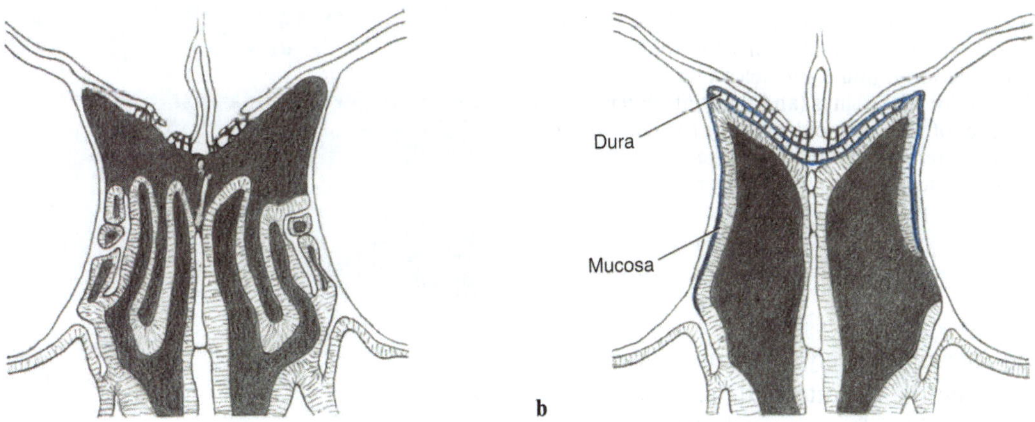

Fig. AS 16a, b. Bilateral extradural duraplasty for a midline fracture of the rhinobase with medially based mucosal flaps (Draf 1980).
a The fracture is exposed by a bilateral ethmoidectomy that spares most of the lateral nasal mucosa.
b The fracture is patched with preserved dura after removal of the upper septal border. The medially based mucosal flaps are fixed with fibrin adhesive

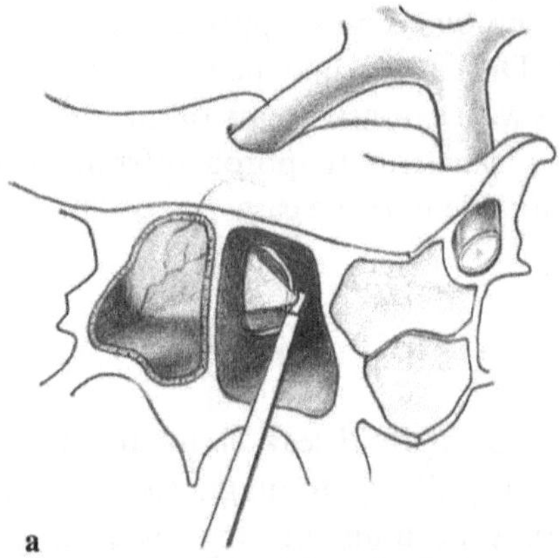

a

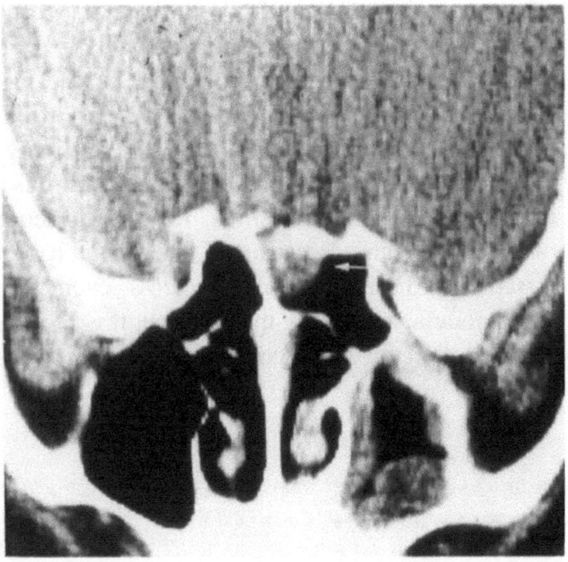

b

Fig. AS 17. a Intraoperative endoscopy of the sphenoid sinus. After external ethmoidectomy the sphenoid sinus is opened anteriorly, and a 30° telescope is used to inspect the interior of the sinus (and the contralateral sinus after removal of the sphenoid septum) for bony defects and possible cerebrospinal fluid leakage.
b Coronal CT scan showing brain herniation through a fracture in the planum sphenoidale

be used intraoperatively to examine the sphenoid sinus on the operated side and also on the contralateral side after removal of the sphenoid septum (Fig. AS 17 a, b). A tentlike bulge of mucosa on the sinus roof or herniating brain tissue offers conclusive evidence of a dural tear, even if a cerebrospinal fluid leak cannot be directly demonstrated (Fig. AS 18).

If cerebrospinal rhinorrhea persists after the primary neurosurgical repair of an anterior basal skull leak, the cause is usually a dural tear in the region of the sphenoid sinus that has not been adequately sealed by the galeal pericranial flap (see p. 140). Rarely, it may also result from cerebrospinal fluid drainage through the auditory tube and nose following a laterobasal fracture, and this injury should be looked for on X-ray films.

The treatment of cerebrospinal fluid leaks in the region of the sphenoid sinus is difficult for several reasons:

1) Because the sphenoid sinus is so deeply situated, its interior is difficult to visualize even with the operating microscope.
2) Because of the basal cisterns surrounding the sinus, cerebrospinal fluid leakage is unusually brisk, making the fixation of sealing material difficult.
3) The removal of slightly mobile bone fragments is contraindicated by the proximity of the internal carotid artery, cavernous sinus, and the 2nd, 3rd, 4th, and 6th cranial nerves. Occasionally bone splinters may be driven into the sphenoid part of the internal carotid artery and may result in an internal carotid-cavernous sinus fistula.

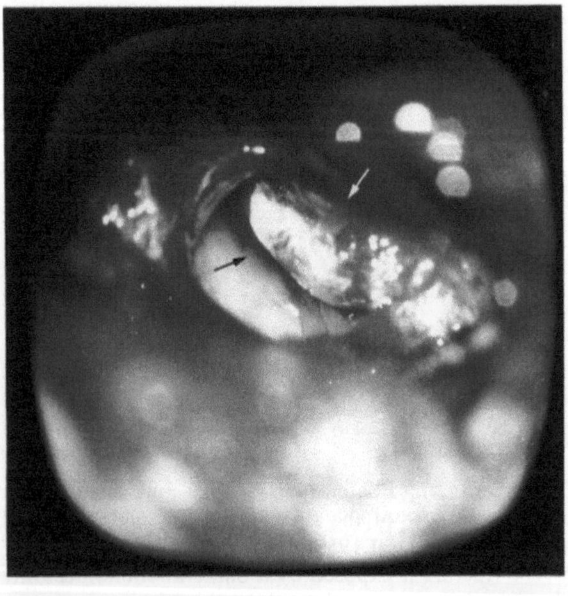

Fig. AS 18. Fronto-orbital exploration of the skull base with endoscopic visualization of the sphenoid sinus cavity, which is found to contain prolapsed brain

For these reasons, the techniques for closing a cerebrospinal fluid leak in the sphenoid sinus differ from those used in other areas of the rhinobase. Besides the actual dural repair, an attempt is made to obliterate the sphenoid sinus with autogenous muscle or fat and to reinforce the closure with mucoperiosteal flaps. Fibrin adhesive has proved especially useful in this area.

The *fascial pouch technique* (Kley 1968, Fig. AS 19 a–c) is indicated for fresh injuries and exploratory procedures in cases where serviceable mucosal flaps cannot be developed in the region of the sphenoid sinus.

The first step in this technique is of prime importance and involves the *total* removal of the mucosa from the sphenoid sinus to prevent the formation of mucosal cysts. Endoscopic control is recommended for this stage of the procedure.

Whereas Wullstein (1953) covered the fracture line with a piece of fascia and filled the sphenoid sinus with a free muscle graft, and Denecke (1956/58) used fibrin sponge, Kley (1967, 1973) removes all the mucosa from the sphenoid sinus, takes a fascia lata graft corresponding to the

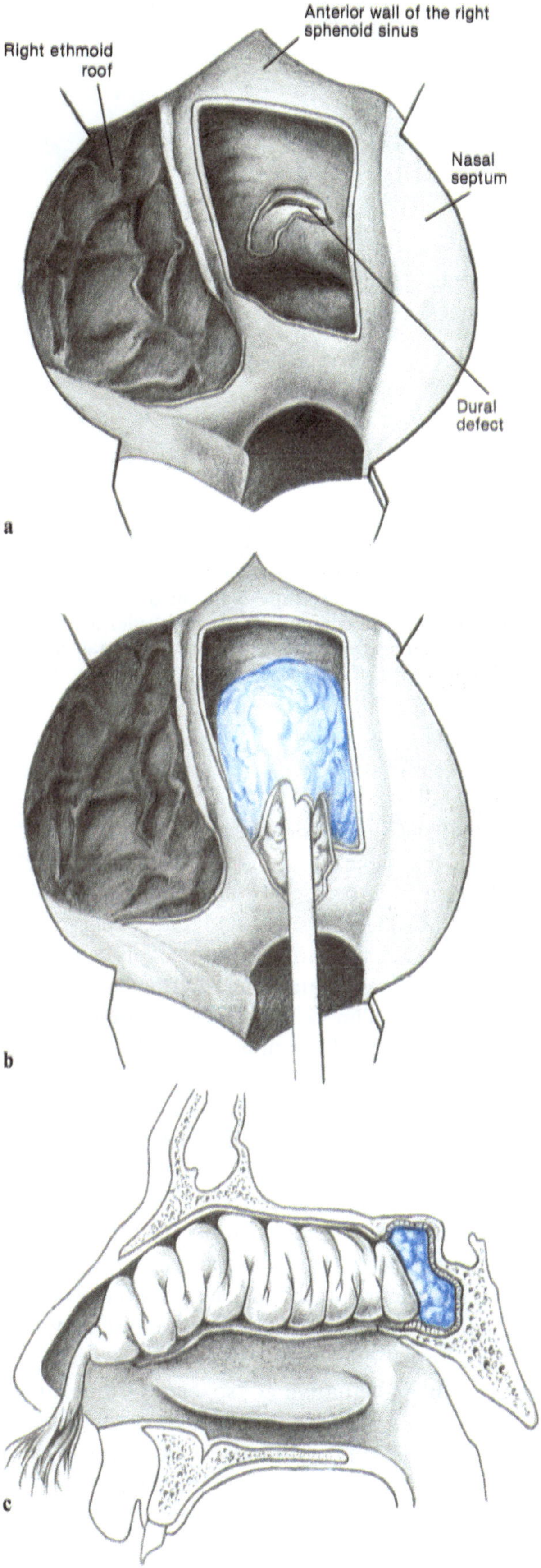

Fig. AS 19 a–c. Transfrontoethmoidal insertion of a fascial pouch for repairing a cerebrospinal fluid leak in the sphenoid sinus (Kley 1967).
a Microsurgical field of vision, anterior view. The anterior wall of the sinus is removed to disclose a cerebrospinal fluid leak through the anterior wall of the sella.
b Microsurgical field of vision, anterior view. After complete removal of the mucosa, a fascial pouch filled with sponge packing is inserted into the sinus and attached with fibrin adhesive.
c Lateral view. The fascial pouch is additionally secured with an intranasal ointment pack. The lower ethmoid cells are left intact to help support the intranasal pack

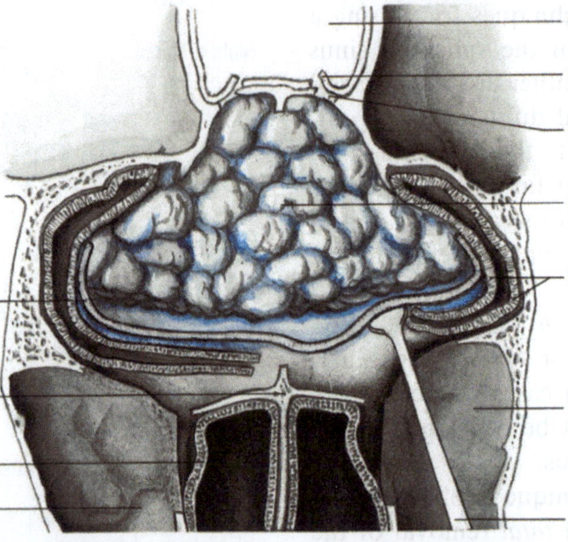

Fig. AS 20. Transfrontoethmoidal dural repair with fat, fascia (preserved dura), and mucosa (Draf 1983). Horizontal section through the upper part of the sphenoid sinus. Bilateral defects in the sphenoid sinus area are approached transethmoidally on both sides after total ethmoidectomy for adequate exposure. Bilateral, laterally based flaps of sphenoid sinus mucosa are formed, and fat grafts are applied over the dural defect with adhesive. The grafts are reinforced with a preserved dural or fascial patch, over which the mucosal flaps are approximated with fibrin adhesive. A cerebrospinal fluid leak through only one sphenoid sinus is approached transethmoidally on the affected side. Care is taken to spare as much of the nasal mucosa as possible

size of the sinus, and packs the graft with dry fibrin sponge in tobacco-pouch fashion outside the operative field. He then inserts the pouch into the sphenoid sinus and soaks the sponge packing with antibiotic solution. This causes the pouch to swell against the interior of the sinus cavity. Penicillin G should not be used because of the danger of seizures. Fascia lata is better for this technique than stored dura because of its superior pliancy. For intranasal packing, good results have been obtained with a 5-cm-wide gauze strip soaked in 10% Xeroform ointment (Osterwald, see p. 132). The advantage of the pouch technique is that it seals off the entire sphenoid cavity, including any minute fracture lines that may not be visible. An even stronger seal is obtainable by attaching the fascial pouch with fibrin adhesive.

A viable alternative to sphenoid sinus duraplasty for gaping bony defects, very severe trauma, or previous neurologic tumor surgery with preservation of most of the sinus mucosa is the unilateral or bilateral fat-fascial-mucosal graft technique (Fig. AS 20). In this technique the anterior wall of the sphenoid sinus is removed, and the mucoperiosteum of the sphenoid sinus is mobilized as a laterally based flap starting at the anterior edge of the sphenoid septum. The entire sphenoid sinus is easily surveyed after the septum is removed. Especially with a widely gaping bone defect, the sometimes copious cerebrospinal fluid leak can be sealed off by applying small fat grafts (5 × 5 mm or smaller) over the defect with fibrin adhesive. Experience has shown that a primary fascial flap applied in this situation is easily washed away by leaking cerebrospinal fluid. After the sphenoid sinus has been filled with the fat grafts, the latter are covered with fascia lata or stored dura, which is supported centrally by the posterior edge of the septum. After another application of fibrin adhesive, the sphenoid mucosal flaps are turned over the lyodura and supported with nasal packing. Any excess sphenoid sinus mucosa is removed.

Techniques of Duraplasty for Comminuted Fractures of the Anterior Skull Base

The indications for the various surgical approaches were described previously (see p. 129).

The Transfrontal Intradural Approach

(Cairns 1937, Dandy 1926, Grant 1923, etc.) (Fig. AS 21 a,b)

The unilateral transfrontal craniotomy may be appropriate for confirmed unilateral frontal comminuted fractures that cannot be treated through a rhinosurgical approach. The great majority of comminuted fractures of the anteri-

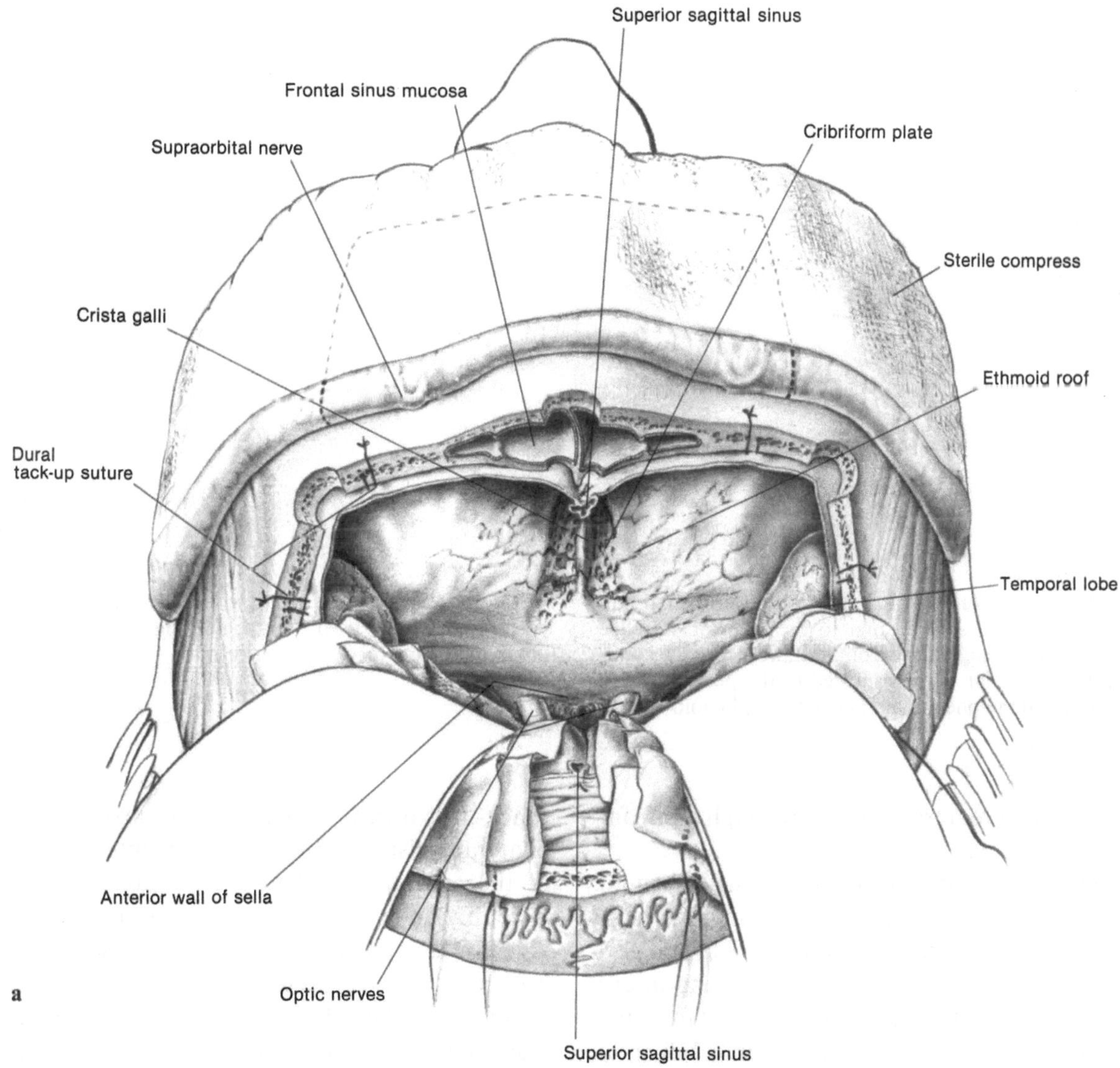

Fig. AS 21 a, b. Transfrontal intradural repair of an extensive dural defect.
a A scalp flap is developed from a bitemporal skin incision, sparing the supraorbital nerves, and an osteoplastic craniotomy is performed using 4 or 5 burr holes. The frontal sinuses are entered. Dural "tack-up" sutures are placed around the bone edges. The superior sagittal sinus is doubly ligated and divided. The falx is cut, and both frontal lobes are retracted until the optic nerves are visualized at their entry into the optic canals

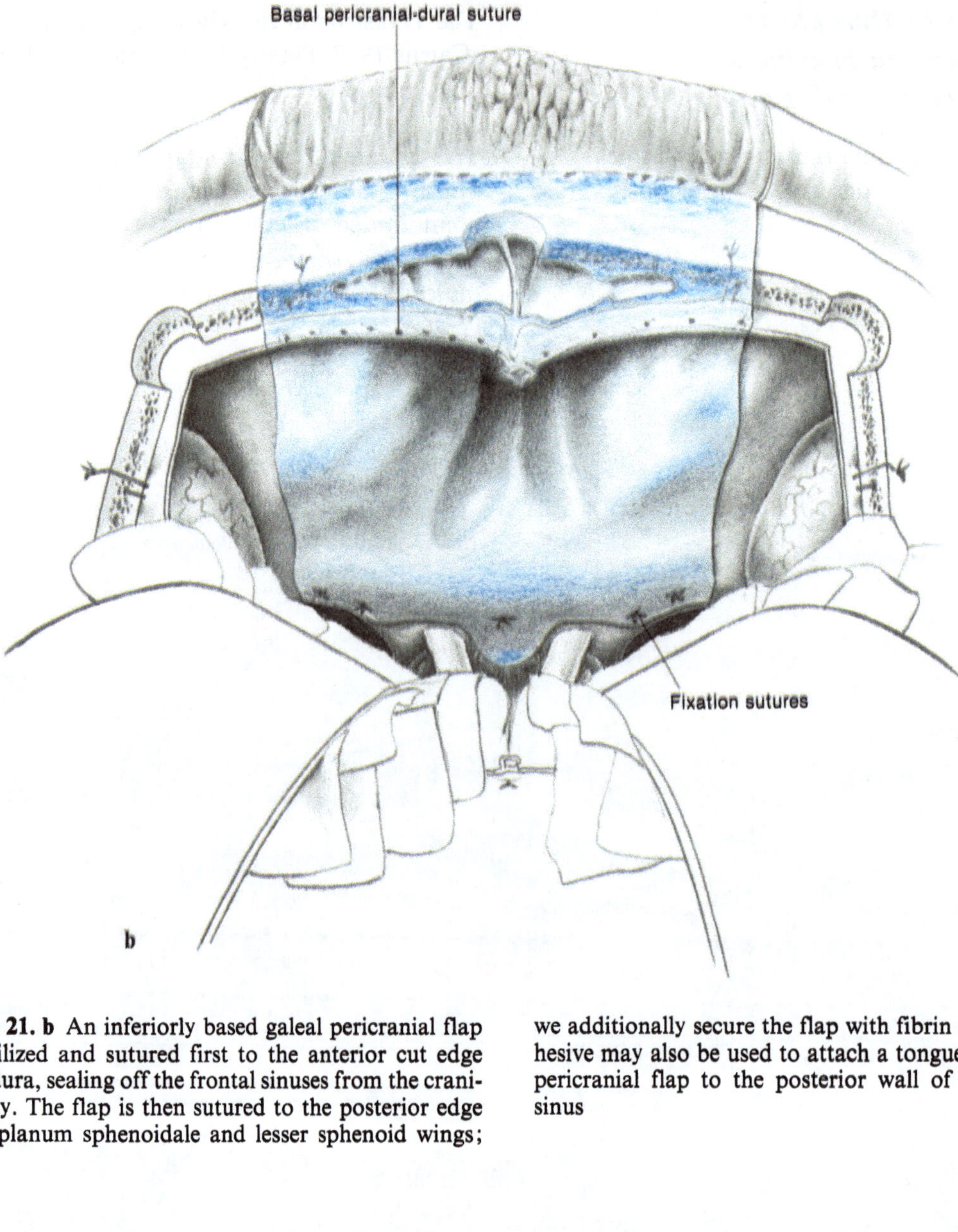

Fig. AS 21. b An inferiorly based galeal pericranial flap is mobilized and sutured first to the anterior cut edge of the dura, sealing off the frontal sinuses from the cranial cavity. The flap is then sutured to the posterior edge of the planum sphenoidale and lesser sphenoid wings; we additionally secure the flap with fibrin adhesive. Adhesive may also be used to attach a tongue of the galeal pericranial flap to the posterior wall of the sphenoid sinus

or skull base require exposure through a bifrontal craniotomy.

A bitemporal coronal incision is made behind the hairline, and the scalp, including the pericranium, is separated from the cranial vault and turned inferiorly over the face, avoiding injury to the supraorbital nerve. Next, four or five burr holes are made in preparation for a bifrontal osteoplastic skull flap. Both frontal sinuses may be entered at this time, especially if the cranium is well pneumatized. As a precaution against postoperative epidural hematoma, the dura is secured up to the bone margins with several "tack-up sutures" spaced 2–3 cm apart. After bilateral incision of the dura at the inferior edge of the craniotomy, the superior sagittal sinus is doubly underrun with ligating sutures and divided. Then the falx cerebri is exposed from both sides and transected in the direction of the crista galli. The inferior sagittal sinus is easily managed with bipolar cautery. Next the frontal lobes of the cerebrum are gently retracted while cerebrospinal fluid is withdrawn, exposing the dural laceration and comminuted fracture of the anterior skull base. The base of the brain is separated microsurgically from the olfactory tract (provided the tract is uninjured) to preserve olfactory sensation. The frontal lobes are protected with moistened cotton paddies. The angle of the optic chiasm, both optic nerves, and the internal carotid artery are also identified and protected with cotton paddies.

An inferiorly based galeal pericranial flap is mobilized to create a barrier between the cranial cavity and the pneumatized spaces of the paranasal sinuses. The flap is first sutured to the inferior edge of the dura in watertight fashion using continuous and interrupted stitches to isolate the opened frontal sinus from the cranial cavity. If the residual frontal sinus is in good condition and drainage to the nose is unimpaired, it will not require any additional measures. But if there is significant trauma to the mucosa and walls of the frontal sinus, obliteration of the sinus is recommended. In this procedure all the mucosa is removed from the frontal sinus and inverted toward the nasal cavity in the area of the ostia. The posterior sinus wall is resected down to the sinus floor, and the residual bony margin is burred away to remove the last vestiges of mucosa. The galeal flap is then turned over the remaining part of the anterior wall and floor of the sinus. Fixation sutures are placed in the dura of the anterior skull base before the galeal flap is brought through the craniotomy opening and tucked into position on the anterior cranial floor. The fixation sutures for the upper edge of the flap on the planum sphenoidale are placed well posteriorly and 1.5 cm from the cut edge of the flap so that the tongue-like apex of the flap can be inserted into the chiasmal angle and at least partially cover the anterior wall of the sella. It is helpful to reinforce the sutures with fibrin adhesive. The frontal lobes are returned to the anterior fossa, and the dura is closed with continuous sutures. The craniotomy flap is replaced at the end of the operation. It is imperative that any adherent frontal sinus mucosa be removed before the cranial flap is replaced, and the corresponding bony areas removed with the diamond burr. This will prevent mucocele formation in the angles between the dura and galeal flap. The repositioned bone flap is secured with several interrupted sutures placed through small drill holes. The craniotomy burr holes are patched with methylmethacrylate to avoid unsightly skin depressions. After insertion of a suction drain, the scalp is restored and closed in layers with interrupted sutures.

The Transfrontal Extradural Approach

(Teachenor 1927, Unterberger 1958, etc.)
(Fig. AS 22a, b)

A bifrontal osteoplastic bone flap is performed as described above, and the dura is progressively freed from one or both sides of the floor of the anterior cranial fossa. This is easily accomplished lateral to the olfactory groove, but it is more difficult within a deep olfactory groove that is lined by thin, firmly adherent dura. It is best to mobilize the dura in a lateral-to-medial direction. Because of the intradural course of the superior sagittal sinus, it should be possible to preserve the sinus when mobilizing the dura; it does not require ligation as in the intradural approach. Any portions of the paranasal sinus mucosa driven into the cranial cavity by the trauma must be removed. The dura is retracted farther posteriorly, severing intact olfactory fibers as required, until all fracture lines are visible. The brain spatulas should be handled with particular care over the medial portion of the lesser sphenoid wing to avoid optic nerve trauma.

After the injured area has been exposed, the anterior skull base is securely covered with a galeal pericranial flap or homologous dural graft. This can also seal off a fracture in the posterior wall of the frontal sinus if required. Retraction is released from the frontal lobes, and the skull flap is replaced. After insertion of a suction drain, the bitemporal incision is closed with all-layer scalp sutures.

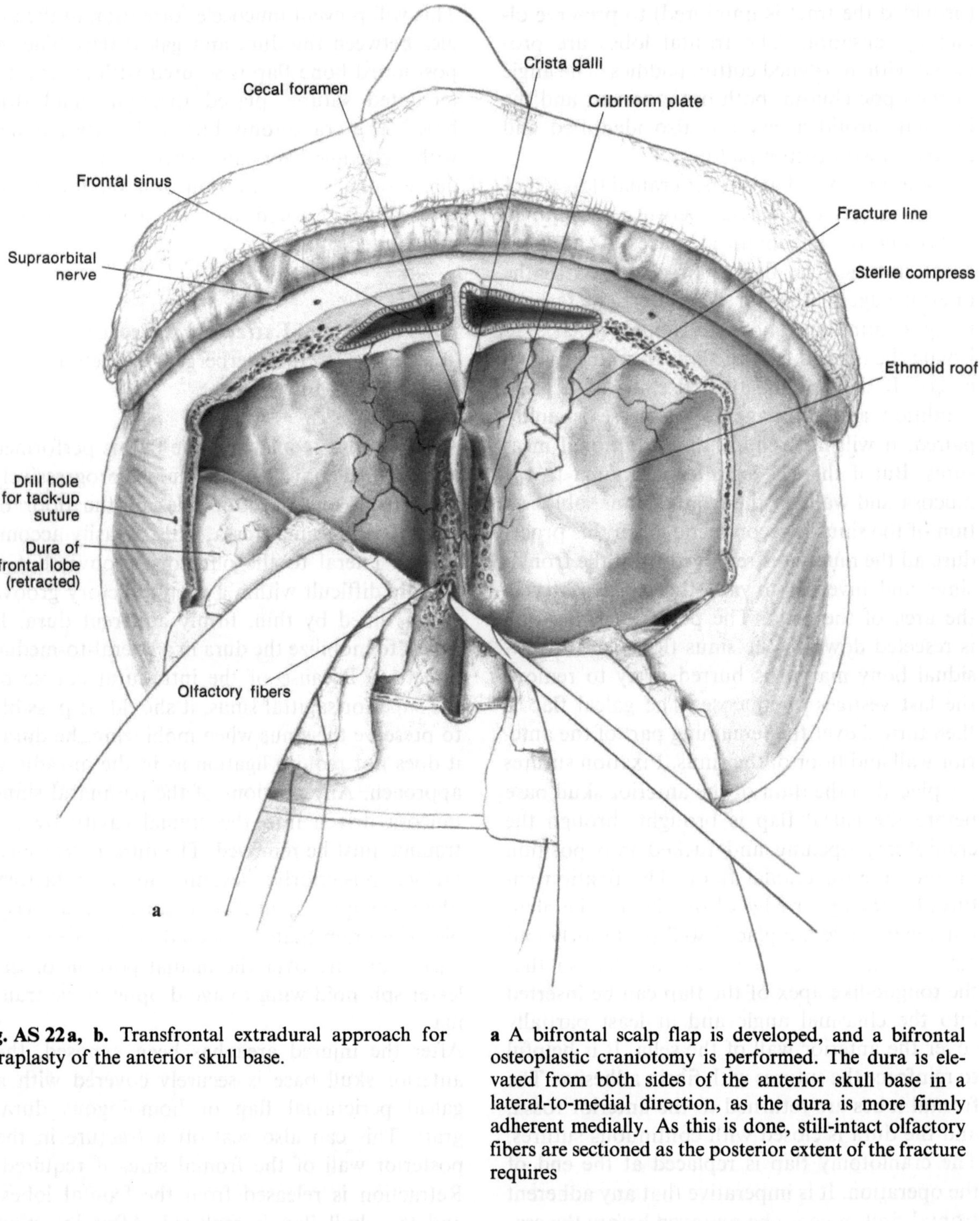

Fig. AS 22 a, b. Transfrontal extradural approach for duraplasty of the anterior skull base.

a A bifrontal scalp flap is developed, and a bifrontal osteoplastic craniotomy is performed. The dura is elevated from both sides of the anterior skull base in a lateral-to-medial direction, as the dura is more firmly adherent medially. As this is done, still-intact olfactory fibers are sectioned as the posterior extent of the fracture requires

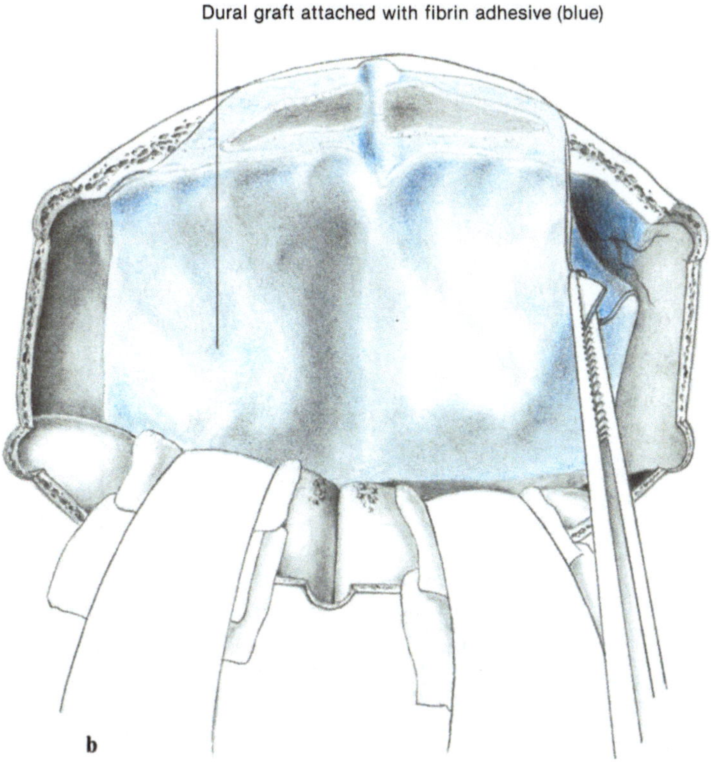

Fig. AS 22. b After complete exposure of the fracture, a dural graft is attached over the frontal sinuses and anterior skull base with adhesive to obtain a watertight seal. A galeal pericranial flap (see Fig. AS 21 b) may also be used

Treatment of Comminuted Fractures of the Lateral Facial Skeleton and Anterolateral Skull Base, Including Dural Injuries (Fig. AS 23 a–g)

Violent trauma to the lateral facial skeleton can fracture the zygoma and produce comminuted fractures of the maxillary sinus, orbit, sphenoid, and temporal squama with associated injuries of the dura and facial soft tissues.

Operative treatment (Fig. AS 23 a–g, 24 a–d) includes wide exposure of the injury and reconstruction of the various tissue layers from within outwards. The existing soft-tissue injury is utilized to create a frontotemporal flap extending downwards over the temporal fossa, in front of the ear, to the anterior border of the sternocleidomastoid muscle. An additional paranasal, infraorbital incision may be needed depending on the extent of soft-tissue and bony injuries. The temporal muscle is freed from the bone. Occasionally it must be temporarily divided at particular sites to gain better exposure. This is followed by the careful debridement and visualization of the infratemporal, pterygopalatine, and pterygoid fossae and the temporary removal of the comminuted lateral orbital rim and lateral portions of the maxillary sinus. After exposure of the dural injury and removal of indriven bone fragments, the dural margins are approximated with interrupted sutures, and all exposed dura is covered with adjacent soft tissues (temporal muscle, temporal fascia, pericranium) or a free dural graft. The latter is tucked under the bony margins and secured with sutures or fibrin adhesive.

If the lateral recess of the frontal sinus has been opened, it is closed by interposing a dural graft between the stripped mucosa and bone, or it may be covered with a galeal pericranial flap. The sphenoid bone fragments are reduced and fixed with wires.

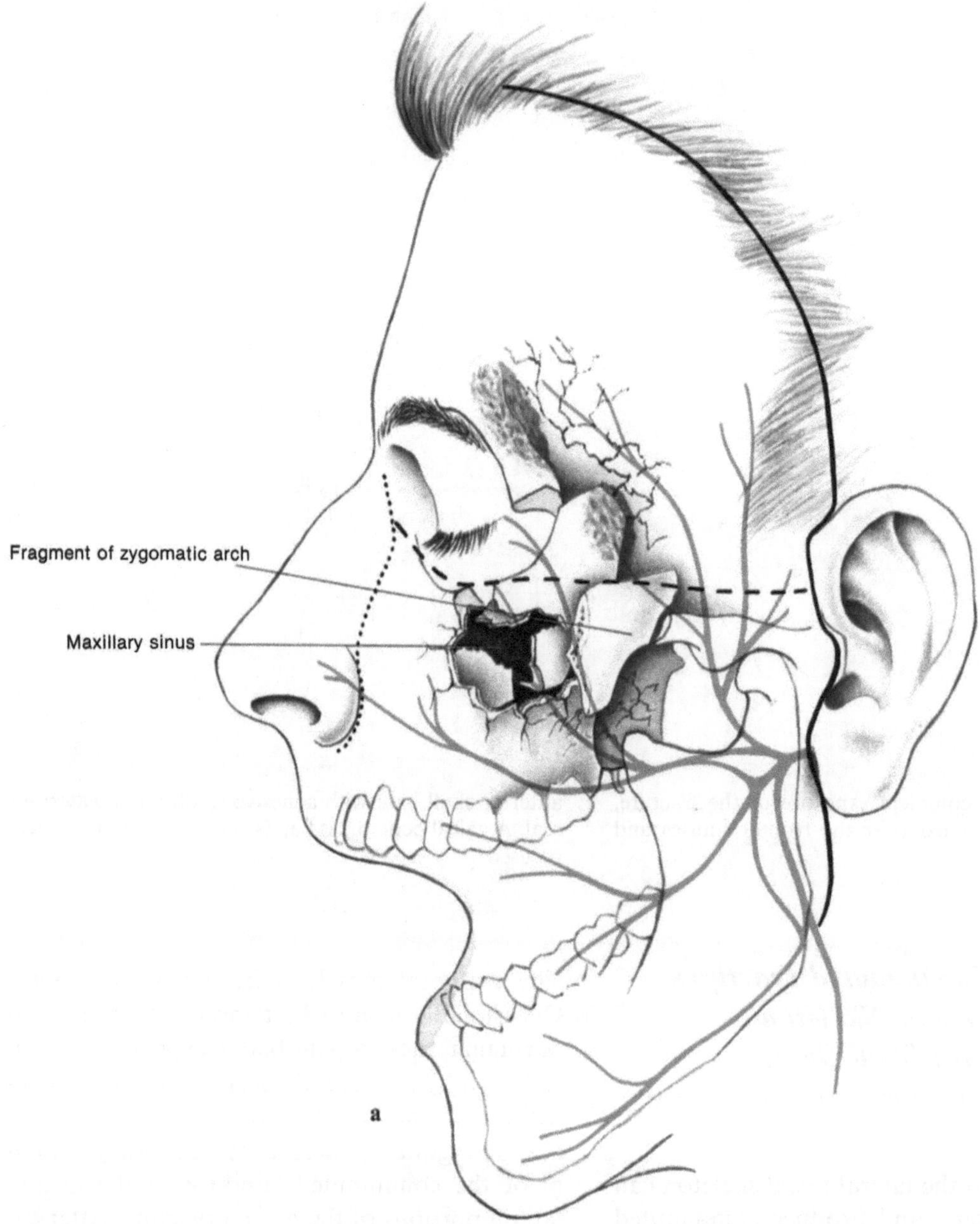

Fig. AS 23a–g. Treatment of comminuted fractures of the lateral facial skeleton and anterolateral skull base, including dural injury.
a Skin incision. The *solid line* indicates the most cosmetically favorable line of incision. The *broken infraorbital line* extending to the zygomatic arch and the *dotted paranasal line* may be necessary because of the configuration of the soft-tissue injury or to gain optimum exposure of the injured area. Care is taken to spare the facial nerve if at all possible.
b Exposure and debridement of the injuries in the lateral facial skeleton. The cranial defect is exposed in the temporal fossa. The dura and periorbita are exposed (see c–e for details).
c A dural tear is closed with simple interrupted sutures.
d With dural tissue loss, the defect is covered with a dural graft and fibrin adhesive.
e If the lateral recess of the frontal sinus has been opened, it is necessary to replace the sinus wall with a dural graft inserted between the mucosa and bone. The cranial vault is restored by wiring the bone fragments together

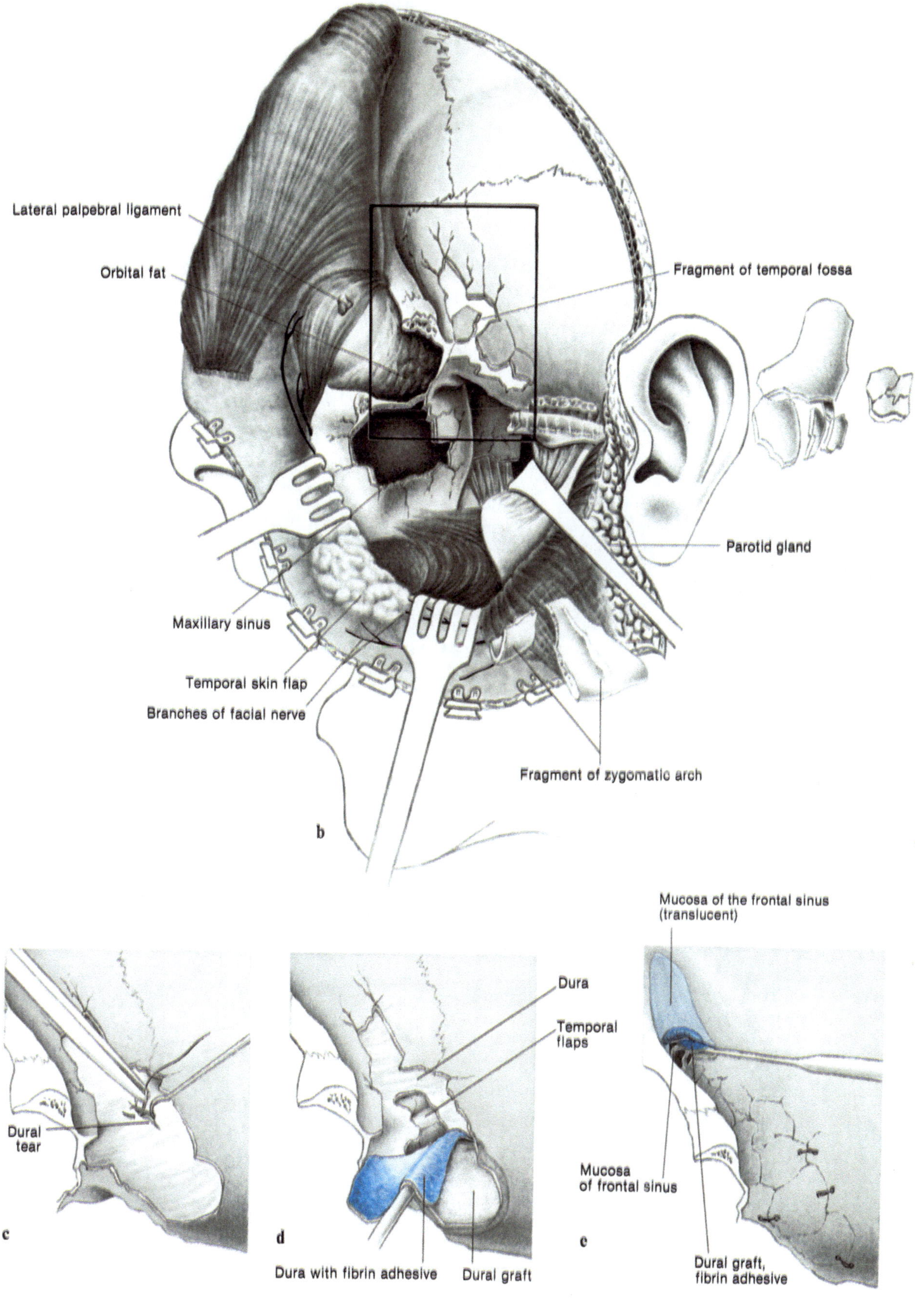
Lateral palpebral ligament
Orbital fat
Fragment of temporal fossa
Parotid gland
Maxillary sinus
Temporal skin flap
Branches of facial nerve
Fragment of zygomatic arch
b
Mucosa of the frontal sinus (translucent)
Dura
Temporal flaps
Dural tear
c
d
Dura with fibrin adhesive
Dural graft
Mucosa of frontal sinus
e
Dural graft, fibrin adhesive

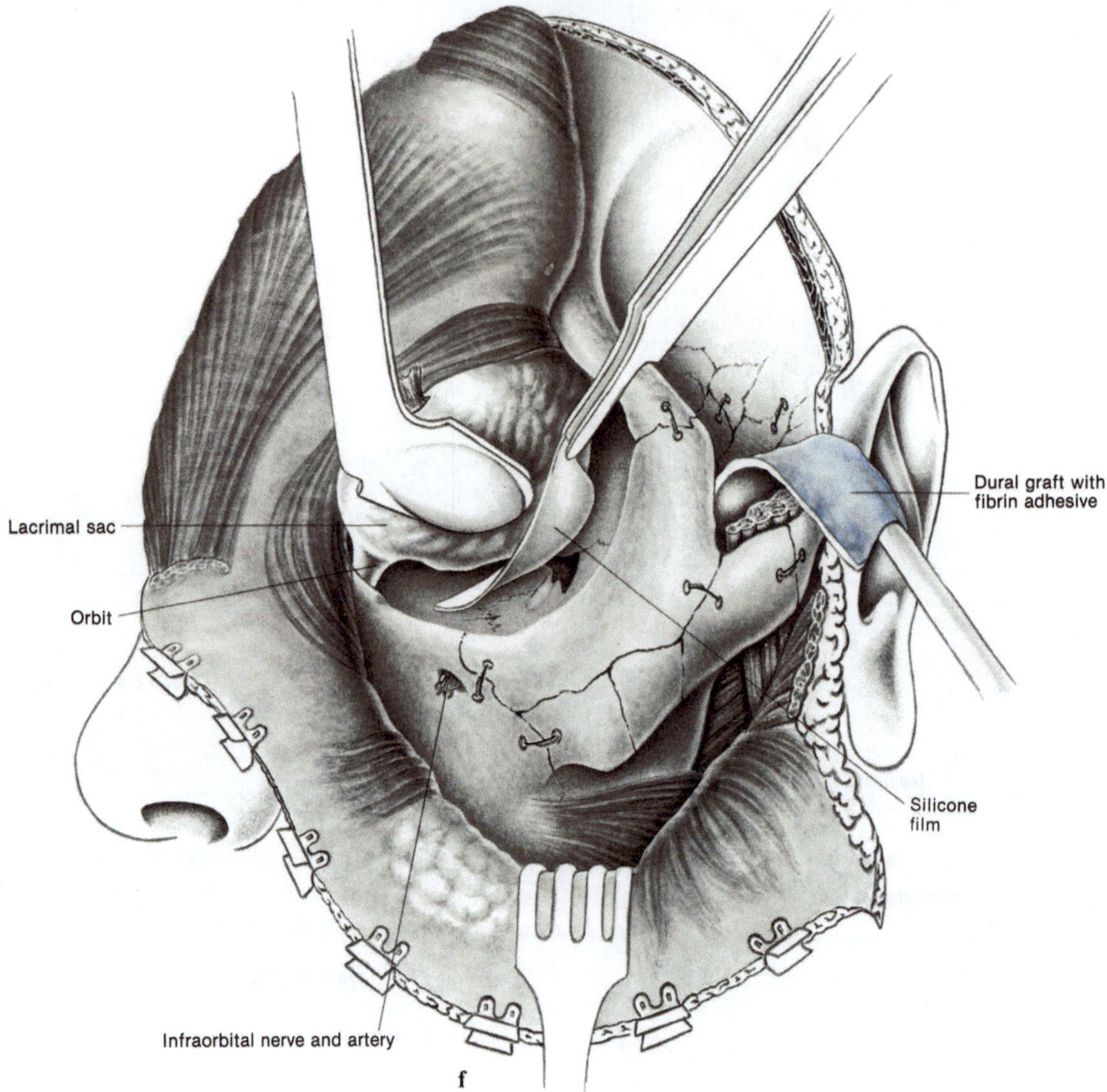

Fig. AS 23. f After treatment of the dural and cerebral injuries, the orbital floor is lined with silicone film. The cranial fracture can be additionally protected with a dural graft. The bone fragments are reapposed with wires, starting from the bony pillars that are still stable

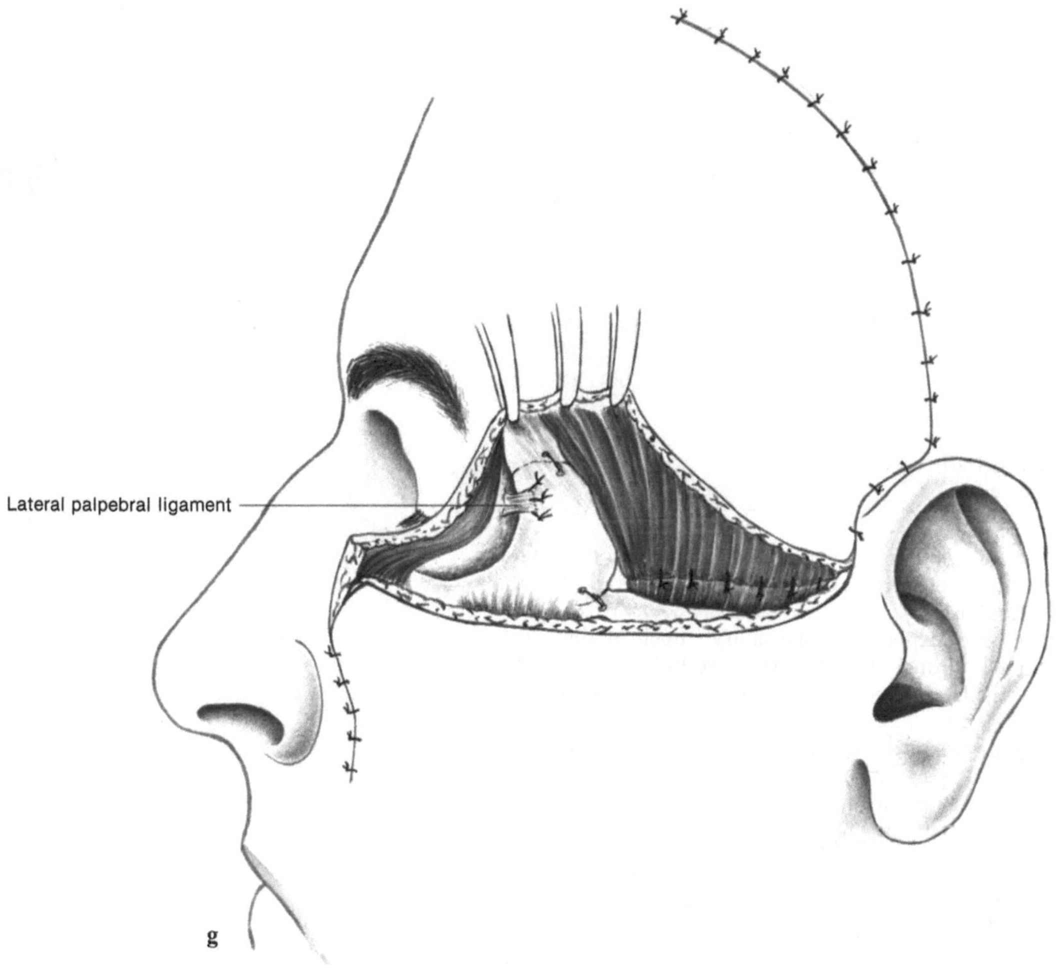

Fig. AS 23. g As a final step, the lateral palpebral ligament is sutured to the lateral orbital rim through drill holes, and the wound is closed in layers

The optic nerve is decompressed as required, and the fragments of the lateral orbital rim are replaced. This is done according to the principle of establishing a stable bony pillar from the periphery of the injury to its center. The zygoma and lateral wall of the maxillary sinus are reapposed with wires. Residual defects in the orbital floor are resurfaced with silicone film. The restored lateral and basal margins of the anterior cranial fossa are additionally covered with a dural graft or with soft tissues. Drill holes are placed in the lateral orbital rim for reattachment of the palpebral ligament. Finally the temporal muscle is repaired, and the wound is closed in layers.

With a comminuted fracture of the maxillary sinus, one should avoid making a window to the inferior nasal meatus if possible so as not to weaken critical points of support for internal fixation. Packing of the antrum is frequently unnecessary, and postoperative transfacial endoscopy may be used to check for inflammatory complications. Fig. AS 24a–d presents a clinical example of this type of injury.

Isolated trauma transmitted to the globe typically produces a *blow-out fracture* of the orbital floor and lamina papyracea, representing a circumscribed injury of the anterolateral skull base (Boenninghaus 1969). A less common result is an *orbital roof fracture* with dural injury. If the

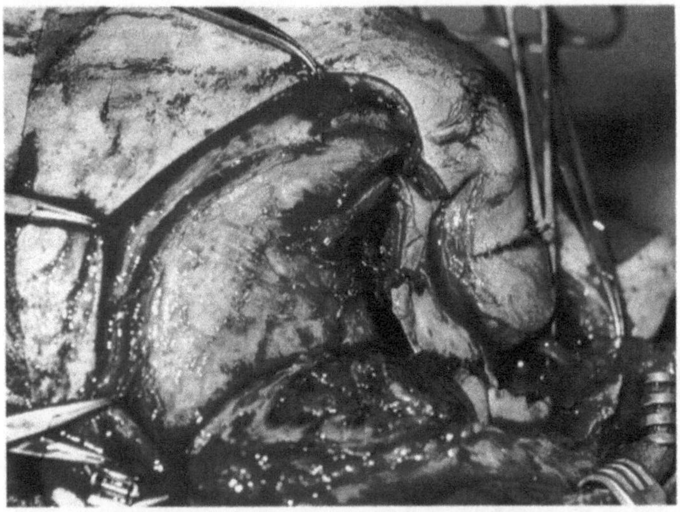

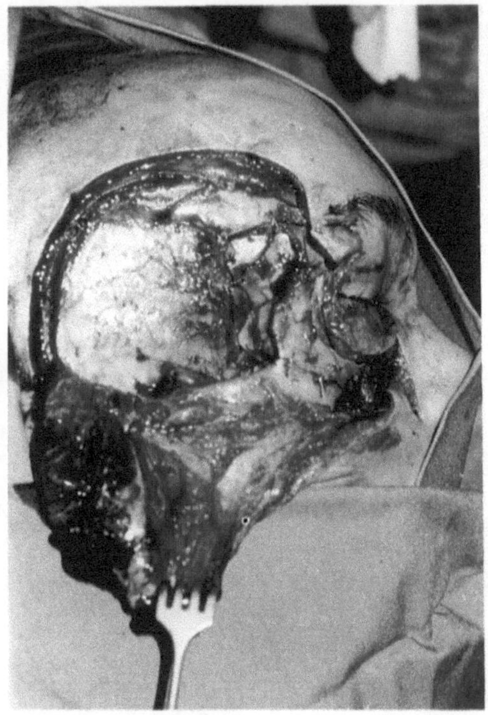

b

Fig. AS 24a–d. Extensive comminuted fracture of the lateral facial skeleton with fracture of the anterolateral skull base and multiple dural tears.
a Situation after exposure of the injury; much of the access was obtained through the traumatic wounds. Comminuted fracture of the lateral and anterior skull base and lateral facial skeleton.
b Status after treatment of the injury from within outward. Duraplasty was performed first, followed by reduction and wiring of the bone fragments and soft-tissue closure.
c The patient at 6 months postoperatively.
d The upper films show opacification and comminution of the posterior paranasal sinuses on the right side. The lower films show the appearance of the sinuses 3 months after treatment of the injury. It was decided not to remove fragments from the ethmoid cells during primary treatment to avoid further weakening of the facial skeleton. The control films confirmed complete re-aeration of the injured sinuses

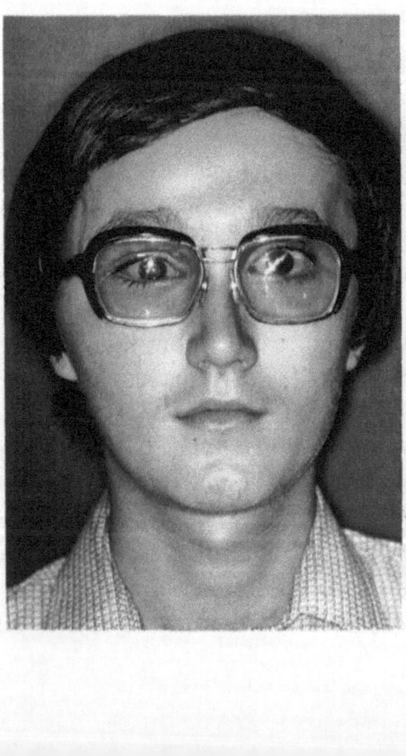

c

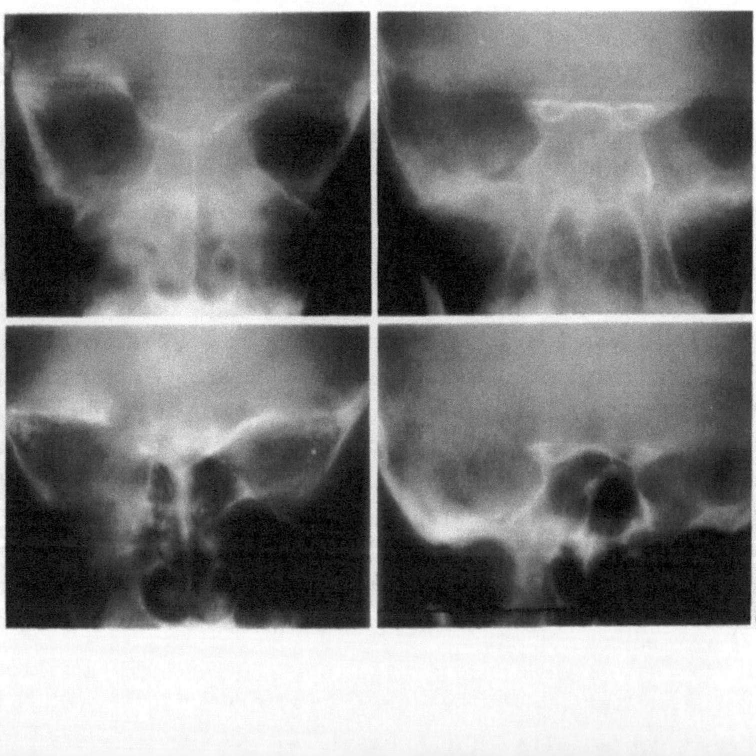

d

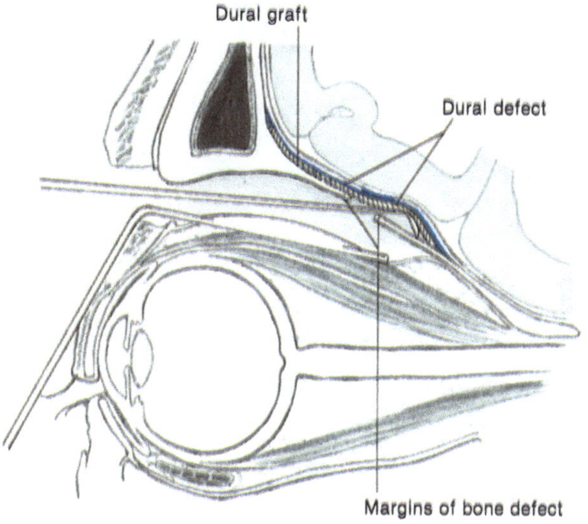

Fig. AS 25. An orbital roof fracture not involving the frontal sinus is exposed through an incision beneath the eyebrow. After release of the oblique and superior rectus muscles, the dura is exposed, and any defect that is found is repaired by inserting a fascial or dural graft

frontal sinus is involved in an orbital roof fracture of this kind, rhinosurgical principles must be applied, following dural repair, to reestablish drainage from the frontal sinus to the nose by exenteration of the ethmoid. If the frontal sinus is not involved, the orbital roof is exposed through a skin incision beneath the brow, and the necessary debridement and duraplasty are performed (Fig. AS 25).

Decompression of the Optic Nerve After Trauma

Introductory Remarks. It is difficult to estimate the true incidence of amaurosis secondary to craniocerebral trauma. Often the effect of the trauma on vision is not recognized because the patient is unconscious (see Brihaye 1981 and accompanying reference list). Confirming vision loss at an early stage and drawing appropriate therapeutic conclusions requires close monitoring of the head-injured patient by an ophthalmologist. An attempt should be made to verify a fracture of the bony optic canal or a retrobulbar hematoma as early as possible by conventional X-ray tomography or, preferably, by CT. The prognosis for visual recovery depends on the mechanism of the injury. If the continuity of the nerve fibers has been disrupted by the shearing action of bone fragments, blindness is immediate and irreversible even with operative treatment. The outlook is more favorable if optic nerve function has been compromised by pressure from bone fragments, by stretching, or by a retrobulbar hematoma. It need hardly be stated that the prognostic differentiation of cases is a very difficult if not impossible task. Because of the inconsistency of results, opinions differ as to the necessity of optic nerve decompression in patients with acute post-traumatic *vision loss* (Brihaye 1981, Dietz 1970, Fukado 1981, Lehnhardt 1973, Schmaltz and Schürmann 1971, etc.). There is greater agreement on the value of surgical exposure of the optic nerve in patients who experience *gradual visual deterioration* after the injury or develop vision problems several days, weeks, or even months later. Brihaye (1981) notes the possibility of secondary optic nerve compression by a traumatic aneurysm of the internal carotid artery, arachnoiditis, or callus formation in the bony optic canal. The delay between the traumatic event and the deterioration of vision proves that the continuity of the optic nerve is intact and implies a better chance of improvement after decompression. While only a relative indication for optic nerve decompression exists in cases of primary amaurosis, we feel that the indication is absolute in cases where post-traumatic vision loss is progressive. The decision for decompression is facilitated if an operation is already necessary due to a frontobasal fracture. Fukado (1981) states that the earlier surgical intervention is undertaken, the better the prognosis for visual recovery. He also notes that visual improvement is possible even after a period of months. The bony optic canal can be opened by the extracranial transethmoidal route as well as through the intracranial transfrontal intradural approach.

If no other indication exists for opening the cranium, we prefer the extracranial, transethmoidal optic nerve decompression, as it involves less operative stress for the patient.

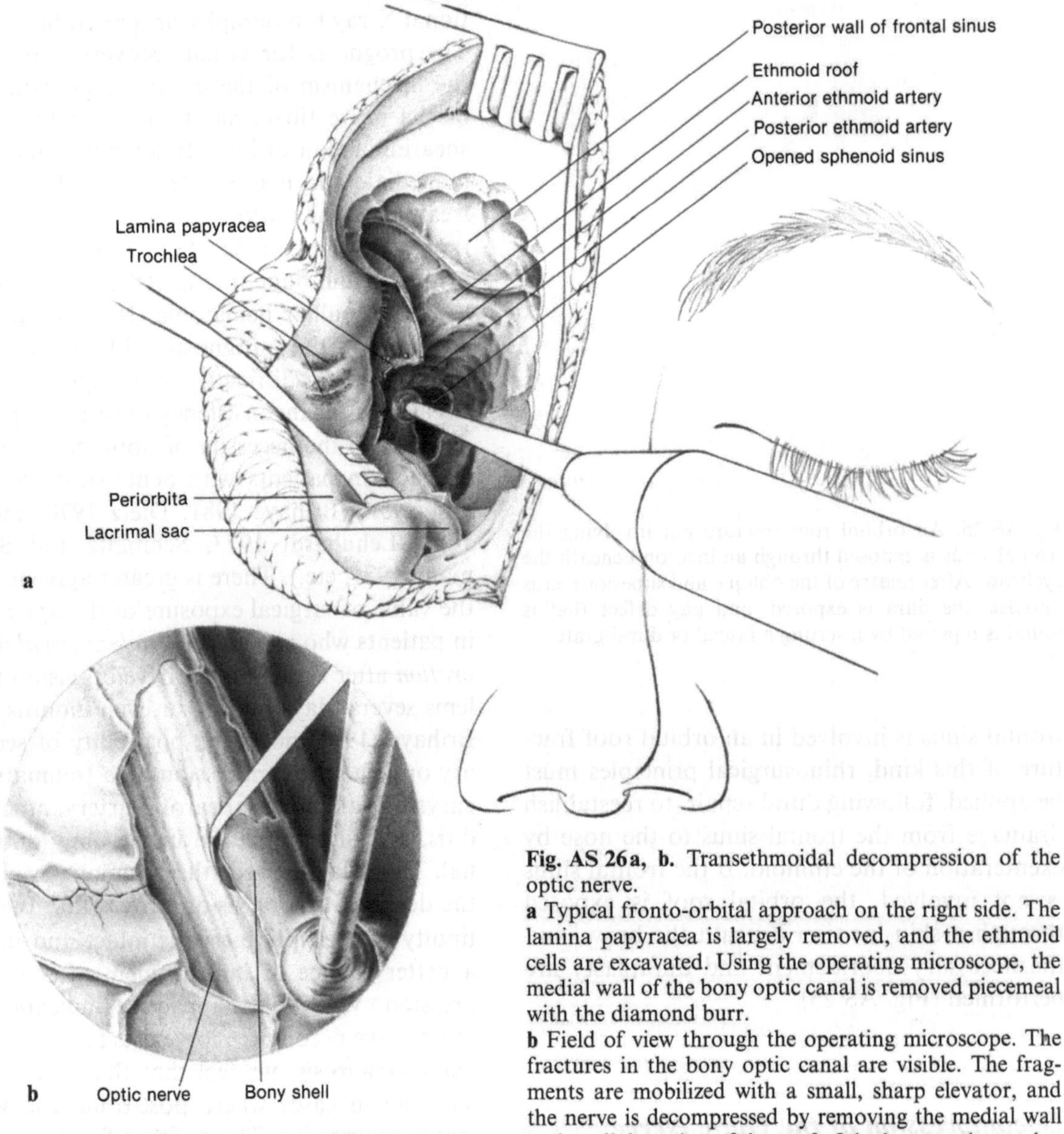

Fig. AS 26a, b. Transethmoidal decompression of the optic nerve.
a Typical fronto-orbital approach on the right side. The lamina papyracea is largely removed, and the ethmoid cells are excavated. Using the operating microscope, the medial wall of the bony optic canal is removed piecemeal with the diamond burr.
b Field of view through the operating microscope. The fractures in the bony optic canal are visible. The fragments are mobilized with a small, sharp elevator, and the nerve is decompressed by removing the medial wall and medial portion of the roof of the bony optic canal

Based on our experience with microsurgical exposure of the optic nerve by various routes, we do not believe that the procedure should cause additional optic nerve damage when performed by an experienced surgeon. Thus we consider the range of indications for the procedure to be relatively broad.

Technique of Transethmoidal Optic Nerve Decompression
(Fig. AS 26a, b)

The nerve is approached through an incision beneath the brow, like that used for external ethmoidectomy. The frontal process of the maxilla is removed, the floor of the frontal sinus is opened, and the ethmoid cells are exposed and exenterated along the cranial base. The la-

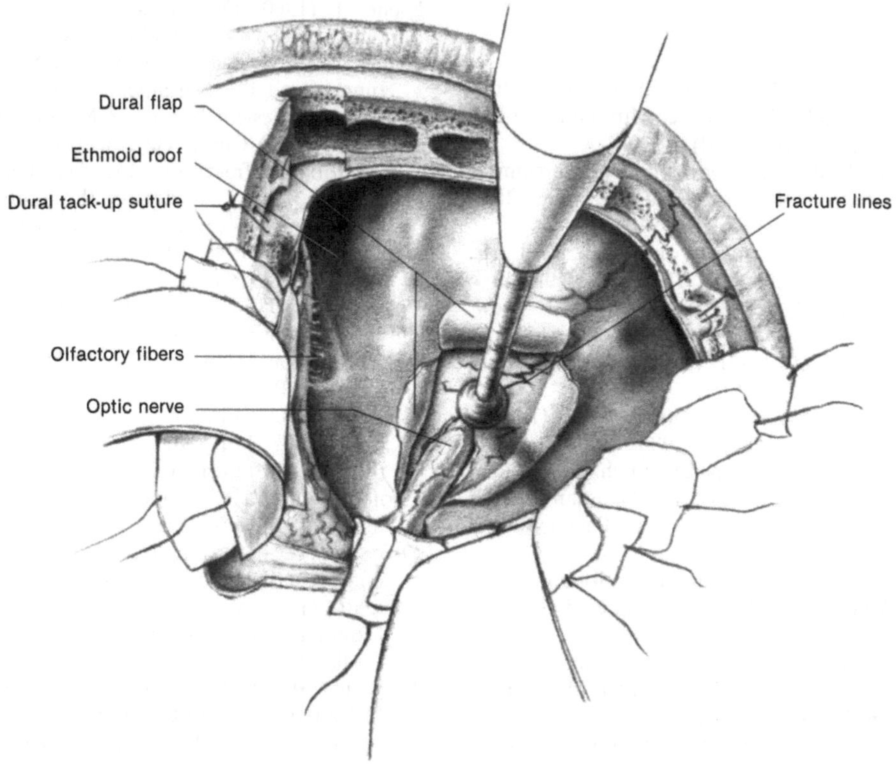

Fig. AS 27. Transfrontal intradural decompression of the optic nerve. The drawing shows the right orbital roof and the site of entry of the right optic nerve into the orbit. The bony optic canal is unroofed with the diamond burr. Both the dura of the anterior skull base and the optic nerve sheath are incised

mina papyracea is removed to the orbital apex to gain access to the anteromedial border of the bony optic canal. It should be noted that when the ethmoid is extensively pneumatized, the optic nerve may traverse the posterior ethmoid cells without a bony sheath. Dehiscence of the optic canal also may be encountered in the sphenoid sinus. Using the operating microscope, the canal is progressively exposed anteriorly to posteriorly by removing the medial wall and medial portion of the canal roof. Bone fragments are removed. Fukado (1981), in contrast to other authors (Lehnhardt 1973), recommends splitting the dural sheath of the optic nerve at the end of the procedure.

Technique of Transfrontal Intradural Optic Nerve Decompression

(Fig. AS 27)

A unilateral or bilateral frontal craniotomy is performed, depending on the need for concomitant treatment of a frontobasal injury. The dura is opened, the frontal lobe is retracted with a brain spatula over protective cotton paddies, and the entry of the optic nerve into the bony canal is dissected free. After elevation of the overlying dura, the optic canal is progressively unroofed with a burr, bone fragments are removed, and, when the exposure reaches the orbital apex, a slit is cut in the dural sheath of the nerve. If the paranasal sinus system remains closed, no further measures are needed. But if the paranasal sinuses are found to communicate with the optic nerve or with the cranial cavity at the end of the operation, the communication must be sealed off with a dural graft.

References

Berendes J (1956) Doppelter autoplastischer Verschluß grösserer Duradefekte in Nähe der Mittellinie bei Liquorrhoea nasalis. HNO (Berl) 6:220

Berendes J (1959) Diskussionsbemerkung 42. Versammlung südwstdtsch HNO-Ärzte Bad Dürkheim 26.–27.09.1958. Z Laryng Rhinol 38:1910

Bock WJ (1983) Schädel-Hirnverletzungen. In: Dietz H, Umbach W, Wüllenweber (eds) Klinische Neurochirurgie, vol 2, pp 399–422. Thieme, Stuttgart New York

Boenninghaus HG (1960) Die Behandlung der Schädelbasisbrücke. Thieme, Stuttgart

Boenninghaus HG (1969) Blow out-fracture des Orbitadaches. Laryng Rhinol 48:395–398

Boenninghaus HG (1974) Die operative Behandlung von Verletzungen der Rhinobasis. In: Naumannn HH (ed) Head and neck surgery, vol 1. Thieme, New York

Bohner J, Hesse W (1989) Albumin/Präalbumin-Quotient zur Diagnostik der Liquorrhoe. Lab med 13:193

Brandt C (1959) Zur Röntgendiagnostik der Liquorfisteln und Pneumatocelen, insbesondere der vorderen Schädelgrube. Röfo 91:182

Brihaye J (1981) Transcranial decompression of optic nerve after trauma. In: Samii M, Jannetta PJ (ed) The Cranial Nerves. Springer, Berlin Heidelberg New York, pp 116–124

Burmeister H (1962) Erfahrungen mit lyophilisierter Dura mater. Zbl Neurochir 22:209

Burmeister H (1962) Zur Frage des intra- oder extraduralen Duraverschlusses bei frontobasalen Schädelverletzungen. Zbl Chir 87:297

Cairns H (1937) Injuries of the frontal and ethmoidal sinusses with special reference to cerebrospinal rhinorrhoea and aeroceles. J Laryng 52:589

Crawford H (1957) Dura replacement. An experimental study of derma autografts and preserved dura homografts. Plast Reconstr Surg 19:299

Dandy WE (1926) Pneumocephalus (intracranial pneumatocele or aerocele). Arch Surg 12:299

Denecke HJ (1956/58) Zur Diagnose und operativen Behandlung von Liquorfisteln im Bereich von Keilbeinhöhle und Hypophyse mit permanenter Liquorrhoe nach perkutaner transethmoidaler Hypophysenausschaltung. HNO (Berl) 6:152

Dietz H (1966) Die frontobasale Schädelhirnverletzung. Thesis, University of Mainz

Dietz H (1970) Die frontobasale Schädelhirnverletzung. Springer, Berlin Heidelberg New York

Draf W (1980) Erfahrungen mit der Technik der Fibrinklebung in der Hals-Nasen-Ohrenchirurgie. Laryng Rhinol Otol 59:99–107

Draf W, Samii M (1983) Fronto-Basal Injuries – Principles in Diagnosis and Treatment. In: Samii M and Brihaye J, Traumatology of the Skull Base. Springer Berlin Heidelberg New York, pp 61–69

Dumas G, Laignel-Cavastine J (1914) Les variations des pression du liquide cephalorachidien dans leurs rapports avec les emotions. Encephale 9:19–21

Escher F (1960) Die frontobasalen Schädelhirnverletzungen. Schweiz Med Wschr: 1481

Escher F (1967) Die frontobasalen Schädelhirnverletzungen und die Nasennebenhöhlenverletzungen im mittleren Gesichtsbereich. Z Militärmed 44:141

Escher F (1969) Clinic, classification and treatment of frontobasal fractures. In: Hamberger CA and Wersäll J (ed) Disorders of the Skull Base Region. Proceedings of the tenth Nobel Symposium Stockholm August 1968. Almquist & Wiksell, Stockholm: Wiley, New York, pp 343–352

Fukado Y (1981) Microsurgical transethmoidal optic nerve decompression: Experience in 700 cases. In: Samii M and Janetta PJ (ed) The Cranial Nerves. Springer, Berlin Heidelberg New York, pp 125–128

Grant FC (1923) Intracranial aerocele following a fracture of the skull (Report of a case with review of the literature) Surg Gynec Obstet 36:251

Grote W (1966a) Traumatische frontobasale Liquorfisteln. Chirurg 37:103

Grote W (1966b) Traumatische Liquorfisteln im Kindes- und Jugendalter. Z Kinderchir 3:11

Hirsch O (1955) Verschluß einer traumatischen nasalen Liquorrhoe auf endonasalem Weg. Mschr Ohren-Heilk 89:265

Kirschner M (1909) Über die freie Sehnen- und Faszientransplantation. Bruns, Beitr Klin Chir 65:472

Kirschner M (1909) Zur Frage des plastischen Ersatzes der Dura mater. Langenscheidts Arch Klin Chir 91:541

Kley W (1967) Diagnostik und operative Versorgung von Keilbeinhöhlenfrakturen. Laryng Rhinol Otol (Stuttg) 46:469–478

Kley W (1968) Die Unfallchirurgie der Schädelbasis und der pneumatischen Räume. Arch Oto-Rhino-Laryng 191:1–216. (Kongreßbericht 1968)

Kley W (1973) Faszienplastiken im Bereich der vorderen und mittleren Schädelbasis und im Bereich der Nasennebenhöhlen. Laryng Rhinol Otol (Stuttg) 52:255

Kley W (1974) Diskussionsbemerkung zu Scheunemann. In: Naumann HH, Kastenbauer ER (eds) Plastisch-chirurgische Maßnahmen nach frischen Verletzungen. Thieme, Stuttgart, p 81

Krausen AS, Samuel M (1979) Pediatric jaw fractures. Indications for open reduction. Otolaryng Head Neck Surg 87:318–322

Lehnhardt E (1973) Die Dekompression des N. opticus bei Fraktur der Rhinobasis. HNO (Berl) 21:158–160

Mahaley MS, Odom GL (1966) Complication following intrathecal injection of fluorescein. J Neurosurg 25:298

Mees K, Beyer A (1982) Akute neurologische Komplikationen nach intrathekaler Fluoresceininjektion. Laryng Rhinol Otol 61:102–104

Messerklinger W (1972) Nasenendoskopie: Nachweis, Lokalisation und Differentialdiagnose der nasalen Liquorrhoe. HNO (Berl) 20:268–270

Metzger J, Proteau J, Sayec G (1965) Les rhinorrhoes posttraumatiques. Ann Med Leg 45:423

Minnigerode B (1967) Zur Technik der extraduralen rhinochirurgischen Deckung von Liquorfisteln nach frontobasalen Schädelverletzungen. Mschr Ohrenheilk 101:441

Naumann HH (1974) Chirurgie der Nasennebenhöhlen. In: Naumann HH, Kopf- und Halschirurgie, vol 2/1. Thieme, Stuttgart, p. 411
Oberascher G (1988) Cerebrospinal Fluid Otorrhoea – Rhinorrhoea. Salzburg Concent of CSF Diagnosis. Laryng Rhinol Otol 67:375–381
Osterwald L (1977) Personal comunication
Probst Ch (1971) Frontobasale Verletzungen. Huber, Bern
Reisner K, Gosepath J (1973) Schädeltomographie. Thieme, Stuttgart
Rettinger G, Kalender W (1981) Computertomographie bei Erkrankungen des HNO-Bereiches. II. Hochauflösungs-Computertomographie des Gesichtsschädels. HNO 29:364–369
Samii M, Brihaye J (1983) Traumatology of the skull base. Springer, Berlin Heidelberg New York
Samii M, Draf W (1978) Indikation und Versorgung der frontobasalen Liquorfistel aus HNO-chirurgischer und neurochirurgischer Sicht. Laryng Rhinol Otol (Stuttg) 57:689–697
Samii M, Draf W (1983) Fronto-basal Injuries – Principles in Diagnosis and Treatment. In: Traumatology of the Skull Base by M Samii and J Brihaye (Ed) Springer, Berlin Heidelberg New York pp 61–69
Scheunemann H (1974) Prinzipien der Behandlung von offenen Frakturen des Kiefer-Gesichtsschädels. In: Naumann HH, Kastenbauer ER. Plastisch-chirurgische Maßnahmen nach frischen Verletzungen. Thieme, Stuttgart, p 65
Schmaltz B, Schürmann K (1971) Traumatische Optikusschäden. Probleme der Ätiologie und der operativen Behandlung. Klin Monatsbl Augenheilkd 159:33
Schreiner L, Herrmann A (1967) Die operative Behandlung der nasalen Liquorrhoe mit der Septum- und Muschelschleimhaut-Plastik. Arch Ohr-, Nas-Kehlk HK 188:418
Schuchardt K (ed) (1966) Das frische Trauma im Kiefer-Gesichts-Bereich. Fortschr Kiefer- und Gesichtschirurgie vol 11. Thieme, Stuttgart
Seiferth LB (1954) Unfallverletzungen der Nase, der Nebenhöhlen und der Basis der vorderen Schädelgrube. Arch Oto-Rhino-Laryng 165:1
Seiferth LB, Wustrow F (1977) Verletzungen im Bereich der Nase, des Mittelgesichts und seiner Nebenhöhlen sowie frontobasale Verletzungen. In: Berendes, Link, Zöllner (Ed.) Hals-Nasen-Ohren-Heilkunde in Praxis und Klinik. 2. Ed. Vol. 1/I/8 Thieme Stuttgart
Teachenor FR (1927) Intracranial complications of fracture of skull involving frontal sinus. J Amer Med Ass 88:987–989
Theissing G, Theissing HJ (1971) Kurze HNO-Operationslehre, vol 1. Thieme, Stuttgart
Tönnis W, Frowein RA (1952) Liquorfisteln und Pneumatozelen nach Verletzungen der vorderen Schädelbasis. Zbl Neurochir 12:323–347
Unterberger S (1958) Zur Versorgung frontobasaler Verletzungen. Arch Otorhinolaryngol 172:463
Voss O (1936) Die Chirurgie der Schädelbasisfrakturen aufgrund 25jähriger Erfahrungen. Barth, Leipzig
Wallace JD, Wintrauh MI, Mattson RH, Rosnagle R (1972) Status epilepticus as a complication of intrathecal fluorescein. J Neurosurg 36:659
Weickmann F, Steinle HJ (1960) Duraplastik mit Gewebskonserven. Med Bild-Dienst Roche Nr. 9:10
Wullstein HL (1972) Hat Terminologie zur Definition unseres Faches eine praktische Bedeutung? HNO (Berl) 20:259–261
Wullstein HL, Wullstein SR (1953) Die Verletzungen der Rhino- und Otobasis unter dem Gesichtspunkt des pneumatischen Systems im Schädel. Chirurg 41:490

Surgery of Inflammatory Complications in the Region of the Anterior Skull Base

Introductory Remarks. Inflammatory complications in the skull base region can result from paranasal sinus infections or they may develop secondarily after trauma (refs. in Draf 1982, Ganz 1977, Gerlach and Simon 1960). Possible intracranial complications of sinusitis include epidural abscess, meningoencephalitis, subdural abscess, brain abscess, and venous sinus thrombosis (Hermann 1964). These complications may arise through direct extension from the paranasal sinuses, by hematogenous spread, or through osteomyelitis of the frontal bone. Thrombosis of the superior sagittal sinus is uncommon.

The possibility of intracranial complications should be considered whenever sinusitis is diagnosed. CT can be used to demonstrate these complications and assess their response to treatment. Small epidural and subdural abscesses at the skull base may be difficult to identify on CT scans.

Treatment

An essential part of treatment is the eradication of the primary focus in the paranasal sinuses under appropriate antibiotic protection.

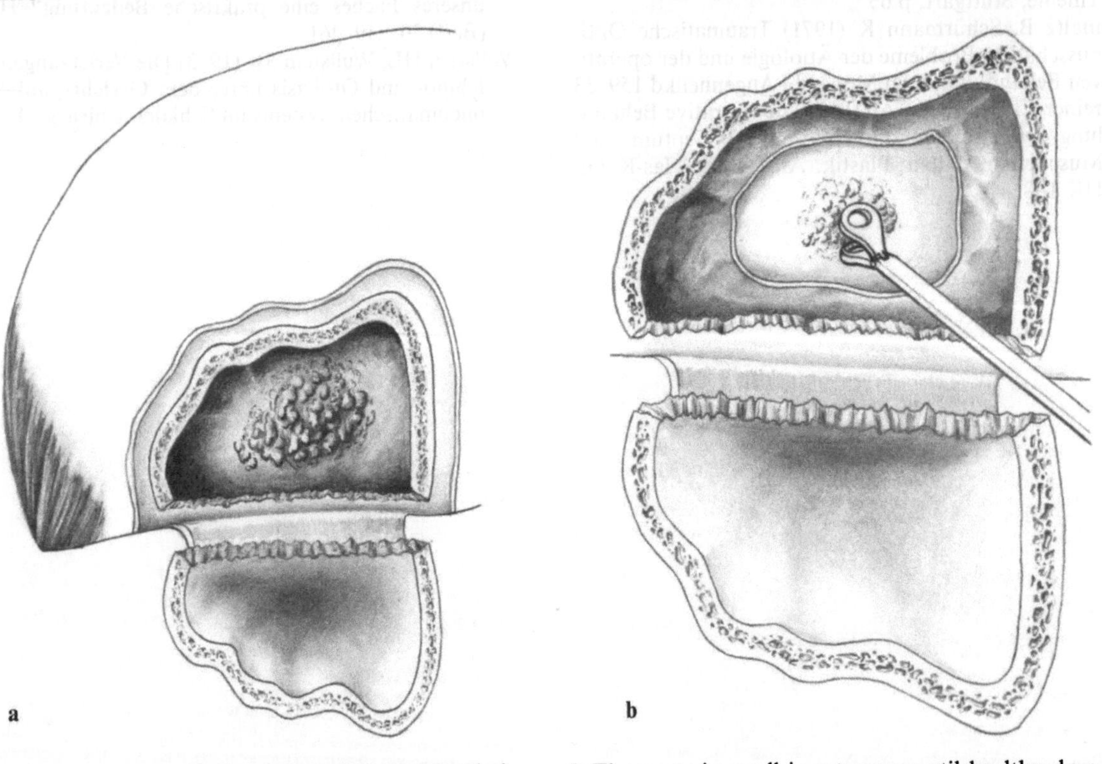

Fig. AS 28 a, b. Osteoplastic exposure of an epidural abscess at the posterior wall of the frontal sinus.
a The frontal sinus is entered through an osteoplastic flap hinged on the periosteum. A granulation layer is visible on the posterior wall, and the exposed dura is palpable beneath it.
b The posterior wall is cut away until healthy dura appears. The granulations are carefully removed tangentially to exclude a dural defect

The *epidural abscess* often produces no clinical symptoms. It may be an incidental finding during rhinosurgical treatment, especially if it is not yet visible on CT scans. If a granulation-filled bony defect of the skull base is found at operation, it is necessary to expose additional bone surrounding the defect. An epidural abscess situated beneath the bone and a dural defect hidden by granulations is excluded by exposing healthy dura on all sides (Fig. AS 28a, b). The layer of granulation tissue on the dura is carefully scraped away with a double curet. If the dura is found to be intact, the sinus operation is concluded in standard fashion.

In cases of *rhinogenic meningitis or meningoencephalitis*, there is disagreement as to the timing of surgery to eradicate the primary focus. While many advocate intensive primary antibiotic treatment for acute meningitis, possibly using intrathecal injections, we and other authors believe that prompt eradication of the primary septic focus offers the best chance for a rapid recovery. Every effort should be made to isolate the causative organism from the cerebrospinal fluid and establish its sensitivity. Having exposed and eradicated the primary focus, the operator exposes the dura at one or more sites and looks for an epidural abscess. If the dura shows obvious inflammatory change, or if a defect is found, it is likely that a subdural abscess has formed. With an intact and normal-appearing dura, the operation may be concluded if CT scans have shown no evidence of a subdural abscess. However, this does not exclude an incipient empyema that is still clinically occult.

If preoperative studies have already confirmed a subdural abscess, rhinosurgical eradication of the primary focus must be accompanied or immediately followed by neurosurgical exposure, irrigation, and possibly several days' drainage of the subdural space.

The problems are illustrated by the following *case report*: An 18-year-old female was admitted with marked systemic symptoms, severe right frontotemporal headache, neck stiffness, and lethargy. ESR on admission was 104/134, leukocyte count was 16,600, and CSF cell content was 400/3. The patient had a 3-week history of a severe generalized infection with fever, purulent bronchitis, bilateral frontal sinusitis, and left maxillary sinusitis. Preoperative CT scans (Fig. AS 29a–c) showed opacification of the frontal sinuses, a right frontal epidural mass (abscess) displacing the brain to the left, a low-density zone in the right temporal area, and widening of the intercerebral fissure as evidence of the subdural empyema. An ear, nose and throat surgeon was called in shortly after admission. The frontal sinuses, ethmoid sinuses, and left maxillary sinus were opened and cleared of disease, and a large epidural abscess was drained. Lack of significant response prompted burr-hole trephination and drainage of the right temporal area. The mass lesion diminished in size, but continued lack of clinical improvement prompted a more extensive trephination on the right side of the superior sagittal sinus and also at the level of the parieto-occipital junction over the lambdoid suture next to the midline. These openings disclosed marked brain swelling, and each yielded a foul-smelling pus that was bacteriologically sterile. The second trephinations were followed by rapid improvement in the patient's general condition and an arrest of the intermittent seizures that had occurred since her admission. Postoperative CT scans (Fig. AS 29d–f) showed an air-filled frontal sinus without further evidence of an intracranial mass, abscess, or empyema.

This case report illustrates the potential for serious intracranial, rhinogenic complications to develop despite the availability of antibiotic therapy. It also demonstrates the inadequacy of eradicating the primary focus when a subdural abscess is already developing. The clinical and CT findings should determine the necessity and extent of further interventional measures.

When *meningitis* results from the *spread of a rhinogenic frontal osteomyelitis*, it is necessary to remove all affected bone in addition to eradicating the primary site of sepsis.

In patients with a *brain abscess*, the trend in neurosurgical treatment is to administer antibiotics and corticosteroids until the abscess is well encapsulated and then surgically extirpate it in a way that minimizes trauma to healthy brain (Carey et al. 1971, Garfield 1969, Le Beau et al. 1973, Meinig et al. 1980, Schiefer and Klinger

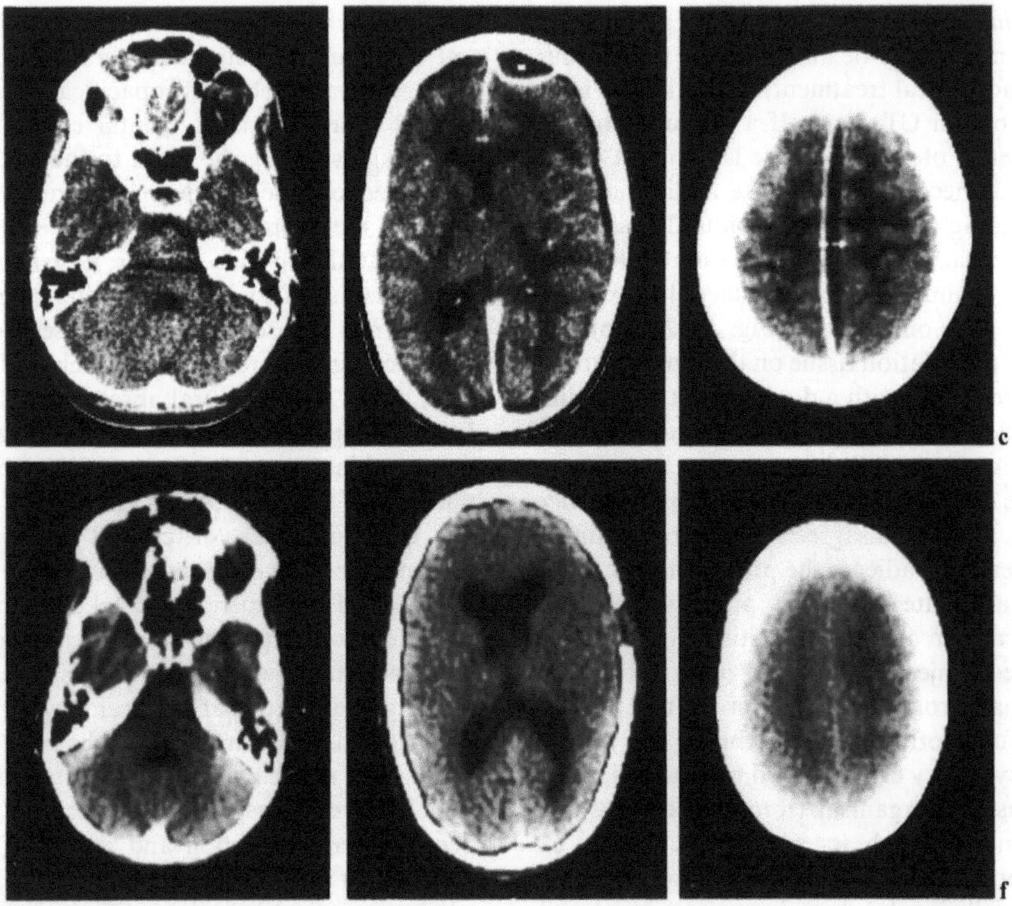

a, b c d, e f

Fig. AS 29a–f. Serial CT scans of a rhinogenic epidural abscess with subdural empyema formation in the right temporal area and interhemispheric fissure.
a-c Preoperative CT scans. **a** Air-fluid level in the frontal sinus. **b** Right frontal epidural abscess with an air-fluid level and a low-density zone in the right temporal area consistent with subdural empyema. **c** Widening of the interhemispheric fissure.
d–f Postoperative CT scans. **d** The frontal sinuses are aerated following rhinosurgical eradication of the infection. **e** The subdural abscess has been evacuated. The trephine opening is visible as a bony defect. **f** The interhemispheric fissure appears normal after frontal and occipital trephination

1978, Wallenfang et al. 1977, 1980, 1981, Zimmermann et al. 1977). It is not unusual for brain abscesses to resolve completely with conservative therapy. If the brain abscess is in proximity to the skull base, it may be acceptable in emergencies for the ear, nose and throat surgeon to drain the abscess, provided he does not have to go through healthy brain tissue. But in these cases as well, we feel it is best to await encapsulation and then remove the encephalic infectious focus completely together with the capsule. Despite advances in diagnosis and conservative treatment (antibiotics, corticosteroids), it has not been possible to reduce the overall mortality from brain abscesses much below 40%. But when the abscess proceeds to a chronic stage with a stable capsule, the mortality falls to about 10% in cases managed by surgical excision (Wallenfang et al. 1981).

In the presence of an unresolving infectious swelling of the face and of septic fever, the angular vein may need to be ligated in order to prevent spreading of the infectious process to the brain. Often in this situation the angular vein

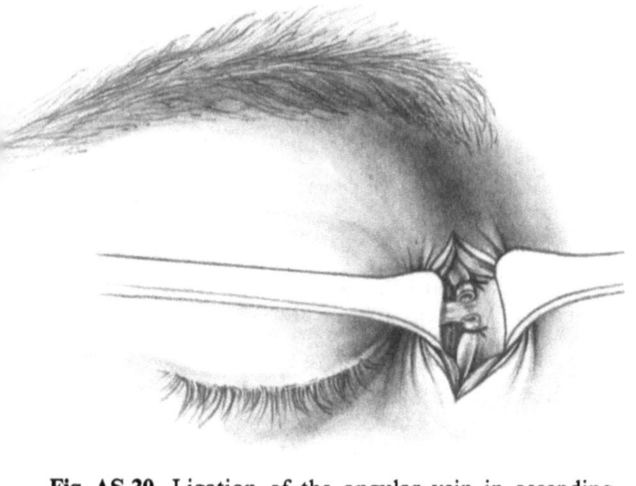

Fig. AS 30. Ligation of the angular vein in ascending thrombosis to prevent cavernous sinus thrombosis. The vessel is exposed through an incision made between the inner canthus of the eye and bony nasal dorsum. It is somewhat shorter than that used for an external ethmoidectomy

contains a septic thrombus. The angular vein may be approached through the same skin incision used to reach the ethmoidal cells (Fig. AS 30).

Thrombosis of the superior sagittal sinus also can result from the direct spread of infection from the frontal sinus. Surgical treatment consists of exposing the sagittal sinus by piecemeal removal of the overlying bone to the area where the channel is still carrying blood, ligating the sinus, and evacuating it. Care is taken to preserve drainage in the posterior third of the superior sagittal sinus. This is necessary to prevent severe venous stasis with cerebral edema and life-threatening neurologic disturbances.

Thrombosis of the cavernous sinus results from the spread of paranasal sinus disease via the pterygopalatine fossa or via the jugular vein and diploic venous channels. It is characterized by progressive impairment of consciousness and orbital symptoms such as lid edema, proptosis, and chemosis. Prompt eradication of the causative paranasal sinus lesion is imperative. Occasionally the pterygopalatine fossa must be widely decompressed by removing the posterior wall of the maxillary sinus. Most authors reject more extensive surgical measures owing to the generally favorable response to antibiotics.

In the exceptional cases where this therapy is unsuccessful, it is necessary to expose the cavernous sinus externally and aspirate it after opening the ethmoid labyrinth and sphenoid sinus.

Mucoceles and pyoceles occur in all paranasal sinuses but are most common in the frontal sinuses. Their basic pathoanatomic features are the same. They occur when inflammatory processes, scarring, or trauma obstruct drainage from the sinus ostium, leading to the retention of mucosal secretions with erosion of the surrounding bony structures by pressure atrophy. The sac may develop in the direction of the orbit, creating a pseudotumor that displaces the globe and may affect its mobility. In other cases the sac may erode through the skull base, allowing the mucosal epithelium to encroach upon the dura. A sac developing toward the nose can cause partial obstruction of the nasal cavity. Mucoceles of the sphenoid sinus can cause sudden blindness as a result of optic nerve compression

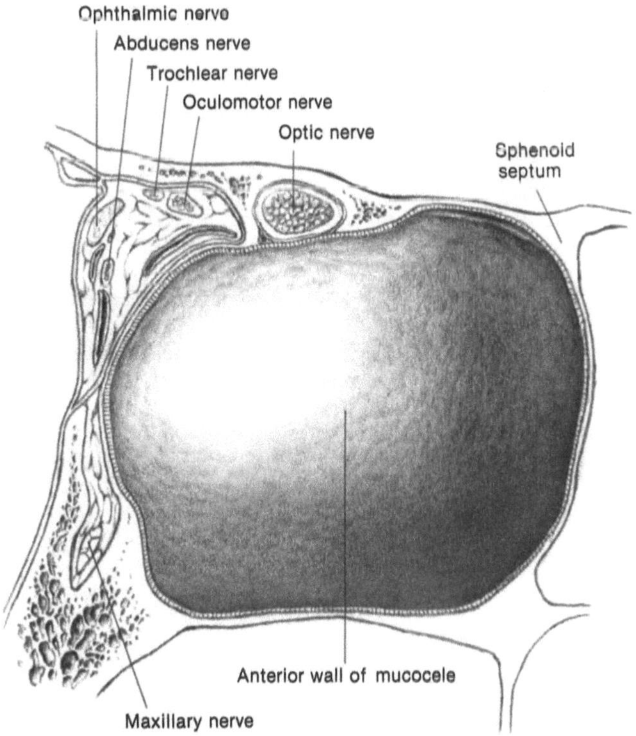

Fig. AS 31. Space-occupying mucocele of the sphenoid sinus (anterior view of the right sphenoid sinus). The mucocele causes compression of surrounding structures, especially the optic nerve

(Blum and Larson 1973, etc.). Extremely large sphenoid sinus mucoceles may produce the clinical picture of a mass lesion of the sella (Fig. AS 31). Two surgical treatment methods are available:

1) The affected paranasal sinus is opened, the pyocele sac is removed in toto, and adequate drainage is established from the affected sinus to the nose.
2) A portion of the sac wall is resected, leaving the epithelium alone, to create a simple blind sac that, like its parent sinus, communicates with the nasal cavity. Especially with large sphenoid sinus mucoceles, this procedure, performed as a transnasal sphenoidotomy with wide drainage of the sphenoid sinus, is preferred over the more extensive transfrontal intradural operation.

References

Blum EMM, Larson A (1973) Mucocele of the sphenoid sinus with sudden blindness. Laryngoscope 83:2042

Carey ME, Chou SN, French LA (1971) Longterm neurological residua in patients surviving brain abscess with surgery. J Neurosurg 34:652–656

Draf W (1982) Die chirurgische Behandlung entzündlicher Erkrankungen der Nasennebenhöhlen. Arch Otorhinolaryngol 235:133–305 (Kongressbericht 1982)

Ganz H (1977) Komplikationen der unspezifischen Nasen- und Nebenhöhlenentzündungen. In: Berendes J, Link R, Zöllner F (eds) Hals-Nasen-Ohren-Heilkunde in Praxis und Kinik, 2nd edn, vol 1/I. Thieme, Stuttgart, p 14.1–14.37

Garfield J (1969) Management of supratentorial intracranial abscess. A review of 200 cases. Br Med J 2:7–11

Gerlach J, Simon G (1960) Erkennung, Differentialdiagnose und Behandlung der Geschwülste und Entzündungen der Schädelknochen einschließlich Orbita. In: Krenkel W, Olivecrona H, Tönnis W (eds) Handbuch der Neurochirurgie vol IV/I. Springer, Berlin Heidelberg New York

Herrmann A (1964) Entzündliche Hirnkomplikationen von 1953–1963 anhand des Krankengutes der Univ HNO-Klinik. München Mschr Ohrenheilk 98:241–243

Le Beau J, Creissard P, Harispe L, Redondo A (1973) Surgical treatment of brain abscess and subdural empyema. J Neurosurg 38:198–203

Meinig G, Reulen HJ, Simon RS, Schürmann K (1980) Clinical, chemical and CT evaluation of short-term and long-term antiedematous therapy with dexamethasone and diuretics. In: Cervos-Navarro J, Ferszt R: Brain edema: pathology and therapy. Ist International Ernst Reuter Symposium, Berlin, Sept. 12–15, 1979. Raven, New York

Schiefer W, Klinger M (1978) Aspects of modern brain abscess diagnosis and treatment. Neurosurg Rev 1/2:37–45

Wallenfang Th, Reulen HJ, Schindling H (1977) Investigation on the prognosis of brain abscess. In: Wüllenweber R, Brock M: Advances in Neurosurg, Vol 4:296–299. Springer, Berlin Heidelberg New York

Wallenfang Th, Bohl J, Kretzschmar K (1980) Evolution of Brain Abscess in Cats. Formation of Capsule and Resolution of Brain Edema. Neurosurg Rev 3:101–111

Wallenfang Th, Reulen HJ, Schünemann K (1981) Therapy of Brain Abscess. In: Advances in Neurosurg, Vol 9: Brain Abscess and Meningitis. Subarachnoid Hemorrhage: Timing, Problems. Edited by W Schiefer, M Klinger, M Brock. Springer, Berlin Heidelberg New York

Zimmermann RA, Bilaniuk LT, Shipkin PM, Gilden DH, Murtagh F (1977) Evolution of cerebral abscess: Correlation of clinical features with computed tomography. Neurol (Minneap) 27:14–19

Surgery of Space-Occupying Lesions of the Anterior Skull Base

Introductory Remarks. Tumors of the anterior skull base can arise from the frontal sinus, the ethmoid cells, the sphenoid sinus, and even from the maxillary sinus, from which they can spread toward the inside of the skull. Invasion may occur through the posterior wall or floor of the frontal sinus, the ethmoid roof, the cribriform plate, the planum sphenoidale, or the tuberculum sellae.

It is noteworthy that tumors arising in the paranasal sinuses can attain considerable size before producing *clinical signs.* Invasion of the anterior cranial fossa may remain clinically silent for some time. Progressive anosmia; deep, dull facial pain; epistaxis; trigeminal nerve irritation; and ophthalmologic symptoms should raise suspicion of a tumor in the region of the anterior skull base. *Endoscopy of the upper respiratory tract*, including examination of the roof of the nasopharynx with modern optical instrumentation, has contributed greatly to the early diagnosis of nasal and paranasal sinus tumors and to the determination of their extent (Fig. AS 32). Even a moderate-size tumor in the middle meatus can obstruct drainage from the paranasal sinuses, leading to swelling of the mucosa. Tomograms and CT scans are not always able to differentiate polypous mucosal swelling from actual tumor growth. Endoscopic biopsies from the nose, the paranasal sinuses, and the pharyngeal roof can serve to establish tumor extent when formulating a plan for operative treatment. In addition, CT scans are indispensable for determining the extent of possible intracranial spread. It appears that radionuclide bone scans can be helpful in differentiating reactive mucosal swelling from neoplastic disease (Frey et al. 1981 a, b).

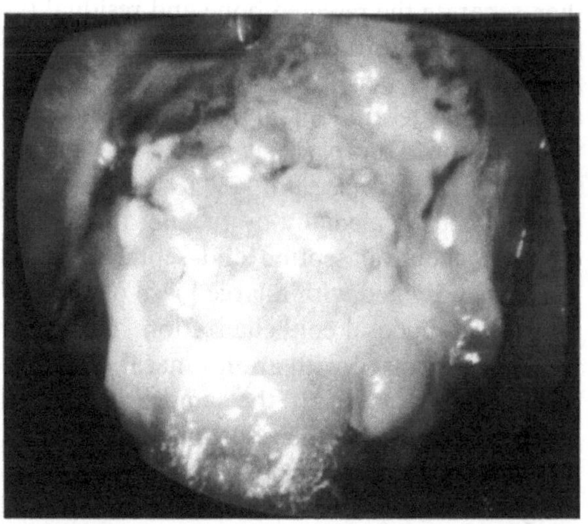

Fig. AS 32. Nasal endoscopy on the left side: an ethmoid carcinoma is visible in the middle meatus, below the middle turbinate

Tumor surgery of the anterior skull base is a subject of interdisciplinary concern. Many of the problems encountered by a surgeon of *one* specialty who enters areas of neighboring speciality can be solved by interdisciplinary understanding and by the formulation of a common surgical concept. By integrating the operative techniques of multiple specialties and applying microsurgical technique, it is possible to minimize tissue trauma during surgery and significantly reduce postoperative morbidity and mortality. This justifies the utilization of radical as well as palliative surgical treatments.

A *basic difference* exists in the approach to the *surgical management of benign and malignant tumors*. With *benign tumors*, the goal is to effect a complete removal while preserving the function of surrounding structures as much as possible. *Malignancies*, on the other hand, require an en bloc resection that includes adequate margins of healthy tissue. *Malignant tumors are considered to be operable* only if radical extirpation is feasible. In some circumstances this may re-

quire a unilateral sacrifice of vision, or the surgeon may have to ligate one of the internal carotid arteries, having first confirmed an adequate collateral flow. If a malignant tumor has invaded the area of the cavernous sinus and pterygopalatine fossa, we believe that radical removal is no longer an option. The same applies to cases in which radical extirpation would necessitate a bilateral sacrifice of vision.
With slow-growing malignancies and very extensive benign lesions, a *palliative operation* that removes only a portion of the tumor is justified in selected cases where the operation would offer a reasonable prospect of prolonging life or temporarily maintaining its quality.

General Operative Techniques

Extracranial Approach to the Anterior Skull Base

Introductory Remarks. A *malignant tumor* of the paranasal sinuses that has caused little or no bony destruction of the anterior skull base is exposed through the extracranial fronto-orbital approach. The bony skull base and adjacent involved dura are resected with adequate margins, and the *dura is grafted from below*. A *benign*, relatively extensive tumor can be approached by this route if it appears likely that it has not breached the dura. If dural penetration has occurred, there is a good chance that a portion of the tumor's blood supply is intracranial and that the lesion is in direct contact with vital centers. In this latter case, an intracranial exposure is indicated. If a malignant tumor has invaded the orbit, orbital exenteration is necessary. This will create sufficient room for performing an extensive resection of the anterior skull base and dura through the transfacial route with good visualization of basal brain structures.

Operative Technique

Extracranial Approach to the Anterior Skull Base with Preservation of the Orbital Contents and Lacrimal Ducts
(Fig. AS 33a-c)

The extracranial approach may be unilateral or bilateral. The incision starts beneath the eyebrow and extends paranasally toward the upper lip, its length depending on the extent of the tumor (Moure 1922). If maxillectomy is indicated, the exposure is extended laterally with a subciliary incision (Zange 1959). The soft tissues and periosteum, including the periorbita, are stripped from the bone, and the lacrimal sac is freed. Following removal of the lateral margin of the nasal bone, anterior ethmoid margin, and the lower portion of the anterior wall and floor of the frontal sinus, the tumor is exposed in stages by resecting the ethmoid cells and by opening the sphenoid sinus as required. If the tumor is benign, one should attempt to preserve as much mucosa as possible. A malignant tumor is resected with a generous margin of mucosa on all sides. Usually it is necessary to remove a piece of the tumor so that the portion adherent to the skull base can be clearly visualized for dissection. We use a burr to cut completely around the tumor through the bony skull base, using the operating microscope as required, and then separate the resected bone and residual tumor from the dura. If a malignant growth is found to have penetrated the bony skull base, an appropriate amount of dura is included in the resection. Duraplasty is carried out as previously described (see pp. 131–138). The dural graft is secured medially by tucking it between the osteochondral septum and septal mucosa. The cavity is lined with a large piece of silicone film to aid mucosal epithelialization. The duraplasty is supported with an intranasal ointment pack for 2–3 weeks. If the lamina papyracea has been included in the resection, care is taken that the pack does not exert undue pressure on the globe. With preservation of the frontal sinus mucosa, a silicone tube should be placed to establish adequate external drainage. Then the periosteum is closed with sutures. The skin is

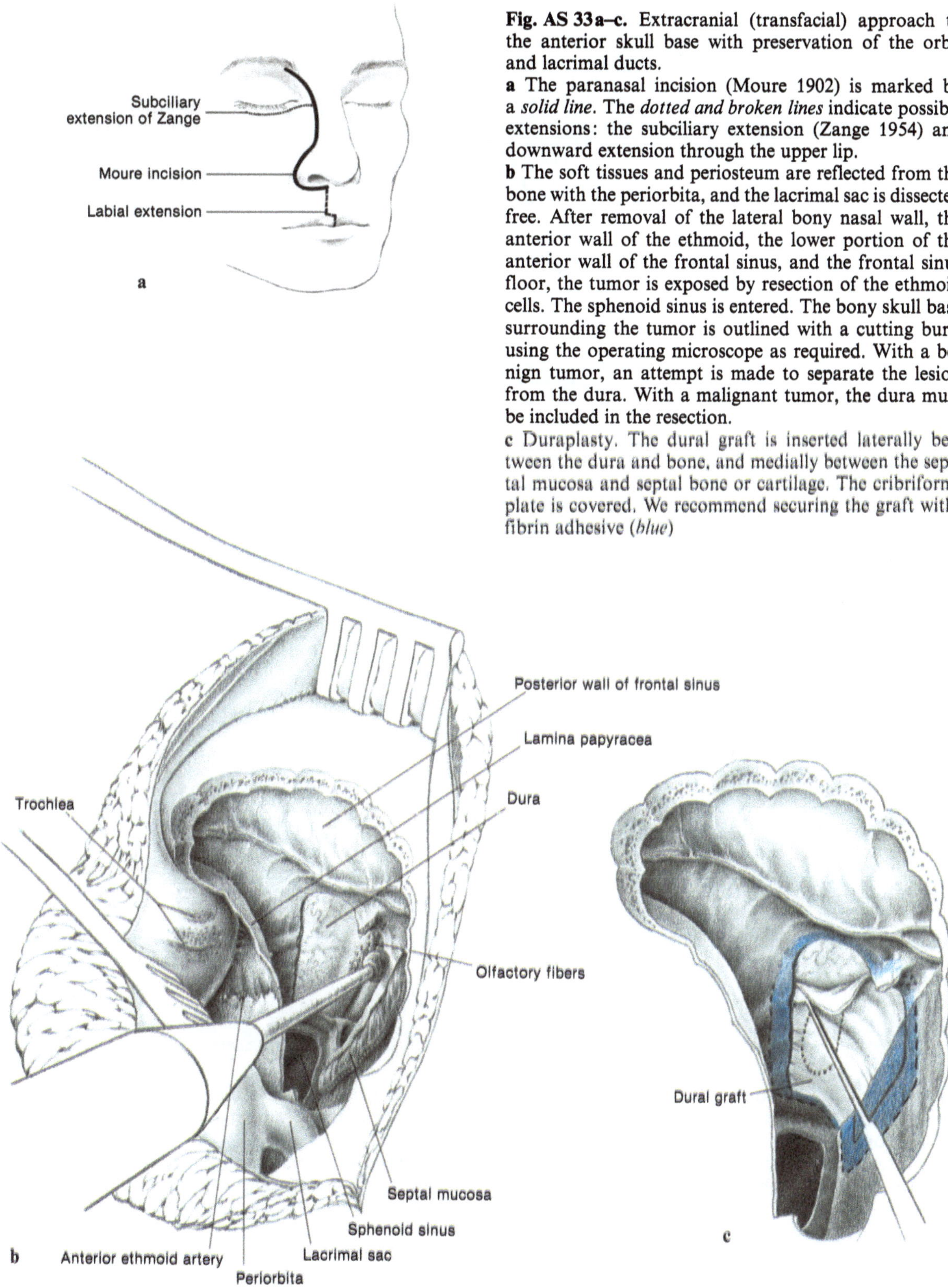

Fig. AS 33a–c. Extracranial (transfacial) approach to the anterior skull base with preservation of the orbit and lacrimal ducts.

a The paranasal incision (Moure 1902) is marked by a *solid line*. The *dotted and broken lines* indicate possible extensions: the subciliary extension (Zange 1954) and downward extension through the upper lip.

b The soft tissues and periosteum are reflected from the bone with the periorbita, and the lacrimal sac is dissected free. After removal of the lateral bony nasal wall, the anterior wall of the ethmoid, the lower portion of the anterior wall of the frontal sinus, and the frontal sinus floor, the tumor is exposed by resection of the ethmoid cells. The sphenoid sinus is entered. The bony skull base surrounding the tumor is outlined with a cutting burr, using the operating microscope as required. With a benign tumor, an attempt is made to separate the lesion from the dura. With a malignant tumor, the dura must be included in the resection.

c Duraplasty. The dural graft is inserted laterally between the dura and bone, and medially between the septal mucosa and septal bone or cartilage. The cribriform plate is covered. We recommend securing the graft with fibrin adhesive (*blue*)

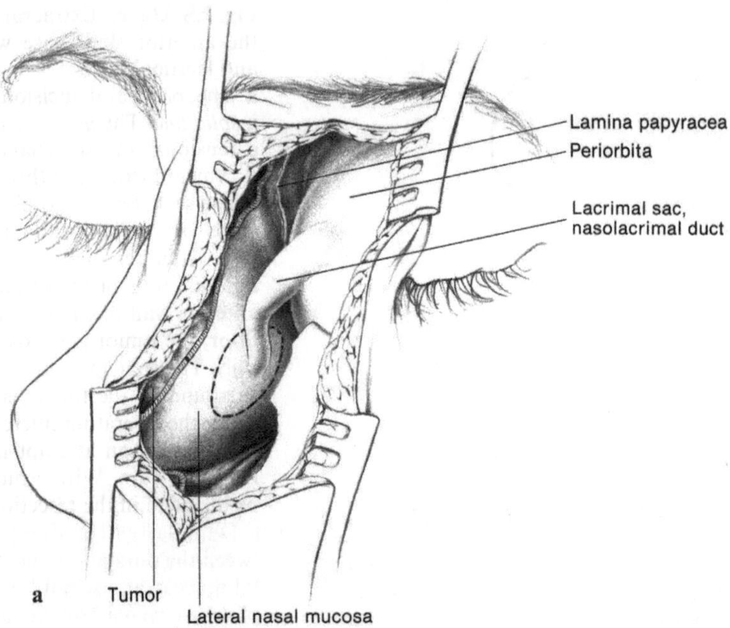

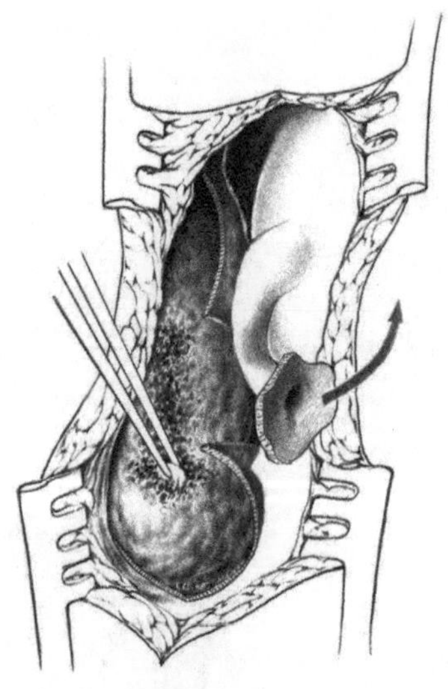

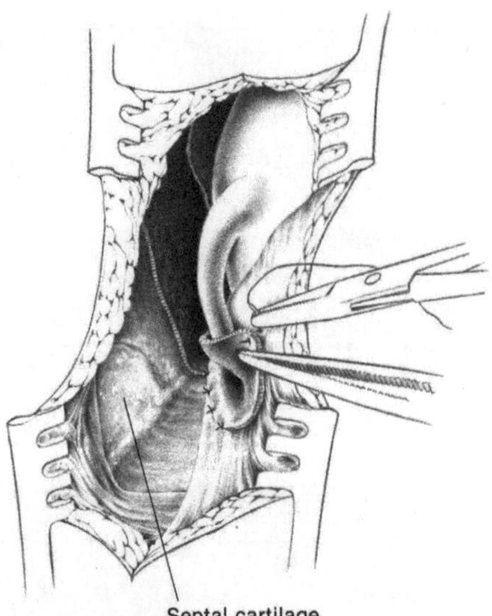

Fig. AS 34a–c. Preservation of lacrimal drainage in nasal and paranasal sinus tumor resections (Draf 1980). If large portions of the nasal mucosa and maxilla must be included in the resection, the orifice of the nasolacrimal duct is outlined with a scalpel in the nasal mucosa.

b The mobilized ductal orifice is retracted to the side. The tumor in the nasal cavity is removed with the surrounding mucosa.
c At the end of the operation, the stump of the nasolacrimal duct is sutured into the cheek flap with the opening directed nasally. Care is taken to avoid kinking of the duct

closed by intracutaneous suture to obtain a minimal scar.

Not infrequently, it is possible to *preserve the lacrimal ducts* in this procedure to avoid troublesome postoperative dacryorrhea. With highly situated benign tumors, the lacrimal sac and nasolacrimal duct are easily spared through careful dissection. If the tumor resection must include a significant portion of the nasal mucosa and maxilla, the drainage of tear fluid can be preserved by the following technique: A funnel-shaped cut is made around the orifice of the nasolacrimal duct in the nasal mucosa, freeing it so that the duct and lacrimal sac can be held to one side with a holding suture during the rest of the procedure (Fig. AS 34a–c). When the resection has been completed, the funnel-shaped stump is opened up and sutured into the reflected soft tissues of the cheek. We have found that the functional results of this transfer are favorable. If the orifice cannot be preserved, the nasolacrimal duct is resected as far back as necessary to enable the lacrimal sac to drain directly into the surgical cavity. It is beneficial to irrigate the nasolacrimal tract for several days postoperatively.

Extracranial Approach to the Anterior Skull Base with Unilateral Orbital Exenteration
(Fig. AS 35a–f)

The skin incision for this approach (Dieffenbach 1848, Fergusson 1857, Weber 1859, Moure 1902, Zange 1959) is shown in Fig. AS 35a. The paranasal incision extends a variable distance toward the upper lip, depending on the tumor extent. The lip is split if necessary, darting the incision to improve the cosmetic result. With ethmoid tumors, the extent of involvement of the medial canthus and orbit will determine how much of the upper and lower lids will have to be sacrificed. If the resection includes only the skin near the canthus, the remaining skin can be used to line the orbital cavity following the exenteration. The cheek flap is developed according to the degree of tumor extent. The tumor is encompassed from below by removing the anteroinferior wall and floor of the frontal sinus, the lateral nasal wall, and a portion of the frontal process of the maxillary bone and anterior wall of the maxillary sinus. The periosteum is incised around the superior orbital margin and freed. The optic nerve and the blood vessels entering the orbital apex are cut with curved scissors and coagulated with bipolar cautery so that the orbital contents can be included in the surgical specimen. This is followed by a partial or complete maxilloethmoidectomy, as circumstances require.

With maxillary and ethmoid tumors that have penetrated the orbit, intraoperative frozen-section examinations of the ethmoid roof mucosa may be positive for tumor even if there was no radiographic or clinical evidence of skull base infiltration prior to surgery. It is possible in such cases to follow orbital exenteration with resection of the adjacent anterior skull base from below, possibly including the cribriform plate and contralateral ethmoid roof. After removal of the frontal sinus floor and lateral bony nasal wall and exenteration of the ethmoid, the adjacent anterior skull base can be readily evaluated. The lateral nasal wall is resected medially to the nasal root. The area of the skull base involved by tumor is then outlined with a diamond burr. The maximum anteroposterior extent of the bone resection is from the anterior margin of the crista galli reaching to about the middle of the roof of the sphenoid sinus. The resection may be extended laterally to include the orbital roof as required. The exposed dura is adequately mobilized with a small elevator about the circumference of the bony resection defect; microsurgical dissection has proved useful at this stage. To guard against infection, the rest of the field should be packed off with cotton paddies before the dura is incised. In the area of the crista galli it is especially important that the dura be adequately elevated on both sides. If the basal skull base resection extends far anteriorly, the superior sagittal sinus is doubly underrun and ligated. The dura is resected in stepwise fashion, pulling it downward with a sharp hook or fine forceps to avoid brain injury. Before any area of the dura is incised, that area and the vessels within it are first coagulated with bipolar current to reduce bleeding. The incision

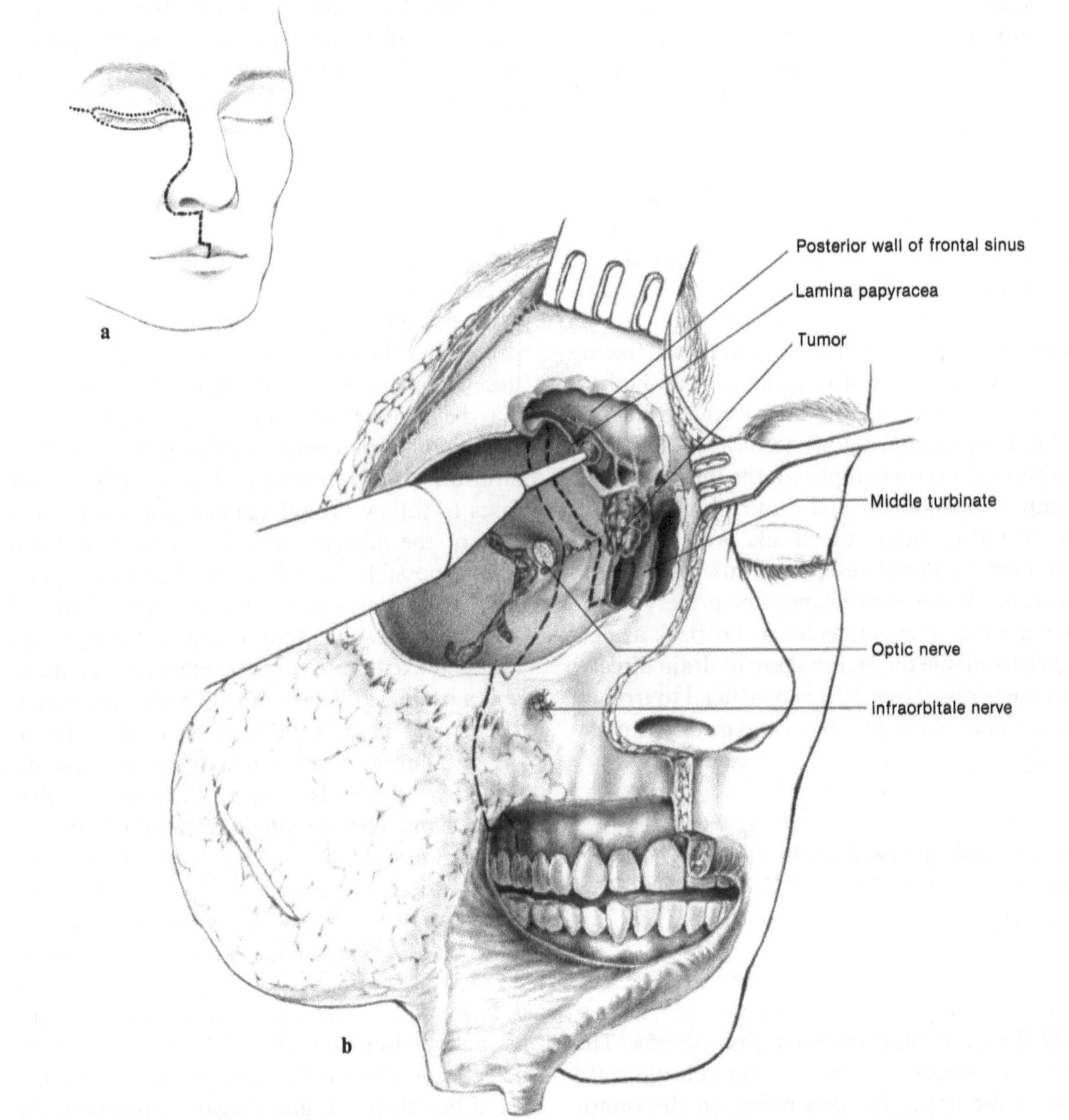

Fig. AS 35a–f. Extracranial approach to the anterior skull base with unilateral orbital exenteration.

a The incision for orbital exenteration surrounds the ciliary margin. The paranasal incision may extend down through the upper lip, according to oncologic requirements.

b The tumor is widely resected with an adequate margin of surrounding bone; an en bloc resection is preferred. The *broken lines* indicate the extent of the bone resection for ethmoidectomy and maxillectomy. The orbital contents are removed. The skull base around the tumor is resected with a burr, making sure to obtain adequate margins.

c The dura of the anterior cranial fossa is exposed widely on the tumor side, less widely on the opposite site, and the crista galli is removed following elevation of the dura. A small elevator is used to mobilize the dura beyond the cut edges of the bone. The sphenoid sinus is opened. The *broken line* shows the extent of the dural resection.

d Before the dura is incised, the site is packed off with cottonoid, and the incision lines are cauterized. Then the dura is pulled downward with a forceps, incised, and resected.

e The dural defect is repaired with a dural graft inserted between the bone and dura; medially it may be tucked between the septal mucosa and septal bone

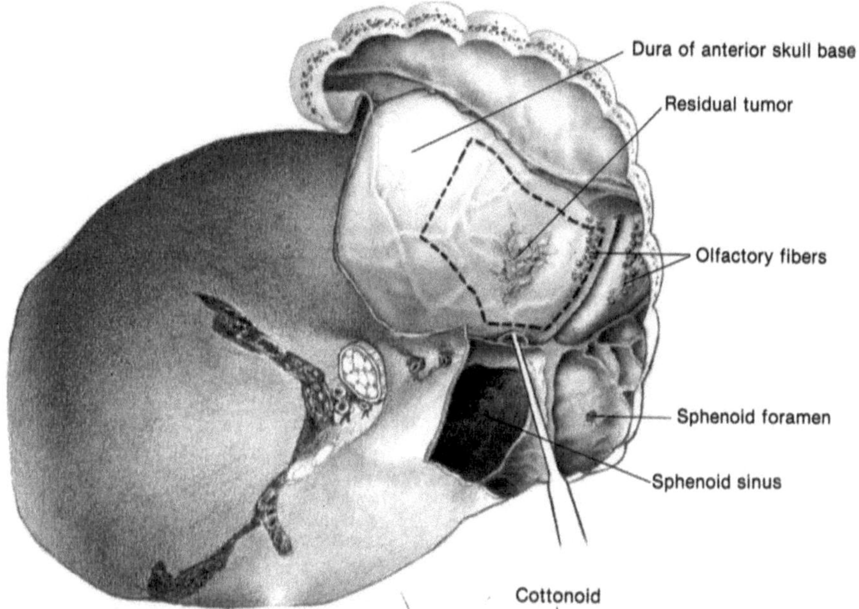
Dura of anterior skull base
Residual tumor
Olfactory fibers
Sphenoid foramen
Sphenoid sinus

c

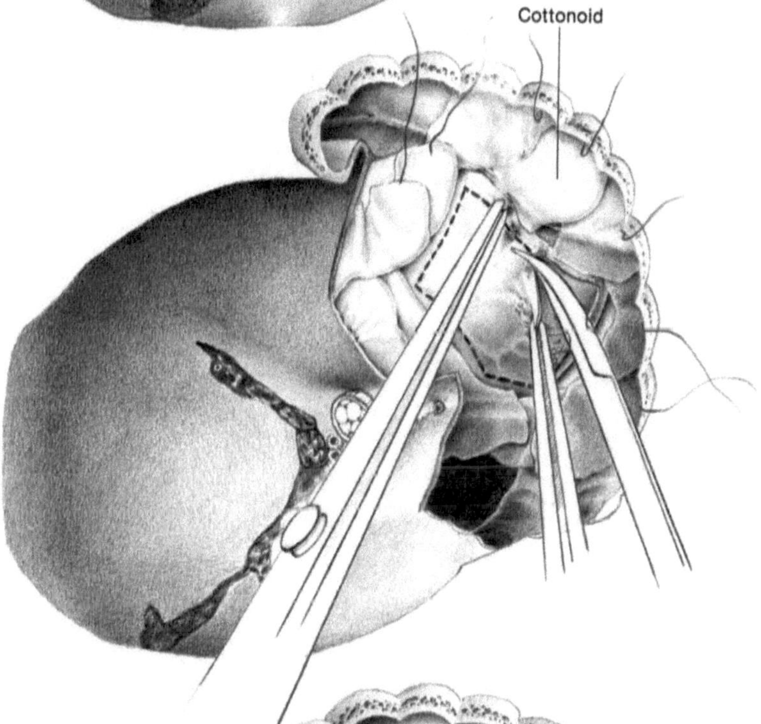
Cottonoid

d

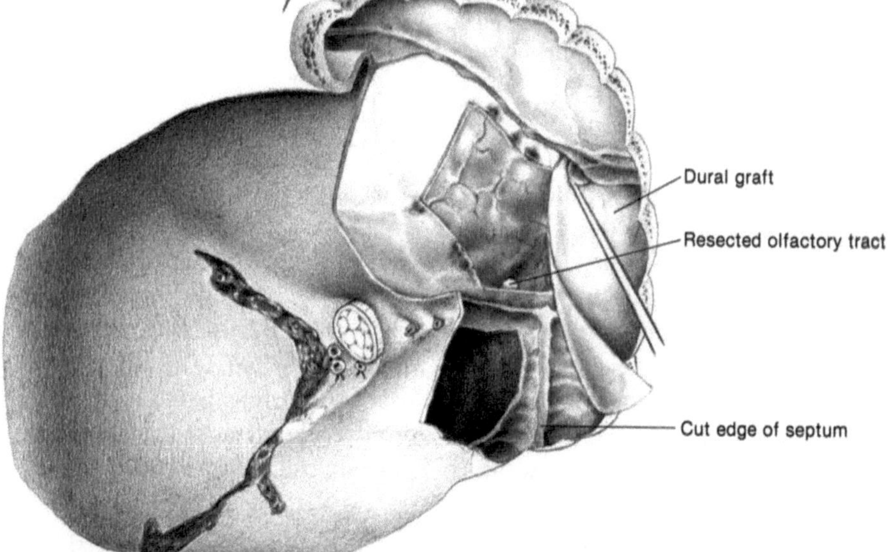
Dural graft
Resected olfactory tract
Cut edge of septum

e

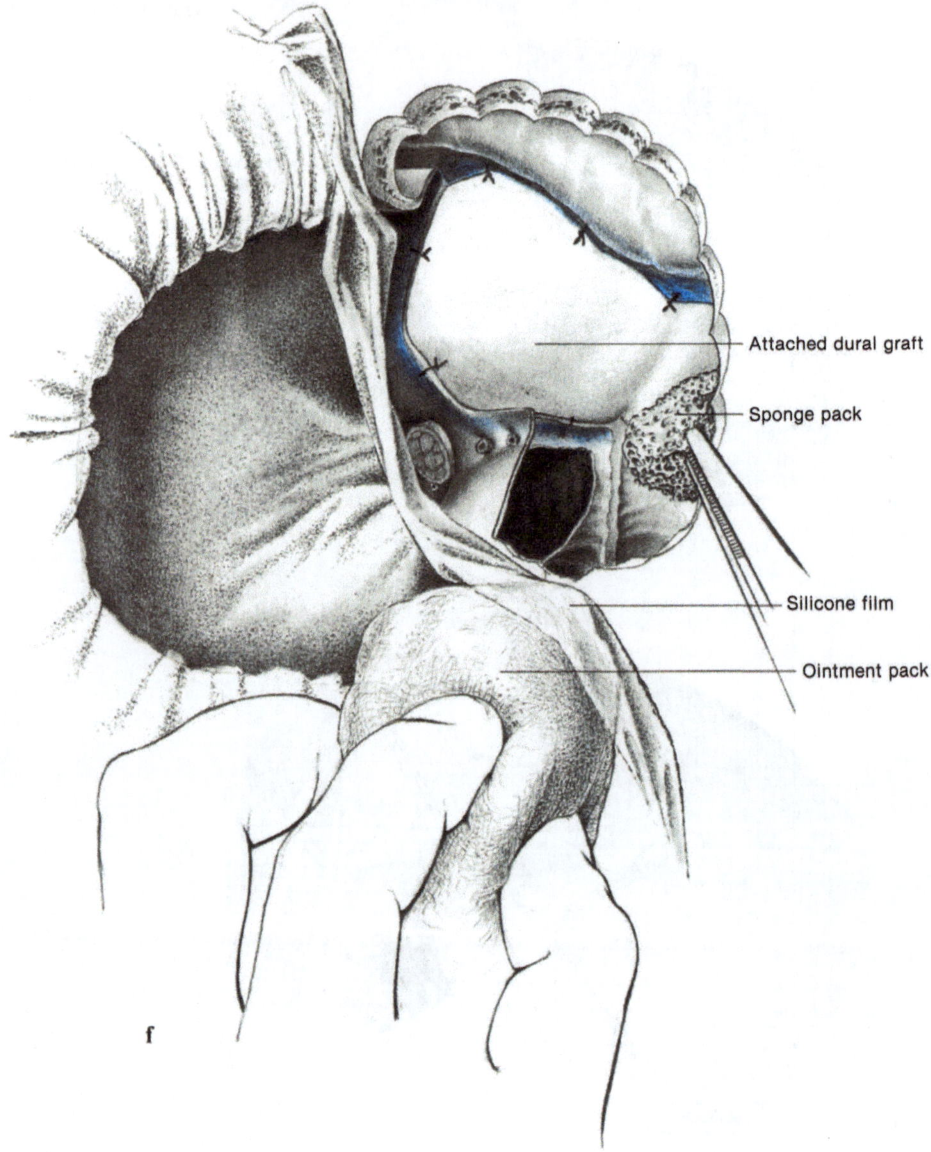

Fig. AS 35. f The graft is secured with fibrin adhesive and a few sutures and is covered with sponge packing. Finally the entire surgical cavity is lined with silicone film to promote mucosal epithelialization; the film is held in place with an ointment pack

is started at the anterior limit of the craniectomy so that the resection can proceed with a clear view of the base of the frontal lobe. Bleeding cerebral cortical vessels are coagulated. The resected piece of dura is labeled and sent for histologic evaluation, and the defect is patched with a suitably trimmed piece of stored dura tucked between the bone and dural margins. The graft is secured with fibrin adhesive and a few all-layer sutures, which may be placed through fine drill holes in the bone. The graft is covered with sponge packing, the entire cavity is lined with silicone film, and the duraplasty is supported with a maxillo-orbital ointment pack for 14 days, if possible, until it has become stable. The basal skull defect patched with the lyophilized dura will become epithelialized from the remaining mucosal margins. Within a few weeks the

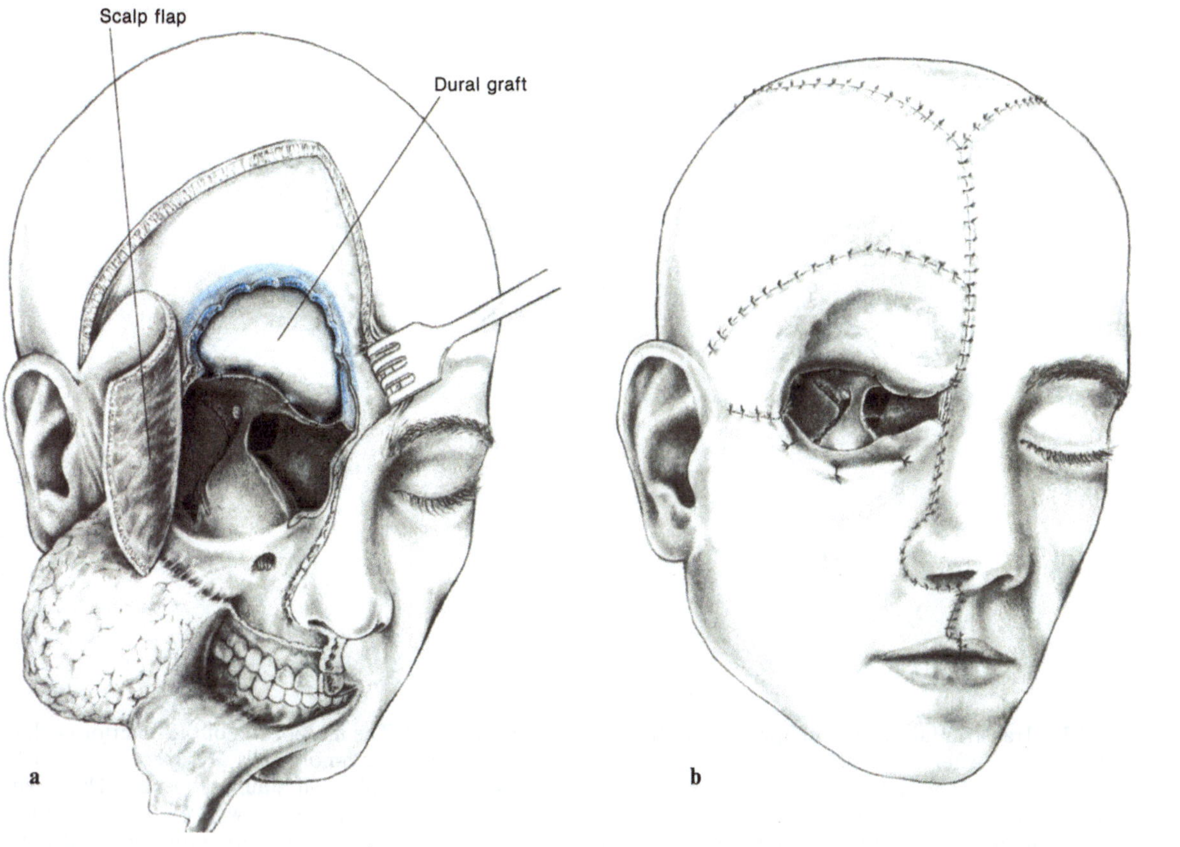

Fig. AS 36a, b. Epithelialization of the skull base and orbit with the aid of a forehead scalp flap.
a Situation after tumor removal and dissection of the forehead scalp flap.
b The scalp flap is sutured in place to cover the duraplasty. Its donor site is covered by advancing other scalp flaps

initially sagging dural graft will become transformed into a flat, firm sheet of scar tissue. If the resection of the anterior skull base extends beyond the ethmoid roof and cribriform plate, a forehead or scalp flap conforming to the size of the cranial defect should be advanced to provide stable coverage of the duraplasty and achieve epithelialization of the remaining orbital and ethmoid roof. The donor area of the scalp flap can be covered with split-thickness skin or by the advancement of other scalp flaps (Fig. AS 36a, b, Shah and Galicich 1977).

Intracranial Approach to the Anterior Skull Base

Introductory Remarks. A distinction is made between the intracranial, primarily extradural approach as described by Unterberger (1958) and others for the treatment of frontobasal injuries (see p. 141) and the intracranial, intradural route. Lesions of the anterior skull base that are largely outside the dura can be exposed extradurally by elevating the dura. This involves division of the olfactory fibers at their site of emergence from the cribriform plate, and one cannot always avoid the creation of small dural rents. Lesions that arise from the dura itself or lesions that have penetrated the dura, such as meningiomas, are an indication for the transfrontal intradural exposure.

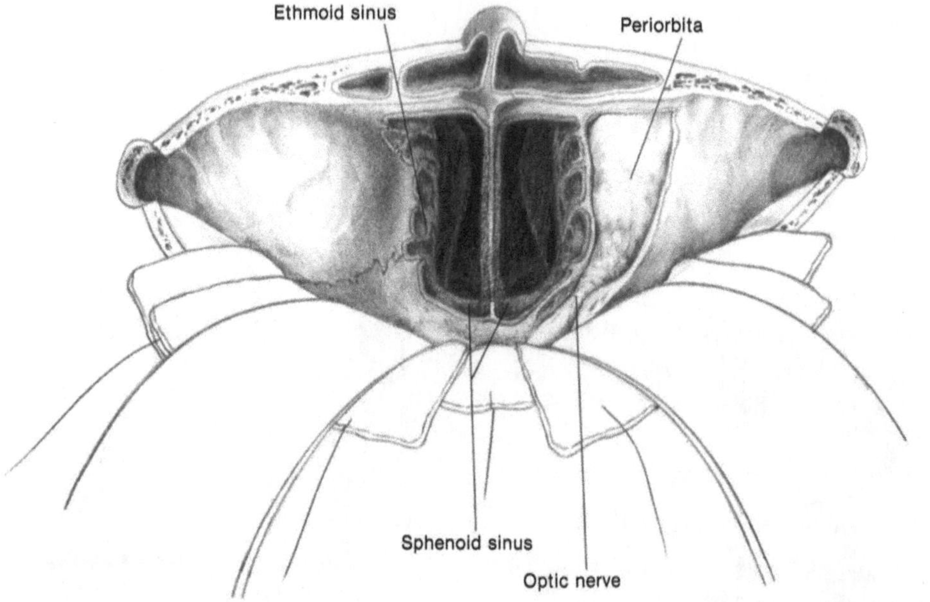

Fig. AS 37. Transfrontal extradural approach to the anterior skull base. After bifrontal craniotomy the anterior skull base is exposed extradurally to the minor sphenoid wings. The falx is divided, sparing the superior sagittal sinus. On the midline the dura is mobilized to within several millimeters of the posterior limit of the bony optic canal. The intracranial part of the optic nerve is not visualized. The midportion of the anterior skull base is removed, the ethmoid cells are exenterated on both sides, and the sphenoid sinus is opened. The clivus is reached along the posterior wall of the sinus. On the right side the optic nerve is decompressed, and the medial part of the orbital roof is removed, sparing the periorbita and the dural sheath of the optic nerve

Operative Technique

The Transfrontal Extradural Approach (Fig. AS 37)

A bitemporal coronal incision is made, a scalp flap is developed (see p. 139), and a unilateral or bilateral frontal osteoplastic craniotomy is performed whose extent depends on the size of the tumor. If the tumor is situated on the midline, the dura is mobilized on both sides of the crista galli and is elevated from the cribriform plate using sharp dissection as required. If necessary, the dura can be mobilized bilaterally as far back as the lesser sphenoid wings and tuberculum sellae to gain broad exposure of the anterior skull base. This approach also gives good exposure of the frontal sinus, ethmoid cells, and sphenoid sinus (possibly with removal of the crista galli) and of the optic canal and superior aspect of the orbital contents (see p. 141). The optic chiasm with the intradural portion of the optic nerve is not visualized. Lesions extending to the clivus are accessible by dissecting along the posterior wall of the sphenoid sinus or anterior wall of the sella. If a small dural defect is created, the cranial cavity can be sealed off from the paranasal sinuses with a dural graft (see Fig. AS 22b) or free fascial graft. Larger defects are more effectively sealed with a galeal pericranial flap (see Fig. AS 21b). The need for a multilayer reconstruction will depend on the size of the defect in the bony skull base (see p. 174). If the bone resection extends beyond the cribriform plate and ethmoid roof on both sides, it usually will be necessary to stabilize the skull base with measures that go beyond a simple duraplasty.

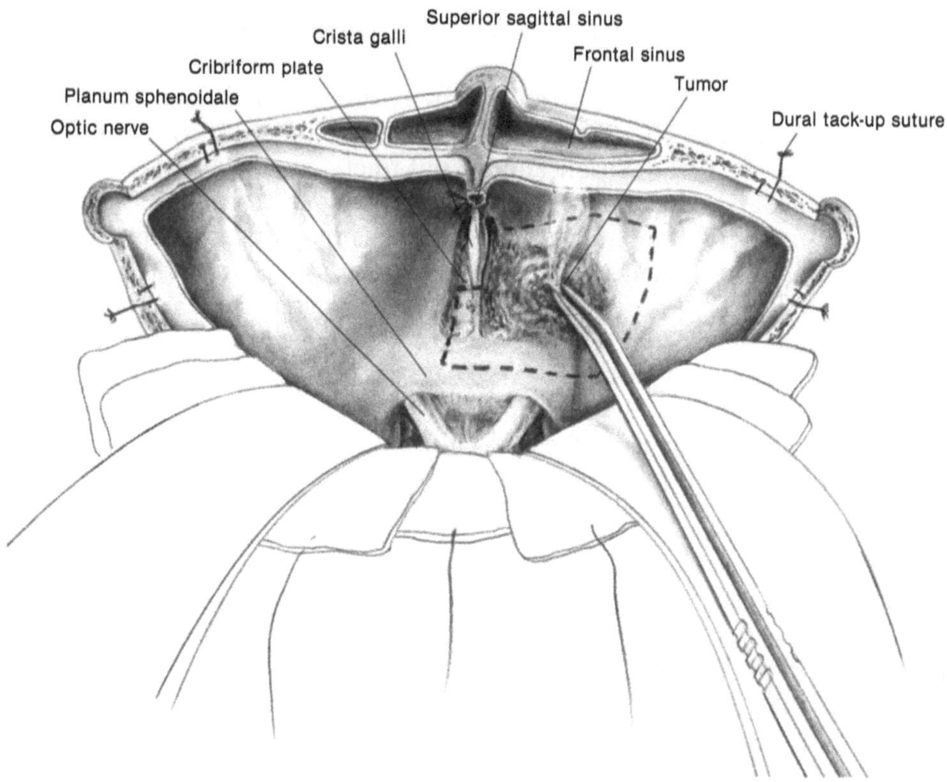

Fig. AS 38. Transfrontal intradural approach to the anterior skull base. Bifrontal craniotomy is performed, and the superior sagittal sinus is doubly ligated and divided. Both frontal lobes are retracted. The tumor is removed down to the skull base. The *broken line* shows the extent of the dural and skull base resection. The optic chiasm and intradural portion of the optic nerve can be visualized in this approach

The Transfrontal Intradural Approach
(Fig. AS 38)

The skull is opened with a unilateral or bilateral frontal craniotomy. The dura is opened from the lateral side, working toward the superior sagittal sinus, which is doubly underrun and ligated. The frontal lobes are gently retracted while cerebrospinal fluid is drained. The frontal lobes are protected with cotton paddies before the self-retaining brain spatula is introduced. The intradural portion of the tumor is exposed and progressively isolated. The tumor capsule is incised, and tumor is removed down to the level of the skull base, using bipolar cautery as the resection proceeds. At this time it will be possible to delineate the involved area of dura on the skull base. That part of the dura is resected with an adequate margin. Any extensions of tumor into the nose, paranasal sinuses, or orbit are removed as required. The operation concludes with a duraplasty or skull base reconstruction (see p. 174). Repair of the dura and replacement of the skull flap are the same as in the treatment of comminuted anterior basal skull fractures (see p. 139).

Combined Intra- and Extracranial (Craniofacial) Approach to the Anterior Skull Base

Introductory Remarks. The craniofacial approach to the anterior skull base was first described by Ketcham et al. (1963). Since then it has been used by numerous authors, often in modified form (Clifford 1980, Derome 1972,

Donald 1981, Guggenheim and Kleitsch 1967, Johns et al. 1981, Ketcham et al. 1966, 1969, Krekorian and Kempe 1969, Littlewood and Maisels 1970, Schramm et al. 1979, Shah and Galicich 1977, Sisson et al. 1976, Wilson and Westbury 1973). Supance and Seid used a craniofacial procedure in 1981 for the removal of an undifferentiated ethmoid carcinoma in a 14-year-old boy.

Although many tumors can be completely removed through a *single* approach (either extracranial or intracranial), especially if they are benign, it may be appropriate to combine the extra- and intracranial approaches in *one* stage for the following reasons:

1) To ensure the radical, en bloc resection of a malignant neoplasm or a benign tumor recurrence.
2) To ensure the complete resection of tumors that have equal intra- and extracranial extents.
3) To reduce, through better exposure, concomitant injuries to the skull base region opposite the surgical cavity.

Microsurgical techniques are additionally recommended as a means of preserving function and facilitating reconstruction. They can improve the prognosis of malignancies and decrease the likelihood of benign tumor recurrence. The nature of the tumor and its primary localization will determine whether the extra- or intracranial part of the operation is done first. One must also consider the degree to which preoperative clinical and radiologic studies have been able to establish the tumor extent. With *malignancies of the upper paranasal sinuses and orbit*, the tumor can be encompassed from below initially, and the surgeon can mark the area of involvement of the skull base. This can shorten the duration of the intracranial part of the procedure and lower the risk of infection. The next phase involves the intracranial, intradural resection of the anterior skull base and affected dura and of involved adjacent portions of the frontal lobe if required. The skull base is then removed en bloc with the total specimen. If it is known preoperatively which portion of the anterior skull base has to be resected, the surgeon may perform the cranial part of the operation first. This is true even in the case of a primary intracranial tumor that has spread to the skull base and invaded the upper paranasal sinus tract.

With very extensive, benign intra/extracranial tumors that are not completely resectable, a two-stage, palliative craniofacial resection should be considered before signs of cerebral compression and irreversible cranial nerve damage appear.

Operative Technique
(Fig. AS 39a–i)

We reemphasize that the sequence of the operative steps may be varied as circumstances require.

1) Intracranial, Intradural Part of the Operation

A bilaterally based scalp flap is developed in the supraorbital region from a bifrontal coronal incision. Burr holes are placed, and a bifrontal craniotomy or craniectomy is performed, depending on the nature and extent of the tumor and the degree of frontal sinus involvement. Benign tumors are usually exposed through an osteoplastic craniotomy. The dura is incised, and the superior sagittal sinus is doubly ligated and divided together with the falx. With malignant tumors, the dural incision is placed higher (farther away from the pathological process) than with benign lesions. The frontal lobes are covered with cotton paddies and gently retracted while cerebrospinal fluid is drained. This permits exposure of the entire anterior skull base up to the optic chiasm.

With a *malignant tumor*, the involved dura and bony skull base are resected with adequate margins, and the bloc is displaced inferiorly toward the paranasal sinuses. Portions of the posterior and anterior frontal sinus walls and orbital contents are also resected as required.

With a *benign tumor* that does not involve the dura extensively, the dura is separated bilateral-

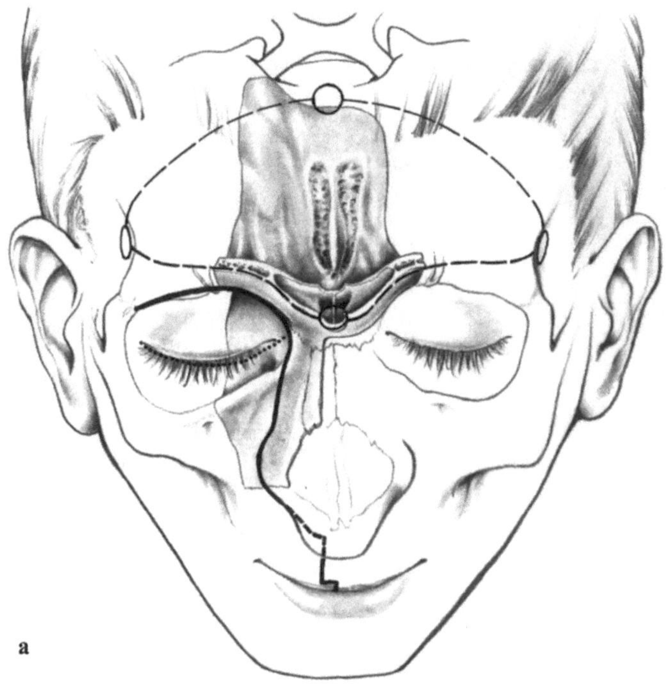

a

Fig. AS 39a–i. Craniofacial approach to the anterior skull base.
a–c *Intracranial, intradural part of the operation* (tumor removal). **a** The *broken line* in the frontal area indicates the extent of the bifrontal craniotomy or craniectomy. The burr hole sites are shown. The facial incision (——) is shown for the case where orbital exenteration is not required. The *dotted line* shows the subciliary extension that would be needed for orbital exenteration

ly from the crista galli and from the lateral margins of the cribriform plate to create a pair of laterally based dural flaps. These flaps will later be used to form the caudal layer of the skull base reconstruction. The flaps having been raised, the involved area of the bony skull base is resected with a burr and displaced inferiorly en bloc with the tumor. If the skull base is not to be closed until after the extracranial part of the operation, the communication between the cranial cavity and paranasal sinuses is temporarily occluded with a dural graft and cotton paddies as a precaution against infection.

2) Extracranial Part of the Operation

The second stage of the operation corresponds to the extracranial approach to the anterior skull base described earlier. The nature and extent of the tumor will determine whether the orbit on the affected side is respected or exenterated. After the tumor has been encompassed transfacially, it is delivered in one piece through the facial wound along with the inferiorly displaced intracranial structures.

3) Three-Layer Reconstruction of the Skull Base

While smaller defects of the bony anterior skull base are satisfactorily repaired in two layers with dura or dural graft covered by a galeal pericranial flap, it is safer in more extensive bone resections to interpose a stabilizing layer of methylmethacrylate between the dural layer and galeal flap (Draf and Samii 1977).

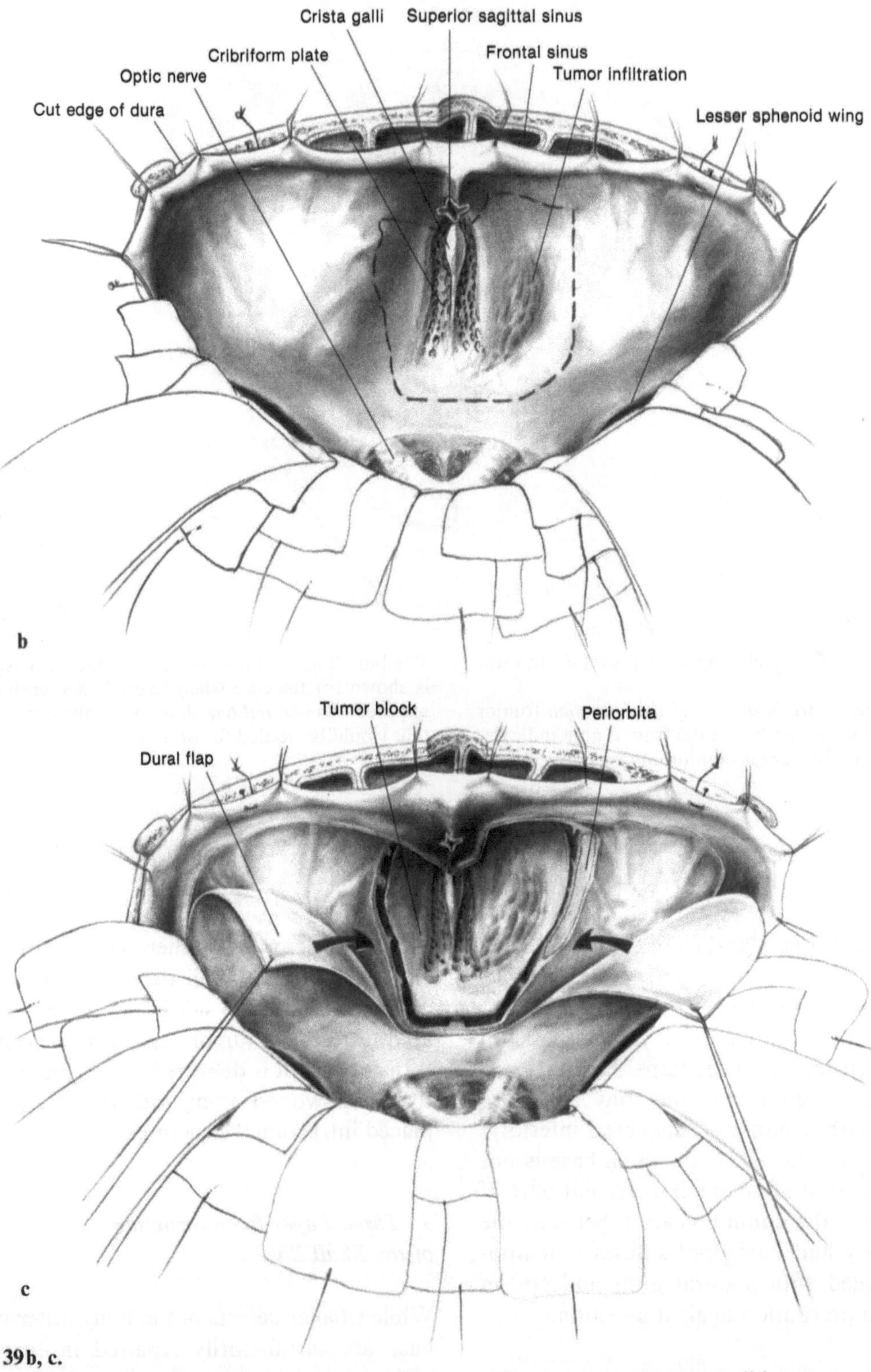

Fig. AS 39b, c.

b After bifrontal craniotomy, ligation of the superior sagittal sinus, and incision of the dura, the frontal lobes are retracted back to the minor sphenoid wings and optic nerves. Tumor infiltration of the dura is apparent over the right ethmoid roof. The *broken line* shows the extent of the dural and osseous skull base resection.

c The dura and adjacent skull base are resected around the tumor and displaced caudally. Lateral dural flaps are created and will be rotated medially for skull base resurfacing

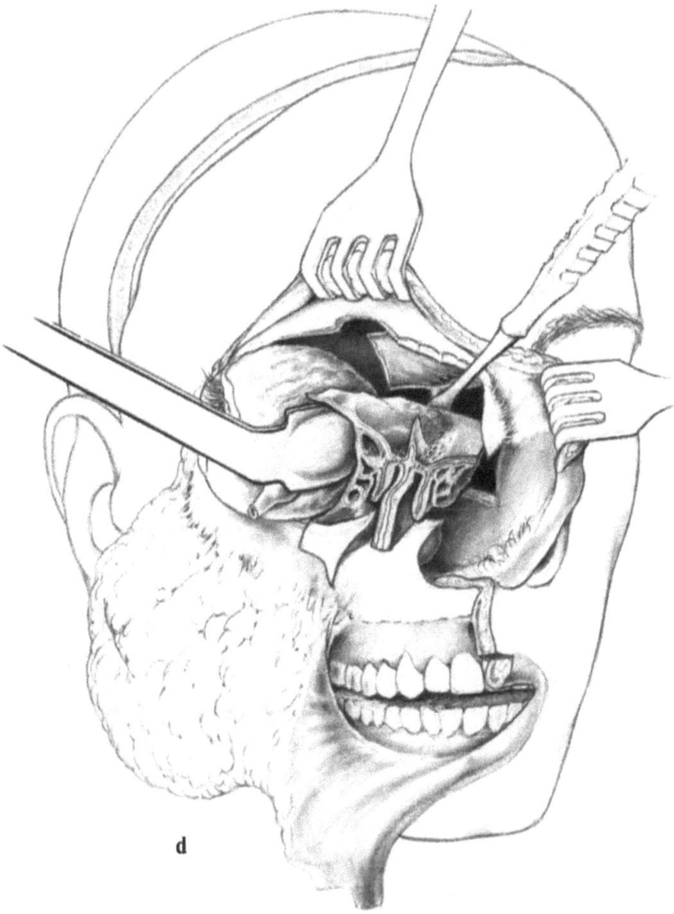

Fig. AS 39. d In the *second, facial part of the operation* the tumor block is delivered through the facial wound with the adjacent portions of the paranasal sinuses. The specimen may or may not include the orbital contents, depending on the tumor extent and histology.

If the *dura* of the anterior skull base is intact, it is easily reapproximated at the midline with simple interrupted sutures. If both the dura and bone have been resected, the dura can be mobilized on both sides to create unilateral or bilateral, posteriorly based rotation flaps that can be apposed over the part of the skull base in continuity with the nose and paranasal sinuses. The residual lateral gap in the skull base can be sealed off from the orbit with a patch of lyophilized dura.

In rare cases the resection of the skull base and dura is so extensive that the lowermost layer of the reconstruction cannot be formed by dura. In these cases it is possible to divide the outer *aponeurotic layer* of the reflected *temporal muscle* at the level of the zygomatic arch and strip it upward. To optimize the blood supply to this fibrous tissue band, about 2 cm of it is left attached to the muscle superiorly. After partial removal of the temporal squama, the band can be transposed to cover the anterior skull base to the midline. This may be done on both sides in extreme cases, especially if pericranium is not available as a covering for the methylmethacrylate.

With skull base tumors that originate from the skin or have infiltrated large cutaneous areas from deeper levels and thus necessitate a concomitant resection of the facial soft tissues, the

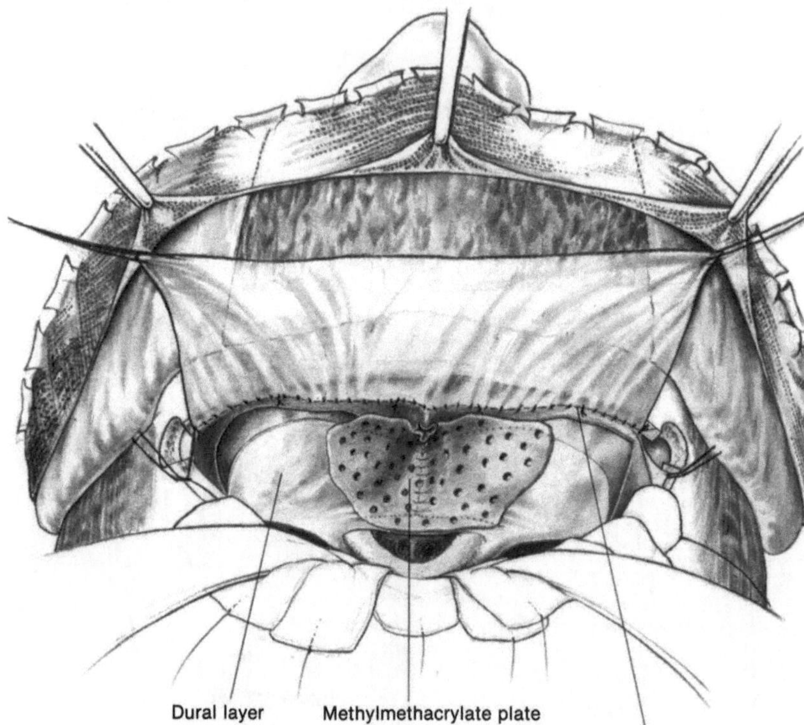

e

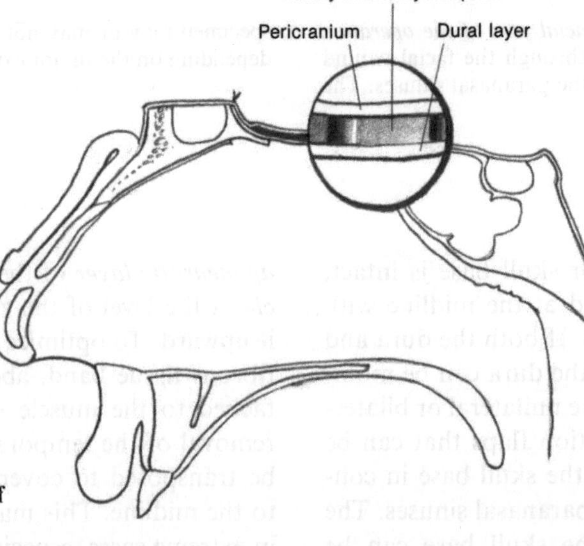

f

Fig. AS 39e–i. *Three-layer reconstruction of the skull base.*
e If possible, the dura of the anterior skull base is used to make rotation flaps that form the caudal layer of the reconstruction. This layer is covered by a suitably molded methylmethacrylate implant that overlaps the osseous defect. The implant is perforated for scar tissue ingrowth. The innermost layer is formed by swinging an inferiorly based galeal pericranial flap over the plastic implant. The flap is first sutured to the inferior dural margin and then fixed to the minor sphenoid wings with fibrin adhesive and posterior fixation sutures. **f** Sagittal section of the three-layer cranioplasty showing the relative positions of the dural layer, the plastic implant, and the galeal pericranial flap. This technique surrounds the plastic implant with viable tissue on all sides

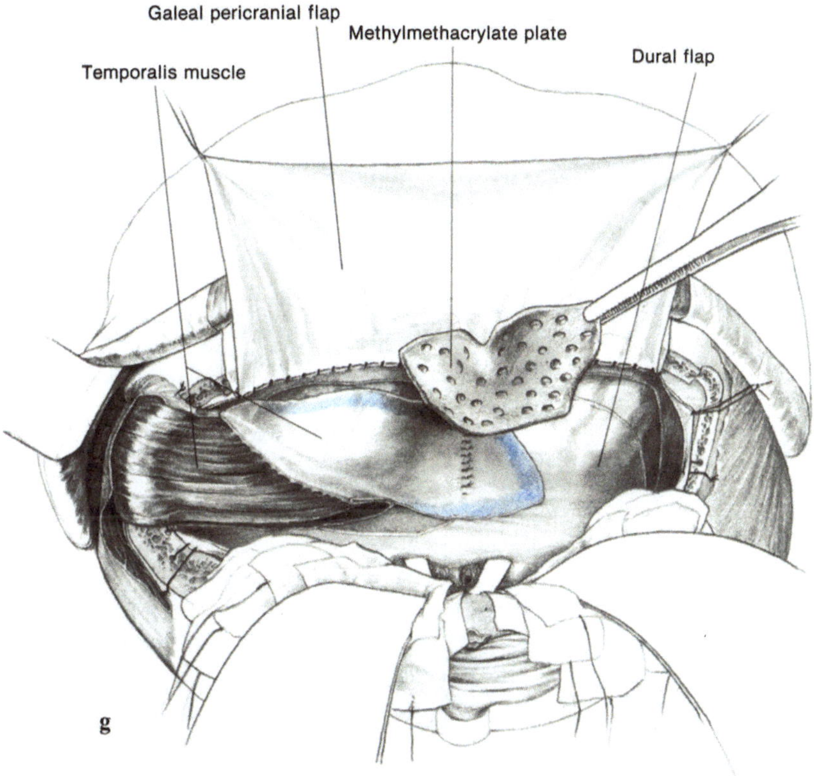

g

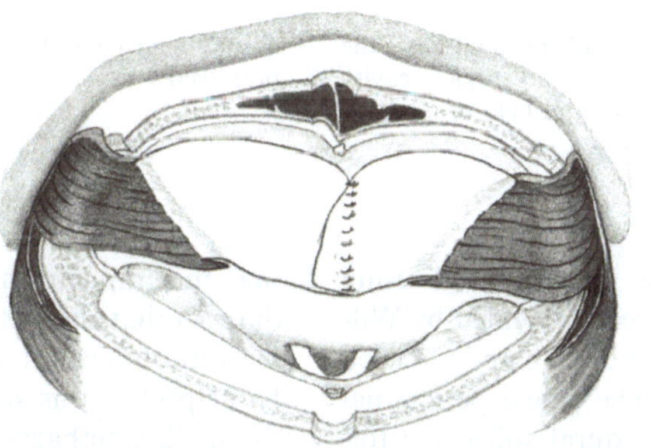

h

Fig. AS 39. g, h In extreme cases where it is necessary to resect up to 2/3 of the anterior skull base and overlying dura, the caudal layer of the reconstruction may consist of temporal muscle instead of dura. The outer aponeurotic layer is stripped upward, effectively doubling the muscle length. A portion of the temporal bone is removed, and the muscle flap is attached to the skull base with adhesive and additionally fixed with sutures. Retraction of the muscle is prevented by fixing it to the bone margins. If a galeal pericranial flap is not available for covering the plastic plate, the contralateral temporal muscle may be mobilized as a substitute

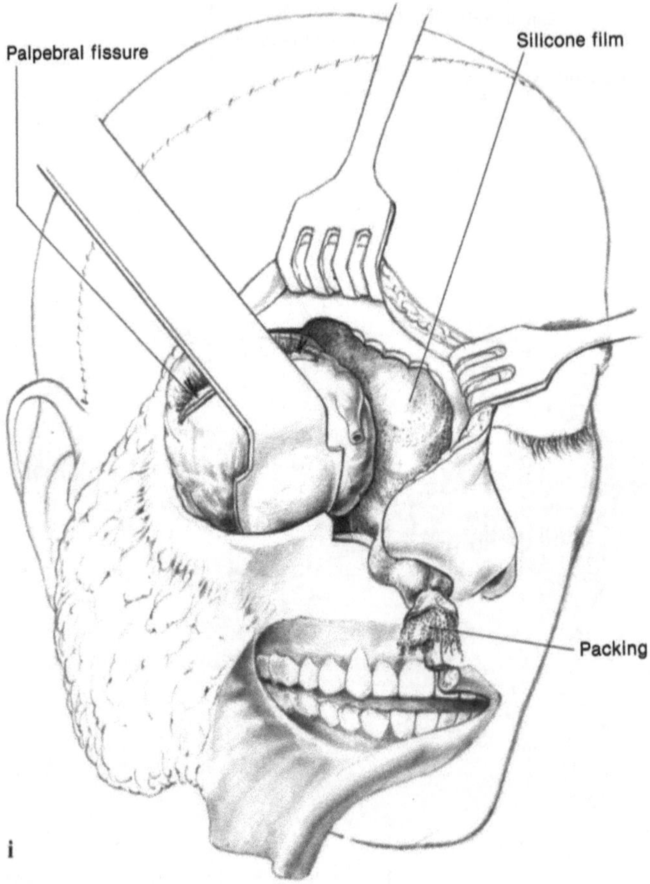

Fig. AS 39. i After reconstruction of the skull base, the scalp flap is replaced and sutured. The surgical cavity is lined transfacially with silicone film held in place by an ointment pack. Here the orbital contents have been preserved

orbit and skull base are reconstructed using *forehead or scalp flaps* as recommended by Wilson and Westbury (1973) and Shah and Galicich (1977) (Fig. AS 36a, b). The galeal pericranial flap also provides a good dural substitute following more extensive dural resections.

Unlike other authors (Schramm et al. 1979), we try to avoid using free skin grafts or pedicled skin flaps as the caudal layer for skull base reconstructions. Not infrequently, this is followed by a crusting that is unpleasant for the patient.

Next the *methylmethacrylate implant* is inserted as the *intermediate layer* of the reconstruction. It is individually molded to conform to the defect and should overlap all the margins of the basal skull defect. In the final phase of hardening, the implant should be elevated from the dura so that the latter is not damaged by polymerization heat; irrigation with cold saline can be helpful at this stage. Before it is implanted, the methylmethacrylate is perforated with drill holes to achieve the desired cicatrization.

Derome (1972) reconstruct the skull base defect with cortical and cancellous bone from the iliac crest and ribs. We feel that this somewhat more involved alternative is justified only in exceptional cases.

Finally the *innermost layer* of the reconstruction is formed from an inferiorly based galeal pericranial flap. The base of the flap is first attached to the caudal dural margin, and after fixation sutures are placed in the planum sphenoidale and lesser sphenoid wing, the flap is drawn as far back over the skull base as possible and sutured to the cranial dural margin. If a skull flap exists, it is replaced after first carefully removing any frontal sinus mucosa from the flap and freshening the bone with a burr to prevent secondary infection and mucocele formation. The burr holes for the craniotomy are patched with methylmethacrylate. Craniectomy defects are similarly repaired. After the scalp has been repositioned and sutured, the inferior aspect of the skull base is inspected transfacially, the surgical cavity in the facial skeleton is lined with silicone to aid mucosal reepithelialization, packing is inserted, and the facial soft tissues are closed.

Surgery of Space-Occupying Lesions of the Orbit and Adjacent Skull Base

Introductory Remarks. Because advanced tumors of the skull base produce a mass lesion in the orbit, and because primary tumors of the orbit can spread to involve the cranial base, surgical approaches to the orbit form an integral part of skull base surgery. Orbital involvement is manifested clinically by the gradual development of proptosis, visual deterioration, and disturbances of ocular motility.
The choice of operative treatment depends on the extent of skull base involvement and on the location of the tumor in the orbit (Henderson 1980).

Operative Technique

Basically the following *surgical approaches* are available (Fig. AS 40):

1) Simple Orbitotomy

This is an anterior approach to the orbit through an incision along the bony orbital margin. Its course in the anterior part of the orbit depends on the site of the tumor.

Following incision of the skin, the periosteum is incised at the orbital margin and progressively mobilized. Opening of Tenon's capsule should be delayed until the time of tumor removal to avoid the troublesome herniation of orbital fat. If necessary, the portion of the skull base adjacent to the orbit can be resected with the tumor. The dura may be included in the resection, necessitating a subsequent duraplasty. The periorbita is closed with interrupted sutures and a dural graft to avoid orbital fat adhesions with restricted ocular motility.

2) Transmaxillary Orbitotomy
(A. Seiffert 1926, O. Hirsch 1929)

The transmaxillary approach is appropriate for circumscribed lesions affecting both the maxillary sinus and orbit, for excisional biopsies, for the complete removal of circumscribed benign masses such as retrobulbar hemangiomas and cysts (Denecke 1954), and for decompression in endocrine ophthalmopathy (Hirsch 1929). With lesions that have spread to the skull base, this approach permits no more than an excisional biopsy as a basis for further treatment planning.

3) Bony Orbitotomy

a) The *transfrontoethmoidal approach through the paranasal sinuses* is used for exposures of the medial orbital wall and medial part of the orbital roof. The approach is like that for an external frontoethmoidectomy, as might be performed for optic nerve decompression (see p. 150 and Fig. AS 26a, b). After reflection of the soft tissues and periosteum, the anterior ethmoid margin and lateral bony nasal wall are partially resected, the lacrimal sac is displaced laterally, and the lamina papyracea and orbital roof are resected with the tumor, simultaneously removing the periorbita and portions of the orbital contents as required. The resection may be continued in this way to the orbital apex. An effort is made at the end of the procedure to restore the mobilized trochlea of the superior

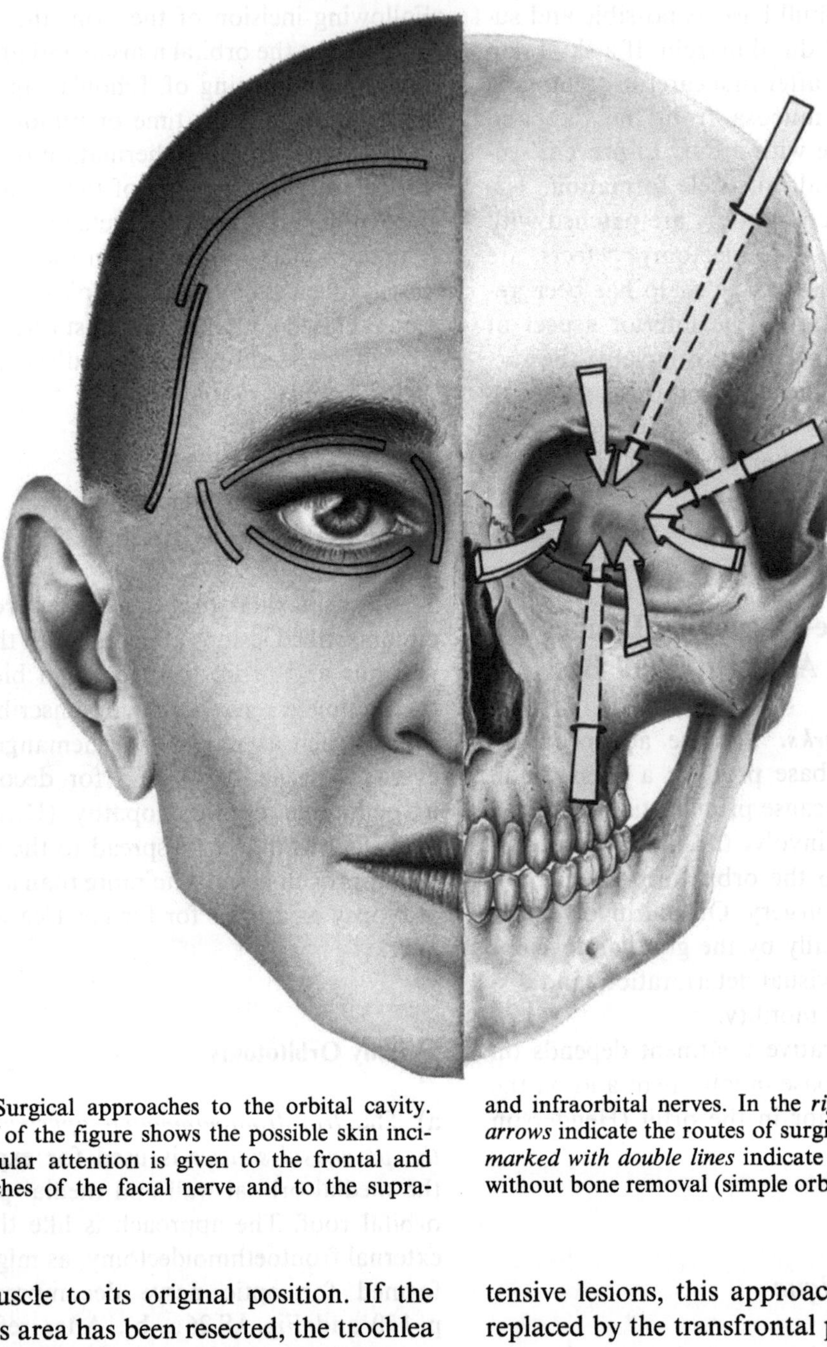

Fig. AS 40. Surgical approaches to the orbital cavity. The *left half* of the figure shows the possible skin incisions. Particular attention is given to the frontal and ocular branches of the facial nerve and to the supra- and infraorbital nerves. In the *right half* of the figure, *arrows* indicate the routes of surgical access. The *arrows marked with double lines* indicate the direct approaches without bone removal (simple orbitotomy)

oblique muscle to its original position. If the bone in this area has been resected, the trochlea is fixed to the periosteum of the frontal bone (Draf 1982).

b) The *lateral bony orbitotomy* (Krönlein 1938), originally proposed for the removal of orbital dermoid cysts, can be extended by carrying the incision behind the frontal hairline, osteotomizing the body of the zygomatic arch, and performing microsurgical exploration of the orbit (Jones 1970). Portions of the lateral skull base can be resected through this approach. For extensive lesions, this approach has been largely replaced by the transfrontal procedure.

4) Transfrontal Intracranial Approach to the Orbit

This technique gives wide exposure of the anterior skull base on one side. It is chiefly indicated for retrobulbar orbital neoplasms, even when confined to the orbit, for orbital tumors with extensive invasion of the anterior and lateral

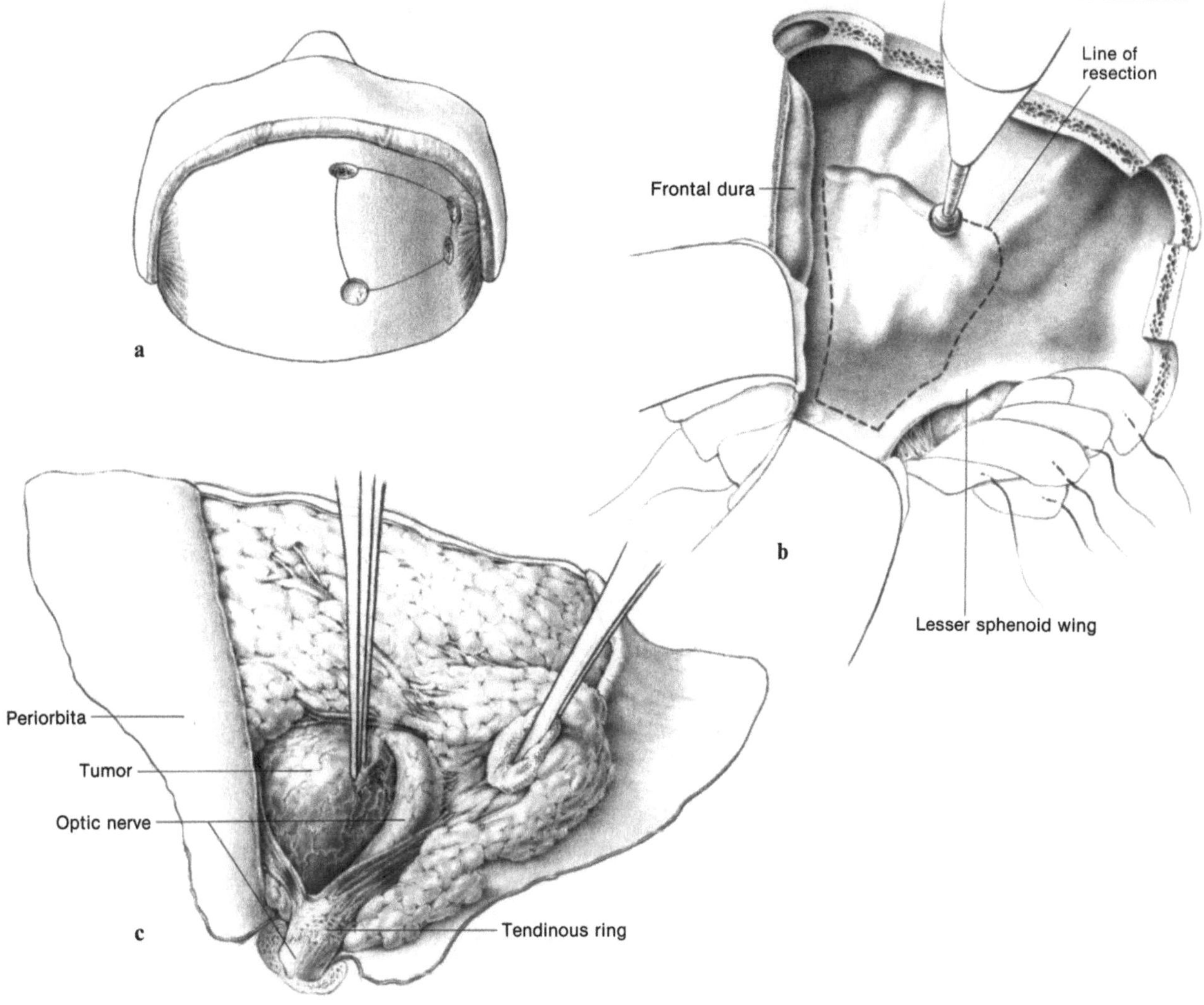

Fig. AS 41 a–f. Transfrontal *extradural* approach to the orbit.
a A scalp flap is developed from a bitemporal coronal incision, and a unilateral frontotemporal craniotomy is performed.
b The anterior skull base and orbital roof are exposed extradurally on one side.
c The periorbita is incised in trapdoor fashion and reflected to the side, exposing the tumor in the periorbital fat. Here the tumor is causing optic nerve displacement. The tumor capsule is coagulated with bipolar forceps before it is opened.

skull base, and also for tumors that have invaded the orbit from the skull base (Brenner et al. 1967, Schürmann 1968, 1974, Schürmann and Voth 1972, Valencak et al. 1970). The approach is rarely used for the operative treatment of endocrine ophthalmopathy (Naffziger 1941), as the transmaxillary or transethmoidal procedure is more suitable.

The Transfrontal Extradural Approach
(Fig. AS 41 a–f)

Usually a unilateral frontotemporal craniotomy is performed after elevating a bitemporal scalp flap with an incision behind the hairline. After removal of the craniotomy flap, the skull base is exposed *extradurally* with successive retraction of the frontal lobe. Depending on the tumor extent, the orbital portion of the anterior skull base can be explored to the orbital apex and the medial border of the optic canal. It is

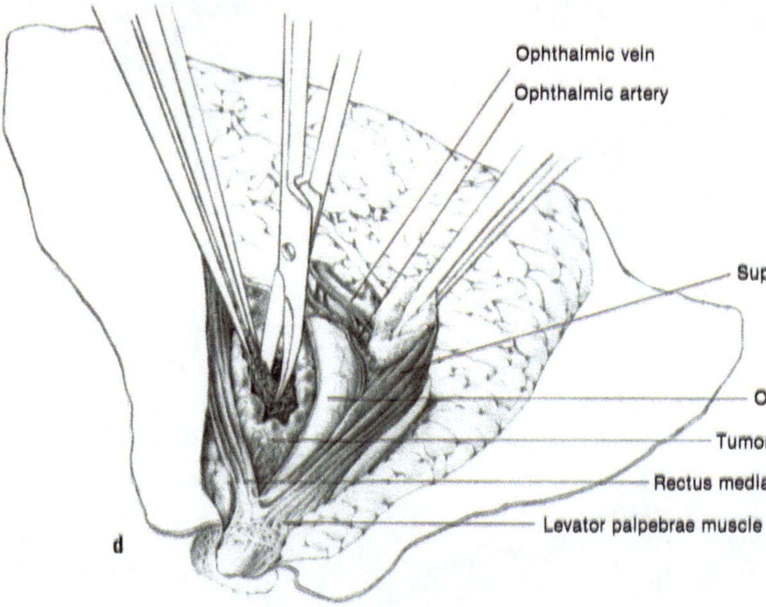

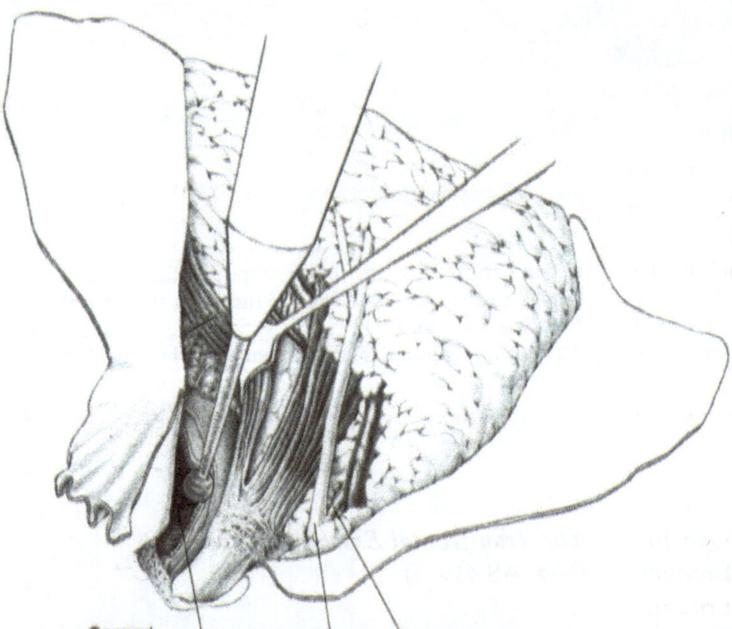

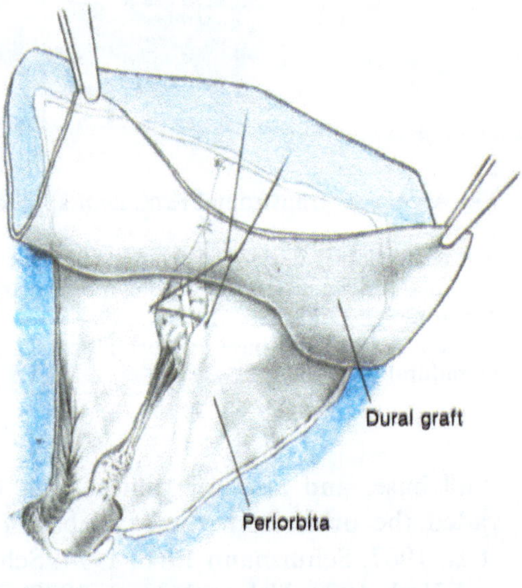

Fig. AS 41 d–f.
d Bipolar coagulation is alternated with piecemeal enucleation of the tumor. **e** Status after tumor removal. Occasionally the sphenoid sinus is opened. The optic nerve has returned spontaneously to its normal position. **f** The periorbital flaps are replaced and sutured, and the sphenoid sinus is closed. The orbital roof is covered with a dural graft

possible to remove the anterior skull base posteriorly along the lesser sphenoid wing to the anterior clinoid process. The bony orbital margins should be adequately resected before the periorbita is opened, for afterward this is made difficult by herniating fat. Once exposure is achieved, tumors are enucleated and their capsule removed. Communications formed between the cranial cavity and paranasal sinuses must be closed to prevent ascending infection. After removal of the tumor, the optic nerve will return to its normal position. The periorbital flap is turned back into place, and the orbit is additionally covered with a dural graft.

With an *optic sheath meningioma*, it is of interest to determine 1) whether the sheath tumor has infiltrated the optic nerve and 2) whether the tumor has spread beyond the optic canal into the intracranial space. Unfortunately, these questions cannot always be answered preoperatively by CT and MRI examinations. The extradural approach to the orbit is preferred, as it permits the optic canal to be opened extradurally if required. If the tumor also envelops the intradural portion of the optic nerve, it will be necessary to open the dura to remove all the tumor.

Optic sheath meningioma may be of the expansive or infiltrating type. In either case the prognosis is doubtful with regard to improving or even preserving the vision that remains.

The total removal of an infiltrating sheath meningioma cannot be accomplished without sacrifice of the optic nerve (Fig. AS 42a,b). If the nerve is merely compressed by the tumor, we use microsurgical dissection in an attempt to preserve remaining vision.

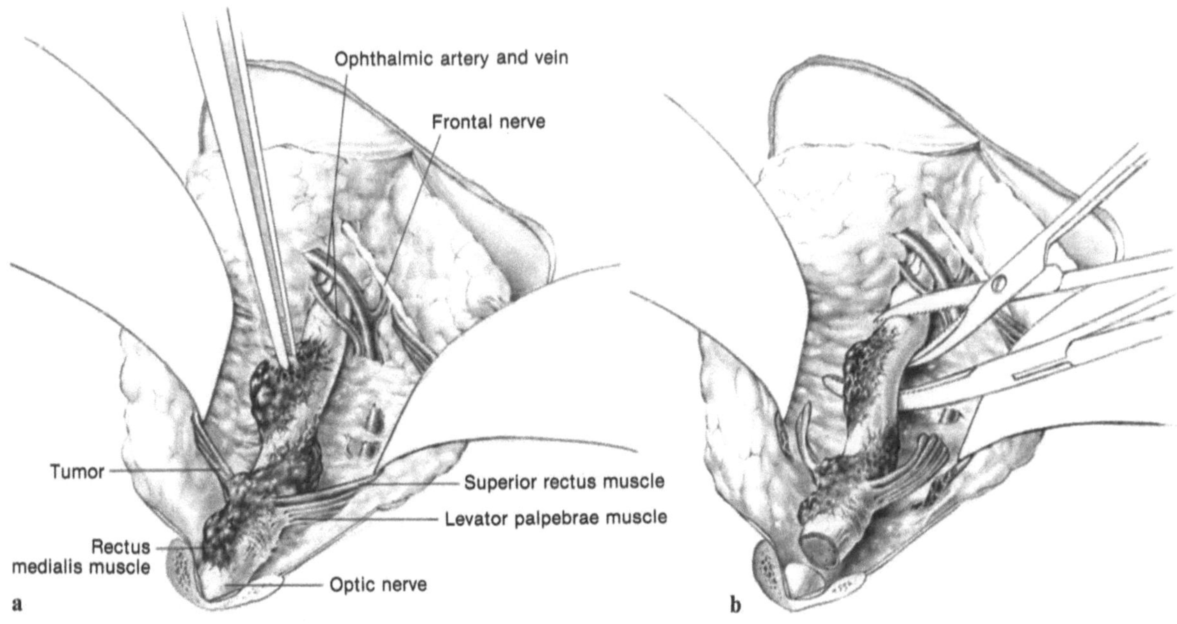

Fig. AS 42a, b. Transfrontal extradural exposure and resection of an optic nerve infiltrated by a sheath meningioma.
a Optic nerve with the infiltrating tumor, exposed by opening the optic canal in the retrobulbar space.
b The optic nerve has already been resected proximally with a margin of normal tissue, and the distal portion is being transected with microscissors

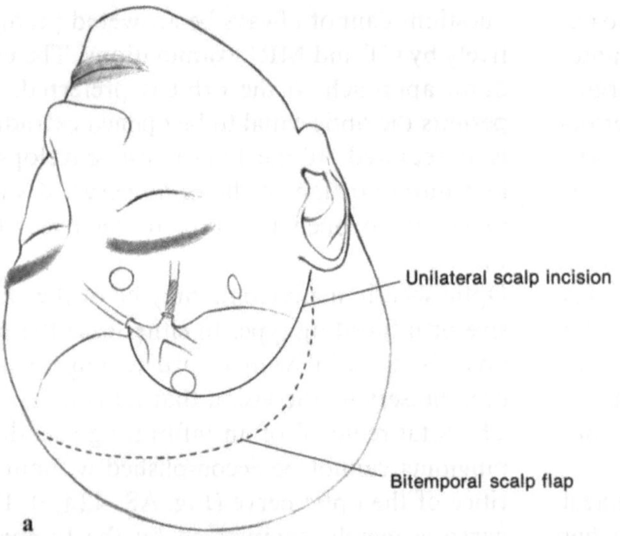

a

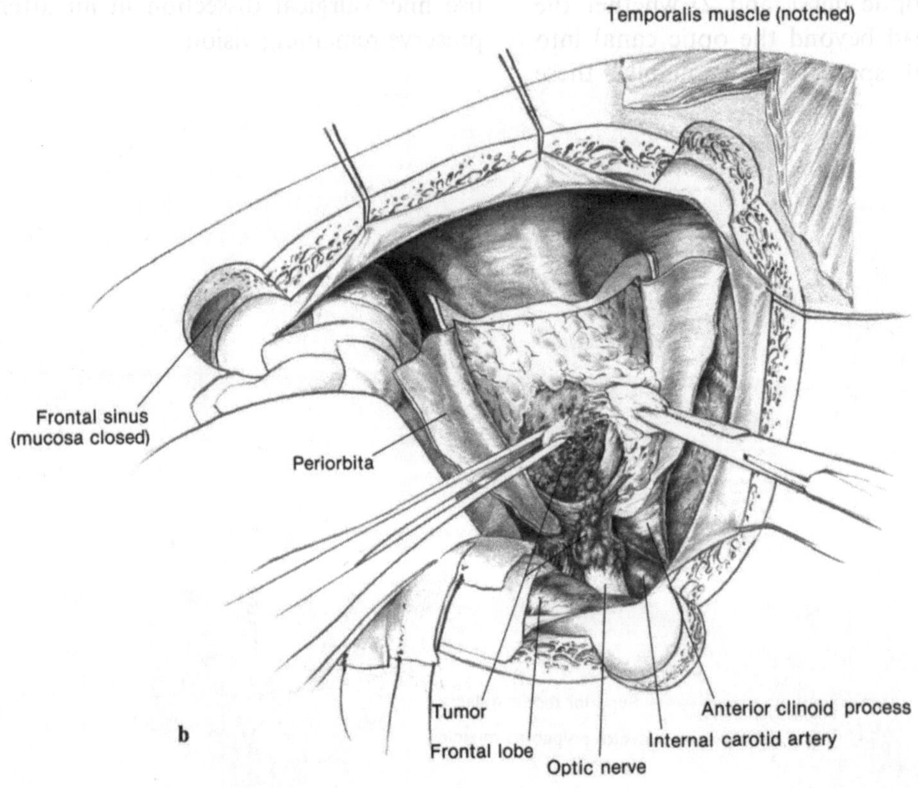

b

Fig. AS 43a, b. Transfrontotemporal intradural orbitotomy.
a The drawing shows the burr hole sites, the unilateral scalp incision, and the more cosmetically favorable bitemporal scalp flap.
b The orbit is opened intradurally. This also permits good visualization of the intradural course of the optic nerve and internal carotid artery

The Extended Transfrontotemporal Intradural Approach
(Fig. AS 43a,b)

The intradural approach is preferred for attacking orbital tumors that have a significant intradural component and for primary intradural tumors that have invaded the orbit.
The skin may be opened unilaterally with the classic frontotemporal incision or with the more cosmetically acceptable bitemporal incision behind the hairline.
After dissection of the skin flap, three burr holes are made. The anterior inferior burr hole is placed next to the midline, as close to the border of the frontal sinus as possible. It may be necessary to include a very large frontal sinus in the craniotomy to avoid a large bony ledge at the junction with the orbit. The posterior inferior burr hole is placed over the root of the zygoma and the edge of the superolateral orbital rim. The temporal muscle is split in line with its fibers and stripped from the bone sufficiently to allow placement of this hole. A curved bony channel is cut back from that point into the infratemporal fossa to provide the deepest possible access to the basal part of the middle cranial fossa. The superior burr hole is placed about 4 cm above the two lower holes to create a bone flap with rounded margins. As in the extradural approach, the lesser sphenoid wing is partially resected after elevation of the frontotemporal dura. The dura is then opened with a basal, curved frontotemporal incision. Cerebrospinal fluid is drained so that the lateral portion of the frontal lobe and anterior pole of the temporal lobe can be retracted farther posteriorly without tension, giving wide exposure of the posterior and lateral borders of the orbit. At this time the intracranial portion of the tumor is removed. Intraorbital tumor is exposed by incising the dura along the course of the optic nerve over the anterior skull base and raising a pair of trap-door flaps. The bony orbital margin can now be resected as needed, according to the tumor extent. In some cases it is necessary to open the optic canal with the diamond burr, avoiding injury to the lateral wall of the sphenoid sinus and to the posterior ethmoid cells. If this bone must be removed for oncologic reasons, the defect must be securely covered with a galeal pericranial flap or stored dura. The rest of the dissection corresponds to the transfrontal extradural approach.

Special Operative Techniques

Introductory Remarks. The pathology of space-occupying lesions of the skull base is highly diverse, and the different types of tumor present the surgeon with unique problems. The highly vascular tumors, for example, require a more extensive diagnostic workup that may include superselective angiography. Preoperative angiographic assessment of collateral flow via the circulus arteriosus is necessary when a radical operation is proposed that will involve sacrifice of the internal carotid artery.
Pathoanatomic classification can be difficult in cases that are not evaluated by preoperative biopsy. Intraoperative frozen section examinations are of only limited value. Table 4 from Batsakis (1979) makes it easier for the surgeon to evaluate rare tumors of the skull base and draw appropriate therapeutic conclusions. Because a number of tumors require *special techniques of surgical dissection*, we have supplemented our discussion of general operative technique with a presentation of case reports illustrating the special surgical problems that are associated with different tumors. Hommerich (1977) presents a comprehensive literature survey on benign tumors of the nose and paranasal sinuses with possible extension to the anterior skull base, and Wustrow (1977) presents a similar survey on malignancies. Tumors of the nasopharynx are reviewed by Zehm (1977), and Zülch (1955/1956) gives a detailed discussion of intracranial tumors that involve the skull base. Details on incidence, pathology, clinical presentation, and therapeutic guidelines may be found in these studies; here we shall limit our attention to problems of surgical technique.

Table 4. Tumors of the Facial Bones and Skull: A Histological Classification (Batsakis 1979)

Type	Benign	Malignant
Hematopoietic and reticulo-endothelial	Histiocytosis	Plasmacytoma Myeloma Malignant lymphoma Histiocytosis
Chondrogenic	Osteochondroma Chondroma Chondroblastoma Chondromyxoid fibroma	Chondrosarcoma Differentiated Dedifferentiated Mesenchymal
Osteogenic	Osteoma Osteoid osteoma Osteoblastoma	Osteogenic sarcoma Endosteal Parosteal Periosteal
Fibrogenic	Fibroma Ossifying Nonossifying Desmoplastic fibroma ? Fibromyxoma	Fibrosarcoma
Odontogenic	Myxoma	? Myxosarcoma
Notochordal	–	Chordoma Conventional Chondrogenic
Vascular	Hemangioma	Angiosarcoma Hemangiopericytoma
Lipogenic	? Lipoma	? Liposarcoma
Neurogenic	Neurilemmoma Neurofibroma	Neurogenous sarcoma Primary and secondary neuroectodermal tumors
Disputed origin	Giant cell granuloma "Brown" tumor Cherubism Giant cell tumor Benign fibrous histiocytoma	Malignant giant cell tumor Ewing's sarcoma Malignant fibrous histiocytoma

Surgery of Benign Space-Occupying Lesions of the Anterior Skull Base

Cavernous Hemangioma of the Orbit

It cannot always be determined from pathoanatomic criteria whether a vascular tumor is in fact a malformation or a true neoplasm. We know, however, that malformations can give rise to true neoplasms, which are described as "dysontogenetic" (Hommerich 1977). The cavernous hemangioma is a ubiquitous tumor that is characterized histologically by enlarged capillary spaces. This accounts for the profuse bleeding tendency of these tumors, which compounds the technical difficulty of their removal. Cavernous hemangiomas present clinically as painless

Fig. AS 44a–f. Cavernous hemangioma of the orbit.
a CT contrast scan shows a large, vascular, retrobulbar tumor of the left orbit.
b Status after microsurgical transfrontal extradural orbitotomy. The orbital fat is dissected away from the tumor. (*1*) Fundus, (*2*) periorbital fat, (*3*) lateral rectus muscle, (*4*) brain spatula.
c The neoplasm is progressively mobilized; using bipolar cautery to control bleeding. The ciliary nerve is dissected off the tumor. (*1*) Tumor, (*2*) periorbital fat, (*3*) ciliary nerve

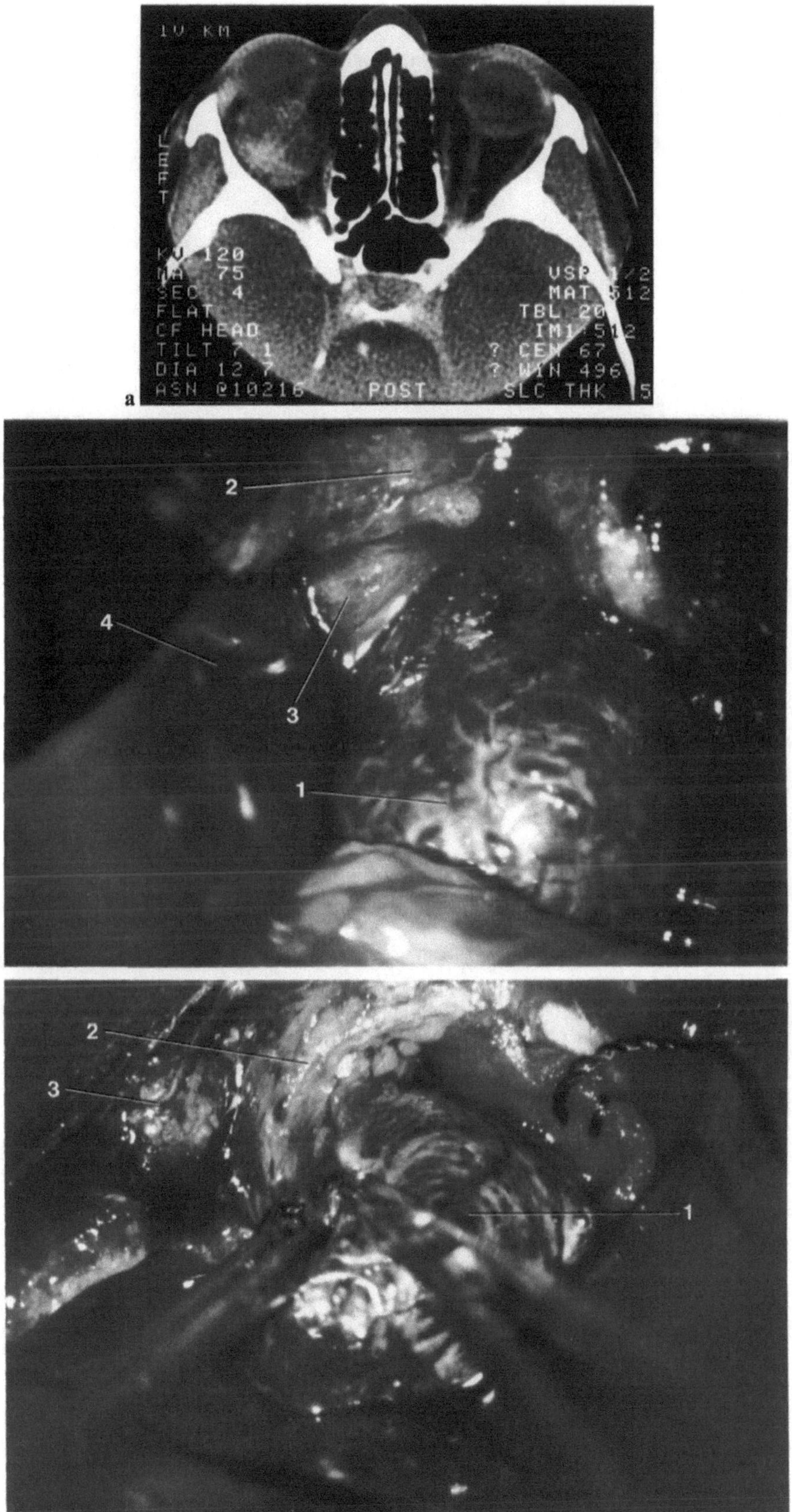
a
b
c
2
4
3
1
2
3
1
FLAT
POST
TBL 20
? CEN 67
? WIN 496

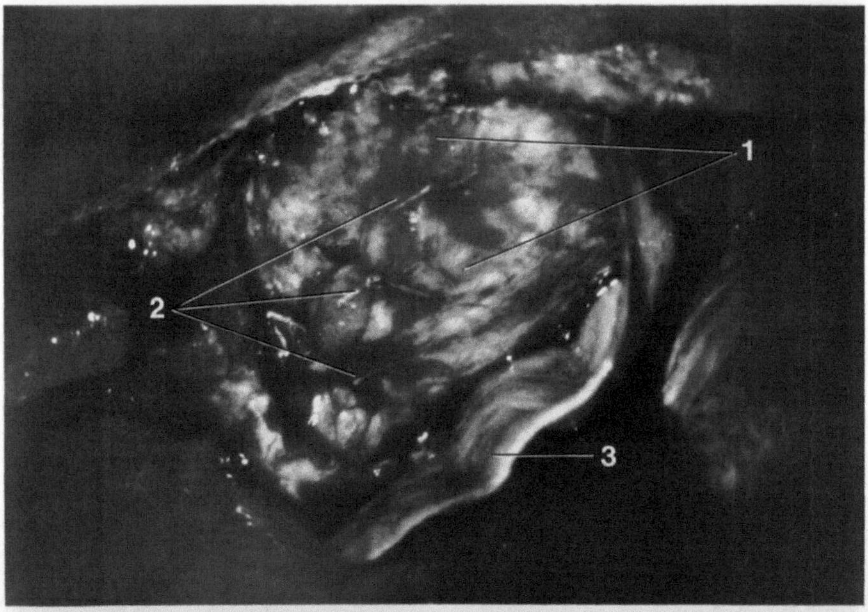

d

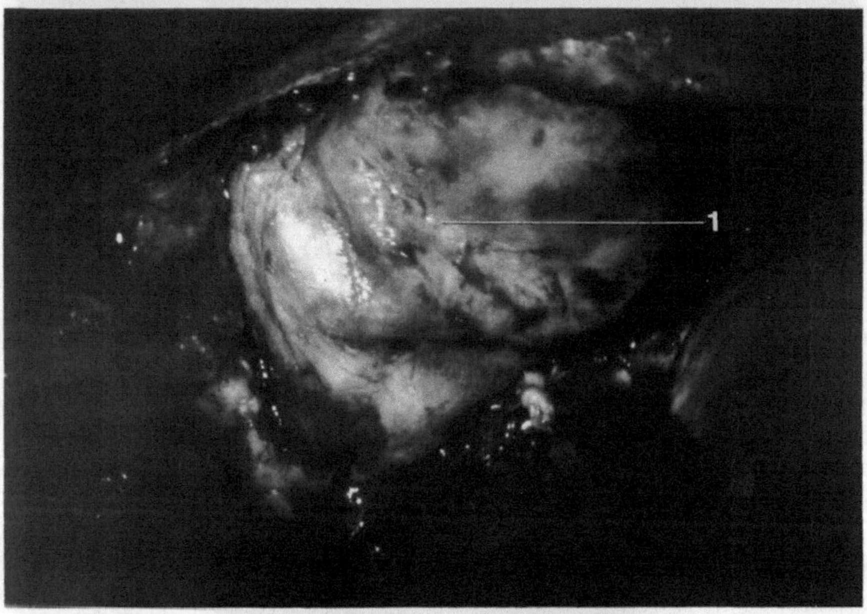

e

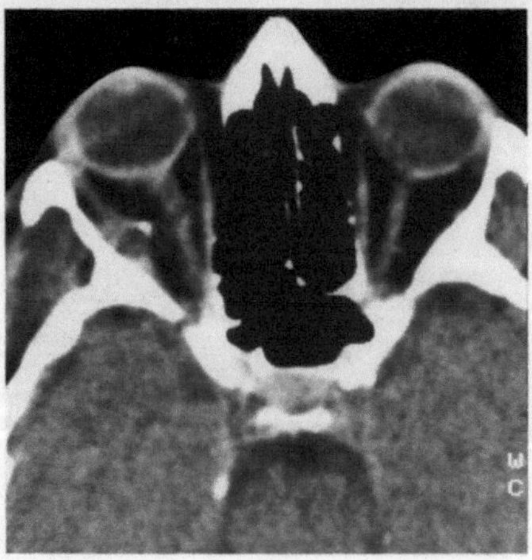

f

masses that cause functional disturbances and bone destruction through pressure on surrounding tissues. This is particularly true in the rare cases with orbital involvement. Surgical intervention is necessary 1) to establish a histologic diagnosis and 2) to correct the disturbances of ocular motility and of vision in extreme cases. The operation itself should not cause any additional injury.

Case Report (Fig. AS 44a–f). The patient had a 3-year history of increasing proptosis of the left eye without subjective visual problems. Ophthalmologic examination disclosed a small arcuate scotoma in the visual field and a proptosis of 5 mm relative to the right side.
Computed axial tomography with contrast enhancement demonstrated a large, smooth, rounded retrobulbar mass that was slightly larger than the globe itself. The contrast uptake was consistent with a highly vascular tumor.
Operative removal was accomplished through an osteoplastic, transcranial, extradural exposure of the anterior skull base with resection of the orbital roof. The neoplasm had a firm capsule that was well demarcated from surrounding tissues, and even the ciliary nerve could be dissected off the tumor capsule without difficulty. The tumor was totally removed without damage to the optic nerve or muscular structures of the orbit. The periorbita was closed with interrupted sutures, and the orbital roof was covered with a dural graft. The lesion was identified histologically as a cavernous hemangioma. The postoperative course was uneventful, ocular motility was normal, and proptosis was relieved. Visual deterioration did not occur.

Fig. AS 44d–f.
d At the end of the procedure Tenon's capsule is closed with simple interrupted sutures. A dural graft is inserted beneath the medial cut edge of the bone. (*1*) Tenon's capsule, (*2*) suture, (*3*) stored dura.
e The bony orbital defect is also covered with a dural graft. (*1*) Lyophilized dura.
f CT scan after 10 days, no longer shows evidence of the tumor. Slight postoperative swelling of retrobulbar structures is still apparent

Comments: A large intraorbital, retrobulbar cavernous hemangioma was removed in toto through a transfrontal extradural approach, using microsurgical techniques to enable preservation of orbital structures. There was no evidence of function impairment following the surgery.

Eosinophilic Granuloma of the Frontal Bone

Introductory Remarks. The majority of authors, according to Hommerich (1977), place eosinophilic granuloma in the class of tumorous reticulohistiocytic systemic diseases and group both the acute form (Abt-Letterer-Siwe syndrome) and the chronic generalized form (Hand-Schueller-Christian disease) under the heading of "histiocytosis X" (Jung and Gutjahr 1977, Lichtenstein 1953). Henderson et al. (1950) state that the term "eosinophilic granuloma" is applicable only in the presence of one or at most two osseous foci. The disease is most prevalent in the first two decades of life. In 62 children with histologically confirmed histiocytosis X, Nebit et al. (1970) found 14 with orbital involvement and the clinical features of paranasal sinus disease. Eosinophilic granuloma often presents as a painful swelling on the head. Occurrence in the ear can mimic otitis media, while occurrence in the frontal sinus can mimic a chronic sinusitis. X-ray films show rounded or irregular "punched-out" osteolytic foci without sclerotic margins (Draf 1974). Radionuclide scans of the skull demonstrate the full extent of the lesion through concentration of the radioisotopes. Because we are dealing with a neoplastic disease whose radiation response is questionable, the treatment of choice is surgical resection with a margin of healthy tissue.

Case Report (Fig. AS 45a–g). A 10-year-old boy presented with a tender swelling in the area of the superolateral orbital margin. CT scans showed a sharply marginated bony defect in the right fronto-orbital area with extension to the lateral orbital roof. Radionuclide scans showed increased uptake over a large area of the superolateral orbital margin; scans in the rest of the skeleton were negative. Under a presumptive di-

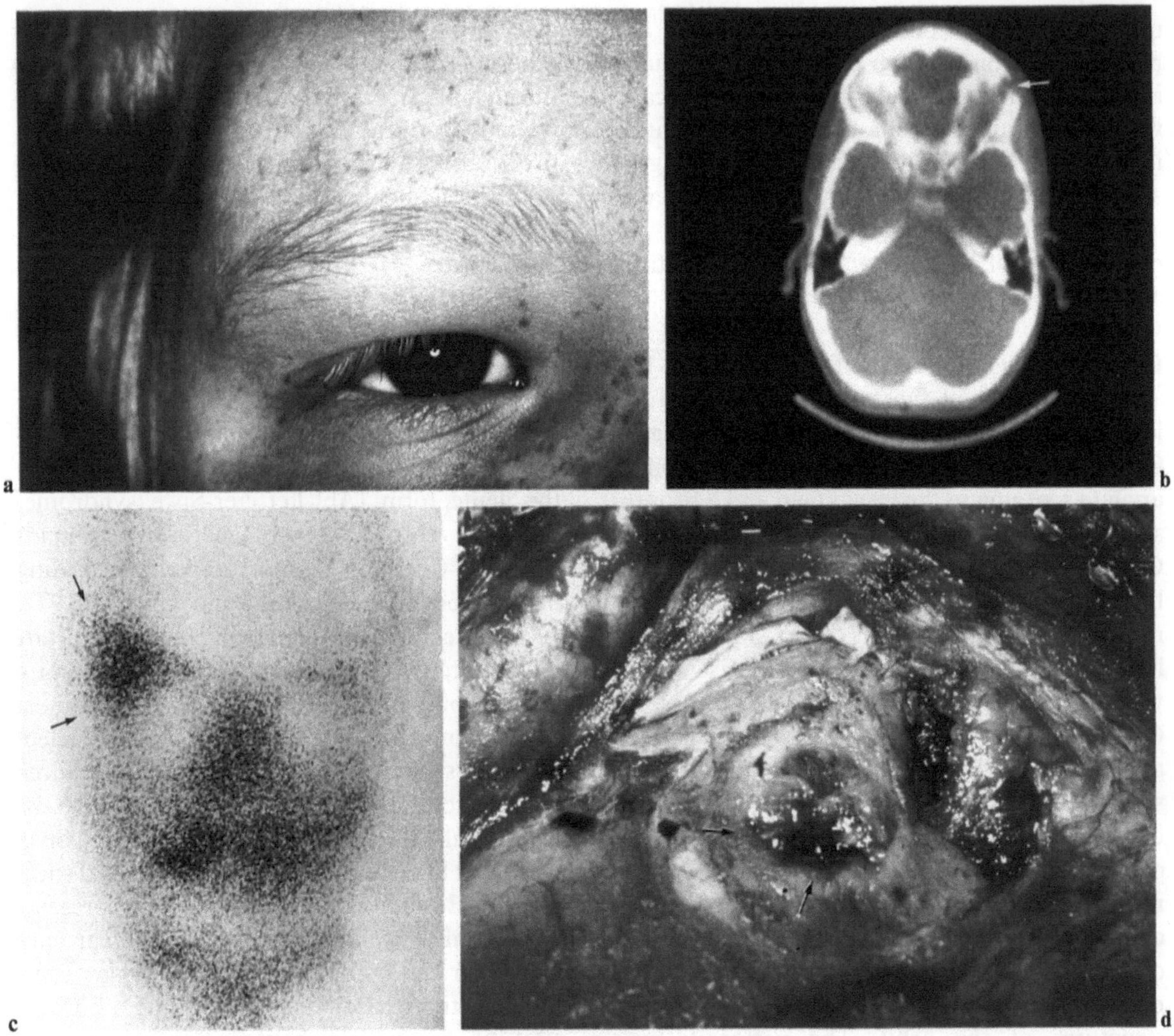

agnosis of eosinophilic granuloma, the osteolytic focus was surgically exposed after developing a right-sided scalp flap from an incision behind the hairline. The involved bone was resected with a 1-cm margin, resulting in a frontotemporal craniectomy with partial resection of the orbital roof and the lateral part of the lesser sphenoid wing. The bony defect was repaired with methylmethacrylate, and the wound healed uneventfully with a minimal scar.

Comments: An eosinophilic granuloma of the anterior skull base was treated by an intracranial extradural craniectomy with immediate methylmethacrylate reconstruction.

Osteoma of the Anterior Skull Base

Introductory Remarks. Osteomas comprise approximately 50% of benign paranasal sinus tumors (Eggston and Wolf 1947). Kastenbauer and Rudert (1968) saw 52 osteomas in 12,000 roentgenograms of the paranasal sinuses (0.44%). Males predominate by 2:1 . The paranasal sinus most commonly affected is the frontal sinus (about 50%–55%), followed by the ethmoid sinus (20%), maxillary sinus (about 5%), sphenoid sinus (about 2%), and nasal cavity (about 0.6%). In 15%–25% of patients, the site of origin can no longer be established by the time of diagnosis (Eckel and Palm 1959, Ganz 1960). According to Zülch (1955) the

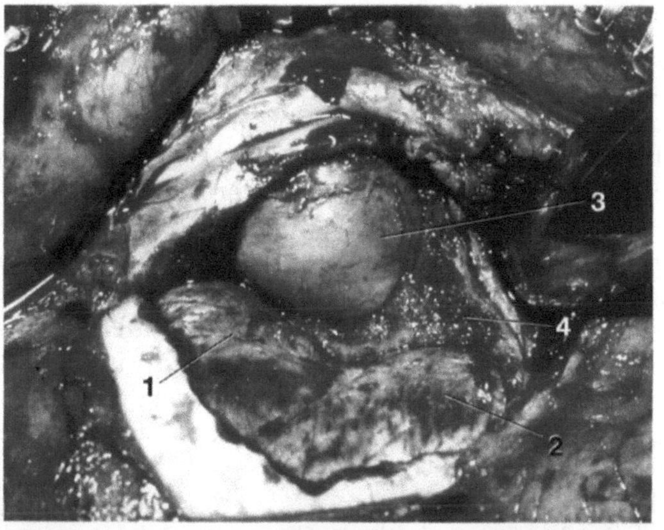

e

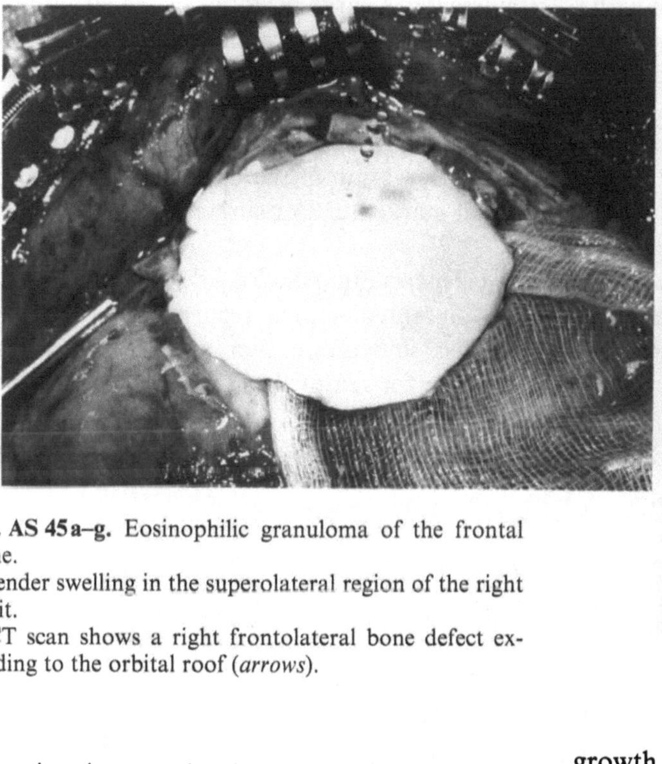
f

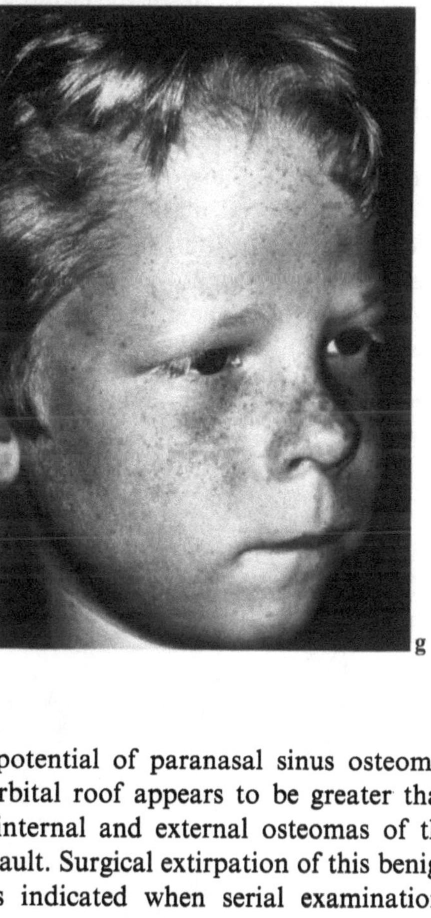
g

Fig. AS 45a–g. Eosinophilic granuloma of the frontal bone.
a Tender swelling in the superolateral region of the right orbit.
b CT scan shows a right frontolateral bone defect extending to the orbital roof (*arrows*).

The pericranium covering the tumor has been resected.
e The tumor resection leaves a frontotemporal craniectomy with exposure of frontal and temporal dura and periorbital tissue. The lateral portion of the minor sphenoid wing has also been partly removed. (*1*) Frontal dura, (*2*) temporal dura, (*3*) periorbita, (*4*) minor sphenoid wing.
f A molded methylmethacrylate plate is inserted. Continuous irrigation on a moist compress is maintained to avoid dural injury. Before definitive attachment, the plate is perforated with drill holes to achieve better scar fixation.
g The boy 2 years after surgery

growth potential of paranasal sinus osteomas of the orbital roof appears to be greater than that of internal and external osteomas of the cranial vault. Surgical extirpation of this benign tumor is indicated when serial examinations demonstrate a marked growth tendency with a clinically symptomatic mass lesion in the paranasal sinuses, anterior cranial fossa, and/or the orbit (refs. in Hommerich 1977). The dissection and resection of these benign neoplasms should be done as atraumatically as possible, with preservation of the mucosae. The minimal bleeding facilitates piecemeal removal with the drill and osteotome. The operating microscope is useful in the region of the skull base. One should not attempt to lift the tumor from its site of origin on the skull base, as this can cause secondary injury with troublesome bleeding. With a tumor having broad attachment to the skull base, all the surrounding bone is resected with an adequate margin. This should virtually eliminate the possibility of recurrence.

Case Report (Fig. AS 46a, b). A 35-year-old woman first noticed a protrusion of the left eye 4 years before consultation. She complained of pain and a gradual decline of visual acuity. On admission, she had proptosis of the left eye with anterior, downward, and lateral displacement of the globe, vision impairment, and left-sided hypesthesia in the distribution of the fifth nerve with a reduced corneal reflex. Optic disc pallor was noted. Rhese films demonstrated a large, smoothly marginated mass of osseous density in the posterior portion of the left orbit that had enveloped the upper half of the optic foramen. On axial CT scans the tumor occupied almost the entire retrobulbar space and had partially invaded the ethmoid labyrinth. The tumor was exposed extradurally through a frontotemporal craniotomy on the left side. It was found to involve portions of the orbital roof and lesser sphenoid wing. The retrobulbar space was opened through piecemeal resection of the orbital and ethmoid margins, and the tumor was removed. The orbital roof was covered with a dural patch, the dura was tacked up to the bone margins, and the bone flap was replaced and fixed with sutures. The burr holes were repaired with methylmethacrylate to prevent indrawing of soft tissues. The histological examination identified the lesion as an osteoma.

Comments: A large osteoma of the left anterior skull base with intracranial and intraorbital extension, ethmoid involvement, optic nerve compression, and proptosis was totally removed through a transcranial, extradural approach with preservation of the optic nerve. Vision improved markedly after surgery.

Case Report (Fig. AS 47a–i). A 23-year-old woman presented with a recurrence of osteoma. She had undergone two previous operations elsewhere for removal of an osteoma, the most

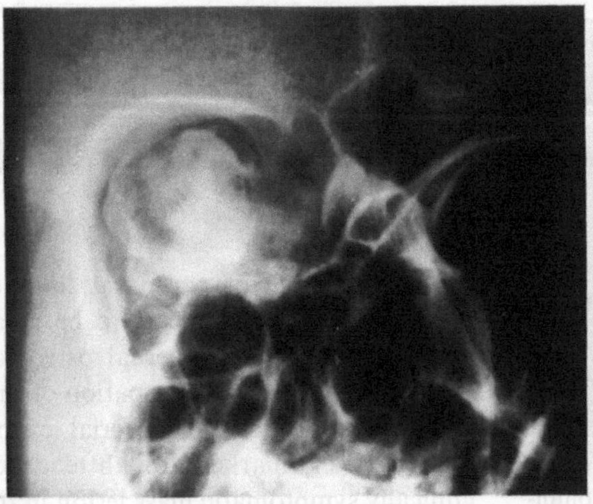

a

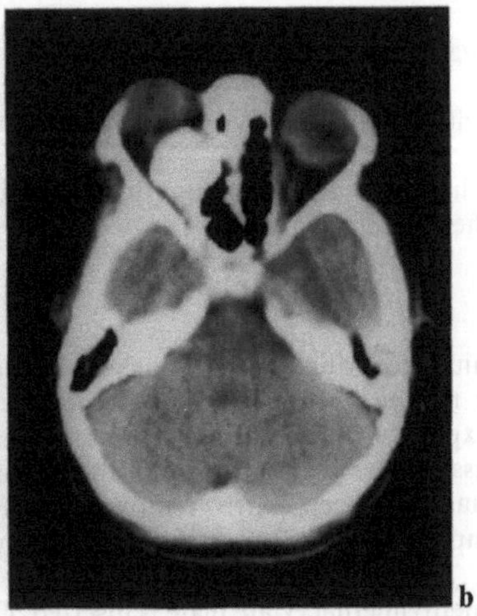

b

Fig. AS 46a, b. Osteoma of the left orbit.
a Large, cloudy, smoothly marginated mass of osseous density projecting into the left orbit. Part of the mass appears to be intracranial and part intraorbital, with involvement of the ethmoid cells. The superior half of the optic foramen is encased by tumor.
b CT scan shows anterior and lateral displacement of the globe, involvement of the left ethmoid cells, and the close proximity of the mass to the optic nerve

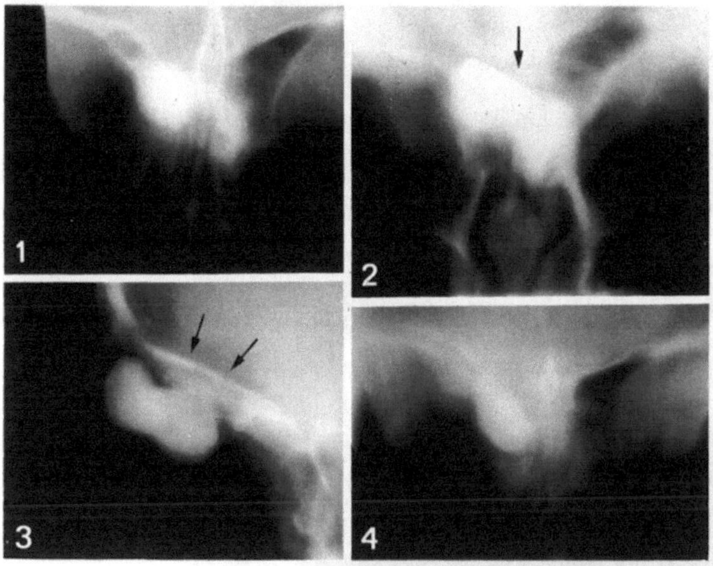

a

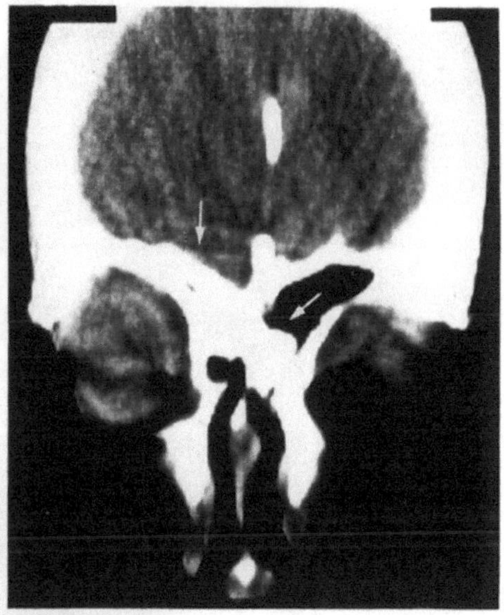

b

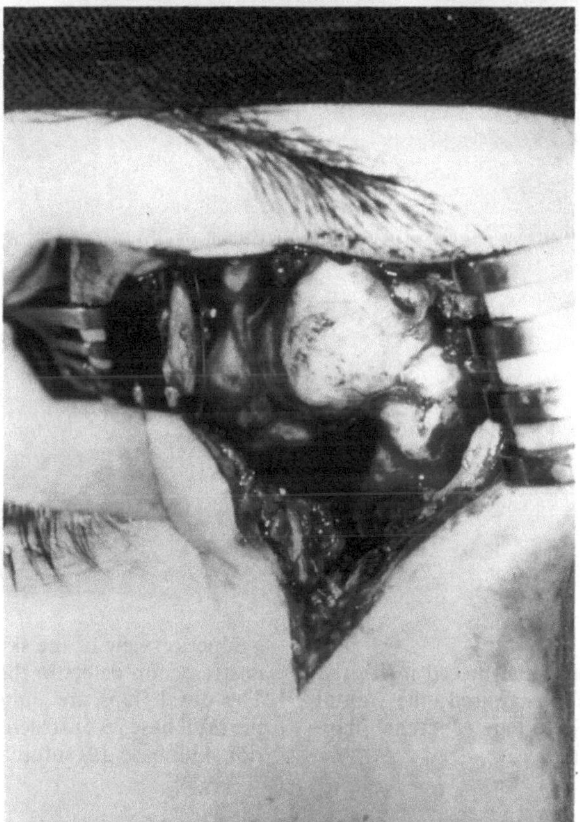

c

Fig. AS 47 a–i. Recurrent osteoma of the anterior skull base.
a (*1–4*) Tomograms of the anterior skull base showing the tumor extent in the ethmoid sinuses and frontal sinus with broad involvement of the anterior skull base (*arrows*).
b Tumor extent on the coronal CT scan (*arrows*).
c The tumor was extirpated through a combined craniofacial approach. First an incision beneath the brow was made as for a transfacial operation on the frontal and ethmoid sinuses, and the tumor was exposed bilaterally in the ethmoid sinuses

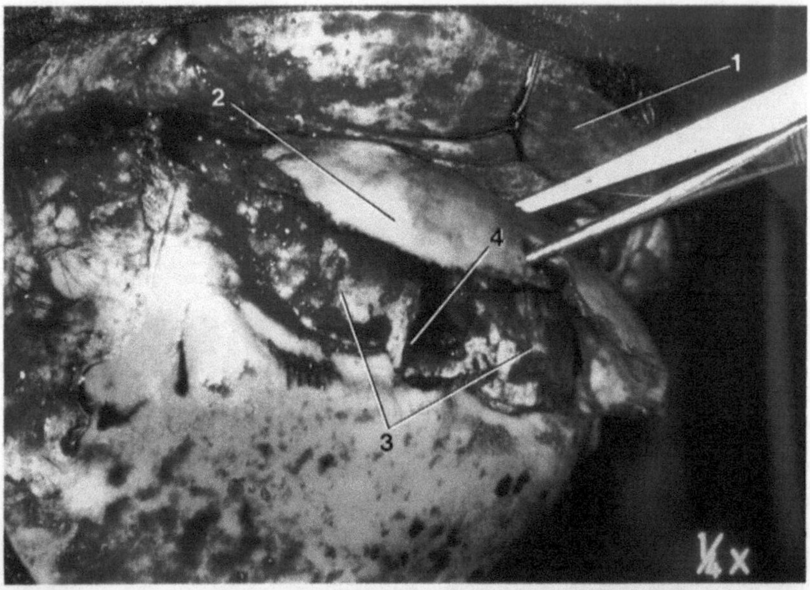

d

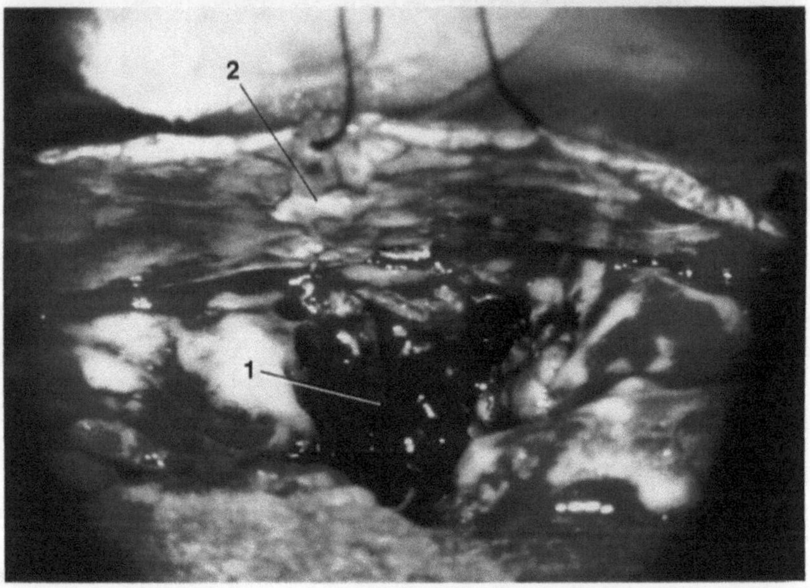

e

Fig. AS 47 d, e.
d Superior view: The scalp has been turned inferiorly, and the craniotomy flap has been raised; the frontal dura and falx are visible. (*1*) Scalp flap, (*2*) cranial flap, (*3*) frontal dura, (*4*) falx cerebri.

e Superior view of the skull base after craniotomy. The postresection defect in the anterior skull base is visible. The dural flaps are united to form the first layer of the skull base reconstruction. (*1*) Bony defect in the anterior skull base, (*2*) suture line for the dural flaps

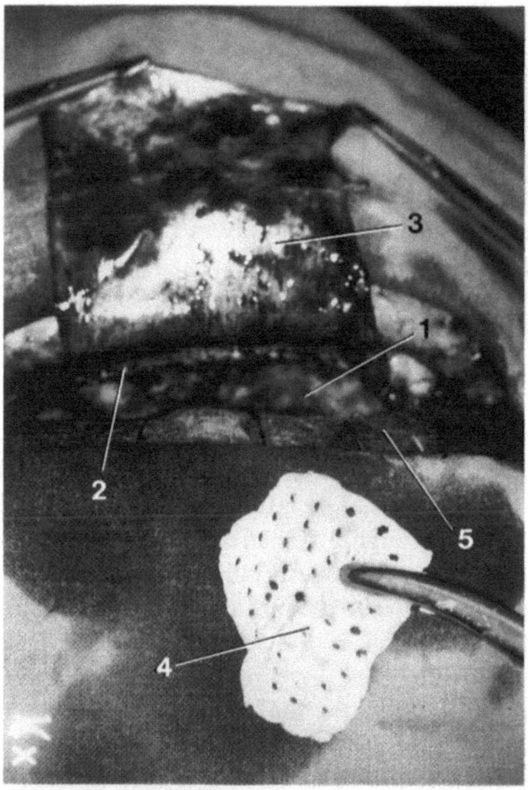

f

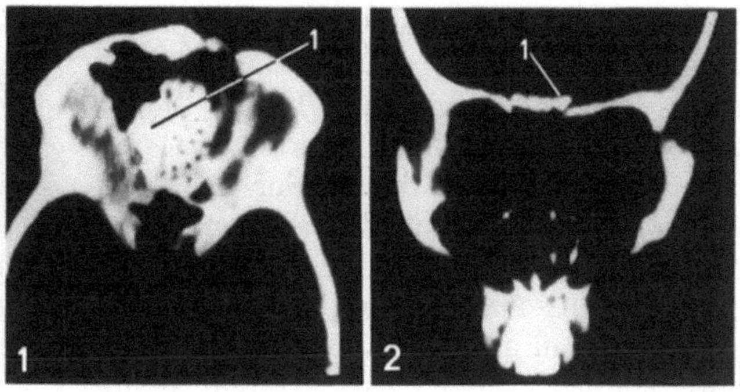

h

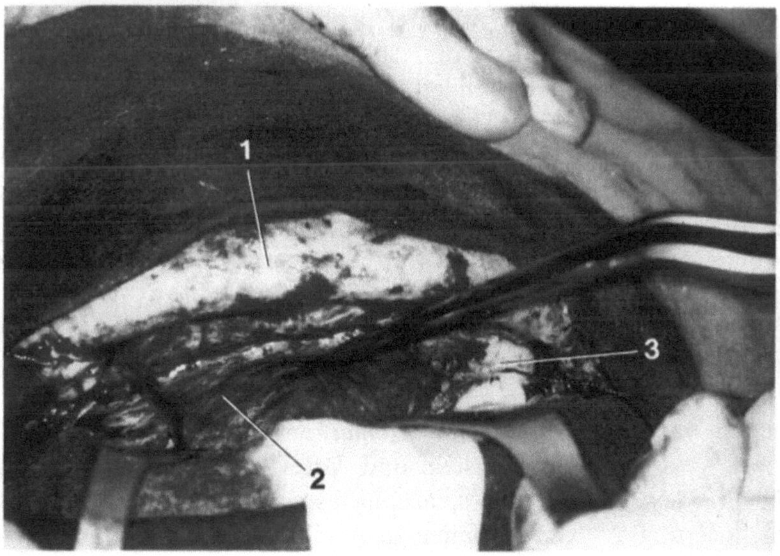

g

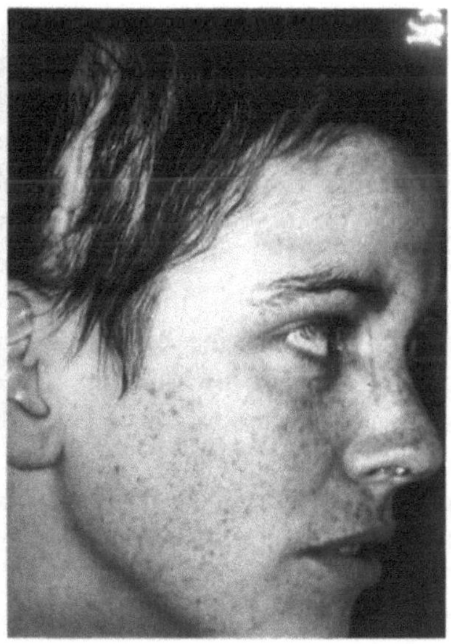

Fig. AS 47f–h.
f The base of the galeal pericranial flap is sutured to the anterior basal dural margin, and a methylmethacrylate plate is molded to the bony defect; the plate is perforated for scar ingrowth. (*1*) Dural flaps on the cranial floor, (*2*) dural-pericranial suture line, (*3*) galeal pericranial flap, (*4*) methylmethacrylate, (*5*) retracted frontal lobe.

g The galeal flap has been reflected over the plastic implant and sutured into place. It covers almost the entire anterior skull base. Note that the implant is surrounded on all sides by living tissue. (*1*) Basal part of galeal flap covering the frontal sinuses, (*2*) part of galeal flap covering the methylmethacrylate, (*3*) retracted frontal lobe.
h (*1* + *2*) Postoperative axial and coronal CT scans showing the plastic implant. (*1*) Methylmetacrylat.
i The patient 3 months after surgery

recent via an intracranial-extradural approach (Unterberger; see p. 141) with duraplasty.
Preoperative tomograms and CT scans showed the bilateral extent of the recurrent osteoma, which widely involved the anterior skull base. Because we were dealing with a second recurrence, we elected the combined craniofacial approach to the anterior skull base through an incision beneath the right eyebrow and a bitemporal coronal incision. After exposure of the ethmoid, the anterior pole of the osteoma was visualized. The ethmoid cells were removed, and the necessary line of resection was marked on the skull base transfacially with a punch and drill.
The rhinosurgical part of the operation was performed first so that the extent of the skull base resection around the tumor could be established.
The intracranial part of the operation then commenced with a bifrontal craniotomy. The frontal sinus was opened, followed by a bilateral frontobasal incision of the dura with double suture ligation of the superior sagittal sinus. The falx was divided and the anterior cranial fossa exposed by frontal lobe retraction. The olfactory tract was cauterized with bipolar forceps and divided to expose the planum sphenoidale and optic nerves. A pair of laterally based dural flaps were raised, uncovering the crista galli and the bone resection marks made previously. At this point the bone block was outlined with a cutting burr in the anterior part of the planum sphenoidale, the crista galli and midportion of the anterior skull base including the cribriform plate were resected, and the specimen was removed.
The skull base was reconstructed in three layers by reapproximating the dural flaps, inserting a suitably molded, perforated methylmethacrylate implant, and covering the implant with an inferiorly based galeal pericranial flap. Then the bone flap was replaced, the burr holes patched with methylmethacrylate, and the scalp flap closed over a suction drain. To conclude the operation, the skull base was examined transnasally with an endoscope, the nasal surgical cavity was lined with silicone film, an intranasal ointment pack was inserted, and the facial incision was closed with intracutaneous sutures. The patient was discharged 3 weeks later after an uneventful course.
Two years later the patient developed a gradual, mildly painful swelling in the middle of the forehead. Reexposure of this area disclosed a small mucocele situated epidurally in the middle and inferior portion of the osteoplastic bone flap. It was easily removed without altering the contour of the forehead, and the calvarium was smoothed with a drill.

Comments: A 23-year-old woman had her second recurrence of an osteoma broadly attached to the skull base. The latest attempt at removal had been through a transfrontal extradural approach. The third operation involved a craniofacial, intradural exposure that permitted complete extirpation of the lesion. The skull base was reconstructed in three layers with dura, methylmethacrylate, and a galeal pericranial flap.
The occurrence of a circumscribed mucocele two years later probably resulted from a small amount of residual frontal sinus mucosa that had been left on the bone flap in the first operation. This complication proves the importance of carefully removing all residual paranasal sinus mucosa from the bone flap, preferably with a drill.
Seven years after surgery the patient remains free of disease.

Fibrous Bone Dysplasia

Introductory Remarks. Lichtenstein (1938) and Lichtenstein and Jaffe (1942) describe fibrous bone dysplasia as a specific anomaly of osseous development in which normal bone is replaced by fibrous tissue, within which new bony trabeculae are formed. The disease may be localized (monostotic form) or it may occur at multiple sites (polyostotic form).
Fibrous bone dysplasia is a systemic disease that most often affects younger patients. Operative treatment is indicated when the cosmetic deformity leads to psychologic changes, and intra- and extracranial spread of the tumor lead to pain and loss of function.

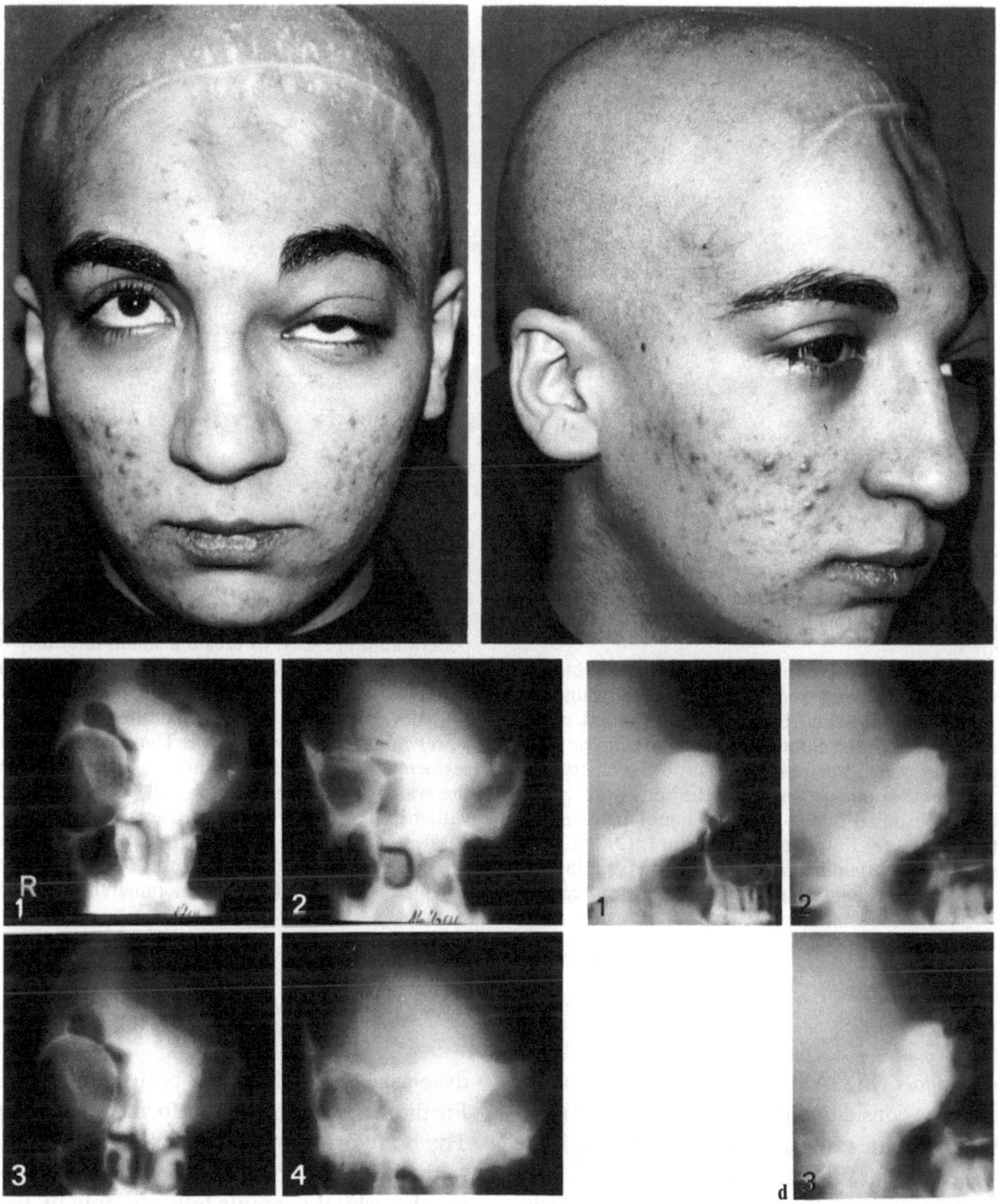

Fig. AS 48 a–q. Extensive fibrous dysplasia with anterior skull base involvement in a 19-year-old female. Operative treatment was elected for functional and cosmetic reasons. The patient had had two previous operations 10 years earlier.

a, b Patient presented with cosmetic deformity, progressive visual impairment in the left eye with proptosis and downward displacement of the globe, and history of long-standing headaches.

c, d AP and lateral tomograms show the tumor mass extending forward from the cranial vault to the anterior clinoid process and down into the clivus

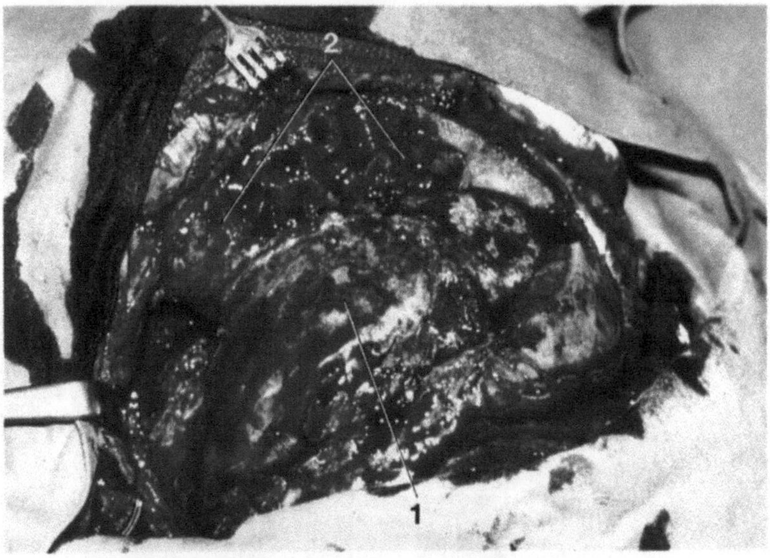

e

Fig. AS 48e–h.
e Bifrontal left temporal craniectomy is done, exposing a wide area of the dura. Both frontal sinuses are largely obliterated by the tumor. (*1*) Dura, (*2*) frontal sinuses (*arrows*).
f Complete tumor excision necessitated almost total removal of both lateral and superior orbital walls and 2/3 of the anterior skull base including the left minor sphenoid wing to the clinoid processes; the upper paranasal sinus system was resected far into the clivus. The portions of the optic nerves within the bony optic canals had to be exposed due to bilateral tumor involvement of the canals. (*1*) Retracted frontal dura, (*2*) left optic nerve, (*3*) right optic nerve, (*4*) exposed left periorbita, (*5*) view into the exenterated sphenoid sinus and middle and posterior ethmoid cells, (*6*) clivus, (*7*) view into the left middle cranial fossa.
g *Step one of the reconstruction:* The left periorbita is covered with a dural graft, and the remaining galea and pericranium are used to create a small, inferiorly based flap that is sutured to the basal part of the dura. (*1*) Frontal dura, (*2*) lyophilized dura on the periorbita, (*3*) galeal pericranial flap, (*4*) fixation sutures (*arrows*).
h *Step two of the reconstruction:* The exposed optic nerve segments are covered by returning the frontal dura to the cranial floor. The orbital wall defects are patched with methylmethacrylate, which is covered medially with nasal mucosa. The galeal pericranial flap has been sutured into place. (*1*) Frontal dura, (*2*) methylmethacrylate plate, (*3*) sutured galeal pericranial flap

Case Report (Fig. AS 48a–q). Wide surgical excision was considered necessary in a 19-year-old female with an extensive, benign systemic bone disease of the anterior and middle skull base with the histologic features of fibrous dysplasia. The patient had undergone two previous operations 10 years earlier. The main indication for surgery was not so much the cosmetic deformity as the progressive restriction of motility in the left eye and the threat of vision loss.

The tumor extent was established by X-ray tomograms.

Following a bifrontal craniectomy and removal of the involved portions of the calvarium, the tumor was exposed at the skull base. Fibrous dysplasia had obliterated both frontal sinuses. Further dissection was performed extradurally. The bony orbital wall had to be removed down to the healthy portions of the orbital floor, leaving the orbital contents tethered only by the optic nerve. The largely resected sphenoid sinus created a window between the two optic nerves through which the surgeon could look toward the clivus. The lesser wing of the left sphenoid was completely removed, allowing visualization of the middle cranial fossa.

The extensive defect was reconstructed in four steps. First the orbital soft tissues were reinforced with a dural graft. The galea-pericranium still available was used to construct an inferiorly

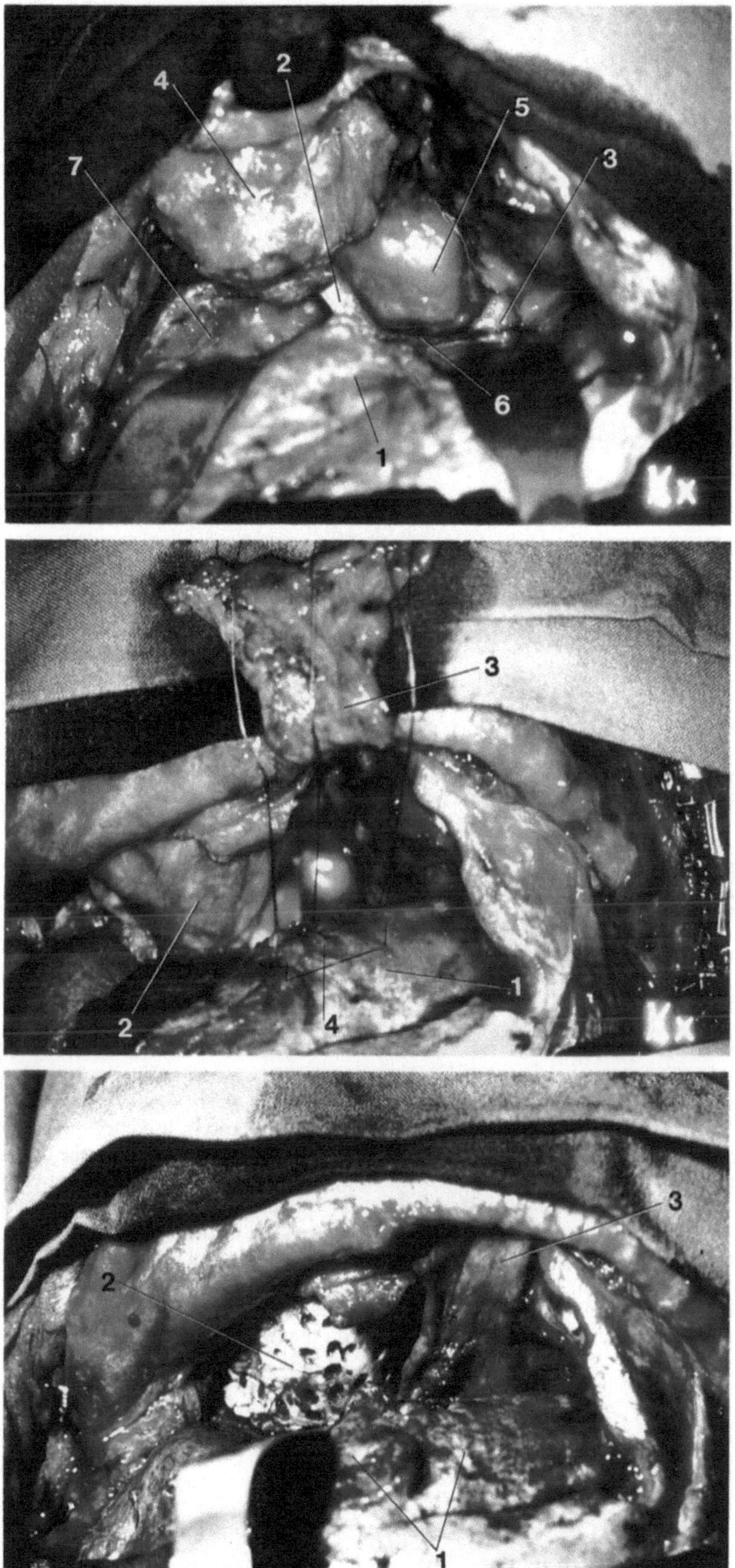

f

g

h

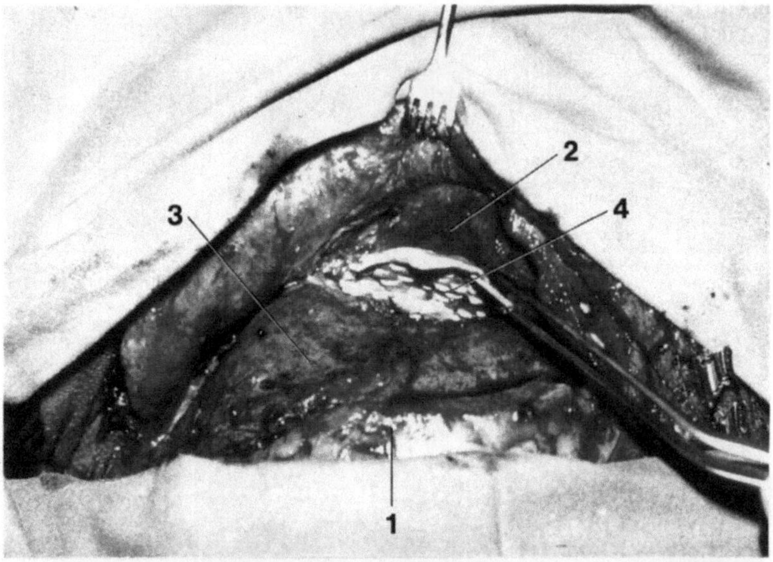

i

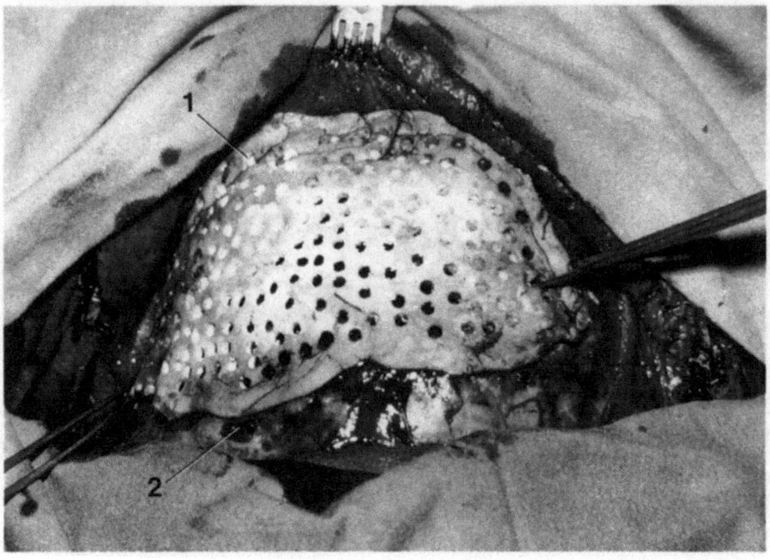

j

Fig. AS 48i–q.
i *Step three of the reconstruction:* The soft-tissue coverage of the orbital implant is reinforced (especially nasally) by overlaying a lateral flap of temporal muscle and the bone defect in the anterior skull base is reconstructed with another methylmethacrylate implant, suitably molded and perforated. It is placed between the pericranium, temporal muscle, and dura. (*1*) Frontal lobe, (*2*) galeal pericranial flap, (*3*) temporal flap (*from the left side*), (*4*) plastic implant.
j *Step four of the reconstruction:* A third methylmethacrylate implant is used to reconstruct the frontal part of the calvarium, including the orbital ridges. (*1*) Orbital ridge area, (*2*) posterior limit of craniotomy.
k, l Plain skull films before (*k*) and after surgery (*l*). The extent of the bone resection is apparent. (*1*) Orbital implant, (*2*) skull base implant, (*3*) cranial vault implant.
m–q Status 4 weeks postoperatively: ocular motility is preserved, the pupils are level, and the levator weakness on the left side has improved

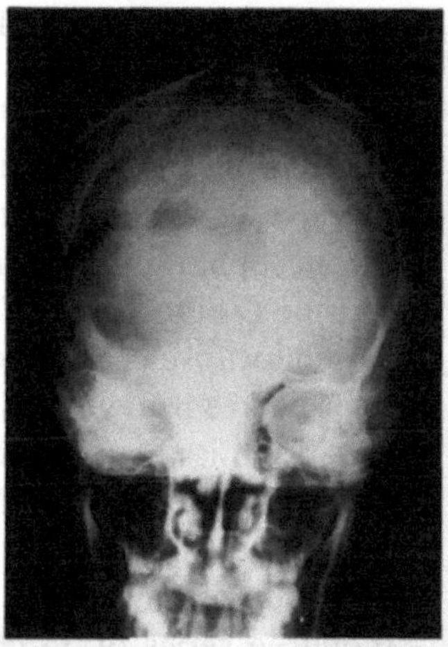
k

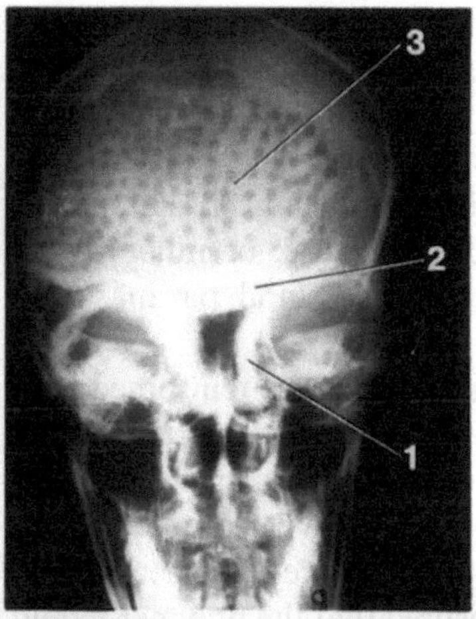

l

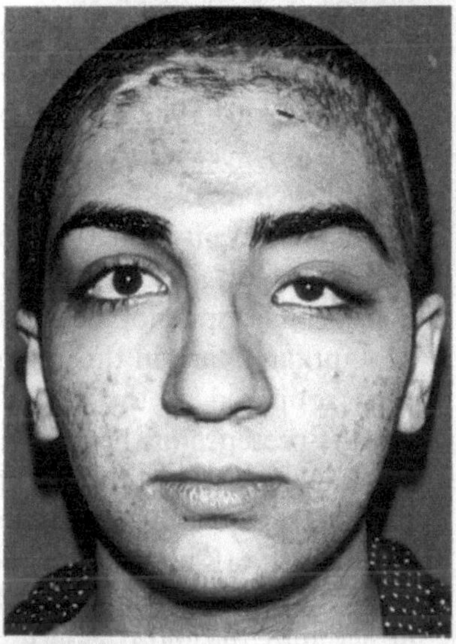
m

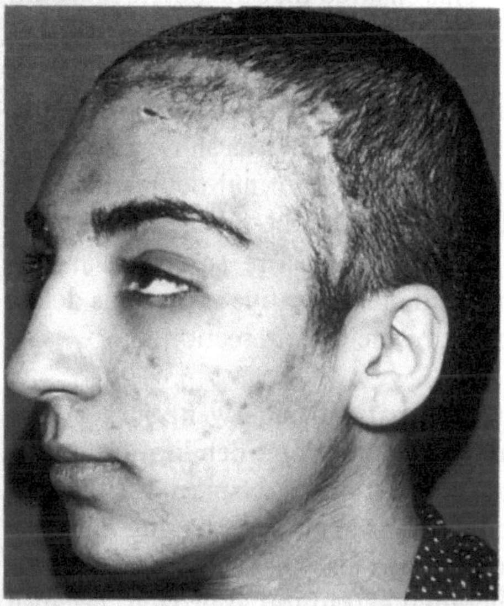
n

o, p
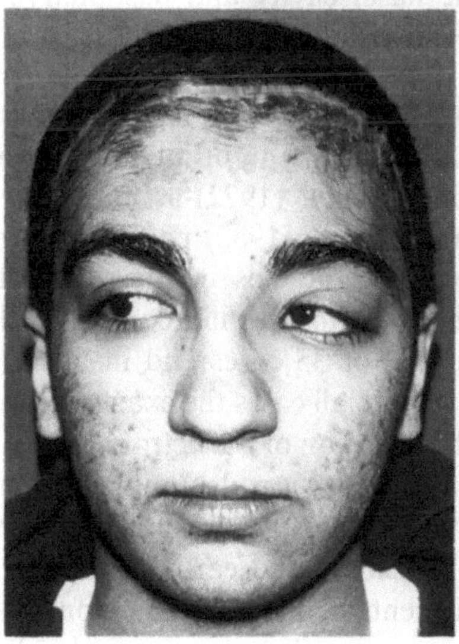

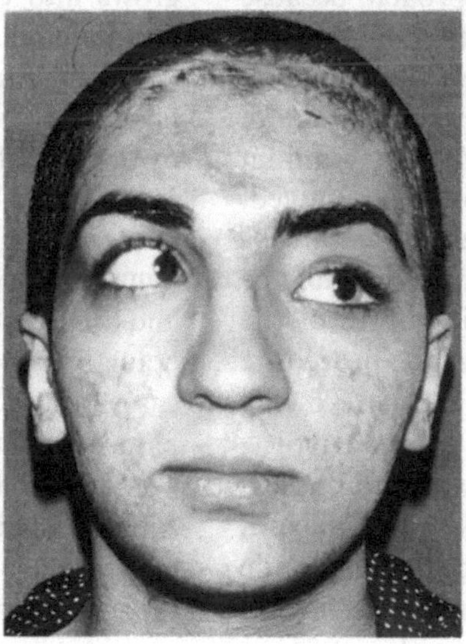

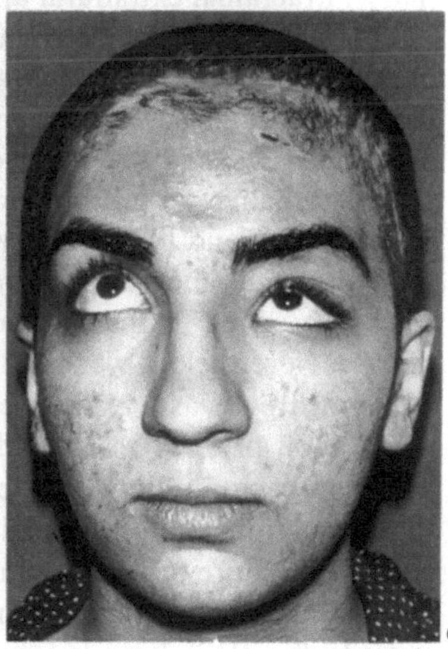
q

based flap. Then the orbital walls were reconstructed with methylmethacrylate. To avoid wound healing disturbance and implant rejection, it is necessary to cover the polymer implant with well-vascularized autogenous tissue such as pericranium, temporal muscle, or mucoperiosteum from the nasal cavity and paranasal sinuses.
Next the anterior skull base was reinforced with a second polymer implant, and the craniectomy was likewise repaired with methylmethacrylate. The implants were multiply perforated with a drill bit to achieve the desired permeation by scar tissue. This ensured that the polymer would be covered on all sides by well-perfused soft tissues.
The patient tolerated the 14-hour operation well. The postoperative photos show a satisfactory esthetic result and normal ocular motility with no displacement of the globe. The levator weakness that existed before surgery was improved. Pre- and postoperative skull films delineate the extent of the bone resection.

Comments: The patient underwent surgery for an extremely disfiguring and debilitating multiple recurrence of a fibrous dysplasia of the calvarium and anterior skull base, having had two previous operations elsewhere. We chose a primary intracranial extradural approach, because the tumor had a substantial intracranial, extradural component, and because the necessary extent of the skull base resection could be more accurately assessed from inside the cranium than externally. All gross tumor was removed. The cosmetic and functional result was satisfying, although another recurrence cannot be ruled out owing to the systemic nature of the disease. Nevertheless, we feel that the procedure is justified even as a palliative measure owing to its good primary result and low morbidity. This approach not only gives extradural access to the anterior skull base but also permits exposure of the entire orbit including the bony optic canal and upper paranasal sinuses. It is also suitable for skull base lesions with extension into the clivus.

Juvenile Nasopharyngeal Angiofibroma

Introductory Remarks. Juvenile nasopharyngeal angiofibroma (JNA) is a highly vascular, locally invasive, cone-shaped tumor that grows beneath the nasopharyngeal mucosa and lacks a true capsule (Zehm 1977). The tumor is covered by a pseudocapsule, however, so mobilization rarely provokes heavy bleeding as long as the pseudocapsule is intact (Neel et al. 1973). This tumor, which is rare in Europe and the United States and more common in the Near East, affects adolescent males almost exclusively, although a series of 35 cases described by Ward et al. (1974) included 3 females. The highest prevalance is between the ages of 14 and 25 years (Krause et al. 1982). The youngest patient to date is a 5-week-old child, reported by Martin and Ehrlich in 1948.
There have been numerous theories concerning the site of origin of JNA, which still remains unclear. The sphenopalatine foramen is an important landmark in this regard. It has not only been proposed as the site of origin for JNA, but the presence of the pterygomaxillary fissure also makes it a portal for tumor extension into the pyterygopalatine, pterygoid, and infratemporal fossae (Krause and Baker 1982, Ward et al. 1974). This histologically benign tumor grows into the nasal cavity and nasopharynx, and fingerlike extensions may invade the orbit, infratemporal fossa, skull base, and cheek. We have seen several instances of bony destruction of the skull base, and apparently this is not as rare as Seid and Vorster (1972) assume. Ward et al. (1974) and Krause (1982) performed systematic angiographic studies in their patients and found extension into the anterior and middle cranial fossae in 7 of 35 cases and in 5 of 14 cases, respectively. In all cases the extension was parasellar in the direction of the petrous bone.
The *symptoms* of JNA are determined by its extent. Impaired nasal respiration and recurrent epistaxis are present in the early stage. Later there is impairment of olfactory function, and certain patterns of growth can cause ocular displacement with visual deterioration, headache, facial deformity, and protrusion of the soft palate. Extension toward the petrous bone is mani-

fested by middle-ear deafness due to effusion in the tympanic cavity and by recurring bouts of otitis.

Tumor extent is established most effectively by CT and by selective angiography. It is useful to determine the extent to which large tumors are supplied by the external and internal carotid arteries of both sides and by the vertebral arteries. It is likely that superselective angiography, including preoperative embolization of the tumor vessels to reduce bleeding at operation, will assume increasing importance (Robarson et al. 1972, Pletcher et al. 1975, Lasjaunias and Berenstein 1987).

Opinions are divided concerning the potential of JNA for spontaneous remission during puberty (Neel et al. 1973). We have never observed this, although there are well-documented cases of regression of residual tumor following nonradical therapy. We agree with many other authors that the *treatment* of choice is operative removal (Neel et al. 1973, Pressmann 1962, Waldman et al. 1981, Ward et al. 1974, Zehm 1977 and accompanying bibliography). There have been reports of good results with primary irradiation (Fitzpatrick et al. 1980). We feel that radiation is acceptable postoperatively in cases where the tumor could not be completely resected. Ward et al. (1974) recommend a dose of 4,500–5,500 rad for this purpose.

The following surgical approaches are available:

1) The transpalatal approach employing a midline or transverse incision of the soft palate. Exposure is most limited toward the paranasal sinuses, skull base, and pterygopalatine fossa.
2) The lateral transmandibular or transzygomatic approach to the temporal and infratemporal fossa. This gives good exposure of tumor extensions in this area but somewhat poorer exposure of the nose and nasopharynx.
3) Craniofacial resection is recommended for tumors that have invaded the anterior skull base (Krekorian and Kempe 1969).
4) The transmaxillary approach. With sufficient bone removal, this affords good exposure of the nose, pterygopalatine fossa, infratemporal fossa, and inferior orbital fissure.
5) The extracranial approach through an extended Moure incision is recommended for larger tumors that have not yet invaded the anterior or middle cranial fossa, owing to the good exposure that is obtained.

Zehm (1977), Albrecht (1959), and other authors state that preoperative treatment with hormones is helpful in reducing intraoperative bleeding. Estrogens are said to be more effective in this regard than androgens. Lasjaunias and Berenstein (1987) emphasize the value of preoperative embolization by superselective angiography in controlling bleeding. The efficacy of intraoperative ligation of one or both external carotid arteries or their branches is questionable, although intraoperative ligatures may be placed close to the tumor to reduce its collateral supply.

Case Report (Fig. AS 49a–k). A 15-year-old boy presented with marked impairment of nasal respiration, hyposmia, progressive vision loss in the left eye, and downward displacement of the left globe with mild proptosis. The left nasal cavity and nasopharynx were filled with a firm, knobby tumor that bled heavily when biopsied. Histologic examination identified the lesion as an angiofibroma showing all the features of JNA. CT scans showed an extensive mass that not only filled the left side of the nasal cavity, paranasal sinuses, and nasopharynx but also had eroded through the left parasellar area of the skull base and had invaded the left orbit through the lamina papyracea, causing optic nerve compression. The mass also appeared to have invaded the infratemporal fossa. Carotid angiography showed that the tumor was supplied by both external carotid arteries and by small branches of the left internal carotid via the ophthalmic artery.

Because primary tumor growth extended caudally to the skull base, and because the histologic diagnosis implied that the intracranial portion of the tumor was situated extradurally, the extracranial approach was selected. The procedure was planned, however, so that a craniofacial resection could be carried out if necessary.

With the aid of the operating microscope, the tumor and surrounding mucosa were removed

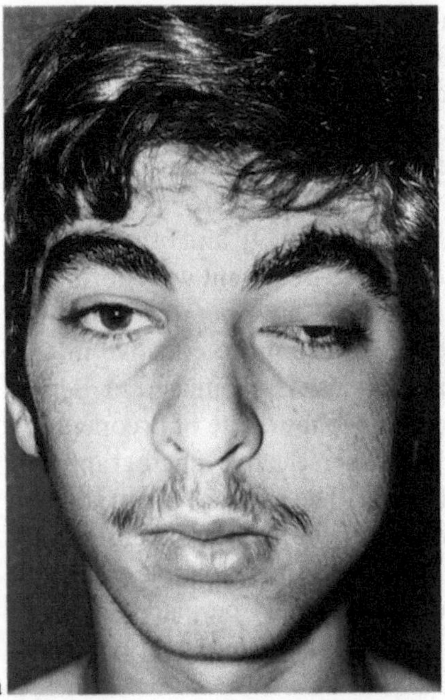

a

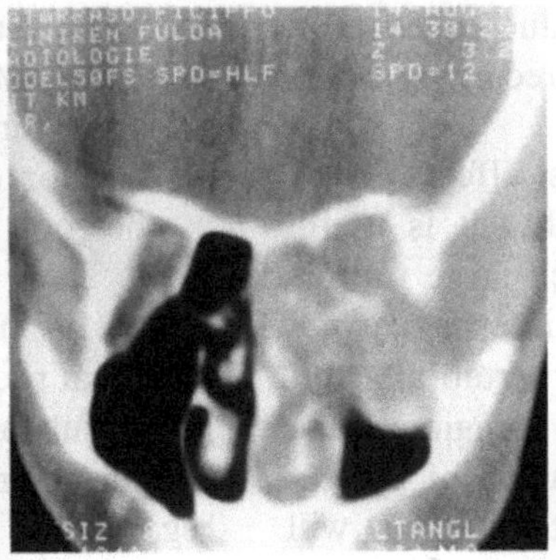

b

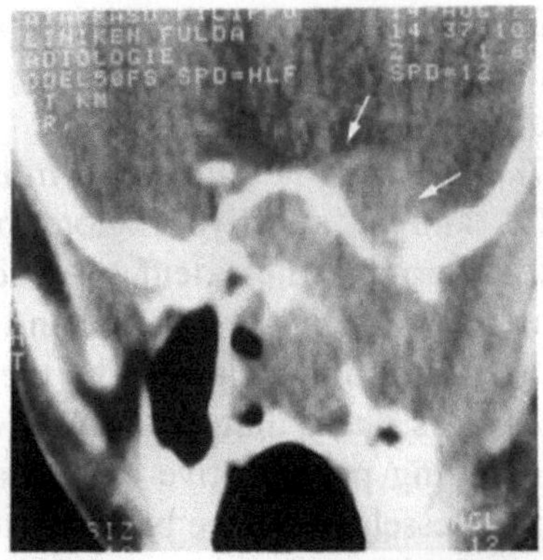

c

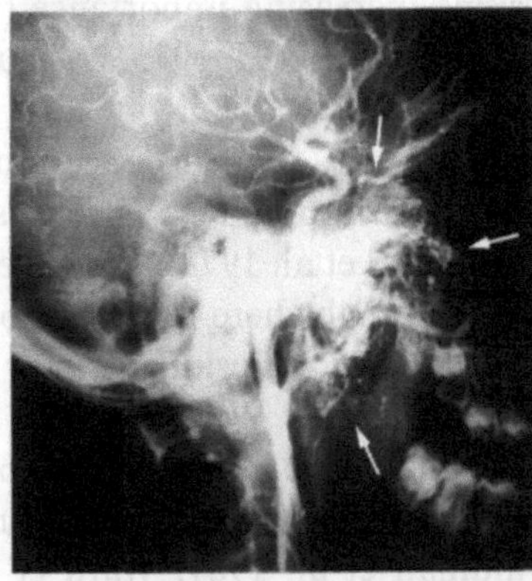

d

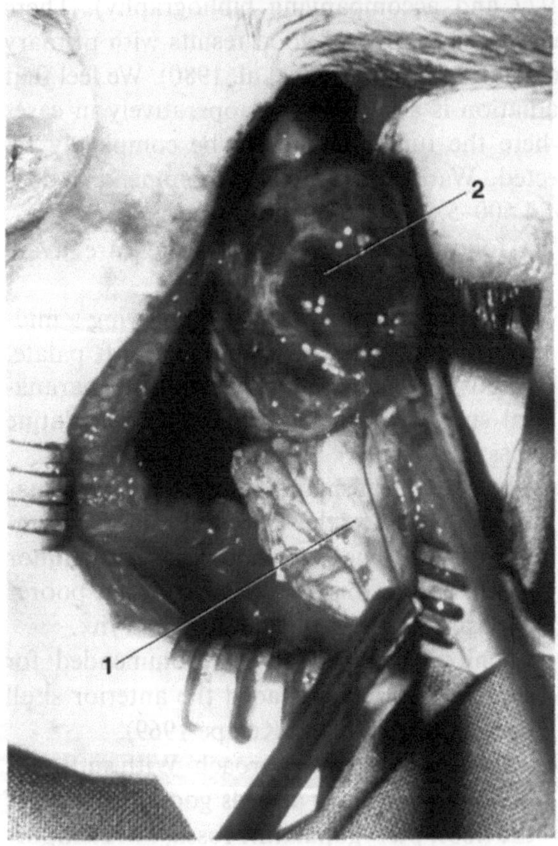

e

Fig. AS 49 a–k. Juvenile nasopharyngeal fibroma in a 15-year-old boy.
a The patient was admitted with impaired nasal respiration, left-sided hyposmia, and an almost complete loss of vision in the left eye with displacement of the globe.
b, c Coronal CT contrast scans. **b** shows the tumor extent in the nasal cavity, maxillary and sphenoid sinuses. **c** demonstrates partial destruction of the skull base (*arrow*) with a small, left parasellar tumor extension and invasion of the pterygopalatine fossa.
d Left carotid angiogram shows the rich tumor blood supply derived from both the external and internal carotid arteries (*arrows*).
e The tumor was exposed through a left paranasal incision. (*1*) Nasal mucosa, (*2*) tumor.
f The tumor specimen with surrounding mucosa.
g Four weeks after surgery ocular displacement is relieved, and the paranasal incision is healed. The incisions to expose the carotid artery and its branches are visible on the sides of the neck.
h The bilateral visual fields. The *shaded area* (I/4) represents the preoperative left visual field, and the *outer rings* (IV/4) represent the postoperative left and right fields.
i Two years later, CT scan shows a large tumor recurrence.
j The recurrence is excised with a margin of macroscopical normal tissue through a combined transmaxillary, transpalatine approach with elevation of a cheek flap. Histologic examination showed positive margins, so surgery was followed by telecobalt irradiation. Despite CT planning of the therapy, exposure was limited to 30 gray to decrease the risk of visual disturbances.
k CT scan 4 1/2 years after the second operation and radiation therapy. The patient has been free of disease for 6 years

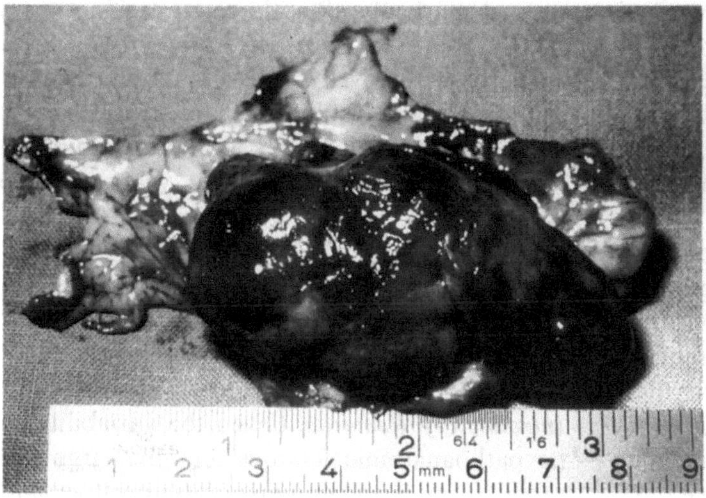

f

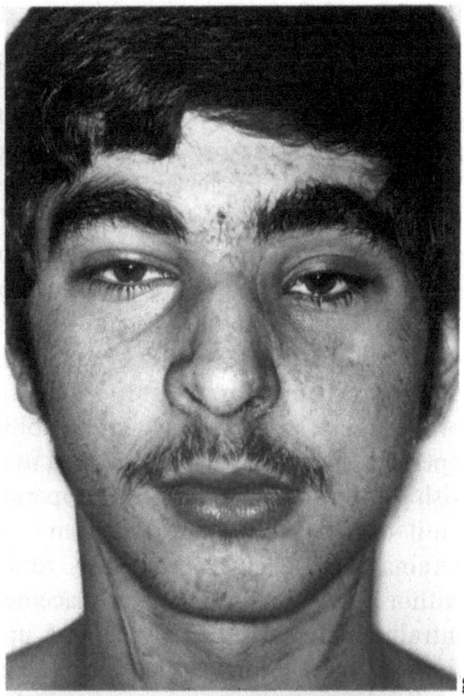

g

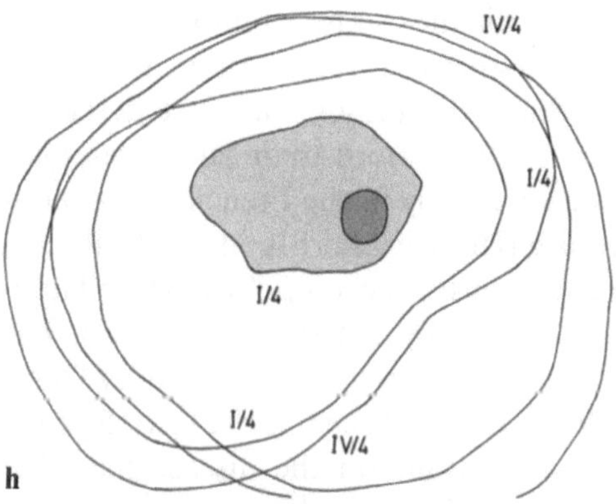

h

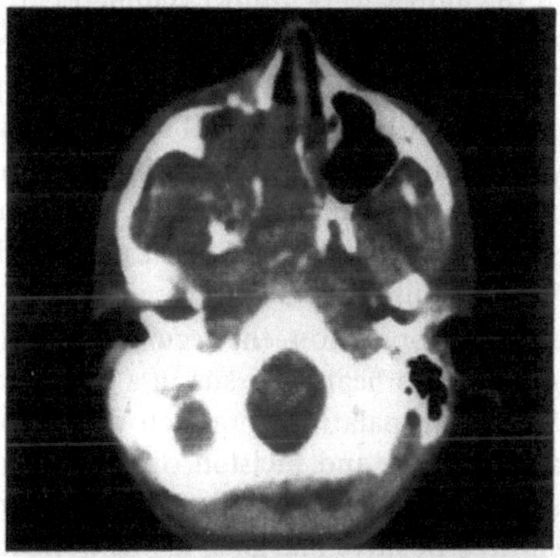

i

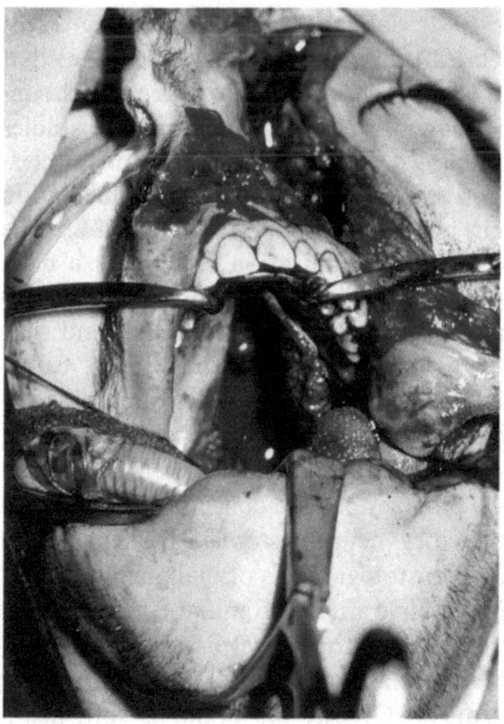

j

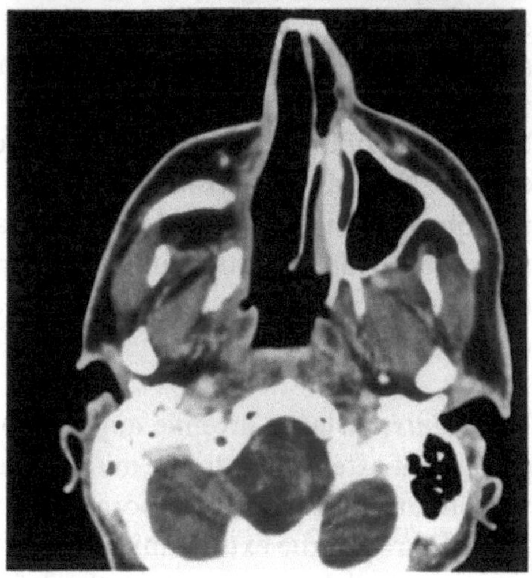

k

through a left paranasal incision as described by Moure (1902, 1922). The parasellar tumor extension was still surrounded in places by a thin bony rim, which was pared from the dura along with the tumor. The optic nerve, which was compressed in the area of the optic foramen, and the globe were exposed and spared. A partial maxillectomy was performed that spared the hard and soft palate. Intraoperative frozen-section examinations confirmed negative margins. Ligating the external carotid branches feeding the tumor at the start of the operation proved remarkably effective in controlling intraoperative bleeding. We were pleased to note that vision improved in the first postoperative days until only a small central scotoma remained. Drainage of tear secretions was reestablished within a few weeks following placement of an intraluminal stent in the remaining upper portions of the lacrimal apparatus. The positions of the globes were almost symmetrical.

About two years after the first operation, a large recurrence developed in the area of the pterygopalatine and infratemporal fossa and nasopharynx, manifested clinically by impaired nasal respiration and swelling of facial soft tissues. The extent of the recurrence was established by CT. Visual acuity in the left eye was unchanged. In a second operation, the recurrence was resected grossly into healthy tissue in a combined transfacial-transpalatine approach with elevation of a cheek flap and incision of the upper lip and soft palate. When histologic examination showed positive margins, it was decided to irradiate the area of the left pterygopalatine fossa and nasopharynx postoperatively with a total of 30 gray. The danger of vision loss and the benignancy of the tumor contraindicated a higher dose. No change of vision was noted on completion of the irradiation. More than six years after the second operation and postoperative radiation, the patient is asymptomatic and free of disease.

Comments: A large juvenile angiofibroma with extradural extension into the middle cranial fossa, left orbit, and infratemporal fossa was removed through the extracranial approach to the anterior skull base. Vision in the left eye improved markedly after the surgery. Two years later a recurrence in the left infratemporal fossa was grossly removed through a combined transfacial-transpalatine approach, and the area was subsequently treated with 30 gray of radiation. The patient is free of disease six years after the second operation.

Olfactory Neuroblastoma (Esthesioneuroblastoma)

Introductory Remarks. Given the variability of its pathoanatomic features and the large age range from 3 to 88 years, false-positive and false-negative diagnosis are common with olfactory neuroblastoma (Löblich 1981, Martin et al. 1983). Since the tumor was first described by Berger in 1924, more than 200 cases have been reported, mostly in the French and American literature (Homzie and Elkon 1980). Recent literature surveys have been published by Hommerich (1977) and by Martin et al. (1983). The fact that 125 of the 160 cases reviewed by Oberman in 1976 were published in the last 15 years, and that publications on the disease have become frequent only in the last few years (Foet et al. 1981, Jahnke et al. 1979, Jung 1981, Löblich 1981, Samii and Draf 1980) proves that special experience is needed to make a pathoanatomic diagnosis. Electron microscopic studies are assuming a growing importance for the classification of these neoplasms and the elucidation of their histologic origin (Löblich 1981). The World Health Organization recognizes a class of paranasal sinus tumors called "olfactory neurogenic (esthesioneurogenic) tumors" and subdivides them into esthesioneurocytoma, esthesioneuroepithelioma, and esthesioneuroblastoma, in order of decreasing differentiation. In the WHO classifiction of central nervous system tumors, these lesions are collectively referred to as "olfactory neuroblastomas." They exhibit few if any histologic signs of malignancy.

As with juvenile angiofibroma, the major symptoms are impaired nasal respiration and recurrent bleeding, although epistaxis appears to be less frequent. Grossly the tumor is soft, has a smooth surface, and is reddish to bluish-gray in color. Extension can produce symptoms of a mass lesion in the orbit and anterior cranial fossa. The disease may also begin with the signs of a brain tumor or meningitis (Becker et al. 1964, Jakumeit 1971, Silcox 1966). In a review of 200 cases, intracranial extension was present in one-fourth of the patients at the time of diagnosis (Martin et al. 1983). Regional metastases can occur in 10%–40% of cases, even after a silent period of years, and distant metastases occur in about 8% of cases, the lungs being the most frequent site.

The *prognosis* is affected less by the histologic classification of the tumor than by its degree of spread when treatment is initiated. There is disagreement as to the most effective form of therapy, due to the limited number of long-term observations on the response of this very rare tumor to current treatment modalities. A statistical evaluation of 133 cases with adequate documentation suggests that surgery and irradiation have equal efficacies in the treatment of smaller intranasal tumors (Martin et al. 1983). With more extensive tumors, combined surgery and irradiation are believed to be superior to either modality applied singly. The combined rhinosurgical-neurosurgical approach has been used in several cases of intracranial extension (Blokmanis 1972, Doyle and Paxton 1971, Sarwa 1979). In these cases we feel that the risk of cerebral necrosis (Baron 1979) and other dangers contraindicate postoperative irradiation that involves exposure of the cerebrum, except in cases of tumor recurrence. Appelblatt (1982) likewise reports that with larger tumors, primary or preoperative irradiation yields less favorable results than craniofacial resection followed if necessary by radiation at recurrence. Cytostatic agents have rarely been used. Walters et al. (1980) and Claux et al. (1979) report favorable experience in this regard and recommend that closer scrutiny be given to chemotherapeutic options.

One should be hesitant about declaring a total remission. Evidence to date indicates that 50% of patients who are 5-year survivors eventually succumb to recurrent or metastatic disease (Skolnik et al. 1966).

Case Report (Fig. AS 50a–h). A 29-year-old woman was referred to us with impaired nasal respiration on the left side. A reddish-gray, lightly bleeding tumor with extension into the nasal vestibule was identified histologically as an esthesioneuroblastoma. CT demonstrated a large tumor of the left nasal cavity that involved portions of the adjacent paranasal sinuses. The neoplasm appeared to arise from the skull base, although there was no objective evidence of bone destruction. Due to the questionable nature of the tumor and the patient's young age, we elected to perform a wide excision that included the surrounding mucosa, the cribriform plate, and the adjacent dura with the olfactory tract. This necessitated a combined craniofacial approach. Since we were able to establish the extent of the skull base resection preoperatively, we performed the intracranial part of the operation first in order to save time and reduce the risk of infection.

The anterior skull base was exposed intradurally through a bifrontal craniotomy. Both olfactory nerves were microsurgically dissected to the anterior angle of the optic chiasm and resected before entering the brain. The bone resection encompassed the cribriform plate, the ethmoid roofs, and a portion of the planum sphenoidale to ensure that the en bloc specimen would include all of the olfactory bulb with its filaments (a potential parent substance). The skull base was reconstructed in three layers consisting, from below upward, of a dural flap, a methylmethacrylate plate molded to the shape of the defect, and a galeal pericranial flap.

After closure of the craniotomy, the facial, extracranial part of the operation was performed through a paranasal incision extending from the medial third of the left eyebrow to the base of the ala nasi. The soft tissues and periosteum were reflected to expose the maxillary process of the frontal bone, the frontal process of the maxilla, and the corresponding portion of the nasal bone. The nasolacrimal duct was displaced laterally behind the lacrimal crest, and the periorbita was separated from the lamina papyracea. After removal of superficial bone, the tumor was encompassed from below by piecemeal removal of the lateral nasal wall and

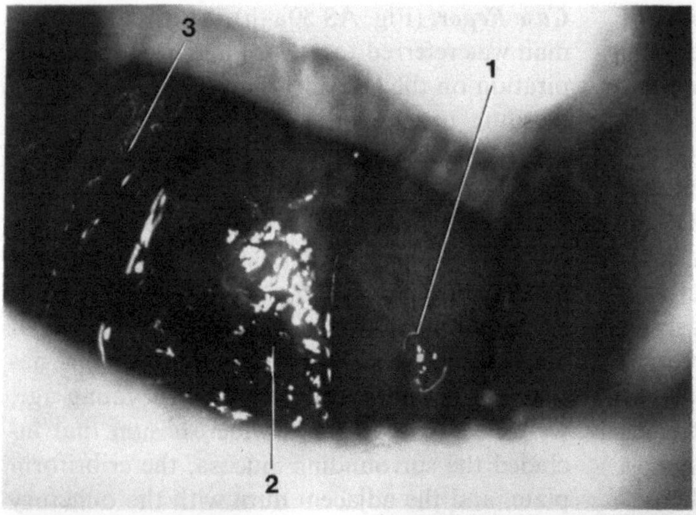

a

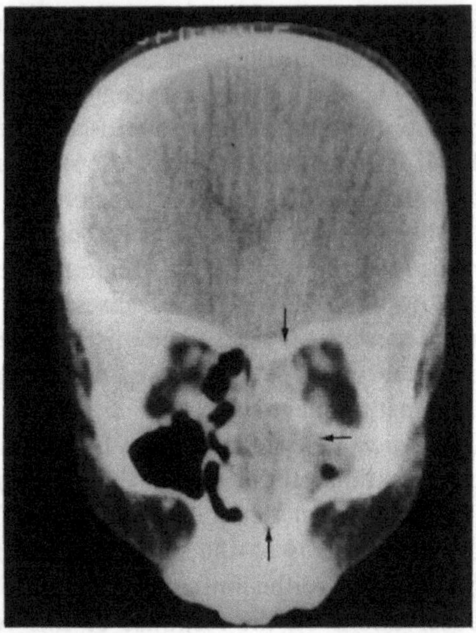

b

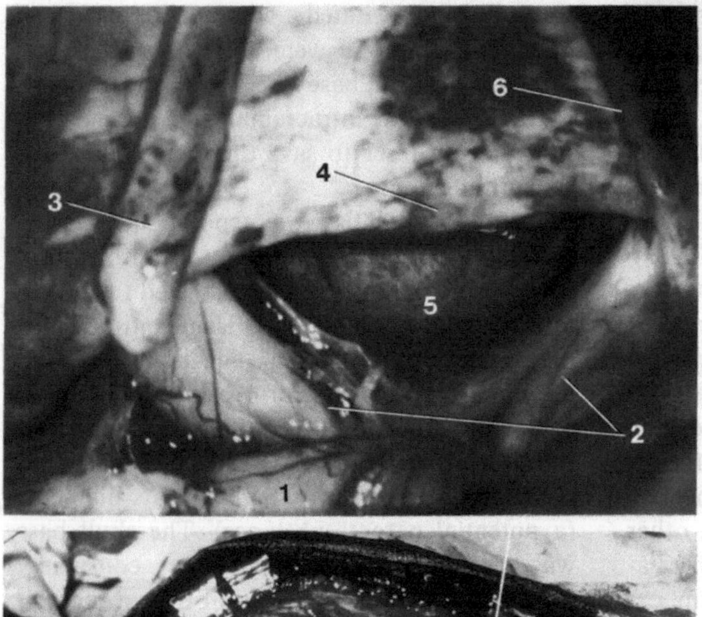

c

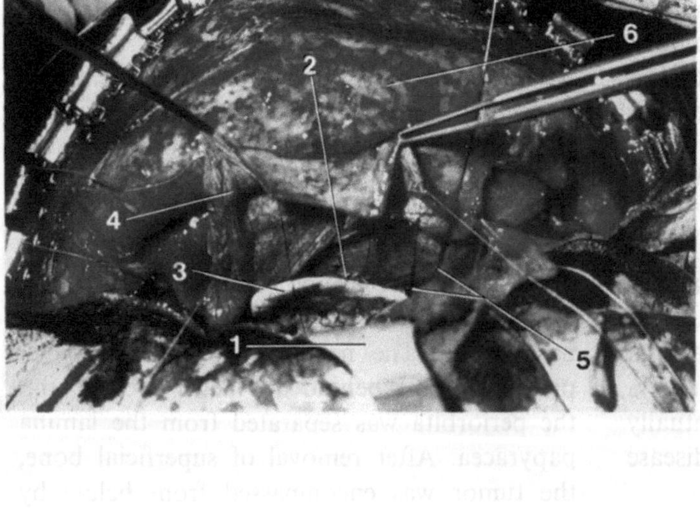

d

Fig. AS 50 a–h. Olfactory neuroblastoma of the left nose and paranasal sinuses with extension to the skull base in a 29-year-old woman.

a Anterior rhinoscopy shows a tumor between the normal-appearing left inferior turbinate and the nasal septum. The growth completely obstructs the nasal passage. (*1*) Left inferior turbinate, (*2*) tumor, (*3*) septum.

b Coronal CT scan. The tumor (*arrows*) totally obstructs the left nasal cavity and has caused opacification of the left ethmoid cells and maxillary sinus. It extends to the skull base but apparently has not caused bone destruction.

c Bifrontal transcranial intradural exposure of the anterior skull base to the anterior angle of the optic chiasm. Microsurgical dissection of both olfactory nerves. The sellar diaphragm is visible deep in the field. The left olfactory nerve is coagulated with bipolar current and sectioned. (*1*) Retracted frontal lobe, (*2*) optic nerves and chiasm, (*3*) severed left olfactory tract, (*4*) tuberculum sellae, (*5*) sellar diaphragm, (*6*) intact right olfactory tract.

d After resection of the midportion of the anterior skull base (cribriform plate and ethmoid roof on both sides), a three-layer basal cranioplasty is performed with dura, methylmethacrylate, and galea-pericranium. (*1*) Brain spatula, (*2*) duraplasty, (*3*) methylmethacrylate, (*4*) galeal pericranial flap, (*5*) fixation sutures, (*6*) scalp flap

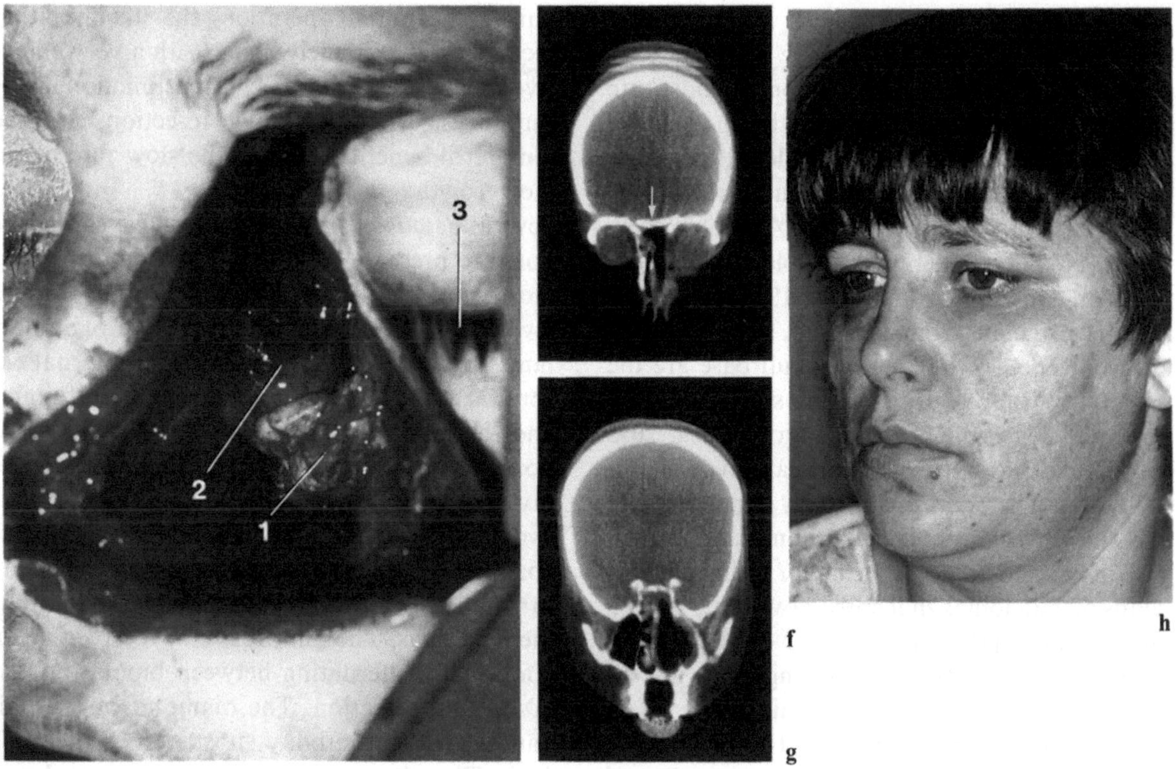

e f g h

Fig. AS 50e–h.
e Facial part of the operation: The tumor is visualized through a left paranasal incision after mobilizing the surrounding mucosa. (*1*) Mucosa, (*2*) tumor, (*3*) left eye. **f, g** Postoperative coronal CT scans. **f** Scan through the posterior part of the operated area with the anterior clinoid process, showing the air-filled surgical cavity lined by a thin layer of scar tissue. **g** The methylmethacrylate implant used to reconstruct the middle anterior skull base is visible (*arrow*).
h The patient 2 1/2 years after surgery

adjacent septum so that an en bloc resection could be achieved. A funnel-shaped cut was made around the tumor-free orifice of the nasolacrimal duct in the inferior meatus, and the orifice was later sutured into the soft tissues of the cheek to provide for lacrimal drainage.
The postoperative course was uncomplicated, and 2 1/2 years later the patient remains asymptomatic (except for anosmia) and free of recurrent disease.

Comments: A large olfactory neuroblastoma with extension to the skull base was removed en bloc through the craniofacial approach along with the adjacent middle anterior skull base. The specimen margins were histologically tumor-free. The nasolacrimal duct was reimplanted into the buccal soft tissues to preserve lacrimal drainage. The postoperative course was uneventful, and 2 1/2 years later the patient remains free of disease.

Meningiomas

Introductory Remarks. Meningiomas constitute the major group of mesodermal "brain tumors" in the current classification (Zülch 1956). The great majority are intracranial, but intracerebral occurrence is extremely rare. Approximately 12%–16% of intracranial neoplasms are meningiomas (Wolman and Path 1969). As these tumors originate from the dura, common sites of occurrence in the anterior skull base are the olfactory grooves, tuberculum sellae, planum sphenoidale, orbital roof, optic sheath, and sphenoid wings. Larger tumors can involve multiple sites. The operative strategy depends upon the site of origin, extent, predominant growth direction, and biologic behavior. The intraosseous meningiomas that spread over a large area of the skull base merit special consideration.
The histologic features of meningiomas are diverse. One classification recognizes five main types, with variants: syncytial, transitional, fibrous, angioblastic, and sarcomatous (Russel and Rubinstein 1971, quoted in Hommerich 1977). Zülch prefers a simpler scheme that recognizes four main types–endotheliomatous, fibromatous, angiomatous, and sarcomatous–although he emphasizes that the first three constitute a uniform group for the clinician in terms of their histologic features and growth behavior.
Primary involvement of the nose or paranasal sinuses by meningiomas is extremely rare compared with the incidence of intracranial occurrence. Hommerich (1977) found only 13 published cases, 4 in the frontal sinus, 3 in the nasal cavity and ethmoid, 2 in the ethmoid, 2 in the maxillary sinus, and 1 each in the nasal cavity and ethmoid. It is our impression that the nose and paranasal sinuses may be involved more frequently by intracranial meningiomas than is suggested by isolated reports in the literature.
We share the opinion of Leroux-Robert et al. (1966) that combined craniofacial approaches are of great potential value for the complete removal of large meningiomas having both intra- and extracranial components. Meningiomas tend to grow slowly, and except for the sarcomatous form, the lesion is clinically and biologically benign. Unless all the tumor is removed during the initial operation, the likelihood of recurrence is extremely high. With a very extensive meningioma that is causing functional disturbances, even a palliative resection can give long-term benefit owing to the slow rate of tumor growth.
Several *details of dissecting technique* should be noted to preserve maximum function during tumor removal. Microsurgical technique should always be used during the exposure of important structures like the optic nerve, internal carotid artery, other cranial nerves, the pituitary, and the pituitary stalk. Also, one should abandon the usual concept of en bloc resection in favor of a piecemeal debulking technique that avoids injury to neighboring structures. Bipolar coagulation has proven very helpful, especially in removing the highly vascular angiomatous meningiomas. The tumor is removed piecemeal, continually alternating between bipolar coagulation and resection. The diamond burr is advantageous in the bony substance of the skull base. The ultrasonic aspirator has proved useful in recent years for rapid tumor reduction. Some authors recommend the use of CO_2 or Nd:YAG lasers for this purpose. When compact bone is reached, all the tumor has been removed. In other cases the bony skull base may have to be resected as far as the nasal mucosa when working from above, or it may be removed together with involved dura from below. Bleeding from bone edges can be controlled with the diamond burr or with bone wax. Flaps may be prepared from uninvolved dura and later used to cover the basal skull defect.
From a *surgical* standpoint, it is useful to classify meningiomas of the anterior skull base into three groups:

1) Meningiomas with predominantly intracranial growth.
2) Meningiomas with predominantly extracranial growth.
3) Meningiomas with intra- and extracranial growth.

Meningiomas with Predominantly Intracranial Extension

Tumors of the olfactory grooves, tuberculum sellae, planum sphenoidale, and sphenoid wing are counted among the predominantly intracranial meningiomas of the anterior skull base.

Olfactory Groove Meningioma

Introductory Remarks. Surprisingly, the neurosurgeon rarely sees these patients with the early symptom of olfactory impairment, and most cases are not diagnosed until the tumor has reached sufficient size to cause visual impairment. Other frequent symptoms are severe headache, mental changes, and occasionally seizures. Erosion of the cribriform plate and hyperostosis of the planum sphenoidale on plain skull films warrant further investigation by CT, MRI, and cerebral angiography. These studies will confirm the diagnosis and establish the extent of the tumor.

While Kempe (1968) and Poppen (1964) favor operative treatment of these lesions through a unilateral frontal exposure with frontal lobectomy, Osemann (1982) prefers a bifrontal craniotomy.

Case Report (Fig. AS 51 a–d). A 59-year-old woman presented with a 2-year history of progressive dementia. Clinical examination disclosed bilateral anosmia and a concentric contraction of the left visual field with visual acuity reduced to 20%. Plain radiographs showed erosion of the cribriform plate, and CT scans demonstrated a large mass lesion suspicious for meningioma. The angiogram showed elevation of the anterior cerebral arteries and pathologic staining of the tumor vessels supplied via the ophthalmic arteries.

The tumor was approached by the transcranial intradural route through a bifrontal craniotomy and exposed by gentle retraction of the frontal lobes. Piecemeal removal of the highly vascular tumor was accomplished by bipolar coagulation and resection. Both anterior cerebral arteries, the optic nerves, and the optic chiasm were microsurgically freed of tumor. After removal of the dura bordering on the tumor, the thickened crista galli and cribriform plate were removed with the diamond burr. The small skull base defect was closed in two layers with a dural graft and a galeal pericranial flap.

The postoperative course was uncomplicated, and CT scans confirmed total tumor removal. One year later the patient was clinically asymp-

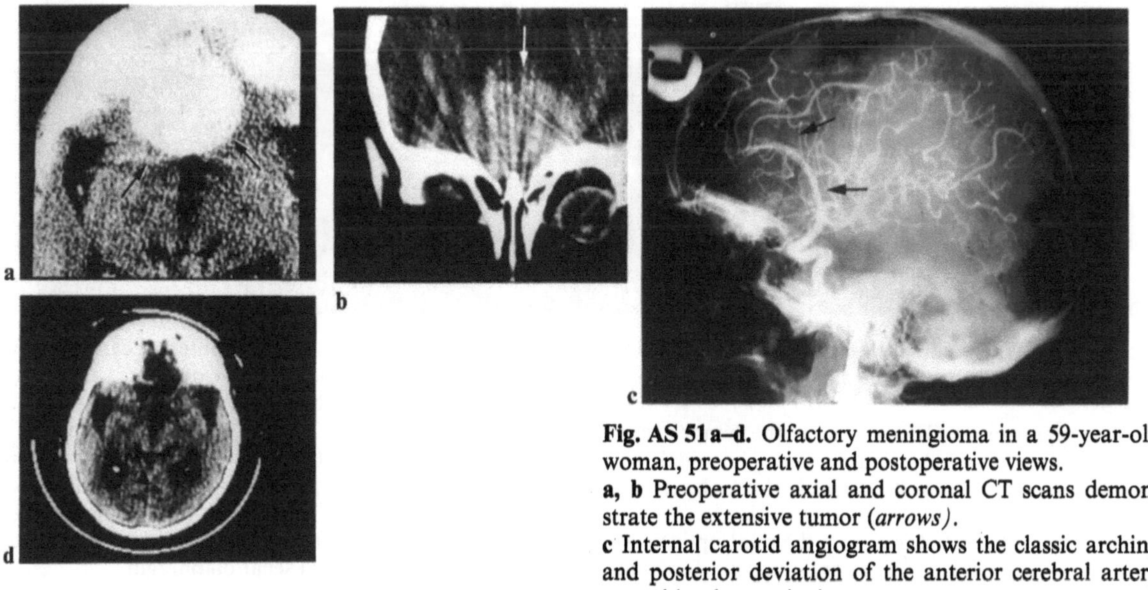

Fig. AS 51 a–d. Olfactory meningioma in a 59-year-old woman, preoperative and postoperative views.
a, b Preoperative axial and coronal CT scans demonstrate the extensive tumor *(arrows)*.
c Internal carotid angiogram shows the classic arching and posterior deviation of the anterior cerebral artery caused by the meningioma.
d Postoperative CT scan confirms complete removal of the tumor through the transfrontal approach

tomatic (except for anosmia) and free of recurrence. The visual disturbance improved markedly.

Comments: A large olfactory groove meningioma compressing the optic chiasm was removed microsurgically through a transfrontal, intradural approach, resulting in good recovery of function.

Tuberculum Sellae-Planum Sphenoidale Meningioma (Fig. AS 52a–f)

A 58-year-old man was diagnosed as having a predominantly intracranial meningioma en plaque of the anterior skull base in the midline area, extending from the tuberculum sellae and planum sphenoidale to the crista galli. The tumor was exposed intradurally through a right frontal craniotomy. The compressed right optic nerve and internal carotid artery were identified and freed from tumor. Then the optic chiasm and left optic nerve, completely encased by tumor, were freed by piecemeal removal of the neoplasm. Residual tumor on the tuberculum

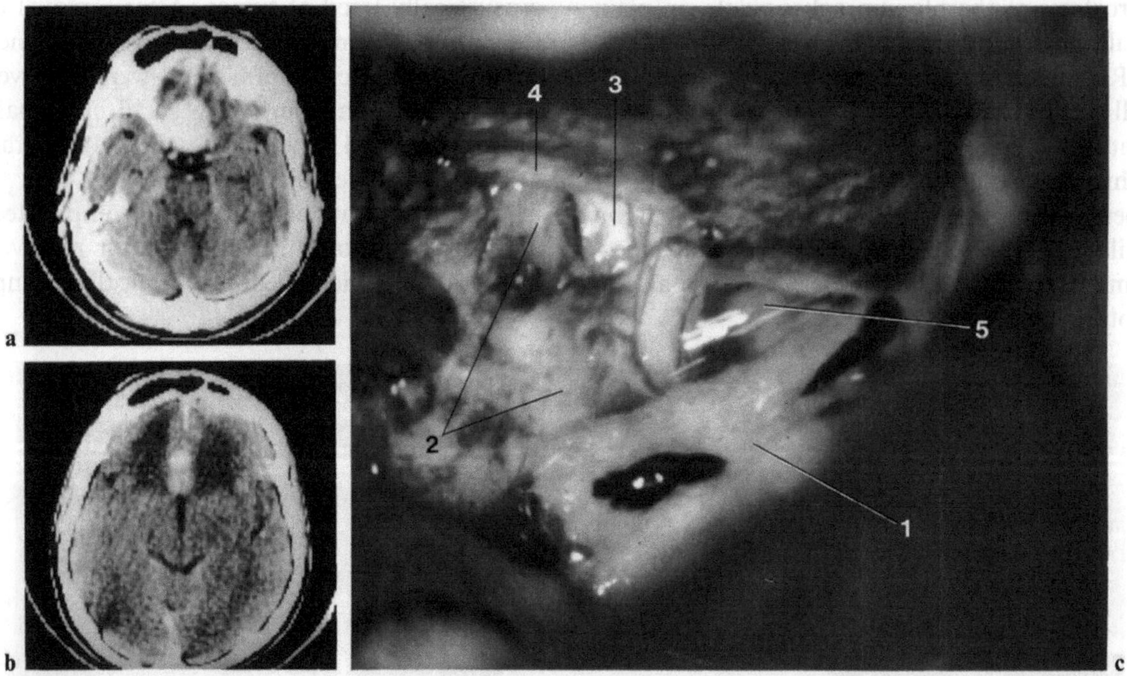

Fig. AS 52a–f. Predominantly intracranial meningioma en plaque involving the midline area of the anterior skull base.
a, b The preoperative CT scans show the tumor arising from the tuberculum sellae and planum sphenoidale and extending to the crista galli. There is marked perifocal edema.
c The tumor is dissected free from the right optic nerve. (*1*) Cotton, (*2*) tumor, (*3*) right optic nerve, (*4*) planum sphenoidale, (*5*) internal carotid artery.
d The right optic nerve and right internal carotid artery have been cleared of tumor. (*1*) Cotton, (*2*) tumor, (*3*) right optic nerve, (*4*) tuberculum sellae, (*5*) right internal carotid artery.
e The anterior angle of the optic chiasm is exposed by piecemeal tumor reduction using bipolar coagulation and scissors resection. (*1*) Cotton, (*2*) tumor, (*3*) right optic nerve, (*4*) right internal carotid artery, (*5*) anterior angle of optic chiasm, (*6*) sellar diaphragm.
f The area of tumor attachment on the skull base is burred away. (*1*) Tumor, (*2*) skull base, (*3*) diamond burr

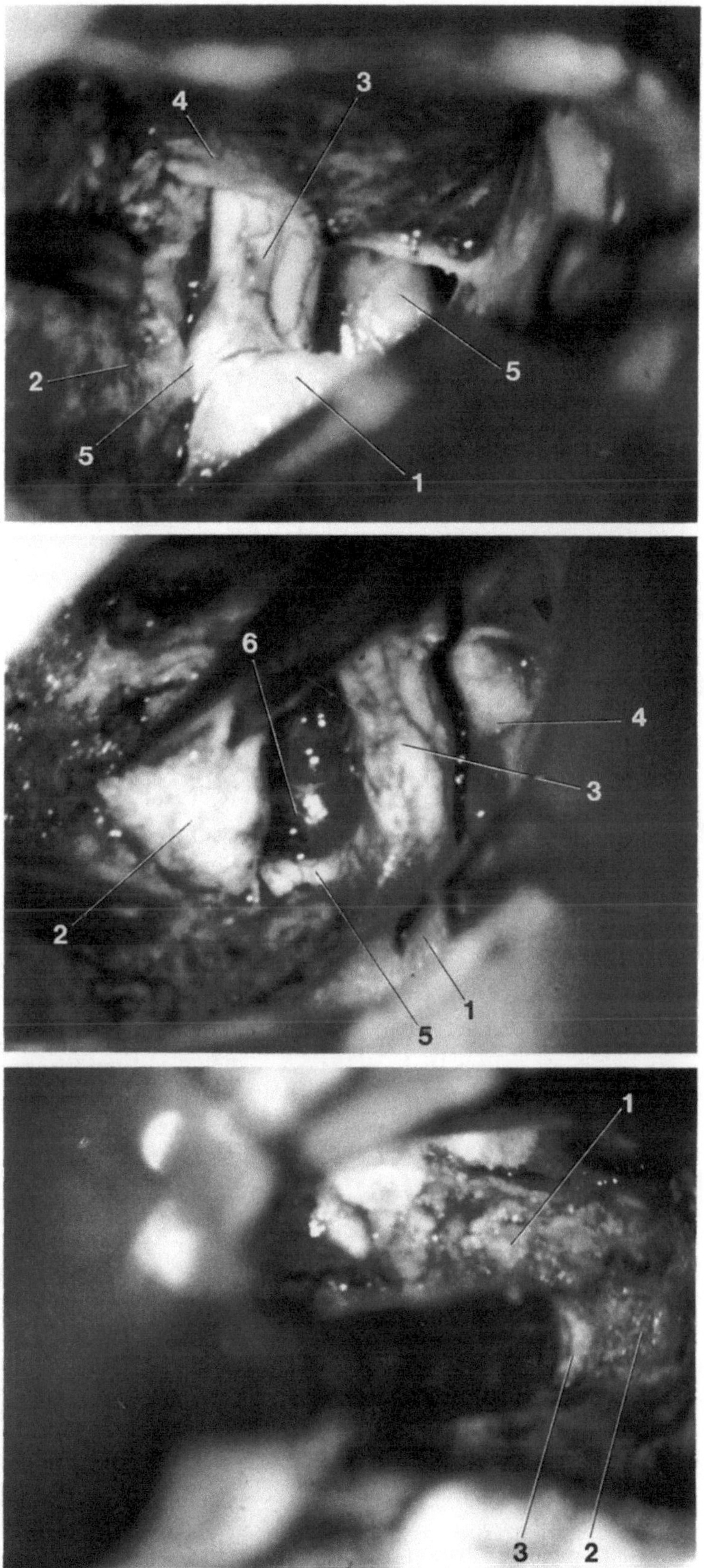

d e f

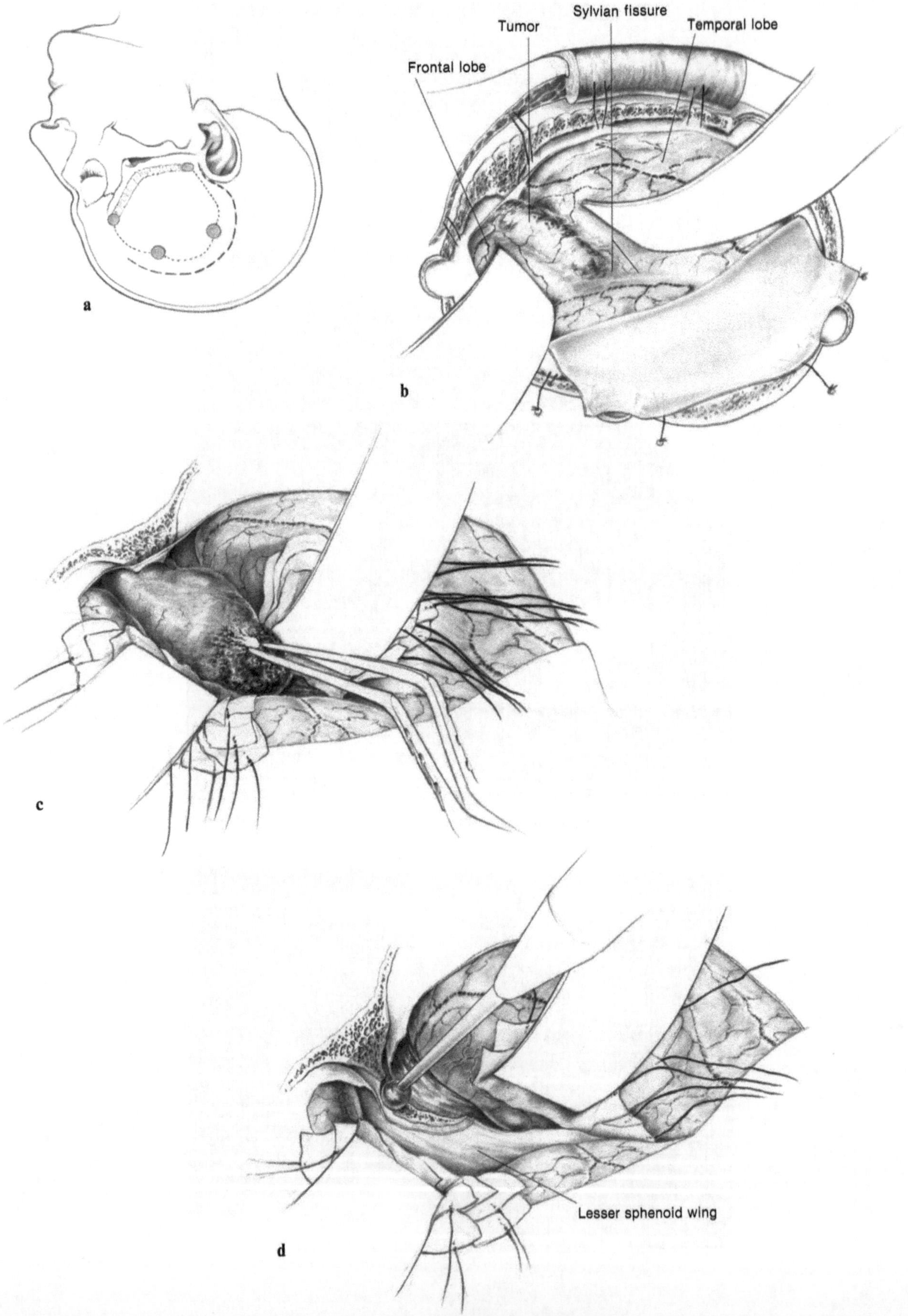
Sylvian fissure
Tumor
Temporal lobe
Frontal lobe
a
b
c
Lesser sphenoid wing
d

Fig. AS 53a–d. Removal of a *lateral* sphenoid wing meningioma.
a Skin incision, burr holes, and osteoplastic craniotomy for the frontotemporal intradural approach (pterional approach).
b The sylvian fissure is opened microsurgically, and the frontal and temporal lobes are retracted to expose the tumor on the minor sphenoid wing.
c Piecemeal tumor resection is alternated with bipolar coagulation.
d Most of the minor sphenoid wing is removed with the area of tumor attachment to ensure a complete resection

sellae and portions of the planum sphenoidale were removed with the diamond burr. The bone defect was closed in two layers with lyophilized dura and a galeal pericranial flap.

Comments: The relations of a large tuberculum sellae-planum sphenoidale meningioma to the optic nerves, chiasm, hypothalamus, and anterior cerebral vessels required precise microsurgical dissection, allowing total tumor removal with preservation of surrounding structures.

Sphenoid Wing Meningioma

Introductory Remarks. Sphenoid wing meningiomas are classified by their location as lateral or medial (Tönnis and Schürmann 1951). While even extensive lateral tumors usually pose no difficulty in terms of surgical access (Fig. AS 53a–d), medial sphenoid wing meningiomas frequently involve important structures like the internal carotid artery and its cerebral branches, the optic nerve, and the brain stem region. This introduces a considerable element of risk and difficulty in their operative removal. In our experience, it is better to open the sylvian fissure and carefully retract the frontal or temporal lobe than undertake a piecemeal removal of the tumor along the skull base. The former technique is less traumatizing in terms of brain compression and allows better visualization of the internal carotid artery and its branches. Opening the sylvian fissure permits the tumor to be approached laterally from above. The lesion is removed piecemeal with the aid of bipolar coagulation. After the tumor has been exenterated, its capsule is carefully dissected off the branches of the middle cerebral artery. The tumor resection is continued along these branches to reach the internal carotid artery, which may be completely embedded in tumor. In that case the vessel is microsurgically dissected free of tumor (Fig. AS 54a–e).

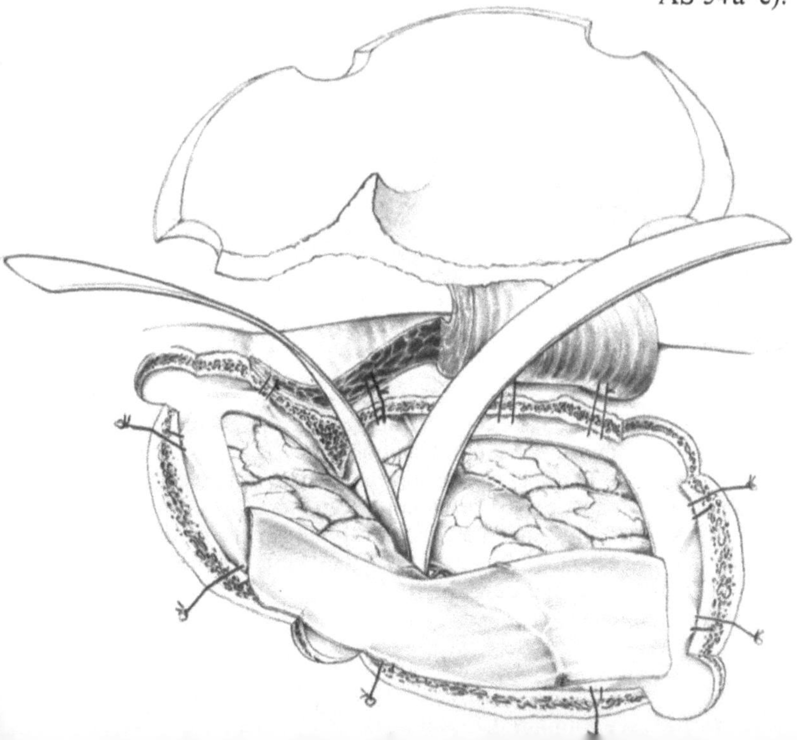

Fig. AS 54a

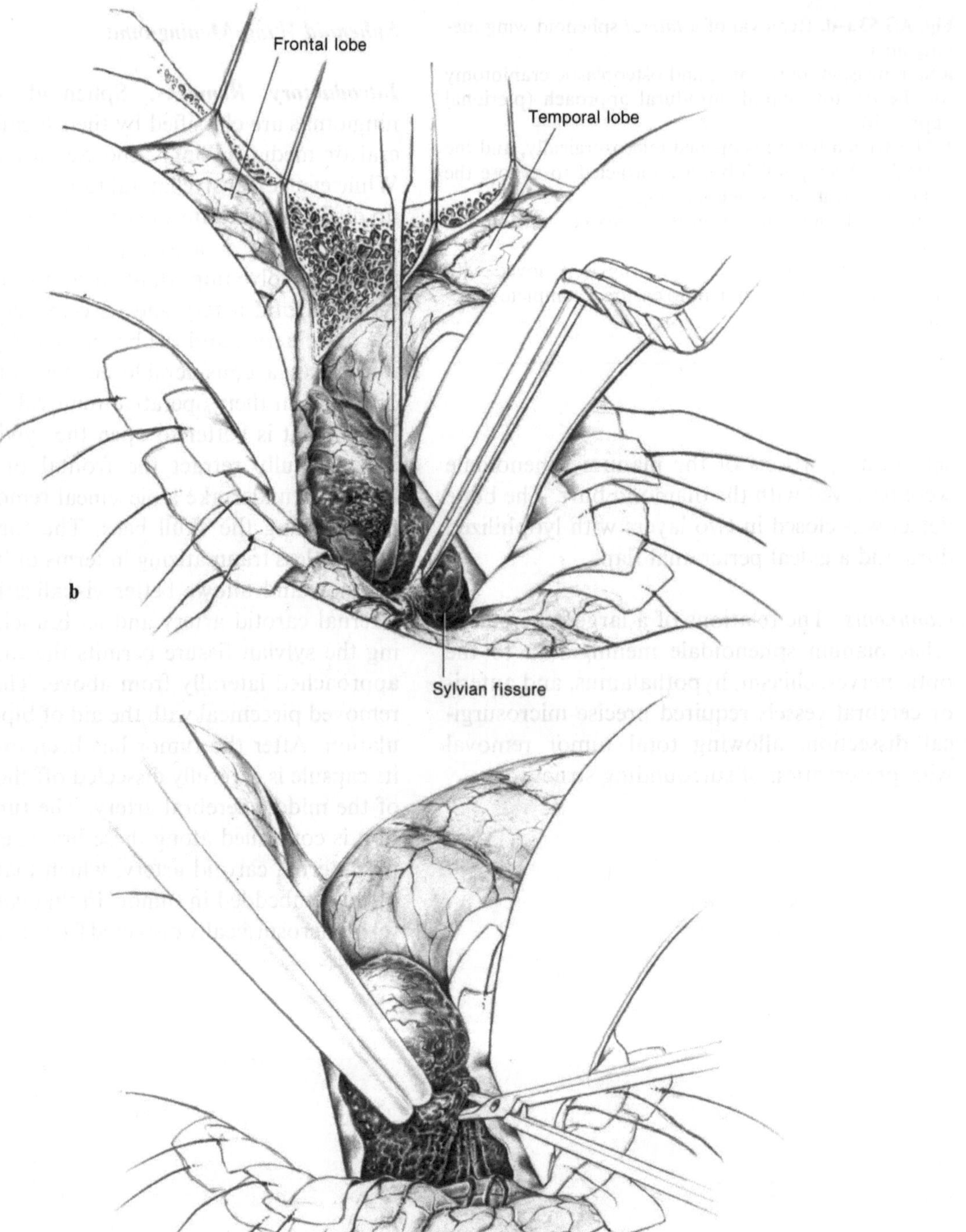

Fig. AS 54a–e. Resection of a *medial* sphenoid wing meningioma.
a After frontotemporal osteoplastic craniotomy, the dura is opened in trap-door fashion, and the tumor is approached through the sylvian fissure.
b, c The tumor is visualized laterally from above and resected piecemeal with the aid of bipolar forceps. The tumor capsule is separated from the middle cerebral artery.
d The resection continues along the middle cerebral artery to the internal carotid.
e The field after complete removal of the neoplasm. The functionally important neurovascular structures have been preserved. The dural attachment of the tumor is resected, the minor sphenoid wing is removed with the diamond burr

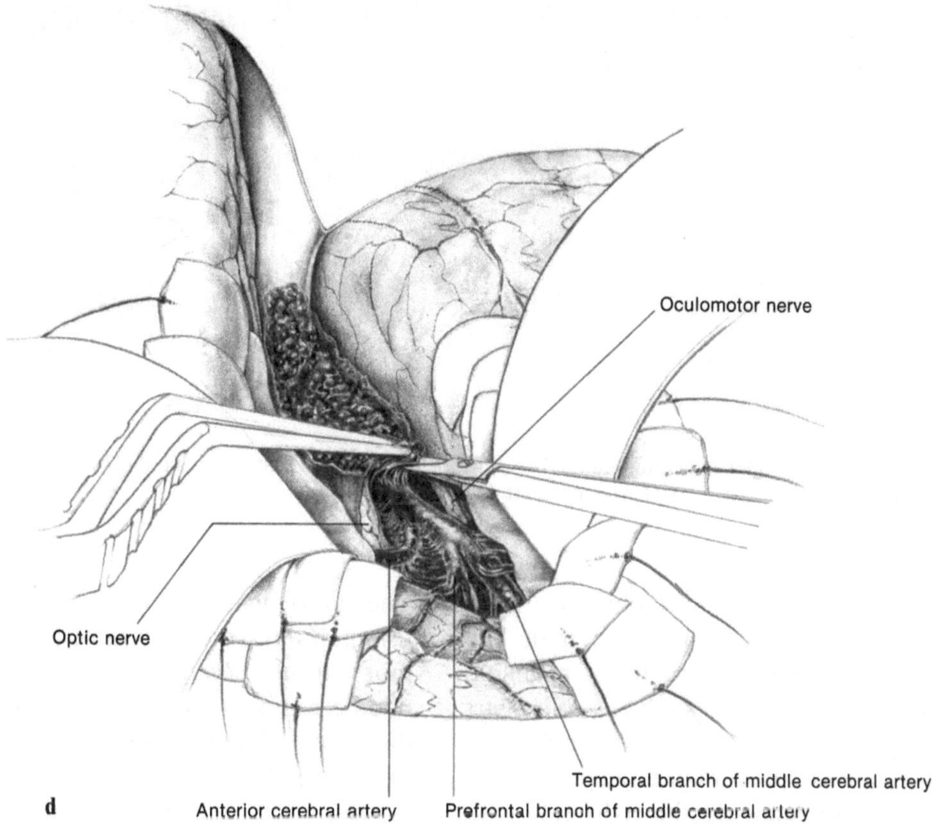
Oculomotor nerve
Optic nerve
Temporal branch of middle cerebral artery
Anterior cerebral artery
Prefrontal branch of middle cerebral artery

d

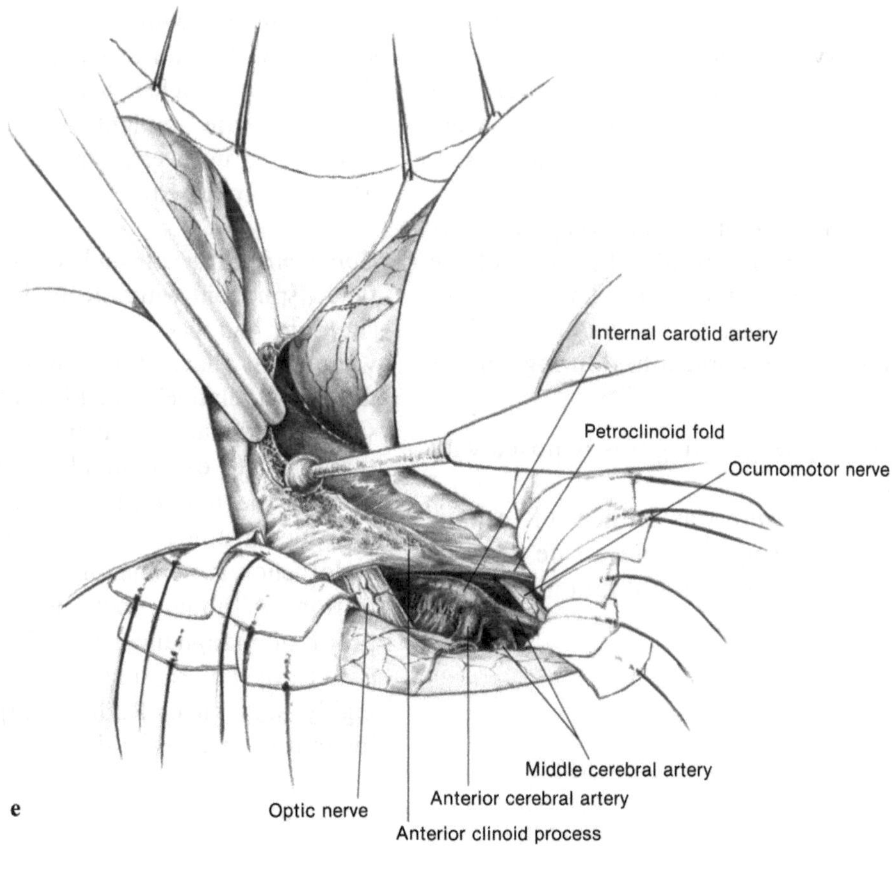
Internal carotid artery
Petroclinoid fold
Ocumomotor nerve
Middle cerebral artery
Optic nerve
Anterior cerebral artery
Anterior clinoid process

e

a, b

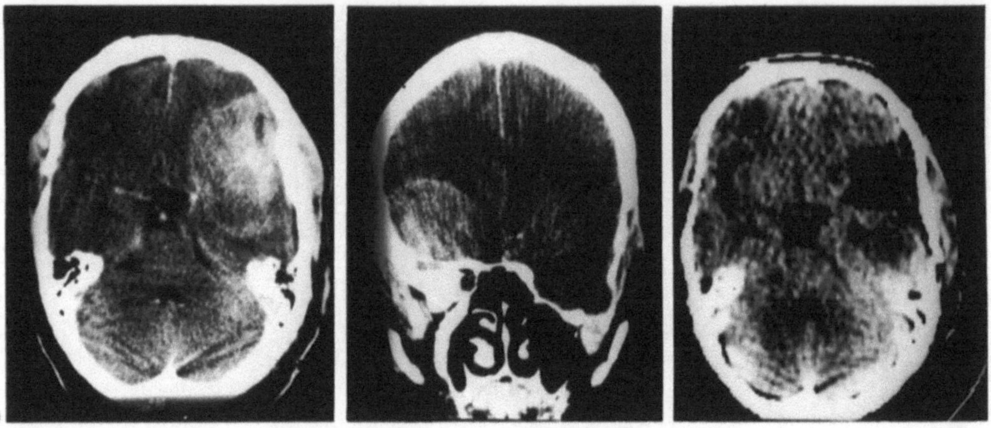

c

Fig. AS 55a–c. Extensive lateral meningioma of the right sphenoid wing on preoperative axial and coronal CT scans (**a, b**) and on an axial CT scan following operative removal (**c**)

Case Report. Lateral sphenoid wing meningioma (Fig. AS 55a–c). A 51-year-old man had previously undergone surgery for a sphenoid wing meningioma of the left skull base. Six years later he complained of a dull headache. CT disclosed an extensive, predominantly lateral sphenoid wing meningioma on the right side with infiltration of the temporal muscle. This was presumed to represent an extracranial extension from a primary intracranial tumor.

Tumor infiltration of the temporal muscle and infratemporal fossa was already evident when the right frontotemporal skin flap was raised. After removal of the extracranial part of the tumor, a frontotemporal craniotomy was performed, exposing the extradural portion of the large intracranial meningioma. Two measures were taken to minimize tension and pressure on the frontal and temporal lobes during further dissection:

1) The lesser sphenoid wing was removed with the diamond burr.
2) The sylvian fissure was opened microsurgically after incising the dura a safe distance from the area of tumor infiltration.

The tumor was then debulked from its center using an ultrasonic aspirator (Cusa). As the tumor capsule became lax, the branches of the middle cerebral artery could be identified, and dissection of the capsule proceeded along the middle cerebral artery branches to the internal carotid artery. At that point it was possible to remove the tumor completely, including its dural attachment, without danger to neighboring structures. The dura was patched with stored dura, the bony defect was repaired with a methylmethacrylate implant, and the soft tissues were closed in layers. The postoperative course was uncomplicated.

Comments: The unusual feature of this case is that a sphenoid wing meningioma of the opposite side had been removed six years earlier, whereupon a large tumor not detectable before developed relatively quickly on the contralateral side. The apparently aggressive growth of this tumor led to extracranial extension with invasion of the temporal muscle. The lesion was identified histologically as a mixed fibromatous-endotheliomatous meningioma with bony infiltration. Although there was no microscopic proof of malignancy, the history and growth pattern of the lesion clearly showed that it was highly aggressive. Radical surgical excision is imperative in cases of this kind.

a, b

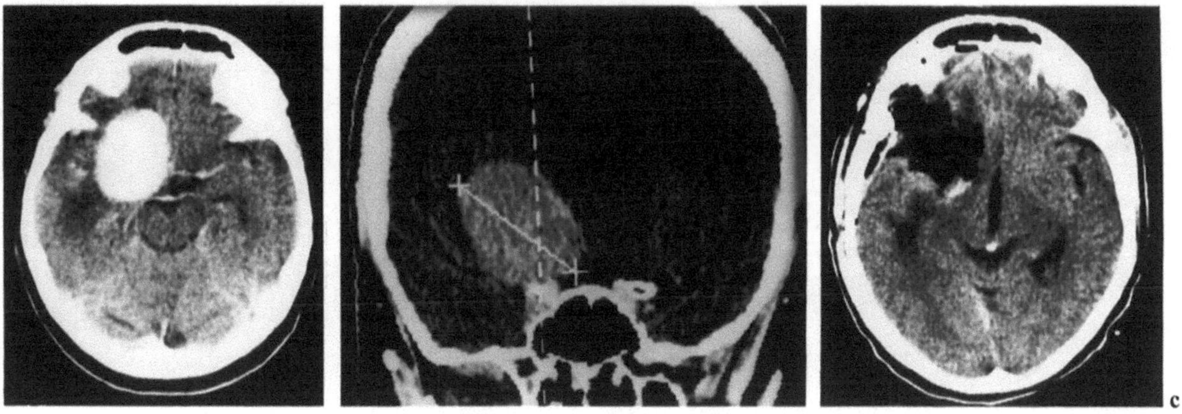

c

Fig. AS 56a–c. Preoperative and postoperative CT scans of a large medial sphenoid wing meningioma that could be totally removed. The histologic diagnosis was endotheliomatous meningioma

Case Report. Medial sphenoid wing meningioma (Fig. AS 56a–c). The patient, a 64-year-old woman, had suffered left-sided headaches for 3 years. Shortly before hospitalization, she experienced transient dizzy spells with loss of consciousness. Two years earlier she experienced transient speech impairment and paralysis of the right arm with remission within a few minutes. On admission we found no neurologic deficits other than a slight paresis of the right arm.

CT scans disclosed a mass lesion that appeared to arise from the left medial sphenoid wing and extended into the anterior and middle cranial fossa. The angiogram showed upward deviation of the middle cerebral artery with displacement of the anterior cerebral artery and a vascular pattern typical of meningioma.

The tumor was exposed through a left frontotemporal craniotomy, removing the lesser sphenoid wing, incising the dura, and opening the sylvian fissure. The tumor was reduced with the ultrasonic aspirator, and the heavily enmeshed middle cerebral artery was microsurgically freed of tumor. Additional tumor was removed along the course of the middle cerebral artery, and the internal carotid artery, also enveloped by tumor, was isolated. It was then possible to remove the meningioma along with its area of attachment. The anterior cerebral artery and the slightly displaced left optic nerve were anatomically and functionally preserved.

The wound was closed in standard fashion. Eighteen days later the patient's general condition was good, she had no neurologic deficits, and she was discharged home.

Comments: The major problem with a medial sphenoid wing meningioma of this type is its close proximity to important structures like the internal carotid artery and its branches, the optic nerve, the oculomotor nerve, and possibly the other motor nerves of the eye. By following the strategy indicated, we were able to safely isolate the internal carotid artery, which was completely encased by tumor, along with functionally important adjacent structures.

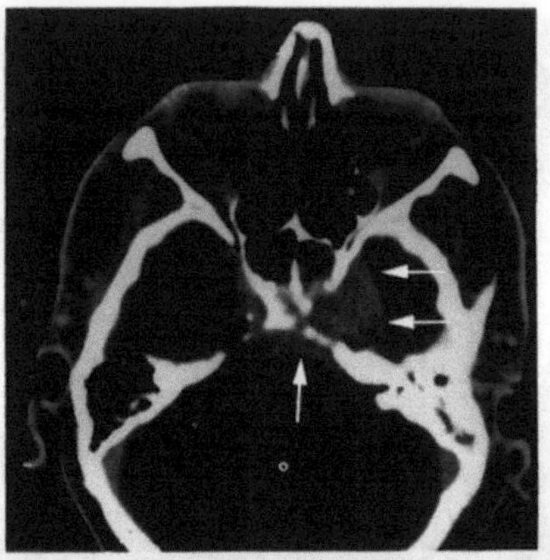

a

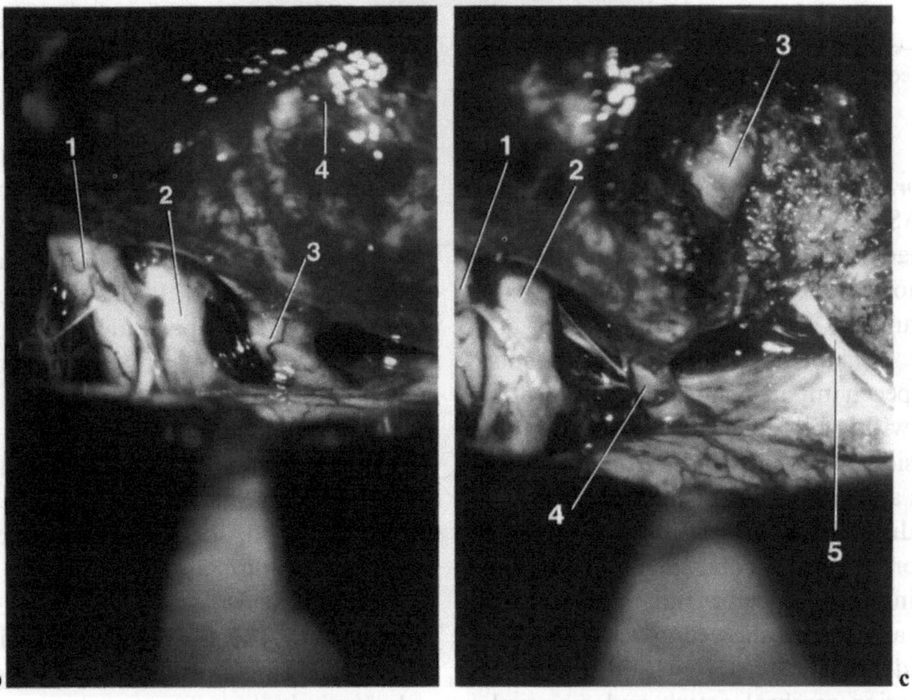

b c

Fig. AS 57a–c. Extensive sphenocavernous meningioma. **a** High-resolution axial CT scan shows the tumor extending from the middle cranial fossa anteriorly into the sphenoid sinus and back into the posterior cranial fossa.
b Exposure of the tumor in the middle cranial fossa and tentorial margin with exposure of the optic nerve, internal carotid artery, and oculomotor nerve. (*1*) Optic nerve, (*2*) internal carotid artery, (*3*) oculomotor nerve, (*4*) tumor.
c Status following extensive resection of the middle skull base, partial resection of the cavernous sinus, and exposure of most of the intracavernous portion of the internal carotid artery. The central stump of the trochlear nerve is visible. (*1*) Optic nerve, (*2*) supraclinoid portion of the internal carotid artery, (*3*) intracavernous portion of the internal carotid artery, (*4*) oculomotor nerve, (*5*) trochlear nerve

Case Report. Sphenocavernous meningioma (Fig. AS 57a–c). A 57-year-old man who was already blind in the left eye as a result of a war injury developed sensory disturbance in the territory of distribution of the right trigeminal nerve. This was accompanied by functional disturbance of the abducens and trochlear nerves. CT scans showed a medially situated mass lesion in the middle cranial fossa with infiltration of the cavernous sinus, penetration of the right sphenoid sinus, and slight extension into the posterior cranial fossa. Vision in the right eye was intact. The mild nature of the clinical symptoms and the preexisting blindness in the left eye complicated the decision whether to operate. After thorough consultation, the patient insisted that we attempt to remove as much of the tumor as possible without compromising the vision that remained. This meant preserving the function of both the optic nerve and the oculomotor nerve, which was certainly enveloped by tumor. Because of the existing left-sided amaurosis, functional preservation of the trochlear and abducens nerves was of minor importance, since diplopia was not a primary concern.

After classic pterional exposure of the tumor on the lesser sphenoid wing and in the middle cranial fossa, the optic nerve and internal carotid artery were exposed medial to the tumor by opening the sylvian fissure and retracting the anterior pole of the temporal lobe posteriorly. The tentorium was incised, and the meningioma was progressively exposed from behind along with the trochlear and trigeminal nerves. As expected, both nerves were infiltrated on all sides by tumor, so they could be sacrificed. The tumor in the cavernous sinus was removed piecemeal, sparing the intracavernous portion of the internal carotid artery. Because of the heavy vascularity of the meningioma, it was necessary to leave behind a thin layer of tumor attachment on the oculomotor nerve; otherwise we would have risked functional loss. Standard wound closure was carried out, and the postoperative course was uneventful. There was no evidence of functional abnormality of either the optic nerve or the oculomotor nerve.

Comments: Subtotal removal of an extensive sphenocavernous meningioma with involvement of the internal carotid artery, oculomotor nerve, and trigeminal nerve was indicated in a patient with preexisting blindness in the left eye in order to preserve the function of the right optic and oculomotor nerves.

Meningiomas with Predominantly Extracranial Extension

For circumscribed, intraosseous, predominantly extracranial meningiomas, the surgical goal is still radical removal. This is usually accomplished through an extradural approach.

Case Report. Meningioma of the lateral anterior skull base (Fig. AS 58a–i). A protrusion above the right eye of a 50-year-old man prompted further diagnostic evaluation. CT scans showed a predominantly extracranial, intraosseous meningioma with involvement of the right frontal sinus and sinus floor, orbital roof, lateral orbital wall, and infratemporal fossa.

The tumor was resected with an adequate margin of normal tissue through a transfrontal extradural approach. The skull, orbital roof, and lateral orbital wall were reconstructed with methylmethacrylate, with a satisfactory cosmetic result.

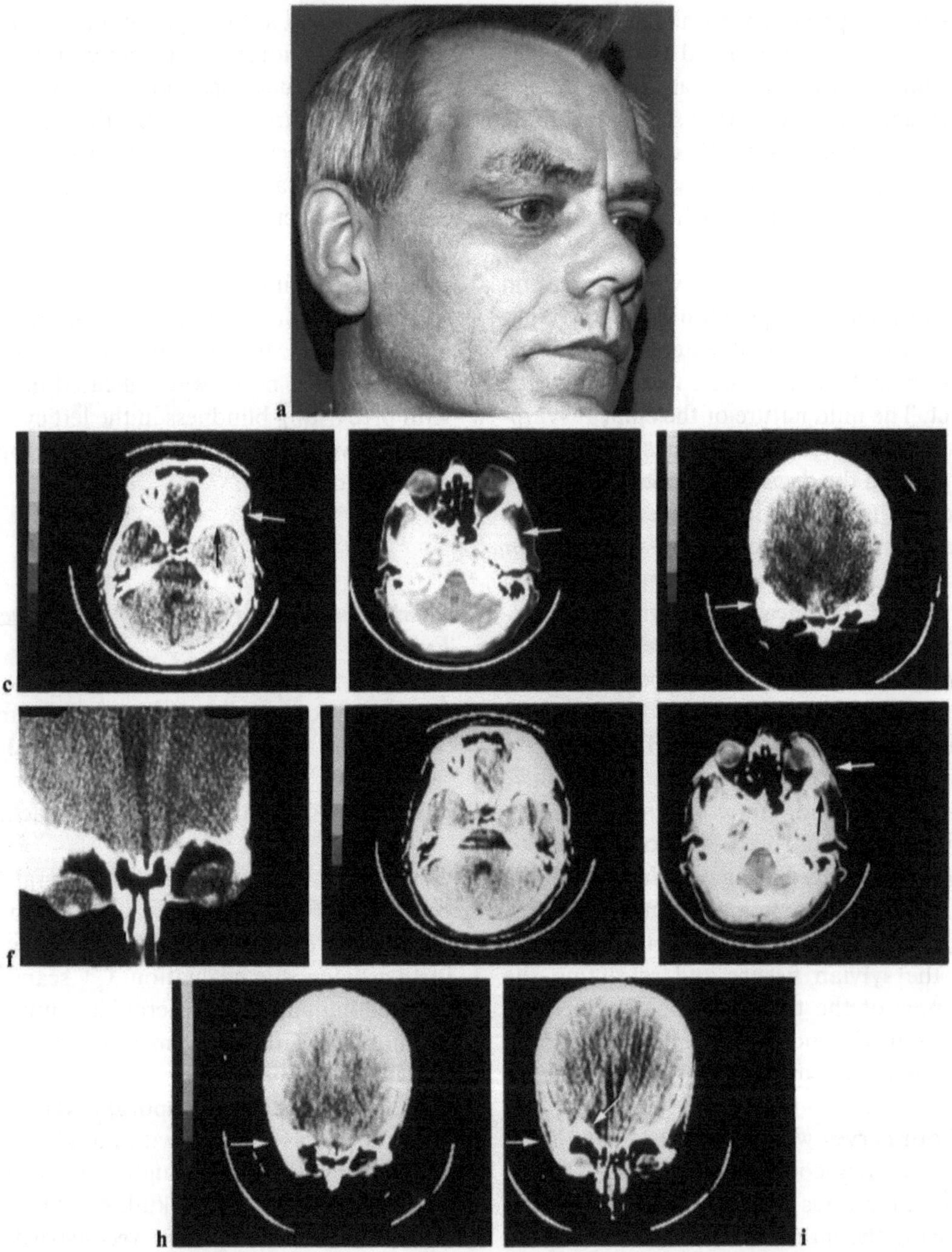

Fig. AS 58 a–i. Predominantly extracranial meningioma of the lateral anterior skull base.
a The extracranial tumor growth is manifested by a swelling in the right frontotemporal area.
b–e CT scans show the tumor extending from the right frontal sinus over the entire orbital roof to the minor sphenoid wing and temporal fossa. The orbit is constricted laterally and from above (*arrows*).
f–i CT scans following intracranial, extradural removal of the neoplasm. The *arrows* mark sites where the cranial and orbital-wall defects were reconstructed with methylmethacrylate

Optic Sheath Meningioma

Introductory Remarks. *Optic sheath meningioma* is an extracranial, retrobulbar meningioma that can invade intracranially through the bony optic canal. An important part of operative strategy is to define the tumor extent along the optic nerves. As this cannot be established preoperatively even with CT, the surgical approach must permit exposure of the entire optic nerve, if necessary, from the chiasm to the globe. It is important to note that tumor can infiltrate between the optic nerve structures. Usually this is manifested clinically by an irreversible amaurosis. If the tumor cannot be separated from the nerves, the optic nerve will have to be sacrificed to obtain a complete tumor removal).

Case Report. Meningioma of the right optic sheath (Fig. AS 59a–c). The patient was admitted with a progressive visual deficit and proptosis of the right eye. CT scans showed a dense mass extending from the orbital apex to the globe. After transfrontal extradural orbitotomy and incision of the periorbita, the tumor was progressively dissected free in a posterior-to-anterior direction. It was dissected off the optic nerve, which was completely encased by tumor, and a total removal was achieved. The lesion was identified histologically as an optic sheath meningioma. The proptosis regressed, but the preexisting amaurosis was irreversible because of prolonged optic nerve compression.

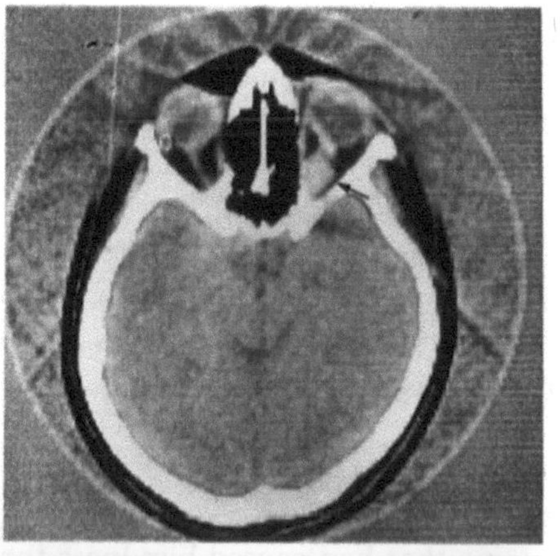
a

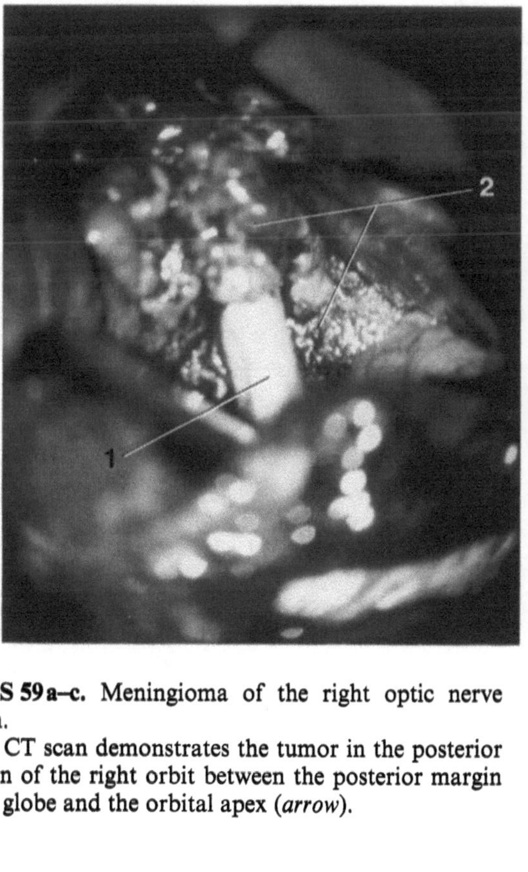

b

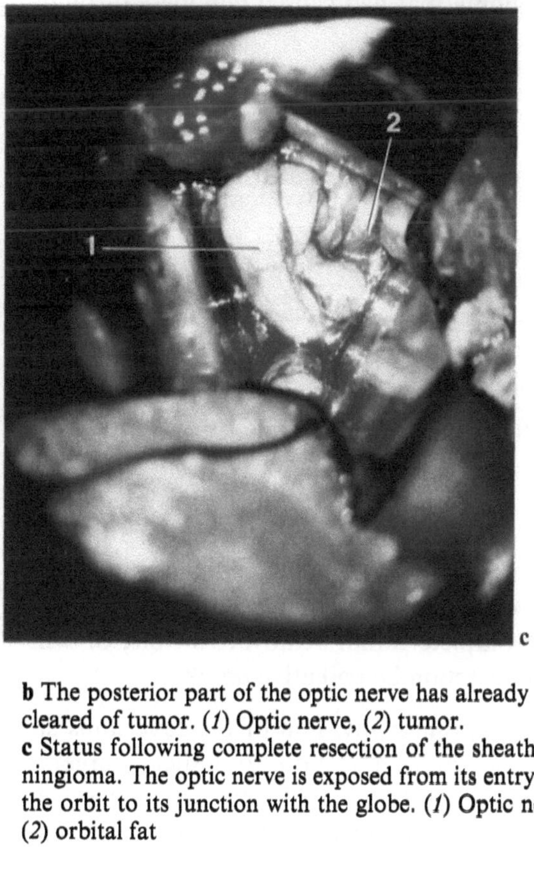

c

Fig. AS 59a–c. Meningioma of the right optic nerve sheath.
a The CT scan demonstrates the tumor in the posterior portion of the right orbit between the posterior margin of the globe and the orbital apex (*arrow*).
b The posterior part of the optic nerve has already been cleared of tumor. (*1*) Optic nerve, (*2*) tumor.
c Status following complete resection of the sheath meningioma. The optic nerve is exposed from its entry into the orbit to its junction with the globe. (*1*) Optic nerve, (*2*) orbital fat

Case Report. Meningioma of the left optic sheath (Fig. AS 60a–d). A 33-year-old woman had a 7-year history of progressive visual deterioration culminating in amaurosis. Axial CT scans with oblique reconstruction showed a dense tumorlike swelling along the course of the optic nerve. The presence of amaurosis despite the small tumor size implied that optic nerve function had been damaged by infiltrative growth.

The tumor was approached through a right frontotemporal osteoplastic craniotomy with extradural exposure of the orbital roof. The orbital roof was removed microsurgically with the diamond burr, and the optic canal was unroofed. The tumor was exposed by incising the dural cuff around the optic nerve. The nerve and surrounding tumor were resected with adequate margins posteriorly and also close to the globe. Salvage of the optic nerve was impossible due to infiltrative growth.

Comments: Total resection of the optic nerve was necessary to remove a small optic sheath meningioma that had caused blindness through infiltrative growth.

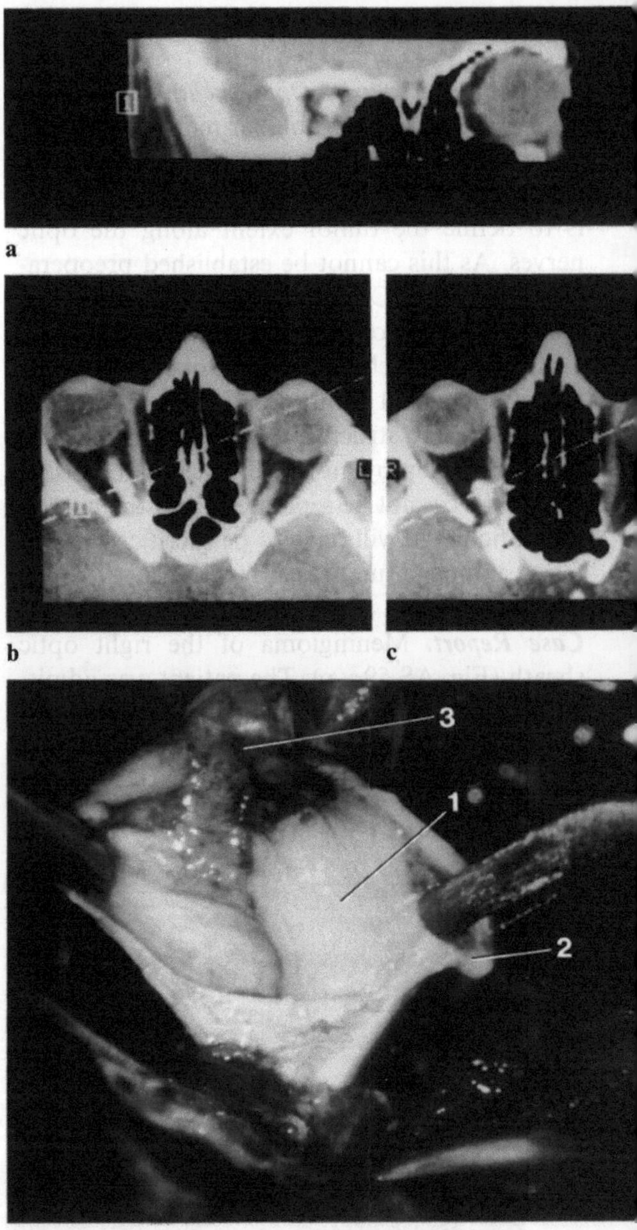

Fig. AS 60a–d. Optic sheath meningioma.
a–c CT scans with axial projection and oblique reconstruction show a dense, spindle-shaped tumor mass along the course of the left optic nerve.
d At operation the dural cuff around the optic nerve is incised. Infiltration of the optic nerve by the tumor is apparent. (*1*) Optic nerve, (*2*) dura, (*3*) tumor

Meningiomas with Intra- and Extracranial Extension

Introductory Remarks. To formulate a surgical treatment plan for meningiomas with intra- and extracranial extension, it is necessary to answer the following questions:

1) What is the extent of involvement of the paranasal sinuses, orbit, and cavernous sinus?
2) Is the intra- or extracranial portion of the tumor beyond the dura accessible through a single approach, or is a combined approach necessary in one or in two stages?
3) Is complete tumor removal feasible, or will the resection be palliative only?

Generally, tumor invasion of the cavernous sinus is a contraindication to radical surgery. Derome and Guiot (1978) and Bonnal et al. (1980) favor a two-stage operation for intraosseous skull base meningiomas that have spread across the midline to involve the paranasal sinuses on both sides. In the first, intracranial part of the operation, the tumor and involved dura are resected, and the defect is repaired with a graft. Three months later the extracranial part of the meningioma is removed with the involved skull base, and the bony defect is closed with free bone grafts. The point at which an intra- or extracranial tumor component located beyond the dura can still be resected through *one* surgical approach is indefinite and depends on the functional importance of structures located between the extra- and intracranial tumor components, and whether those structures might be more easily isolated from the opposite side. When craniofacial resection is indicated for a very large tumor, we perform both parts of the operation in one stage, provided a complete tumor removal is feasible. Based on a broad personal experience, we do not believe that the size of the postresection defect in the anterior skull base poses a significant limitation to a one-stage combined operation. Also, when there is advanced tumor infiltration of the cavernous sinus with amaurosis and loss of oculomotor nerve function on one side, we would advocate resection of the cavernous sinus with preservation of the internal carotid artery. In cases where the internal carotid artery has become infiltrated by tumor in its cavernous portion, a goal for the future is to resect the involved arterial segment and preserve the cerebral blood supply by means of a preoperative intra-extracranial microvascular anastomosis or by appropriate intraoperative vascular surgery.

With very extensive intra-extracranial meningiomas that are not amenable to radical excision, the surgeon should consider performing a two-stage palliative craniofacial tumor resection before the patient develops signs of cerebral compression and irreversible cranial nerve damage.

Case Report. Intraosseous skull base meningioma with extensive intra- and extracranial growth (Fig. AS 61a–d). A 41-year-old woman had undergone a transethmoidal decompression of the right optic nerve 1 year earlier due to visual impairment by an intraosseous skull base meningioma. After transitory improvement, amaurosis of the right eye with proptosis ensued, and the vision in the left eye began to deteriorate. CT showed a mass extending from

a, b

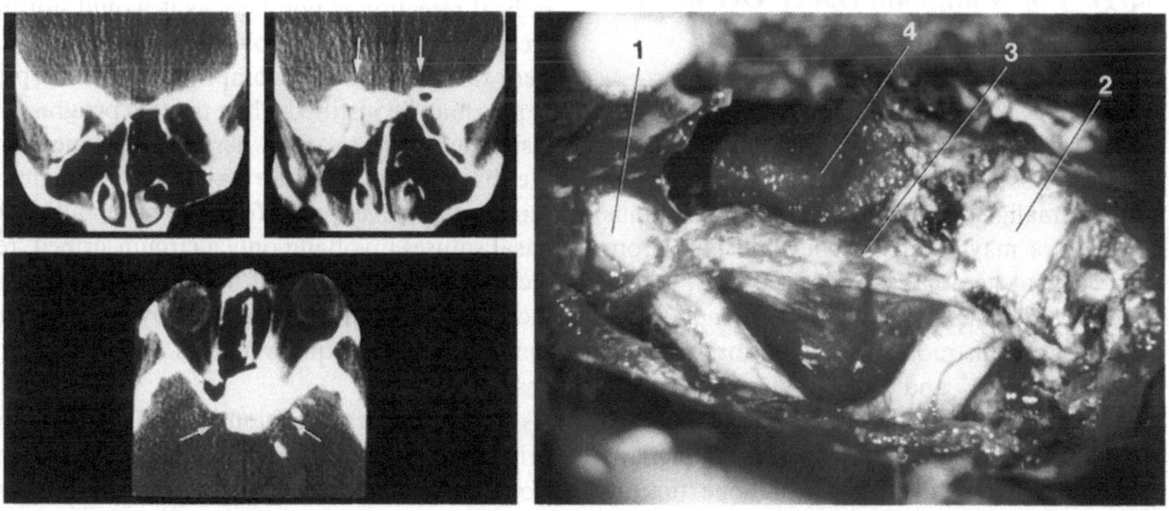

c

d

Fig. AS 61a–d. Intraosseous skull base meningioma with extensive intra- and extracranial growth.
a–c CT scans document tumor extension from the entire right anterior skull base across the midline to the optic nerve on the left side (*arrows*).
d The optic nerves are decompressed bilaterally in their canals. Sponge packing has been inserted into the sphenoid sinus. (*1*) left optic nerve, (*2*) right optic nerve, (*3*) remaining portion of tuberculum sellae, (*4*) sponge packing in sphenoid sinus

the entire right anterior skull base across the midline to the optic nerve on the left side.
A right frontotemporal osteoplastic craniotomy was performed to ensure sufficient intracranial access. The frontal lobe and temporal pole were retracted and the sylvian fissure partially opened to expose the tumor extradurally on the lesser sphenoid wing. Then the optic nerves were decompressed intradurally with the diamond burr. After a dural flap was elevated from the planum sphenoidale, the planum was burred away and the tumor within the sphenoid sinus was removed. The anterior skull base was reconstructed by covering the replaced dural flap with a galeal pericranial flap.

Comments: Palliative resection of an extra-intracranial meningioma with bony infiltration and exophytic growth was indicated because of progressive visual deterioration. The optic nerves were decompressed through a transcranial extra-intradural approach, with removal of the lesser sphenoid wing and large portions of the tumor on the planum sphenoidale and sphenoid sinus.

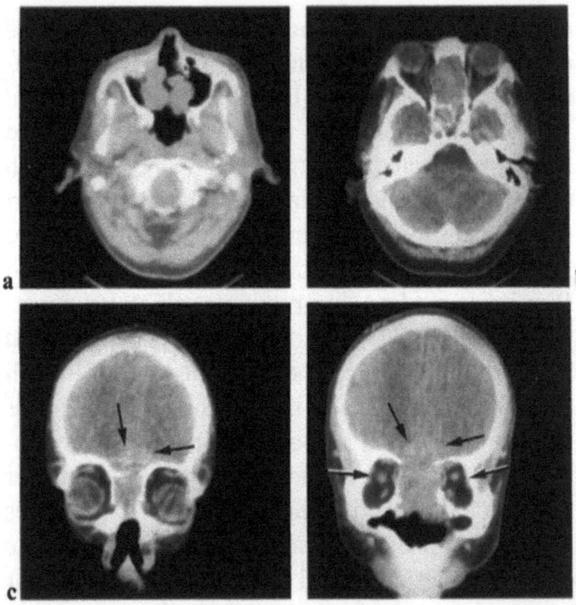

Fig. AS 62a–d. Axial and coronal CT scans of a 41-year-old man with an inoperable squamous cell carcinoma of the paranasal sinuses invading both orbits and the cranial cavity (*arrows*). The patient had undergone two previous operations

Surgery of Malignant Space-Occupying Lesions of the Anterior Skull Base

Introductory Remarks. Malignant tumors of the anterior skull base most commonly originate from the nose and paranasal sinuses. Less frequently, malignant meningiomas and sarcomas of the dura may penetrate the skull base from a primary intracranial site. Occasionally, malignancies of the anterior skull base are metastases originating from more distant tumors such as hypernephroma and melanoma. Wustrow (1977) states that nasal and paranasal sinus tumors account for less than 1% of all malignancies. Only 8% of the 166 facial bone tumors in his series had spread to the dura. Given the rapid growth of malignant tumors, potentially mutilating surgical treatment is indicated only if there is a reasonable chance that the tumor can be completely removed.

With a malignancy that has spread to both orbits and has invaded the cranial cavity through a wide area of the skull base (Fig. AS 62a–d), radical resection is pointless as it would not increase survival or improve the quality of life. Very rarely, surgical decompression of the optic nerves may be justified when there is progressive vision loss due to optic nerve involvement by the disease. On the other hand, with malignant tumors that have spread from the nose and paranasal sinuses involving only a circumscribed, resectable area of the skull base, it is possible to increase the chance of survival by excising the tumor with an adequate margin of surrounding tissue.
As a rule, radical excision is not justified for primary intracranial malignancies with extension to the skull base, because usually the disease involves vital structures. This emphasizes the importance of applying appropriate diagnostic measures, including endoscopy, in symptomatic patients so that an early diagnosis can be established (see p. 128).

Case Report. Adenocarcinoma of both frontal sinuses with involvement of the skull base (Fig. AS 63a–f). Endonasal biopsy in a 58-year-old man with symptoms of chronic frontal sinusitis yielded the surprising diagnosis of adenocarcinoma. The lateral tomogram showed a circumscribed defect in the area of the skull base. The tumor was exposed through an extracranial,

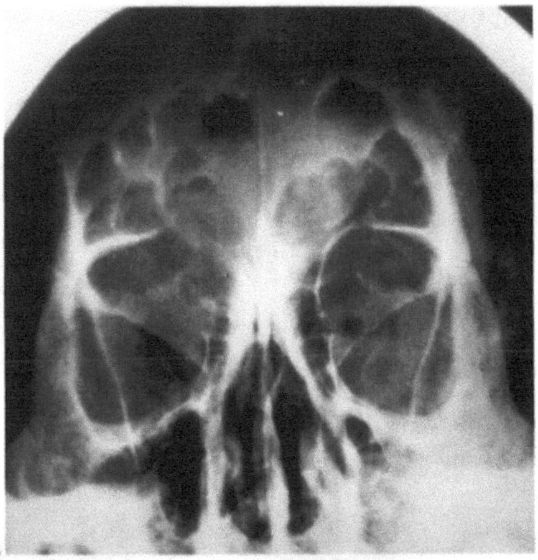
a

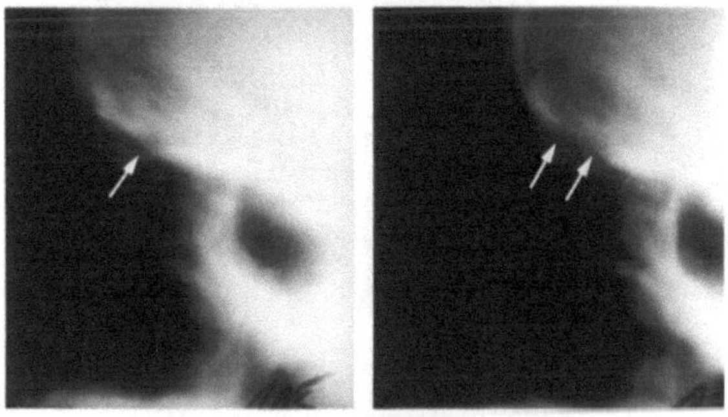
b, c

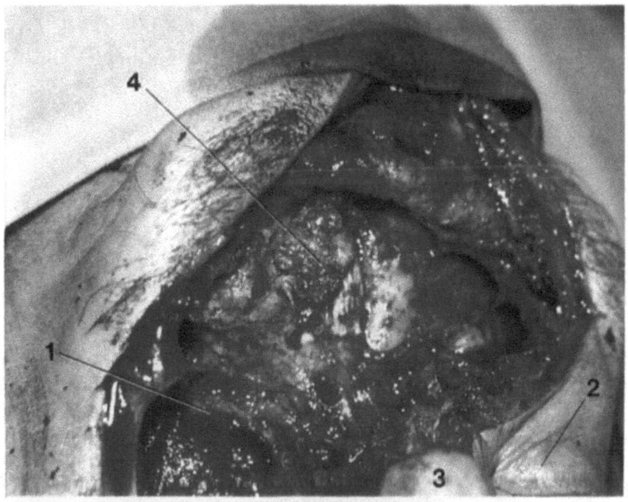

d

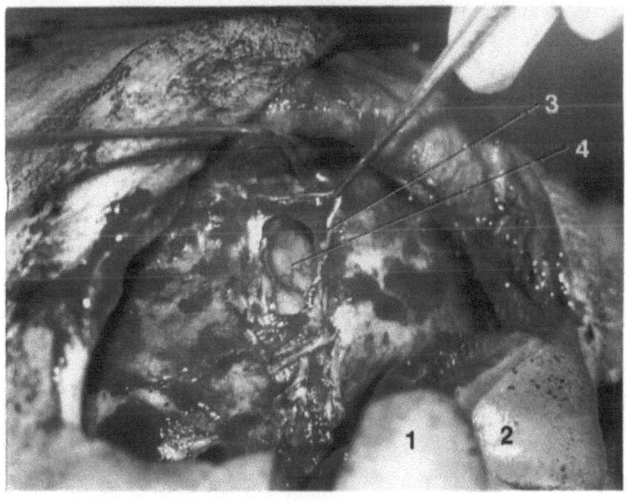

e

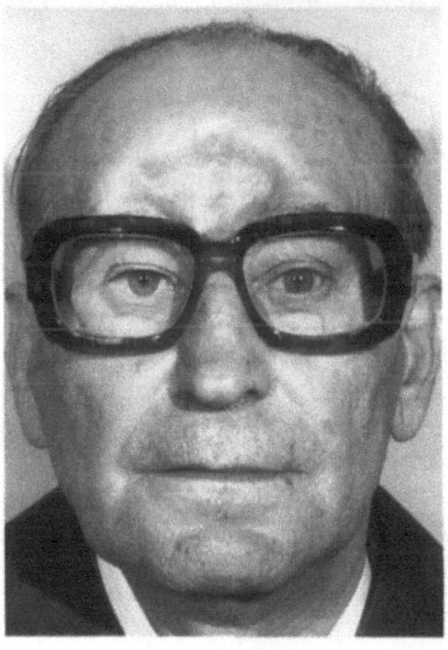
f

Fig. AS 63a–f. Adenocarcinoma of the frontal sinuses with involvement of the skull base.
a Plain film of the paranasal sinuses shows only a diffuse opacity of the frontal sinuses and anterior ethmoid cells, with no apparent bone destruction.
b, c Lateral tomograms disclose circumscribed destruction of the anterior skull base (*arrows*).
d Appearance of the operative field after removal of most of the tumor. Invasion of the right orbit necessitated orbital exenteration. Residual tumor adherent to the dura is visible at the posterior wall of the frontal sinus. (*1*) Right orbital cavity, (*2*) left eye, (*3*) nasal root, (*4*) residual posterior-wall tumor.
e The residual tumor is removed with the overlying dura. Dural penetration has not occurred. The right anterior frontal lobe is visible deep in the field. (*1*) Nasal root, (*2*) left eye, (*3*) dural margin, (*4*) frontal brain.
f The patient 1 year after surgery, with a facial prosthesis

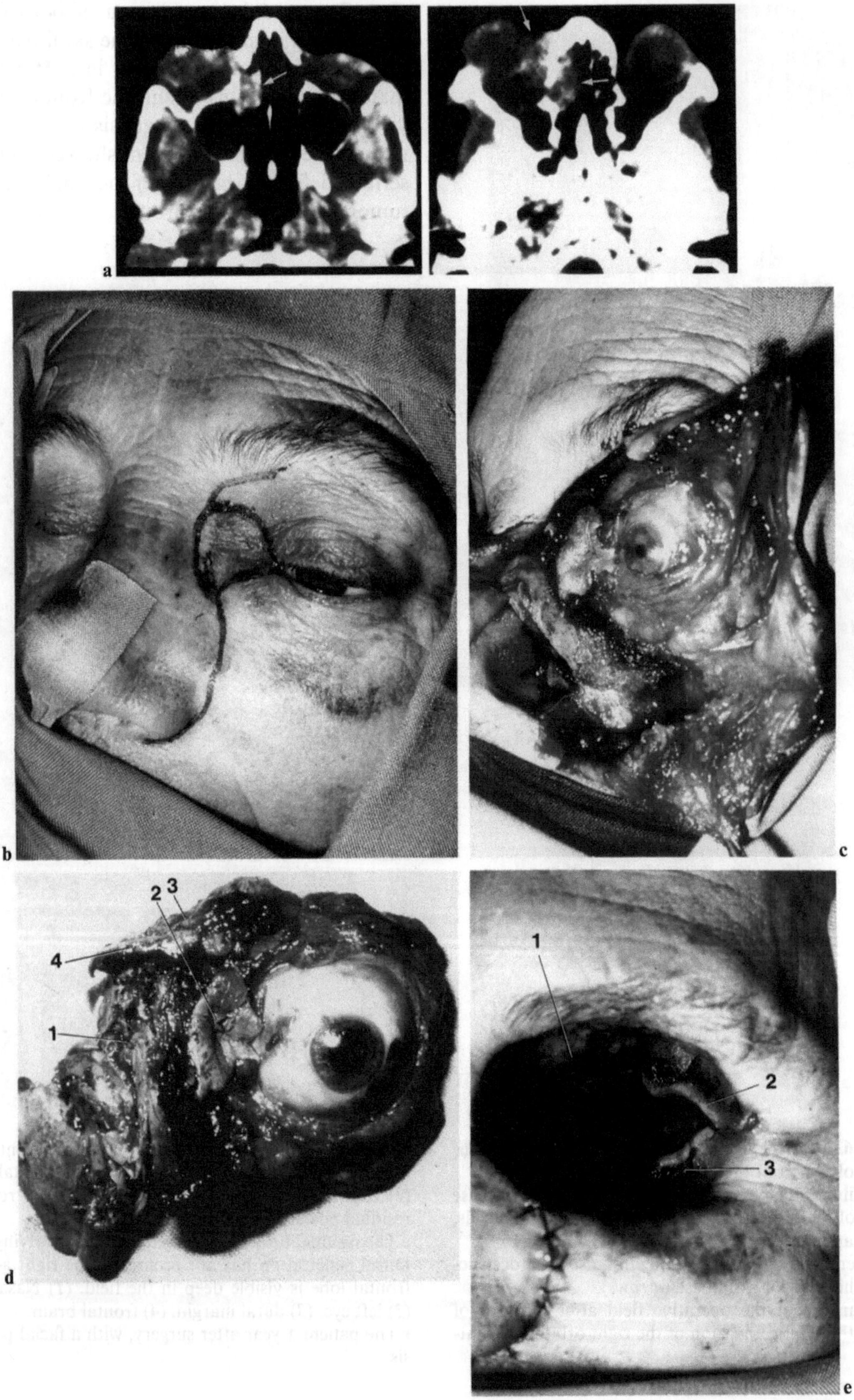
a
b
c
2 3
4
1
d
1
2
3
e

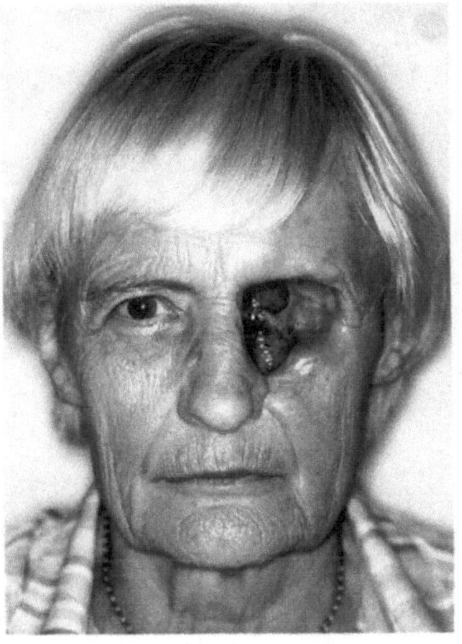

f

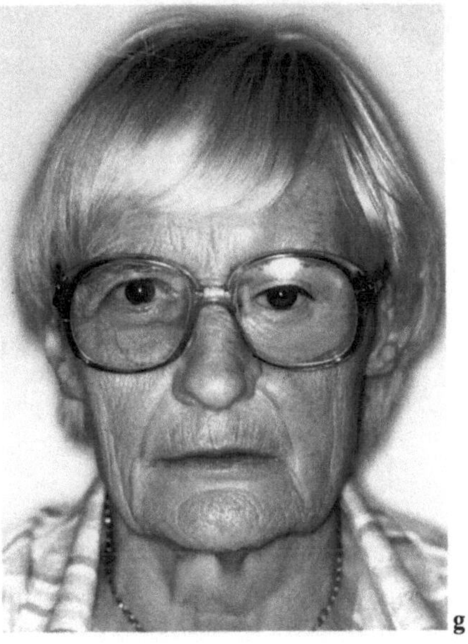

g

Fig. AS 64a–g. Left ethmoid carcinoma with invasion of the left orbit.
a The CT scans show the tumor projecting into the left orbit.
b The carcinoma was exposed through a left paranasal incision, removing the skin directly overlying the tumor.
c The lesion was excised with wide margins, including orbital exenteration.
d The margins of the specimen were histologically negative for tumor. As a precaution, the left ethmoid roof and left cribriform plate were included in the resection. (*1*) Medial ethmoid wall, (*2*) tumor-infiltrated skin, (*3*) dura, (*4*) cut bony edge of the left anterior skull base.
e The preserved palpebral skin was reflected into the orbital cavity. (*1*) Duraplasty, (*2*) lateral part of left upper lid, (*3*) lateral part of left lower lid.
f, g The patient 5 years after surgery, with and without a facial prosthesis

transfronto-orbital approach. The tumor had grown into the orbit, so it was resected in one piece, along with the orbital contents, leaving a small remnant adherent to the dura.
Next the skull base and involved dura were resected with grossly and microscopically tumor-free margins, and the cranial cavity was sealed with a dural graft. Cosmetic rehabilitation was achieved with a facial prosthesis.

Comments: This case illustrates that with a paranasal sinus malignancy whose removal necessitates orbital exenteration, a substantial portion of the skull base and associated dura can be resected *from below* during tumor removal.

Case Report. Left ethmoid carcinoma with invasion of the orbit (Fig. AS 64a–g). A 65-year-old woman was admitted with increasing lateral displacement of the globe and a firm swelling in the medial canthus of the left eye. Excisional biopsy from the tumor, which extended almost to the skin, disclosed squamous cell carcinoma. Radiologic studies showed a relatively extensive ethmoid tumor with invasion of the orbit.
The tumor was exposed through a left paranasal incision with removal of the overlying skin and was removed en bloc with the orbital contents. The bloc specimen included the lateral wall of the ethmoid. Intraoperative histologic examination confirmed tumor-free margins. Although the bony skull base was not infiltrated by the tumor, the left ethmoid roof and left cribriform plate were nevertheless removed as a precaution. The exposed dura was reinforced with a graft, and intact palpebral skin was reflected into the orbital cavity. The tumor bed was irradiated postoperatively with telecobalt. Satisfactory cosmetic rehabilitation was obtained with a facial prosthesis.

Comments: An ethmoid-orbital carcinoma with extension to the skull base was removed en bloc along with the adjacent bony skull base to establish a safety zone. The specimen margins were histologically negative. The patient has been free of disease for five years.

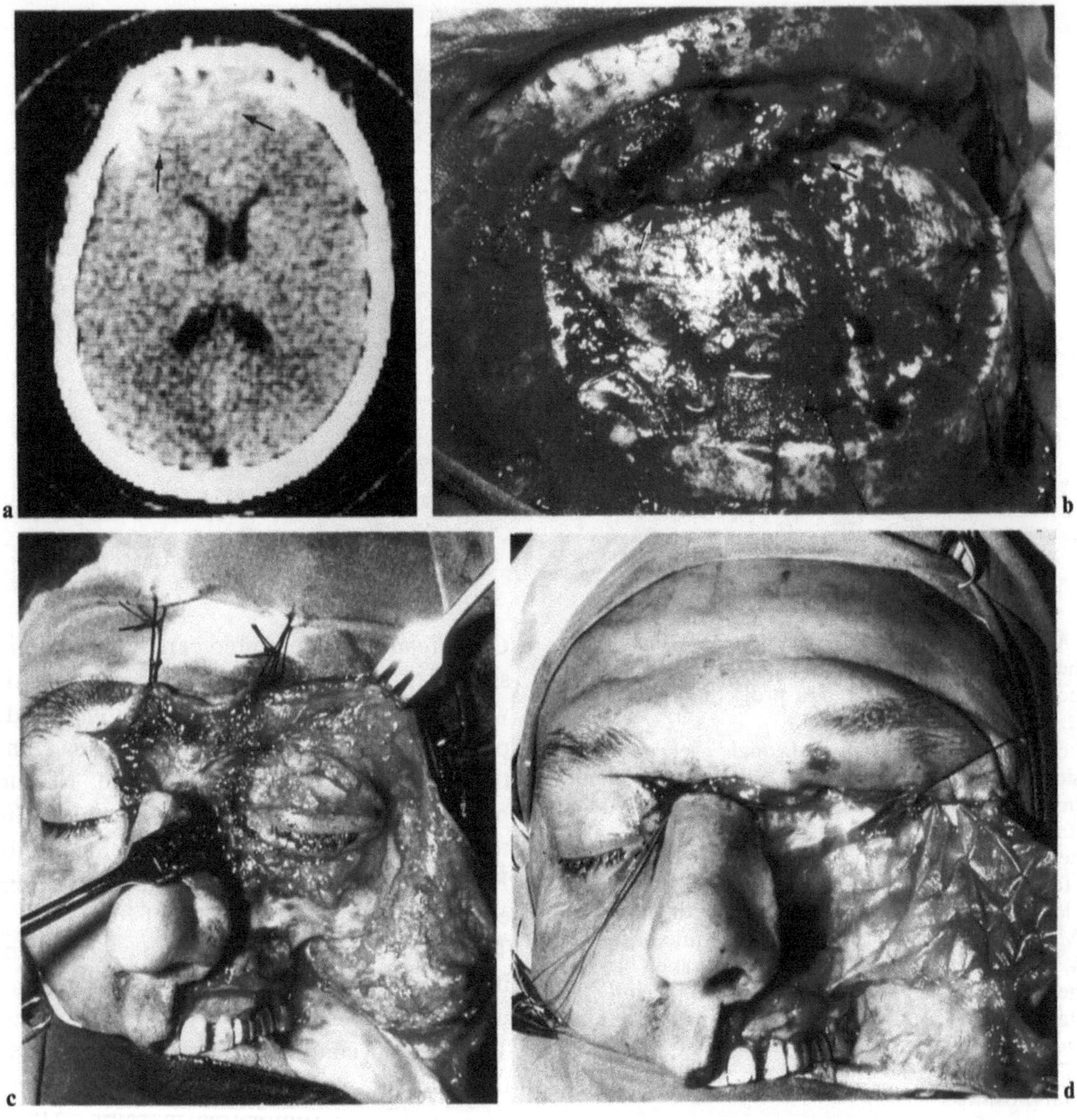

Fig. AS 65 a–f. Extensive ethmoid-frontal sinus carcinoma with invasion of the anterior cranial fossa.
a CT scan shows the intracranial extent of disease (*arrows*).
b Bifrontal craniotomy has been performed, opening the frontal sinus. The tumor is compressing the dura (*arrows*).
c A large cheek flap is mobilized, carrying the incision around the orbital contents.
d Status near completion of the operation. The skull base and frontal cranial vault have been reconstructed with methylmethacrylate and covered internally with a galeal pericranial flap and dura. The palpebral skin was utilized for external coverage. The surface of the cheek flap was covered with a dural graft.
e Status on completion of the operation.
f The patient 6 months after surgery, with a facial prosthesis. Death occurred 1 1/2 years postoperatively due to intracranial metastasis

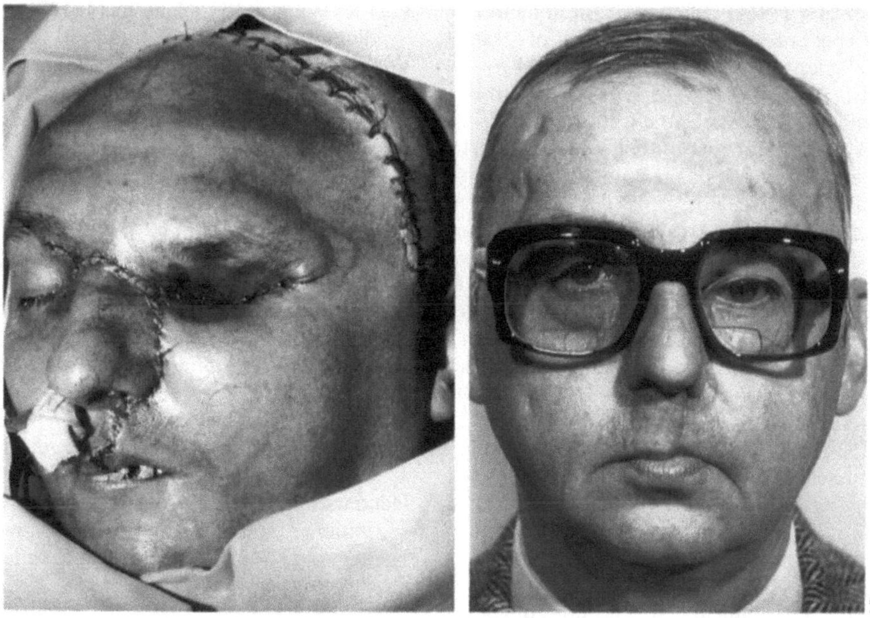

e f

Case Report. Carcinoma of the ethmoid and frontal sinuses (Fig. AS 65a–f). A 55-year-old man had an extensive, predominantly left-sided carcinoma of the ethmoid and frontal sinuses with invasion of the anterior cranial fossa. The extent of the tumor is visible on the CT scan. A carcinoma of this size is resectable only through a combined craniofacial approach. The anterior scalp was mobilized via a bifrontal coronal incision, and a large bifrontal craniotomy was performed. The posterior wall of the frontal sinus was infiltrated by tumor, so the supraorbital ridge could not be spared. After a high dural incision and retraction of the frontal lobes, it was found that the tumor was in broad contact with the dura but did not penetrate it. The dura was excised with a 2-cm margin of normal tissue towards the lesser sphenoid wing and posterior edge of the planum sphenoidale. Then the cranium bordering on the dura was resected, encompassing the entire left anterior skull base and the cribriform plate on the opposite side.
Next the facial soft-tissue flap was mobilized and an incision made around the ciliary margin of the left eye so that the orbital contents could be included in the en bloc resection. Because endoscopy had excluded involvement of the maxillary sinus, the hard palate could be spared. The surgical defect in the bony anterior skull base and left frontal bone was repaired with a methylmethacrylate plate, covered internally by a galeal pericranial flap and externally by palpebral skin. By three weeks the patient was well enough to be discharged. The facial defect was managed with a prosthesis.

Comments: An extensive carcinoma of the ethmoid and frontal sinuses with broad invasion of the anterior cranial fossa was resected en bloc through a craniofacial approach. The skull base was reconstructed in three layers, from within outward, with a galeal pericranial flap, methylmethacrylate, and skin. The patient died 11/2 years post-operatively due to intracranial metastasis.

References

Albrecht R (1959) Die Nasenrachentumoren und ihre Behandlung. Arch Ohren-, Nasen- und Kehlk-Heilk 175:1–68

Appelblatt NH, McClatchey KD (1982) Olfactory neuroblastoma: A retrospective clinicopathologic study. Head Neck Surg 5:108–113

Baron SH (1979) Brain radiation necrosis following treatment of an esthesioneuroblastoma. Laryngoscope 89:214–233

Batsakis JF (1979) Tumors of the head and neck. 2nd edn. Baltimore, Williams and Wilkins

Becker MH, Jacox HW (1964) Olfactory esthesioneuroepithelioma. Experiences in the management of a rare intranasal malignant neoplasm. Radiology 82:77

Berger L, Luc H, Richard H (1924) L'esthesioneuroepitheliance olfactit. Bull Ass Franc Cancer 13:416

Blokmanis A (1972) Estesioneuroepithelioma: A report of two cases and discussion of the management. Can J Otolaryng 1:49

Bonnal I, Thihaut A, Brotchi I (1980) Invading meningeomas of the sphenoid ridge. J Neurosurg 53:587–599

Brenner H, Ossoining K, Valencak E (1967) Orbitaltumoren im Kindesalter. In: Kraus H, Sunder-Plasman M (eds): Berichte des 1. Europäischen Kongresses Pädriatische Neurochirurgie, Verlag der Wiener Medizinischen Akademie

Claux J, Coll J, Vincent P, Ane P (1979) Une forme maligne des tumeur de la placode olfactive. Ann Otolaryngol Chir Cervicofac 28:60

Clifford P (1980) Transcranial-facial approach for tumors of superior paranasal sinusses and orbit. J Royal Soc Med 73:413–419

Derome PJ (1972) Les tumeurs spheno-ethmoidales. Neurochirurgie 18, Suppl 1

Derome PJ (1984) Transbasal approach to tumors invading the base of the skull. In: Schmideck HH, Sweet WH (Ed.) Operative neurosurgical techniques Vol 1, Grune & Stratton, New York, p 357

Derome PJ, Guiot G (1978) Bone problems in meningeomas invading the base of skull. Clinic Neurosurg 25:435–451

Dieffenbach JF (1848) Die Resektion des Oberkiefers und des Unterkiefers. In: Operative Chirurgie Vol. 2. Brockhaus Leipzig, p 33

Donald PJ (1981) Recent advances in paranasal sinus surgery. Head and Neck Surg 4:146–153

Doyle PJ, Paxton HD (1971) Combined surgical approach to esthesioneuroepithelioma. Trans Am Acad Ophthalmol Otolaryngol 75:526

Draf W (1974) Differentialdiagnose der Schädelknochenerkrankungen aus HNO-ärztlicher Sicht. HNO 22:14–23

Draf W (1980) Course Surgery of the Anterior Skull Base Hannover

Draf W (1982) Die chirurgische Behandlung entzündlicher Erkrankungen der Nasennebenhöhlen. Arch Otorhinolaryngol 235:133–305 (Kongressbericht 1982)

Draf W, Samii M (1977) Otorhinolaryngo-neurochirurgische Probleme an der Schädelbasis. Laryngol Rhinol 56:1007–1030

Eckel W, Palm D (1959) Statistische und röntgenologische Untersuchungen zu einigen Fragen des Nebenhöhlenosteoms. Arch Ohr-, Nas- und Kehlk-Heilk 174:440

Eggston AA, Wolff D (1947) Histopathology of the Ear, Nose and Throat Williams & Wilkins, Baltimore

Fergusson (1857) Practical Surgery 4th Ed. London P 668

Fitzpatrick PJ, Briant DR, Berman JM (1980) Nasopharyngeal Angiofibroma. Arch Otolaryngol 106:234–236

Foet K, Wünsch PH, Naujocks J (1981) Zur Differentialdiagnose und Behandlung der Esthesioneuroblastome. Vortrag auf der 52. Jahresversammlung der Deutschen Gesellschaft für Hals-Nasen-Ohren-Heilkunde, Kopf- und Hals-Chirurgie Wiesbaden

Frey KW, Theopold HM, v. Lieven H, Schober M (1981) Scintigraphy in Diagnosis and Observations of Malignant Tumors in Head and Neck. Laryng Rhino Otol (Stuttg) 60:289–293

Frey KW, Theopold HM, Rohloff R, Rauscher J (1981) Scintigraphy and tomography in inflammations and non-malignant tumors in head and neck. Laryng Rhino Otol (Stuttg) 60:294–298

Ganz H (1960) Über Kieferhöhlenosteome. Laryng Rhinol Otol 39:74

Guggenheim P, Kleitsch WP (1967) Combined craniotomy-rhinotomy for ethmoid cancer. Ann Otol (St. Louis) 76:105

Henderson ED, Dahlin DC, Bickel WH (1950) Eosinophilic granuloma of bone. Proc Mayo Clin 25:534

Henderson J (1980) Orbital tumors, 2nd edn. Thieme-Stratton, New York

Hirsch O, Urbanek (1929) Behandlung eines exzessiven Exophtalmus (Basedow) durch Entfernung von Orbitalfett von der Kieferhöhle aus. Wien Laryngo-Rhinol-Ges 05.11.1929

Hommerich KW (1977) Gutartige Geschwülste der Nase und der Nasennebenhöhlen. In: Berendes J, Link R, Zöllner F Hals-Nasen-Ohren Heilk in Praxis und Klinik vol 2/Obere und untere Luftwege II/20 Thieme, Stuttgart

Homzie MJ, Elkon D (1980) Olfactory Esthesioneuroblastoma. Variables predictive of tumor control and recurrence. Cancer 46:2509–2513

Huet PC, Labayle J, Thiband B (1953) Un cas d'angiohistiocytome des fosses nasales. Ann Oto-Laryng (Paris) 70:785

Jahnke V, Theopold HM (1979) Klinik der Olfactoriusneurinome. Arch Otorhinolaryngol 223:433

Jakumeit HD (1971) Neuroblastoma of the olfactory nerve. Acta Neurochir 25:99

Johns ME, Winn RH, McLean WC, Cantrell RE (1981) Pericranial flap for the closure of defects of craniofacial resections. Laryngoscope 91:952–959

Jones BR (1970) Surgical approaches to the orbit. Trans Ophthalmol Soc UK 90:269–308

Jung H, Gutjahr P (1977) Kindliche Malignome im HNO-Berich. In: J Berendes, R Link und F Zöllner. Hals-Nasen-Ohren-Heilk in Praxis und Klinik vol II/2, 22.13./14. Thieme, Stuttgart

Jung H, Lüchtrath H (1981) Das extrakranielle Olfactoriusneuroblastom. Laryngol Rhinol Otol (Stuttg) 60:338

Kastenbauer E, Rudert H (1968) Zur Differentialdiagnose der benignen und semimalignen Tumoren der Nasenscheidenwand. HNO 16:225

Kempe LG (1968) Operative Neurosurgery. vol 1. Springer, Berlin Heidelberg New York

Ketcham AS, Wilkins RH, van Buren JM, Smith RR (1963) A combined intracranial facial approach to the paranasal sinusses. Amer J Surg 106:699

Ketcham AS, Hoye RC, van Buren JM, Johnson RH, Smith RR (1966) Complications of intracranial facial resection for tumors of the paranasal sinusses. Amer J Surg 112:591

Ketcham AS, Hammond WG, Chretien P, van Buren JM (1969) Treatment of advanced cancer of the ethmoid sinusses. Nobel Symposium 10. Almquist and Wiksell Stockholm

Krause ChJ, Baker SR (1982) Extended transantral approach to pterygomaxillary tumors. Ann Otol Laryngol 91:391–398

Krekorian EA, Kempe LG (1969) The combined otolaryngology-neurosurgery approach to extensive benign tumors. Laryngoscope (St. Louis) 79:2086

Krönlein RV (1938) Zur Pathologie und operativen Behandlung der Dermoidzysten der Orbita. Beitr Klin Chir 4:149–163

Lasjaunias P, Berenstein A (1987) Surgical Neuroangiography vol 1. Springer, Berlin, Heidelberg, New York, pp 371–381

Leroux-Robert J, Guiot G, Paquelin F, Pracke H (1966) La propagation des meningiomas dans le massif maxillofacial A propos de 4 observations. Ann otolaryng (Paris) 83:617

Lichtenstein L (1938) Tumoren der vorderen Schädelbasis. Polyostotic fibrous dysplasia. Arch Surg 36:874

Lichtenstein L (1953) Histiocytosis X. Integration of eosinophilic granuloma of bone, Letterer-Siwe and Schüller-Christian-disease as related manifestations of a single nosologic entity. Arch Path (Chicago) 56:84

Lichtenstein L, Jaffe H (1942) Fibrous dysplasia of bone conditions affecting one, several or many bones, the graver cases of which may present abnormal pigmentation of skin, premature sexual development, hyperthyroidism, or still other extraskeletal abnormalities. Arch Path (Chicago) 33:777

Littlewood M, Maisels D (1970) Reconstructive surgery in the intracranial approach to facial malignant disease. Proc Roy Soc Med 63:681

Löblich HJ (1981) Nosologie und Therapie der Ästhesioneuroblastome. Vortrag auf der 64. Jahrestagung der Nordwestdeutschen Vereinigung der Hals-Nasen-Ohrenärzte, Hannover

Martin H, Ehrlich HE, Abels JC (1948) Juvenile nasopharyngeal fibroma. Ann Surg 127:513–536

Martin G, Hennel HD, Kleinsasser O (1983) Neuroblastome des N. olfactorius. HNO 31:20–27

Moure P (1902) quoted by Zange in: Thiel R (1959) Ophthalmologische Operationslehre. Thieme, Leipzig

Moure EI (1922) Technique chirurgicale oto-rhino-laryngologique. Premier fascicule, L'oreille et ses annexes. Libraire Octave Dein, Paris 1922

Naffziger HC (1941) Exophthalmus; some principles of surgical management from neurosurgical aspects. Amer J Ophthal 75:25

Nebit ME Jr, Wolfson JJ, Kuffer SA, Peterson HO (1970) Orbital sclerosis in histiocytosis X. Amer J Roentgenol 110:123

Neel III HB, Whicker JH, Devine DK, Weiland LH (1973) Juvenile angiofibroma: review of 120 cases. Am J Surg 126:547–556

Oberman HA, Rice DH (1976) Olfactory neuroblastomas. Clinicopathologic study. Cancer 38:2494–2502

Osemann RG (1982) Basal frontal meningeomas. In: Schmidek HH, Sweet WH (eds) Operative Neurosurgical techniques, vol. 1. Grune and Stratton, New York, pp 535–559

Pletcher JD, Dedo HH, Newton ThH, Norman D (1975) Preoperative embolization of juvenile angiofibromas of the nasopharynx. Ann Otol 84:740–745

Poppen JL (1964) Operative techniques for removal of olfactory groove and suprasellar meningiomas. Clinical Neurosurgery 11:1–7

Pressman JJ (1962) Nasopharyngeal angiofibroma: Removal with hypothermia. Arch Otolaryngol 76:167

Robarson GH, Biller H, Session DG, Ogura IH (1972) Presurgical internal maxillary artery embolization in juvenile angiofibroma. Laryngoscope 82:1524

Russel DS, Rubinstein LJ (1971) Pathology of Tumors of the Nervous System, 3rd edn. Arnold, London

Samii M, Draf W (1980) Operative Behandlung von Tumoren der vorderen Schädelbasisregion. Course on surgery of the anterior skull base. Hannover

Sarwar M (1979) Primary sellar-parasellar esthesioneuroblastoma. Am J Roentgenol 133:140

Schramm VL, Myers EN, Maroon IC (1979) Anterior skull base surgery for benign and malignant disease. Laryngoscope 89:1077–1091

Schürmann K (1968) Zur operativen Therapie der Orbitatumoren. Vorläufiger Bericht über 57 eigene Fälle. In: Tönnis W (ed) Beiträge zur Neurochirurgie 15, Johann Ambrosius Barth, Leipzig 285–292

Schürmann K (1974) Neurochirurgische Aufgaben in der Orbita. In: Arch Oto-Rhino-Laryng 207: 253–383

Schürmann K, Voth D (1972) Die Bedeutung der transfrontalen Orbitomie für die operative Behandlung der intraorbitalen raumfordernden Prozesse. Ein Erfahrungsbericht über 61 Fälle. In: Roper-Hali MJ, Sautter H, Streiff EB (eds) Advances in Ophthalmology 25. Karger, Basel, 188–239

Seid AB, Vorster WF (1972) Juveniles Hämangiofibrom des Nasenrachens. S Afr Med J 46:517–518

Seiffert A (1926) Zur operativen Behandlung retrobulbärer Eiterungen von der Kieferhöhle aus. Passow-Schäfers Beitr 23:112

Shah JP, Galicich JH (1977) Craniofacial resection for malignant tumors of ethmoid and anterior skull base. Arch Otolaryngol 103:514–517

Silcox LE (1966) Olfactory neuroblastoma. Laryngoscope (St. Louis) 76:665

Sisson GA, Bytell DE, Becker SP et al. (1976) Carcinoma of the paranasal sinusses and cranial-facial resection. J Laryng 1:59–68

Skolnik EM, Massari FS, Tenta LT (1966) Olfactory neuroepithelioma. Arch Otolaryng (Chicago) 84:84

Supance IS, Seid AB (1981) Craniofacial resection for ethmoid carcinoma in children. Int J Pediatric Otorhinolaryngology 3:185–194

Tönnis W, Schürmann K (1951) Meningeome der Keilbeinflügel. Zbl Neurochirur 11:1–13

Tringwald RF (1966) Olfactory placode tumors. Laryngoscope (St. Louis) 76:196
Unterberger S (1958) Zur Versorgung frontobasaler Verletzungen. Arch Ohr Nas Kehlk Heilk 172:463
Valencak E, Brenner H, Ossoining K (1970) Entscheidende Fortschritte in der Diagnostik raumfordernder orbitaler Prozesse. Wien Med Wschr 120:882–883
Waldmann STR, Levine HL, Astor F, Wood BG, Weinstein M, Tucker HM (1981) Surgical experience with nasopharyngeal angiofibroma. Arch Otolaryngol 107:677–682
Walters ThR, Pushparaj N, Ghander AZ (1980) Olfactory neuroblastoma. Response to combination chemotherapy. Arch Otolaryngol 106:242–243
Ward PH, Thompson R, Calcaterra Th, Kadin MR (1974) Juvenile angiofibroma: A more rational therapeutic approach based upon clinical and experimental evidence. Laryngoscope 84:2181–2194
Weber O (1859) Chirurgische Erfahrungen. Berlin
Wilson JSP, Westbury G (1973) Combined craniofacial resection for tumor involving the orbital walls. Br J Plast Surg 26:44–56
Wolman L, Path BF (1969) Extracranial spread of meningeomas. Eye Ear Nose Throat Dig 7:46
Wustrow F (1977) Bösartige Tumoren der Nase und ihrer Nebenhöhlen. In: Berendes J, Link R, Zöllner F (eds) Hals-Nasen-Ohren-Heilkunde in Praxis und Klinik, vol 2/Obere und untere Luftwege II/21. Thieme, Stuttgart
Zange I (1959) Operationen im Bereich der Nase und ihrer Nebenhöhlen. In: Thiel R (ed) Ophthalmologische Operationslehre. Thieme, Leipzig, p 1321
Zehm S (1977) Geschwülste des Nasenrachens. In: Berendes J, Link R, Zöllner F (eds) Hals-Nasen-Ohren-Heilkunde in Praxis und Klinik, vol 2/Obere und untere Luftwege II/23 Thieme, Stuttgart
Zülch KJ (1955) Biologie und Pathologie der Hirngeschwülste. In: Krenkel W, Olivecrona H, Tönnis W (eds) Handbuch der Neurochirurgie, vol 3. Springer, Berlin Göttingen Heidelberg
Zülch KJ (1956) Die Hirngeschwülste, 2nd edn. Barth, Leipzig

Surgery of the Middle Skull Base (MS)

Surgery of Traumatic Lesions of the Middle Skull Base

Introductory Remarks. Trauma to the medial and lateral portions of the middle skull base with injuries to bone, dura, brain, and neurovascular structures can be an indication for operative treatment. Otologic aspects of these injuries have been reviewed in comprehensive survey works by H. B. Boenninghaus (1979), F. Escher (1973), W. Kley (1968, 1976) and other authors. Current neurosurgical guidelines on the treatment of lateral skull base injuries have been published by Becker and Ward (1982), Gillingham et al. (1971), Guleke (1950), Kessel (1969), Metzel (1973, 1980), and Samii and Brihaye (1983). These works are particularly instructive with regard to clinical presentation and evaluation. Here we shall focus on the indications for operative treatment and corresponding techniques that have evolved from years of cooperative experience between the neurosurgical and otorhinolaryngologic specialties.

Immediate or early surgical treatment is indicated for open depressed fractures with or without dural injury and for expanding intracranial mass lesions associated with epidural, subdural, or intracerebral hemorrhage. Less extensive epidural and subdural hemorrhages that stop spontaneously by autotamponade will occasionally resolve with nonoperative treatment. With *intracerebral hemorrhage*, impending brain herniation is the only valid indication for surgical decompression.

Intracerebral hemorrhage can be diagnosed and its course followed by means of computed tomography (CT) (Lanksch et al. 1978) and also by magnetic resonance imaging (MRI), which avoids exposure to ionizing rays. Most hemorrhages will resolve in a few weeks with conservative therapy, especially when corticosteroids are given (Reulen et al. 1980).

Open head injuries with bone comminution, dural laceration, and destruction of the soft-tissue mantle are an indication for immediate, atraumatic surgical treatment proceeding in layers, from within outward, using appropriate ablative and reconstructive measures. This is necessary to ensure a reasonable chance of recovery and to remove the danger of an intracranial mass lesion and infection. Considerable cerebrospinal fluid (CSF) leakage from the ear or through the eustachian tube into the nose and nasopharynx that does not arrest spontaneously is an absolute indication for early surgical intervention.

Secondary surgical treatment may be indicated after the acute trauma effects have subsided to avoid complications and to restore function.

Injury to the infraclinoidal portion of the internal carotid artery by a perforating spicule of bone can result in a *carotid-cavernous fistula.* This shunt is manifested at once by a subjectively disturbing intracranial bruit that is synchronous with the arterial pulse and is perceived as a "noise in the ear." Without prompt treatment, the fistula can lead to proptosis with chemosis, progressive visual loss from pressure on the optic nerve, and ocular motility disturbances as the function of the oculomotor nerves becomes compromised. The bruit can be auscultated over the eye, over the forehead and temporal area, and often along the large blood vessels in the neck. In rare cases the bruit is audible to the unaided ear.

Concerning the *indication for the surgical treatment of CSF leaks*, a basic distinction is drawn between fractures involving the otobase and fractures of the rhinobase (Wullstein 1972) (see p. 129). The pneumatized spaces of the ear normally are not colonized by bacteria, so the risk of an ascending infection is much lower than in the anterior skull base region. It is necessary, then, to differentiate "paradoxical" cerebrospinal rhinorrhea, or CSF leak through the eustachian tube following a laterobasal fracture, from true cerebrospinal rhinorrhea secondary to a frontobasal injury (see also p. 127).

Kley, who stated in 1968 that all but a few laterobasal fractures should be explored in the presence of a transient CSF leak, modified his position in later years. He now agrees with Boenninghaus (1979) that all comminuted laterobasal fractures with a broad gaping fracture line should be surgically exposed, regardless of whether or not the CSF leak stops spontaneously. If the radiologic fracture signs are absent or subtle, a compelling indication for exploration does not exist in patients with healthy ears and a self-limiting CSF leak. If exploration of the middle ear should later prove necessary for audiologic reasons, the otologic procedure should be combined with exploration of the posterior and middle skull base, provided this can be done through a retroauricular transmastoid approach. Before surgical exposure of the lateral skull base is done in a patient with a persistent CSF leak, an attempt should be made to demonstrate the fracture line in the petrous bone radiologically so that it can be decided whether the transcranial or transmastoid approach is more appropriate. There will still be cases where one is compelled to use a combined transcranial-transmastoid approach in one or two stages; this is necessary when the CSF leak persists after the sealing of a radiographically visible fracture. If the spontaneous arrest of CSF discharge prompts the withholding of surgery in the presence of a widely gaping fracture line, significant potential exists for arachnid cyst formation or herniation of dura and brain into the middle ear. Forceful nose blowing in such cases can be sufficient to rupture the usually thin scar, thus facilitating an ascending meningitis. When a CSF leak has been objectively demonstrated in a patient with chronic otitis media, surgical exploration is imperative, regardless of whether the CSF leak stops spontaneously, since the presence of microorganisms in the middle ear cavity poses a serious danger of ascending meningitis through the flimsy dural scar. If it can be established that a chronic otitis media was definitively cured prior to the trauma by tympanoplasty, the therapeutic approach is the same as for patients without ear disease. When early or late meningitis develops secondary to a laterobasal fracture, surgical exploration of the lateral skull base is necessary in all but a very few cases.

Another important measure to *avoid trauma-related complications of laterobasal fractures* is surgical debridement of the ear canal and skull base with removal of skin pieces that have become entrapped between fragments of the roof and posterior wall of the external auditory canal or driven into the middle ear cavity. Otherwise, extensive bone destruction with intracranial complications may ultimately result from the development of a traumatic cholesteatoma. The same danger exists when the external auditory canal has become partially occluded by a displaced bone fragment or by impaction of the mandibular condyle. Rarely, the temporomandibular joint may become displaced centrally into the middle cranial fossa (Pieritz and Schmidseder 1981). It may be necessary in such cases to combine treatment of the mandibular displacement with a duraplasty. Finally, the prophylaxis of infectious complications is aided by the removal of foreign bodies and by reconstructive measures on the middle ear in cases where the tympanic membrane has been torn (tympanoplasty).

Serial CT observations of laterobasal fractures are recommended not only in the presence of intracranial contusions and hemorrhages but also for the early detection of incipient brain abscess. When a brain abscess is confirmed, the primary focus of infection in the ear must be eradicated as a necessary prelude to other therapeutic measures. The brain abscess itself is concurrently treated with antibiotics and corticosteroids. A certain percentage of abscesses will resolve completely with this therapy. Otherwise the abscess is totally removed through the transcranial intradural approach after it has become well encapsulated. Modern pharmacologic treatment methods have virtually eliminated the need for emergency measures such as needle aspiration or partial brain resection, which carry a risk of edema-related tentorial herniation of the temporal lobe. Another advantage of awaiting encapsulation is that it avoids surgery in the acute stage, making it possible to defer operation until a time when the patient's general condition is better and the surgical risk is lessened. We reject exploratory aspirations and incisions of temporal lobe abscesses close to the cerebral cortex during otosurgical procedures.

Secondary operations to improve function after laterobasal fractures are most commonly done to treat a persistent conductive hearing loss, which usually is secondary to a traumatic disruption of the ossicular chain by fracture or dislocation, and to repair a tympanic membrane perforation. The *facial nerve* can become stretched, compressed, or torn at various sites along its intracranial and intratemporal course. If electrophysiologic and clinical observations do not show evidence of spontaneous functional regeneration of the facial nerve over time, an indication exists for operative exposure and repair. Details are presented in the chapter on Facial Nerve Surgery. Concerning the possibility of *trigeminal nerve injury* at the gasserian ganglion or injury to the pre- and postganglionic branches, it has not been possible in the past to bridge trigeminal nerve defects in the middle cranial fossa due to technical limitations. Loss of the first trigeminal nerve division can lead to neuroparalytic keratitis with subsequent corneal opacification and blindness. Because trophic problems preclude corneal transplantation in such cases, an attempt has been made to restore sensation and improve the trophic disturbance of the cornea by interposing a long nerve graft between the great occipital nerve and the frontal nerve (Samii 1972).

Surgical Approaches for Middle Skull Base Trauma

Craniectomy (Extended Burr Hole Trephination)

Introductory Remarks. Around the turn of the century, Krönlein systematically studied the pathoanatomic features of middle meningeal artery hemorrhage and established schematic trephination sites for hemorrhages from the middle meningeal vessels (quoted in Guleke 1950).
Even today, Krönlein's scheme can be recommended for cases of acute epidural hemorrhage with impending herniation in which CT and angiographic methods of localization are unavailable (Fig. MS 1a). In 1973 Bushe proposed various trephination sites for the evacuation of epidural and subdural hematomas (Fig. MS 1b).
Following the accurate radiologic localization of an *epidural hematoma* or intracerebral hemorrhage, we expose the lesion through a selectively placed osteoplastic craniotomy (see Fig. MS 3a–f). With a *chronic subdural hematoma*, we have had good results with evacuation through multiple trephine openings (Moringlane and Samii 1981).

Operative Technique
(Fig. MS 2a, b)

First a vertical skin incision is made in the temporal region, terminating anterior to the tragus of the ear. The scalp is separated from the superficial temporal fascia, followed by vertical division of the fascia, the temporal muscle, and the pericranium with one incision in line with the temporal fibers. The muscular soft tissues and pericranium are stripped from the skull. A burr hole is made at the anterior inferior limit of the temporal squama, as close to the skull base as possible, and the opening is extended anteriorly or posteriorly, depending on the direction of spread of the hematoma. At this time it may be necessary to extend the skin incision in the

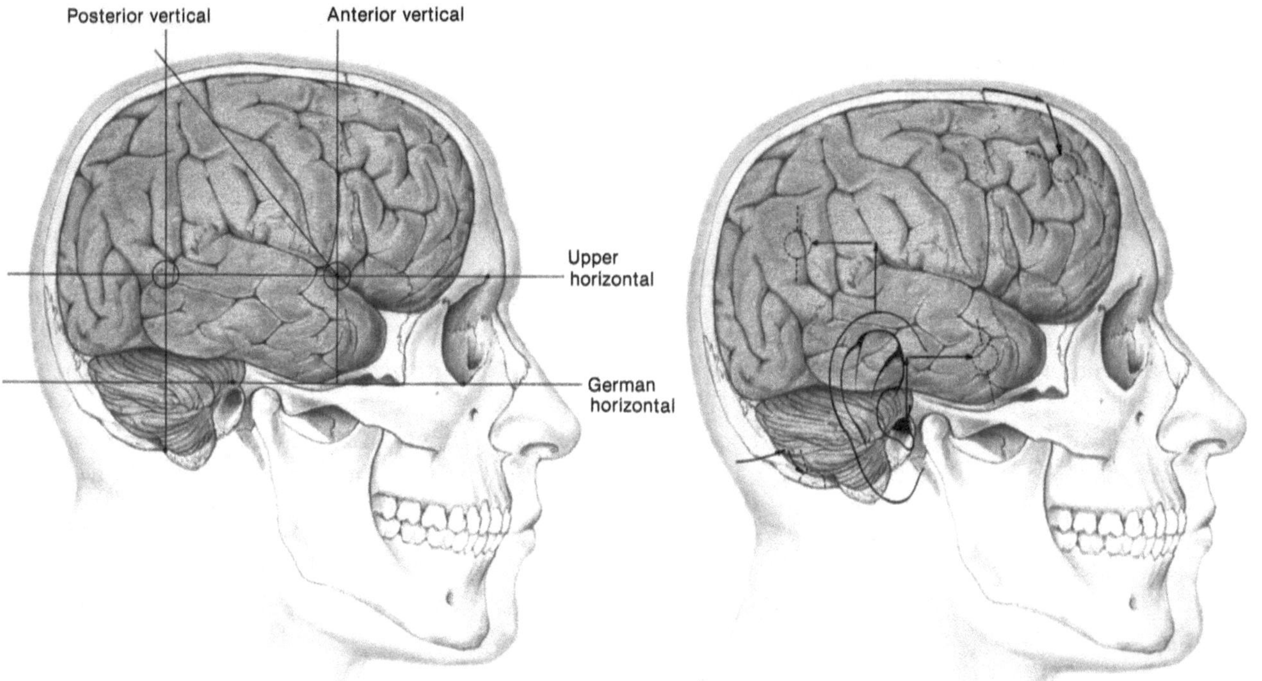

a b

Fig. MS 1. a Krönlein's trephine sites for acute epidural hemorrhage with impending herniation. This scheme is employed when CT and angiography are unavailable as means of localizing the hematoma. The frontal and parietal branches of the middle meningeal artery occur at the points of intersection of the upper and German horizontals with the anterior and posterior verticals, respectively. The upper horizontal passes through the superior orbital margin and runs parallel to the German horizontal, which extends through the inferior orbital margin. The anterior vertical crosses the midpoint of the zygomatic arch; the posterior vertical passes through the posterior border of the mastoid process. These lines serve as guides for burr hole placement for the evacuation of epidural temporal and parietal hematomas. Frontal, occipital, and infratentorial hematomas are not accessible using this scheme.
b Trephine sites for subdural and epidural hematomas, after Bushe (1973). When the hematoma cannot be localized by neuroradiologic methods, Bushe recommends a modified Krönlein scheme using additional frontal and occipital burr holes. The extra trephine sites are indicated

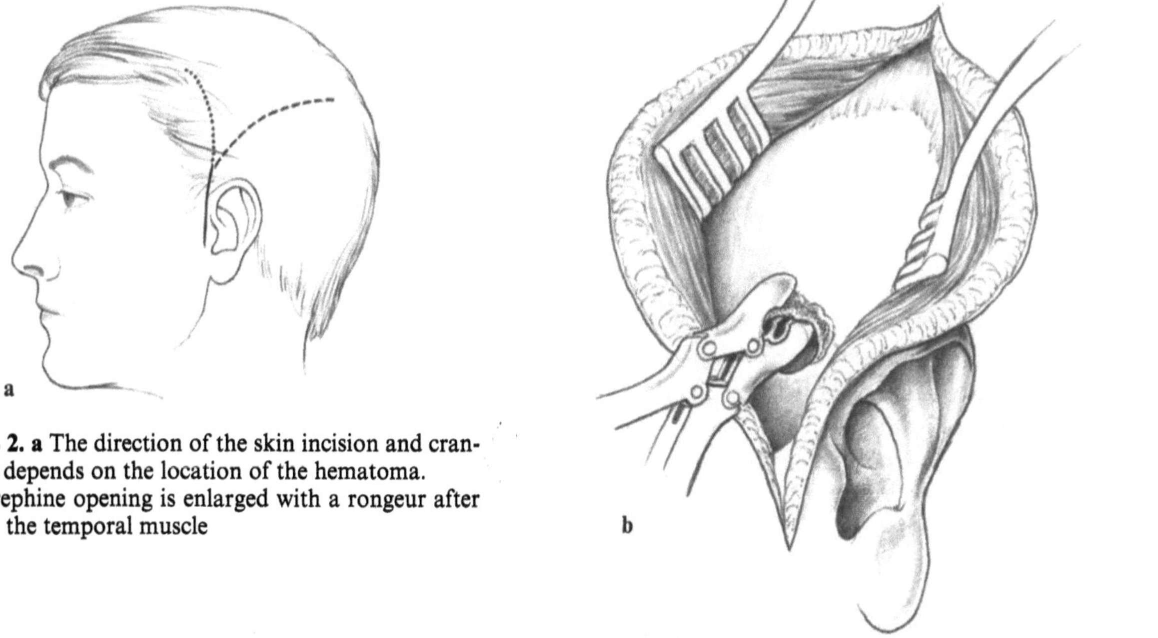

a b

Fig. MS 2. a The direction of the skin incision and craniectomy depends on the location of the hematoma.
b The trephine opening is enlarged with a rongeur after splitting the temporal muscle

same direction in curvilinear fashion. The skin incision is kept behind the hairline if possible.

After removal of the hematoma, the dura is secured to the bone margins with sutures to prevent the reaccumulation of blood. The temporal muscle and its fascia are reapproximated over the bony defect, a subgaleal suction drain is left in place for 1–2 days and the wound is closed in the usual fashion.

With a *chronic subdural hematoma*, the burr-hole technique is as follows: The extent of the hematoma having been established by CT, two burr holes are placed at the anterior and posterior limits of the hematoma through a vertical skin incision 4–5 cm long. The perforations are enlarged to 2–2.5 cm with a rongeur. Following cruciate incision of the dura, the outer hematoma capsule is resected, and the hematoma is progressively evacuated with irrigation and suction. Then the inner hematoma capsule adjacent to the cerebral cortex is resected as completely as possible through the burr hole. A soft Jackson-Pratt silicone drainage tube with multiple openings is introduced without pressure through the posterior burr hole and is connected by tubing to a collecting bag. The dura in both burr holes is closed with simple interrupted sutures, leaving a small opening posteriorly for the tube. The burr holes are patched with methylmethacrylate to avoid unesthetic depressions, and the wound is closed in layers. The tube provides for drainage of residual hematoma and cerebrospinal fluid as the brain reexpands. This process is monitored with serial CT scans. Usually the drainage tube is removed after 8–10 days.

Osteoplastic Craniotomy in Trauma

Introductory Remarks. Except for chronic subdural hematoma, which is evacuated through burr holes, osteoplastic craniotomy is the approach of choice for skull trauma and for all intracranial procedures. The size of the bone flap depends on the extent of the pathology. In a frontal craniotomy for treatment of a frontobasal injury, the bone flap is temporarily removed after the scalp flap has been raised. This contrasts with exposures of the temporal skull and skull base, in which the bone flap is left attached to the temporal muscle. Frontobasal dural defects are covered with an inferiorly based galeal periosteal flap (see p. 140). With a dural defect in the middle skull base region, it is necessary to detach the temporal bone flap completely from the inner fascia of the temporal muscle and create an inferiorly based fascial flap that can be utilized for the duraplasty. When intracranial hemorrhage is present in association with a depressed fracture, the craniotomy should encompass the fracture site to allow elevation of the depressed fragments.

Operative Technique
(Fig. MS 3a–f)

The skin incision may take the form of a temporal flap with a basal pedicle or a scalp flap based frontotemporally, depending on the needed extension and location of the temporal bone flap. If a scalp wound is present, it should be incorporated into the incision. The scalp flap is elevated from the bone, separating it from the temporal muscle and its outer fascia. On the anterior and posterior sides of the proposed bone flap, the temporal muscle is incised in line with its fibers at the junction of the cranial vault and skull base and is mobilized to allow the placement of burr holes. The two inferior burr holes are made between the lateral orbital rim

Fig. MS 3a–f. Osteoplastic craniotomy for trauma.
a Skin incision and burr holes.
b The craniotomy flap is raised to expose the epidural hematoma.
c After reflecting the anteriorly based scalp flap and turning down the craniotomy flap based on the temporal muscle, dural "tack-up"sutures are placed, and the epidural hematoma is identified. Bleeding vessels are controlled with bipolar cautery and suture ligatures, and the epidural hematoma is removed.
d–f Removal of a subdural hematoma. **d** Opening the dura overlying a subdural hematoma. **e** Bleeding cerebral vessels are coagulated. The hematoma is evacuated with its capsule. **f** The dura is closed with interrupted sutures reinforced by a simple running suture line

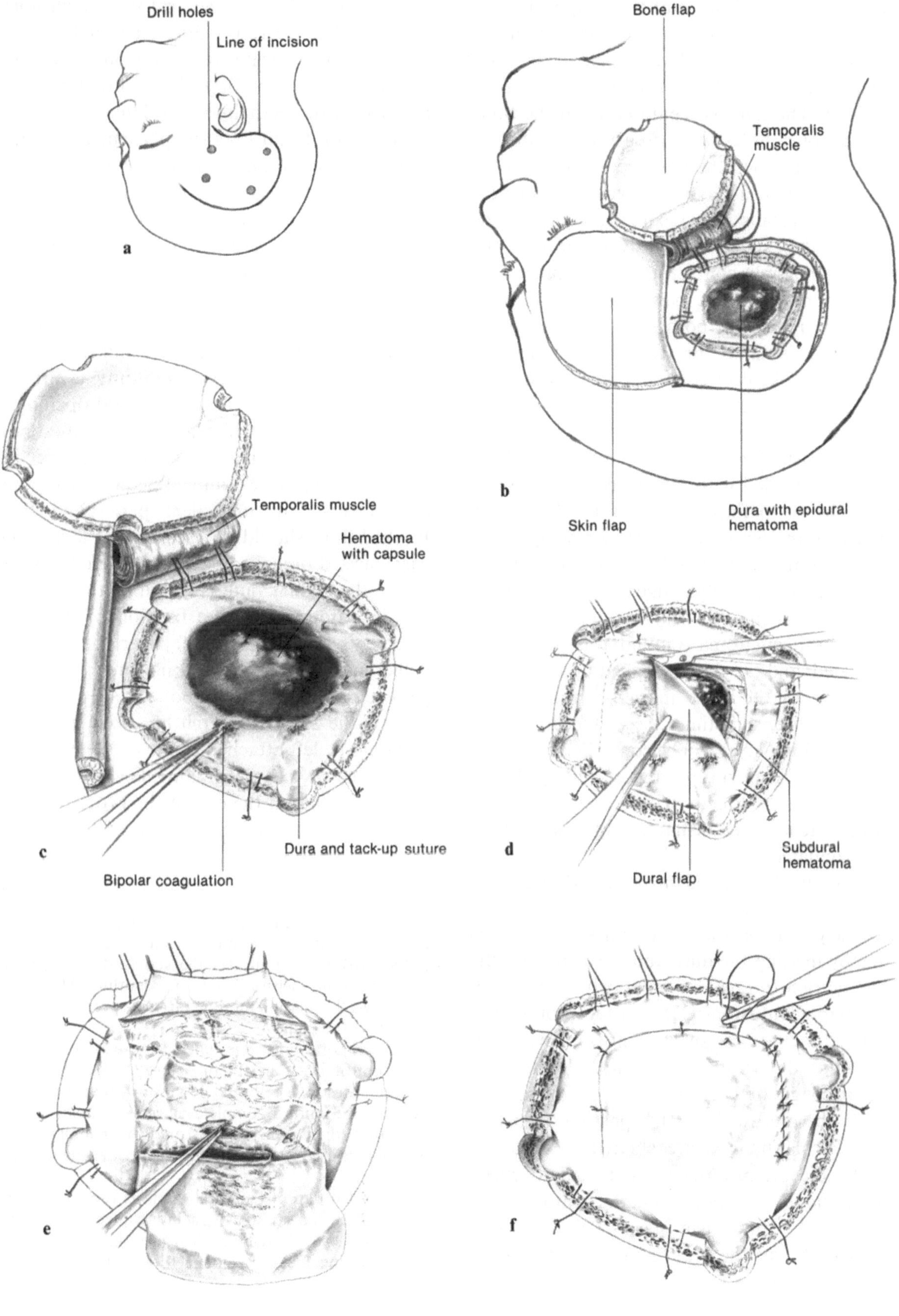
Drill holes
Line of incision
a
Bone flap
Temporalis muscle
b
Skin flap
Dura with epidural hematoma
Temporalis muscle
Hematoma with capsule
c
Dura and tack-up suture
Bipolar coagulation
d
Subdural hematoma
Dural flap
e
f

and the posterior border of the temporal squama. Either one or two perforations are made superiorly in the cranial vault, above the temporal insertion, so that a rounded bone flap is obtained. The dura is separated from the bone between burr holes with a curved elevator or dissector, and then the bone between the openings is cut with a Gigli saw passed from hole to hole by means of a flexible saw guide. The cut should be beveled slightly to provide the broadest possible contact area for replacement of the bone flap. The basal part of the bone flap is narrowed on both sides with rongeurs, avoiding trauma to the temporal muscle, and the flap is broken across the base as it is elevated from the dura. Occasionally the middle meningeal artery traverses the base of the bone flap, causing brisk bleeding when the flap is raised. This is controlled with bipolar cautery or bone wax. The scalp flap as well as the bone flap hinged on the temporal muscle are wrapped in moist compresses and reflected away from the field. The broken rough edge at the base of the craniotomy is smoothed. If nothing more than an epidural hematoma is found, it is completely evacuated, and the dura is tacked up to the soft tissues or to the bone margins through drill holes. Diffuse, sometimes heavy bleeding from the outer dural layer can be controlled by applying dural tack-up sutures and occluding the intradural vessels directly with closely spaced ligating stitches. Any remaining bleeding points are coagulated.

If the trauma has caused *intracerebral contusions and hemorrhage with impending herniation*, it is necessary to open the intradural space. This is done by incising the dura about 5 mm from the bone margin to create a superiorly based trapdoor flap. Contusion-related intracerebral hemorrhagic foci are removed along with irreversibly damaged portions of the brain. Bleeding vessels are coagulated. The medial parts of the temporal lobe are examined for possible transtentorial herniation and are ablated as required. Finally the brain surface is irrigated to check for additional bleeding sites in the contused area that would require hemostasis. The dural flap is replaced over the brain and secured with an interrupted suture line that is oversewn with a simple running suture. Several small drill holes are placed at corresponding sites in the bone flap and bone margins to permit suture fixation of the craniotomy flap. The burr holes are patched with methylmethacrylate. After reattachment of the muscles and placement of a subgaleal suction drain, the scalp is closed with all-layer sutures. Fine cutaneous sutures should be used in the visible part of the incision.

In an *open craniocerebral injury with comminution* (Fig. MS 4a–c), it is necessary to modify the foregoing procedure in accordance with the particular situation. The bone fragments are carefully elevated from the dura and stored, and the defect is enlarged by craniotomy as circumstances require. The traumatic dural opening is enlarged to allow sufficient access to the brain lesion. Losses of dural substance are reconstructed, using for example a pedicled temporal aponeurosis flap or galeal pericranial flap. Banked dura should be used only if local, well vascularized tissue is unavailable. The bony defect in the cranial vault is closed by the progressive insertion and suture fixation of the bone fragments, starting from the periphery of the defect and working toward its center. Residual gaps are obliterated with bone paste and fibrin glue. If the zygomatic arch has been fractured, it should be left attached to the masseter muscle if possible so that the fragments can be turned back into place at the end of the procedure and stabilized by internal fixation. In some cases the

Fig. MS 4a–c. Treatment of an open lateral craniocerebral injury with a comminuted cranial vault fracture.
a The *broken line* indicates the standard, cosmetically favorable scalp incision behind the hairline. The *dotted line* shows the incision modified to incorporate the existing soft-tissue injury.
b The temporal muscle is reflected to expose the skull and dural injury. The fractured zygoma, based on the masseter muscle, is reflected downward. Bone fragments are removed until a complete margin of intact dura is visualized; the fragments are stored for reimplantation. Scissors are used to even-out the lacerated, irregular dural margin.
c A pedicled flap of temporal fascia is turned over the dural defect and secured with interrupted sutures and fibrin adhesive. Osseous defects are obliterated where possible using the stored bone fragments, bone paste, and fibrin glue

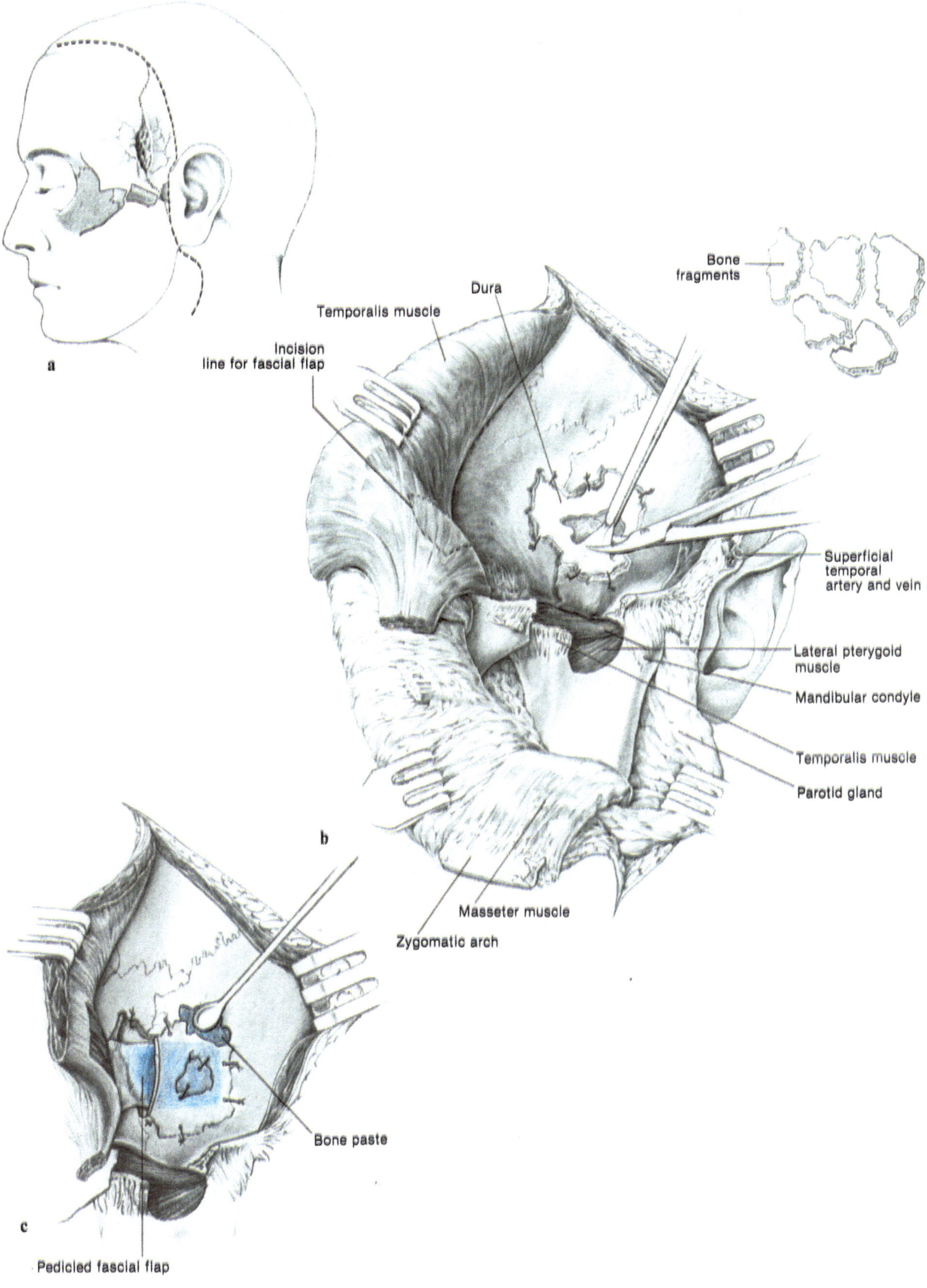
a
Bone fragments
Dura
Temporalis muscle
Incision line for fascial flap
Superficial temporal artery and vein
Lateral pterygoid muscle
Mandibular condyle
Temporalis muscle
Parotid gland
b
Masseter muscle
Zygomatic arch
Bone paste
c
Pedicled fascial flap

cranial vault may be reconstructed at a later stage. This is recommended when the bone fragments cannot be replaced into the defect and the injured area has a risk of infection (Fig. AS 23a–g).

Therapeutic Options in Carotid-Cavernous Fistula

Introductory Remarks. Vascular anatomy of the sellar region: The cavernous sinus and neurovascular structures that traverse it represent an especially critical region of the skull base from a surgical standpoint.

The course of the internal carotid artery in the cavernous sinus is variable and was called the "carotid siphon" by Moniz (1934). Krayenbühl and Yasargil (1965) described seven different siphon configurations based on their angiographic studies: 1) U shape, 2) V shape, 3) arc shape, 4) delta shape, 5) double siphon shape, 6) megasiphon, and 7) dolicosiphon.

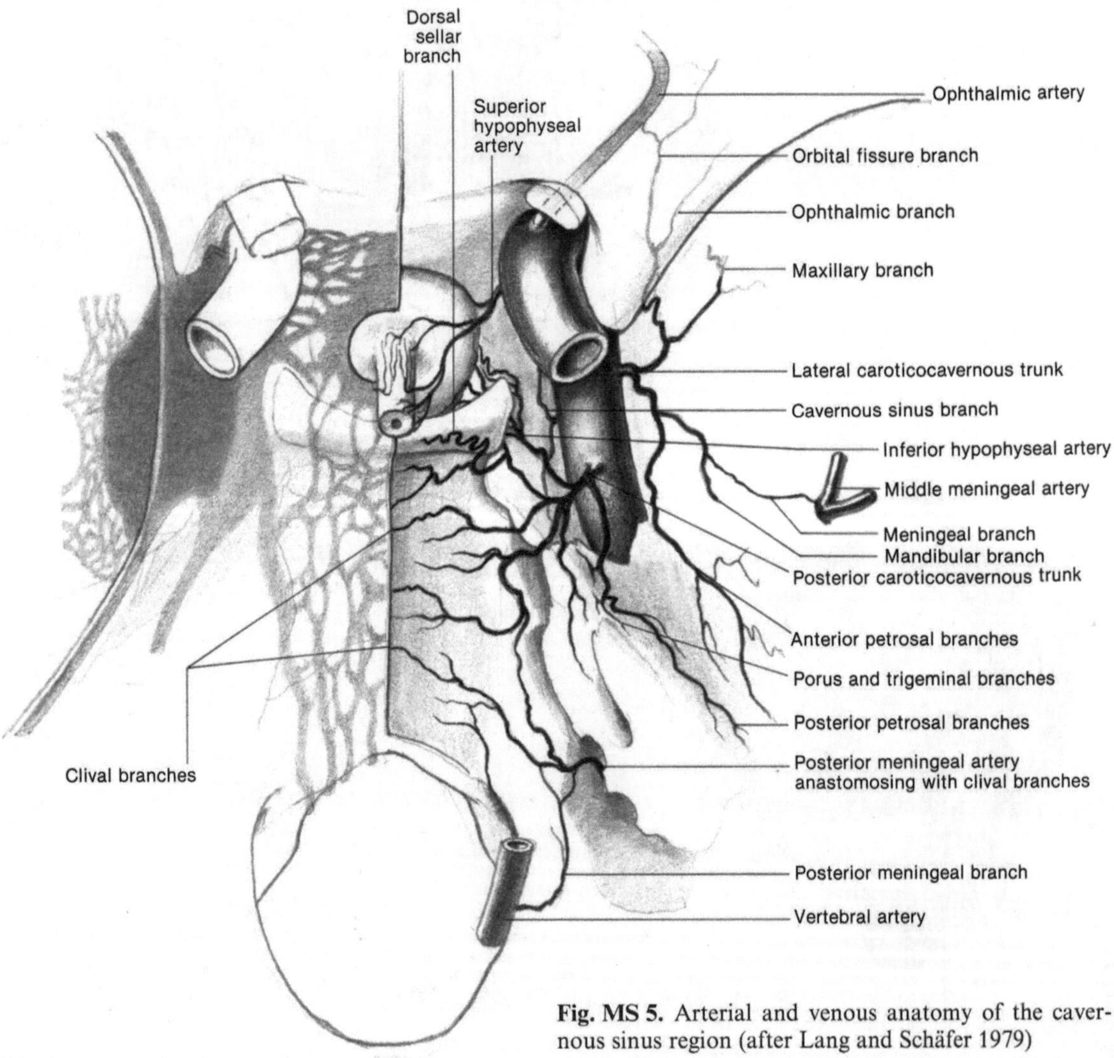

Fig. MS 5. Arterial and venous anatomy of the cavernous sinus region (after Lang and Schäfer 1979)

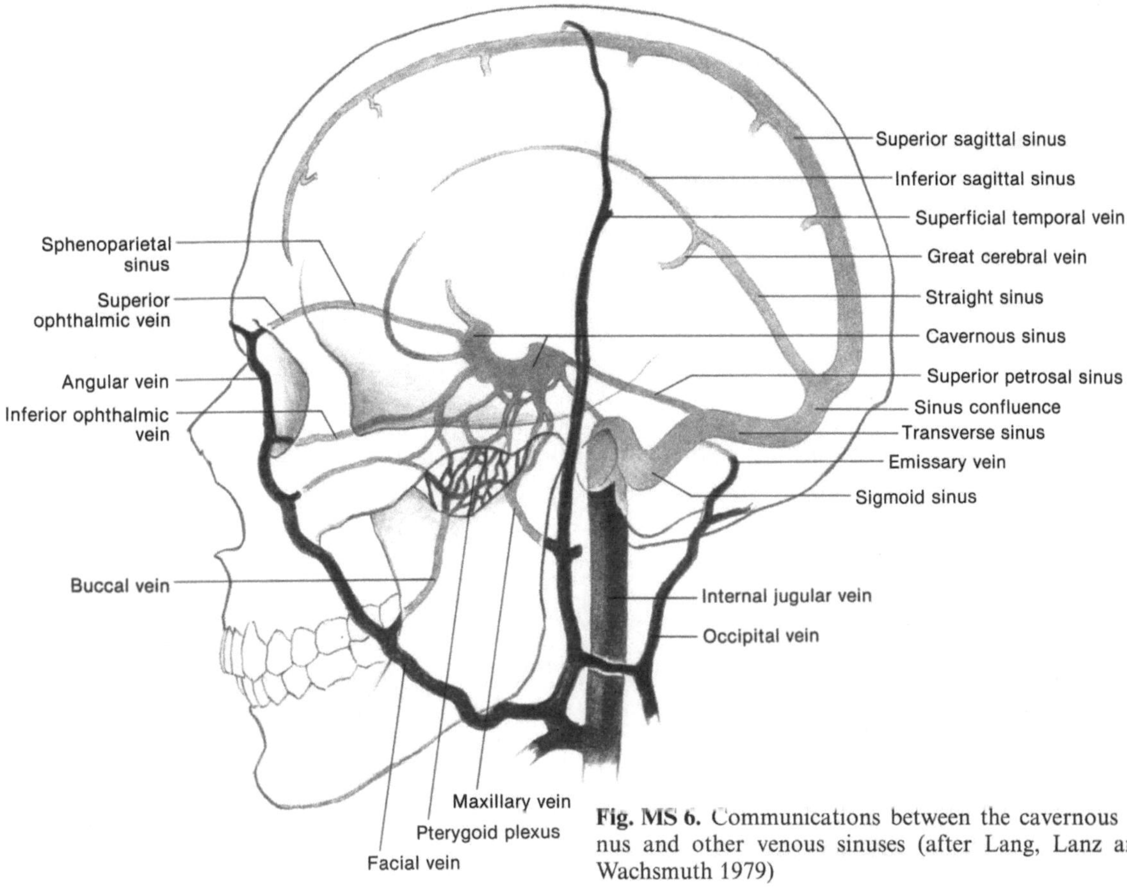

Fig. MS 6. Communications between the cavernous sinus and other venous sinuses (after Lang, Lanz and Wachsmuth 1979)

According to Lang and Schäfer (1976), the carotid artery gives off two to six smaller branches from its intracavernous portion. Two main arterial trunks are usually present – the posterior and the lateral caroticocavernous trunks (Fig. MS 5, superior view of the sellar vascular system).

Lang (1979) states that the venous channel of the cavernous sinus is uniform in about 70% of the adult population and is permeated by 10–60 trabeculae representing remains of the embryonic venous walls. In about 29% of the population the cavernous sinus consists of a variable number of blood-filled lakes (up to 25) that anastomose with one another. In about 4%, thin-walled veins traverse the loculated fibrous tissue compartment. The interspaces are filled with lax fibrous and fatty tissue (Fig. MS 5) (Michailow 1964). The cavernous sinus functions as a central "relay station" for venous drainage of the cranial cavity and communicates directly or indirectly with all of the venous sinuses (Fig. MS 6).

With advances in superselective angiography and with the embolization of traumatic carotid-cavernous fistulae, the microanatomy of this region has assumed increasing practical importance. The treatment of choice depends on the precise localization of the fistula.

Cranial nerves III, IV, V and VI pass through the cavernous sinus, their relative positions changing in the posterior to anterior direction (Fig. MS 7a–d). In the direct frontotemporal approach to the cavernous sinus from the lateral side, Parkinson recommended opening the dura between the trochlear nerve superiorly and the ophthalmic nerve inferiorly ("Parkinson's triangle") in order to minimize the risk of surgical trauma to the cranial nerves.

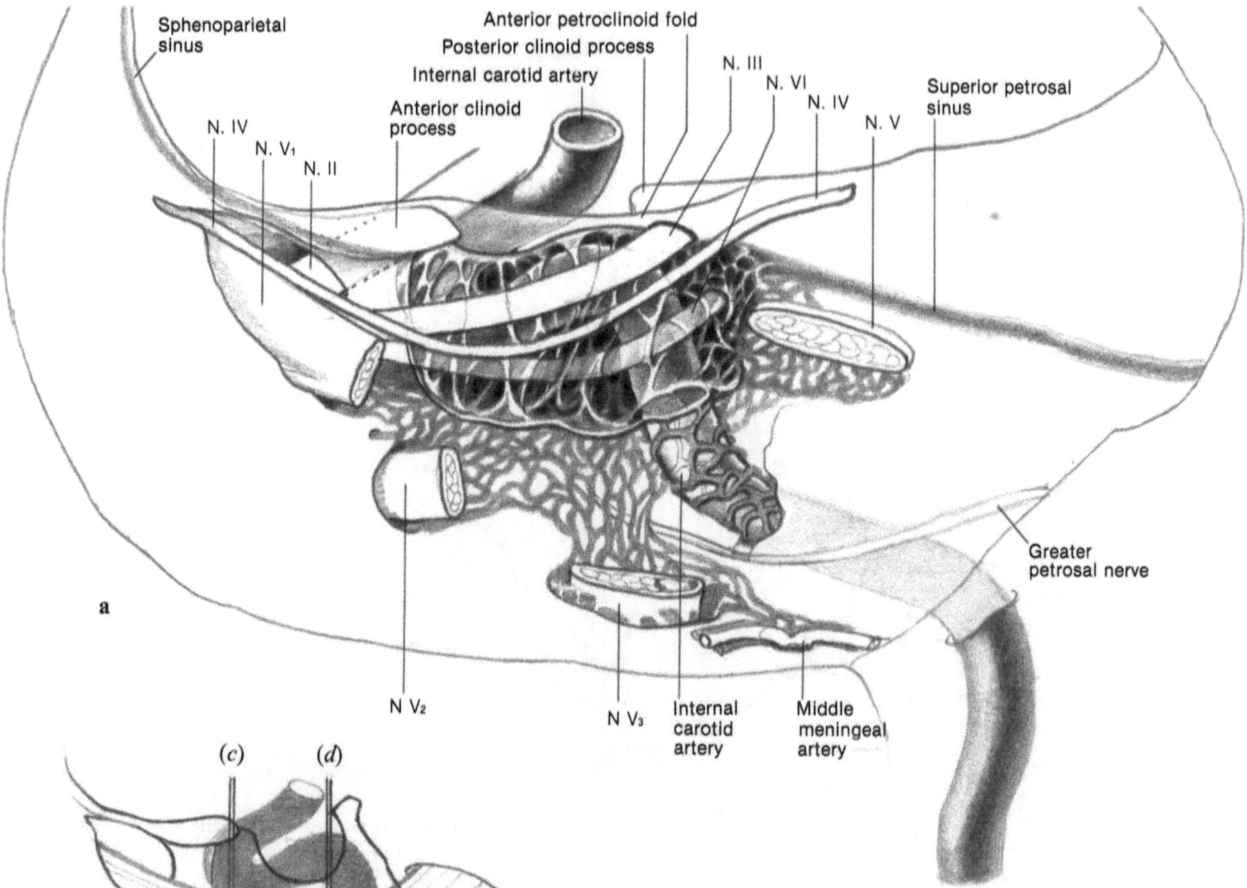

a

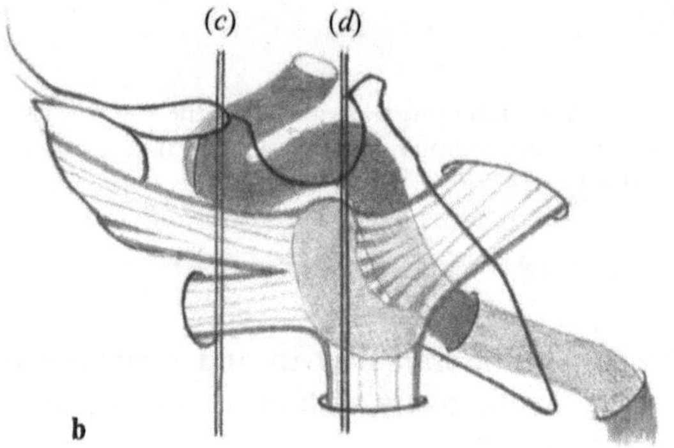

b

Fig. MS 7a–d. Topography of the cavernous sinus from the lateral aspect and in coronal section (after Lang, Lanz and Wachsmuth 1979)

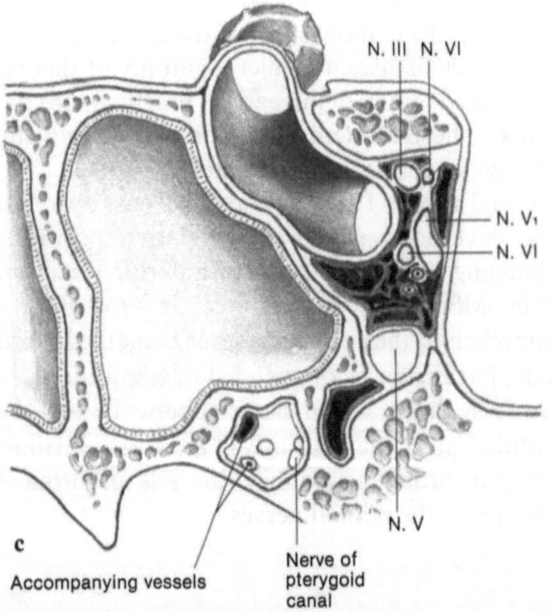

c

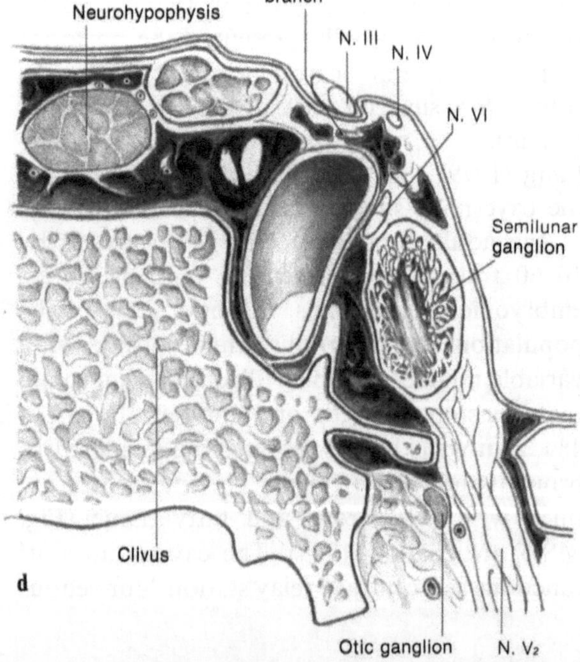

d

Carotid-cavernous fistula was commonly referred to as "carotid-cavernous aneurysm" in the older literature. Reviews have been published by Dandy (1935), Dietrich (1981), Hamby (1933, 1966), and Metzel (1980). Goldhahn (1967) divides the symptoms of carotid-cavernous fistula into three groups according to their frequency:

1) Cardinal symptoms
   a) Bruit synchronous with the arterial pulse
   b) Proptosis (exophthalmos)
   c) Abducens nerve palsy
2) Accessory symptoms
   a) Signs of venous engorgement in the eye
   b) Impaired vision or constricted visual field
   c) Other cranial nerve involvement
3) Rare symptoms
   a) Pulsation of the globe or of venous convolutions
   b) Other ocular symptoms
   c) Headache
   d) Cerebral disturbances
   e) Hemorrhage
   f) Sympathetic nervous system involvement

Differential diagnoses include traumatic aneurysm of the internal carotid artery, nontraumatic aneurysm of the internal carotid artery in the cavernous sinus, vascular malformations of the orbit, cervical carotid-jugular fistula, cavernous sinus thrombosis, orbital encephalocele, and orbital as well as intracranial tumors. The decision when and whether to attempt correction of this arteriovenous shunt is particularly difficult when angiograms show that occlusion of the internal carotid artery does not leave the affected cerebral hemisphere with an adequate collateral supply from the opposite side.

In carotid-cavernous fistula it is important to weigh carefully the patient's symptoms on the one hand and the potential problems that may result from operative treatment on the other hand. Successful elimination of the arteriovenous shunt will improve or even normalize the blood flow to the affected cerebral hemisphere by preventing the premature diversion of arterial flow into the venous system. It will halt the progression of symptoms and allow regression of existing symptoms to some degree. Treatment also has prophylactic value in that it can avert late cardiovascular changes, potentially fatal hemorrhage through the sphenoid sinus, and the severe psychological distress that can result from the disfigurement caused by progressive exophthalmos. Before initiating treatment, the physician must have adequate information on the specific pathoanatomic features of the lesion. Digital compression of the carotid artery at the neck is done to determine what effect occlusion of the common or internal carotid artery will have on symptoms.

Plain X-ray films and tomograms of the anterior and middle skull base, as well as CT scans, may localize the fracture that is responsible for the fistula. Electroencephalography (Nau et al. 1977), cerebral isotope scans, angiography (with and without carotid compression), and new methods of cerebral blood flow measurement with the aid of CT furnish information on the blood flow pattern and functional status in the area of the fistula and in the brain. Doppler ultrasound can supply information on hemodynamic patterns both before and after operation.

Treatment Options

Ligation of the Major Feeding Arteries (Common Carotid, Internal Carotid, and External Carotid and Their Branches)

The vessels are occluded through an intracranial, extracranial, or combined approach. Dandy (1935) and Hamby and Gardner (1933) introduced ligation and clipping of the supraclinoidal internal carotid artery for the management of carotid-cavernous fistula. In all these cases, intracranial ligation was the second step of the operation following carotid ligation in the neck.

Operations in which the fistulous segment of the internal carotid artery is excluded from the circulation are called "trapping" procedures (Fig. MS 8a–c). Intracranial ligation of the internal carotid artery is necessary because if the internal carotid were ligated only in the neck, the fistula would continue to receive substantial

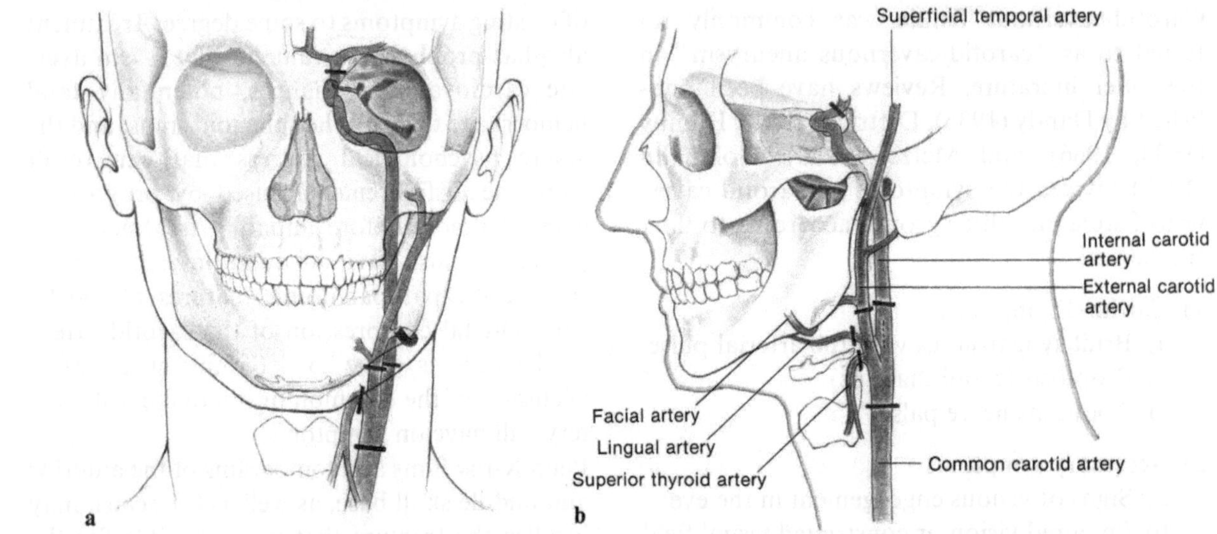

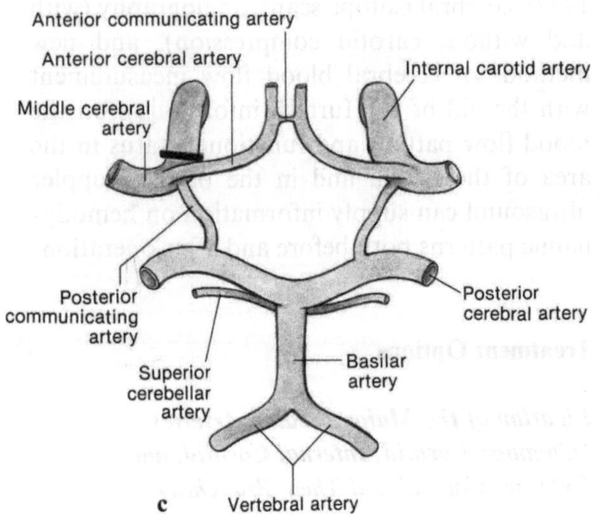

Fig. MS 8 a–c. Technique of the "trapping operation" for treatment of carotid-cavernous fistula. Panels **a** and **b** show the extracranial and intracranial sites for occlusion of the common carotid artery, external carotid artery, superior thyroid artery, and internal carotid artery.
c Collateral connections in the circle of Willis. The internal carotid artery is clipped just before the confluence of the anterior cerebral and posterior communicating arteries

retrograde flow from the circle of Willis via the anterior and posterior communicating arteries – enough to supply the affected cerebral hemisphere and replenish the initially diminished shunt volume of the fistula. The end result of this is a recurrence. Occluding the internal carotid artery only below the origin of the posterior communicating artery does not block collateral flow to the affected hemispheres via the circle of Willis, but it does isolate the fistulous segment from its retrograde supply. This technique relies on an intact collateral circulation through the circle of Willis, however. While Hamby (1964) was able to cure less than one-third of his patients by primary cervical ligation, cures in an additional one-third were achieved by combining cervical ligation with intracranial clipping. Echols and Jackson (1959) reported a 50% cure rate, and Pool and Poots (1965) obtained obliteration in two-thirds of their patients. Krayenbühl (1967) reported a 0% cure rate with improvement in 60%. Friedmann et al. (1970) reported a 25% obliteration rate with the trapping procedure.

Failures resulted from the fact that intracranial clipping of the internal carotid artery did not affect the patency of the ophthalmic artery, whose abundant collateral connections with the ipsilateral and contralateral external carotid arteries permitted retrograde flow into the fistulous segment of the internal carotid, leading to a recurrence of the shunt. Adson (1942) achieved cures in all cases by combining the trapping operation with occlusion of the ophthalmic artery after its origin from the internal carotid. He did not observe visual deterioration. Dandy (1937) was the first to show that ophthalmic artery ligation does not necessarily cause blindness, owing to the development of a collateral circulation.

The question of whether the cervical or intracranial ligation should be performed first in a trapping operation is controversial. There are compelling arguments for and against both alternatives. Cervical ligation of the carotid artery gives rise to a "vascular steal" phenomenon in which arterial blood is diverted from the collateral circulation of the opposite side, causing ischemic deprivation of the ipsilateral hemisphere despite the seemingly adequate capacities of the anterior and posterior communicating arteries. This phenomenon does not occur when the intracranial artery is ligated first.

On the other hand, Pool and Poots (1965) have raised the following objections to primary intracranial ligation:

1) The flow of arterial blood into the cavernous sinus increases because of the pressure rise from the cervical side, both through the fistula itself and
2) through arterial side channels of the internal carotid artery.
3) If the ligation leads to hemiplegia, this is more easily corrected in the neck than intracranially.
4) Cervical ligation alone may be sufficient, obviating the need for further surgery.

Hamby (1964, 1966) tried to avoid the adverse hemodynamic effects of a two-stage ligation by performing the cervical and intracranial ligations in one session, being able to cure 17 of his 18 patients. Nevertheless Stern, Brown, and Alksne (1967) showed that severe complications may follow the one-stage procedure; in fact two of their six patients died, and one developed severe hemiplegia. The remaining three patients were cured.

Aside from the arguments presented above, treatment of carotid-cavernous fistula by internal carotid ligation is problematic in that it is almost impossible to establish a correlation preoperatively between the angiographic capacity of the circle of Willis and the clinically relevant blood flow that is obtained after surgery.

Embolization of the Internal Carotid Artery

Because a direct operation on the fistulous opening was not possible, Brooks (1930) suggested introducing a piece of muscle into the cervical carotid artery and allowing it to embolize to the site of the fistula (Fig. MS 9). The rationale is that a muscle embolus of appropriate size will become firmly lodged in the fistulous opening by the pressure of the arterial current. Hamby and Gardner (1933) marked the muscle embolus with a silver clip for X-ray localization. However, these authors were unable to obtain a definitive cure until they subsequently ligated the internal carotid artery. This led Dandy (1937) to conclude that embolization should be done concurrently with carotid ligation. A major problem inherent to the embolization technique is the difficulty of establishing the exact size of the fistula. This in turn makes it difficult to determine the optimum size and shape of the embolus. If the embolus is too large, it will not reach the fistula and will perform essentially the function of a ligature. If too small, it can pass completely through the fistula and enter into the cavernous sinus, causing a sinus thrombosis. Serious complications such as paralysis, aphasia, or blindness can result if the embolus does not remain lodged in the fistulous opening, but migrates into the supraclinoidal portion of the internal carotid artery or one of its branches. These difficulties prompted Jaeger (1942) to develop a technique in which intracranial clipping of the internal carotid artery is performed as a first step before opening the cervical vessels and introducing the embolus. Isamat et al. (1970) reviewed 89 cases

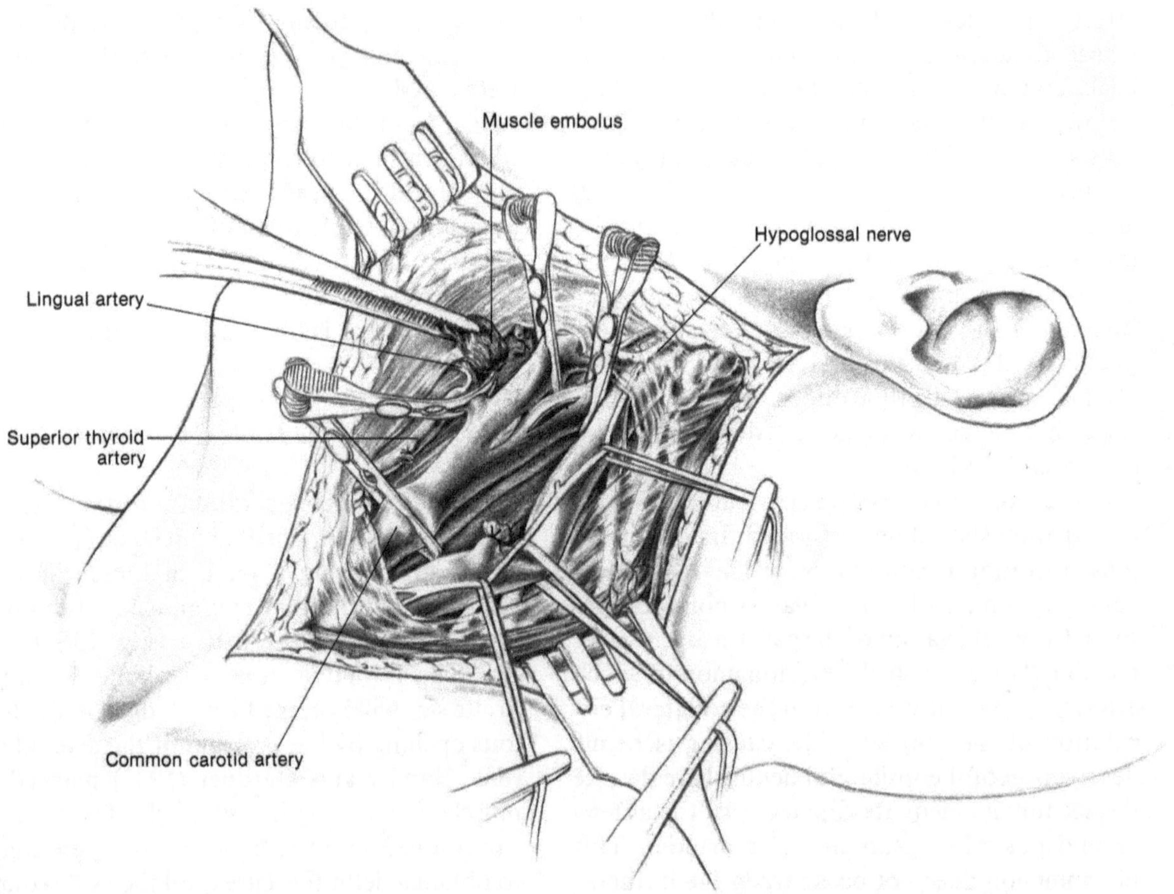

Fig. MS 9. Embolization of the internal carotid artery with a piece of muscle. The carotid bifurcation is exposed, and the internal carotid artery is opened above the bifurcation for insertion of the muscle embolus

of internal carotid artery embolization, with intracranial occlusion done as a first step in 76. The obliteration rate in these cases approached 99%. The "Jaeger maneuver" was further refined by Hamby (1964, 1966): After intracranial clipping of the supraclinoidal internal carotid artery and of the ophthalmic artery if possible, the entire cavernous segment of the internal carotid is embolized with the object of blocking as much arterial inflow as possible. The goal is to block all the ramifications from the cavernous and petrous portions of the internal carotid artery to prevent a recurrence of the fistula through collateral channels. Today this technique is considered one of the most reliable methods for the treatment of carotid-cavernous fistula (Larson and Worman 1968, Noordenbos 1968, Rey et al. 1975, Sedzimir and Occleshaw 1967). Potential complications of the Jaeger and Hamby techniques are cavernous sinus thrombosis with blindness (Krayenbühl 1967), visual disturbances and blindness (Ohta et al. 1973), clip dislodgement and cerebral embolism (Obrador et al. 1974), cerebral ischemia with death or hemiplegia (Besson et al. 1975), and death from paradoxical embolism (McCormick et al. 1976).

A number of authors have modified this embolization technique. Some authors performed the embolization after ligating the internal carotid artery both in the neck and intracranially. Later the *free embolization* technique was introduced in which the carotid-cavernous fistula is occluded while preserving flow through the internal carotid artery (Land and Bucy 1965, Isfort 1967).

In the *controlled embolization* technique, a suture is attached to the muscle embolus before its insertion into the carotid artery, to prevent it from being carried into the cerebral circulation or cavernous sinus. In some circumstances the suture can serve to maintain patency of the arterial lumen. One disadvantage is the danger of thrombosis or embolism from the intraluminal thread. Krayenbühl (1967) used a Foley balloon catheter to advance a muscle strip, with clip and suture attached, into the cavernous portion of the artery, thereby filling the entire fistulous segment. After placement is confirmed by angiography, the common carotid artery is ligated in the neck, anchoring the suture to the ligature.

Fistula Occlusion with the Fogarty Balloon Catheter
(Fig. MS 10)

Prolo and Hanbery (1971) were the first to accomplish the intraluminal occlusion of a carotid-cavernous fistula by means of a Fogarty catheter. This technique, like others, relies on an intact collateral flow through the circle of Willis, since the patency of the internal carotid artery is sacrificed. The balloon catheter is inserted into the common carotid artery and is advanced into the cavernous segment of the internal carotid under image intensifier control. The balloon is filled with contrast medium so that its placement can be monitored. The proximal end of the catheter is secured to the wall of the common carotid artery. Finally the common, internal, and external carotid arteries are ligated in the neck. This balloon technique is a relatively safe and simple method of occluding a carotid-cavernous fistula. Of course, one must take into account the risks and possible complications of the carotid artery ligation, and problems can arise when the catheter has to be inserted through an unusually tortuous vessel (Herrman et al. 1975). Moreover, it is difficult to match the size and position of the balloon accurately to the fistulous opening. Spontaneous deflation of the balloon cannot be ruled out. Finally, it is impossible to say with certainty how the catheter material will be tolerated in the long term. Nevertheless, many authors consider the balloon catheter technique to be the method of choice in patients with an adequate collateral circulation (Chowdhary 1978, Grunert and Sunder-Plassmann 1971, Rougerie et al. 1973, Rupp et al. 1975, Serbinenko 1974).

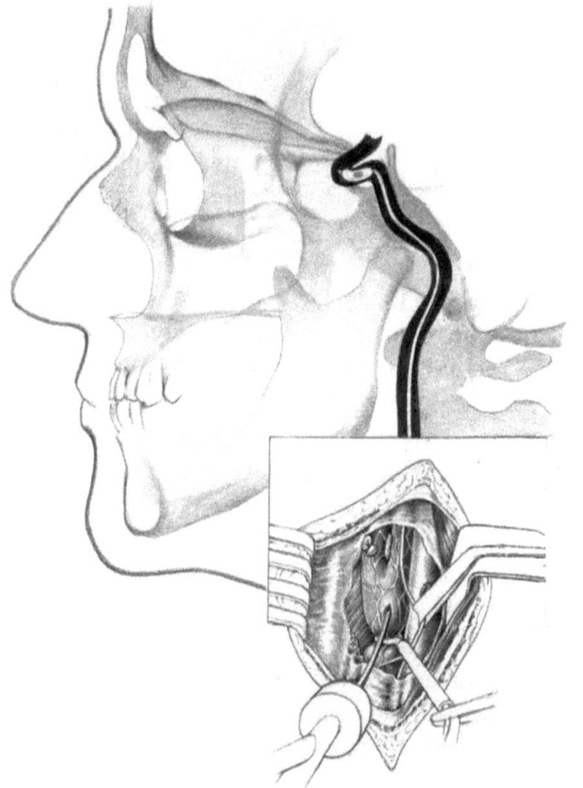

Fig. MS 10. Occlusion of a carotid-cavernous fistula with a Fogarty catheter, which is advanced to the site of the lesion through the cervical portion of the carotid artery

Detachable Balloon Technique
(Fig. MS 11)

In the early 1970s, new superselective micro-catheter techniques employing a detachable balloon were described by Cophignon et al. (1974), Djindjian (1974), and Serbinenko (1971, 1972, 1974). Refinements were introduced by Debrun (1975, 1981, 1982), who in 1981 reported on 54 traumatic carotid-cavernous fistulae that had been treated by this method. In the detachable balloon technique a small latex or silastic balloonis tied to the tip of a microcatheter with a thin latex thread. After reaching its destination, the balloon is released either by traction or by threading a second coaxial catheter over the first catheter and using it to push the balloon off the end of the first catheter. The aperture of the balloon is automatically closed by the elastic thread around its base. The balloon is filled with liquid silicone so that it will retain its dimensions permanently. The silicone mixture solidifies within 5–10 minutes of injection. A recent innovation implies insertion of the balloon catheter through a femoral catheter. This technique employs an "injection chamber" that creates a rapid flow in the guide catheter which propels the uninflated balloon with its tubing to the site of the fistula.

Postoperative arteriograms must show that:

1) The balloon is in the cavernous sinus and outside the internal carotid artery.
2) Contrast medium used for the arteriogram is not leaking into the cavernous sinus.
3) Carotid blood flow is normal.

In the opinion of Debrun and colleagues, the detachable balloon technique has rendered obsolete methods involving the direct occlusion of carotid-cavernous fistulae with solid materials such as beads, lyophilized dura, fibrin sponge, or other substances like isobutylcyanoacrylate, due to the generally poor results of these techniques and the danger of pulmonary embolism.

Thrombosis of Carotid-Cavernous Fistulae
(Mullan 1974, 1982)

Mullan states that deaths from untreated carotid-cavernous fistula are uncommon (3%) and result mainly from severe, uncontrollable epistaxis. Hemiplegia and aphasia are also rare. Progressive ocular complications, on the other hand, arise in 70% of cases. Treatment, therefore, should be directed toward preventing ocular problems but should not involve any mea-

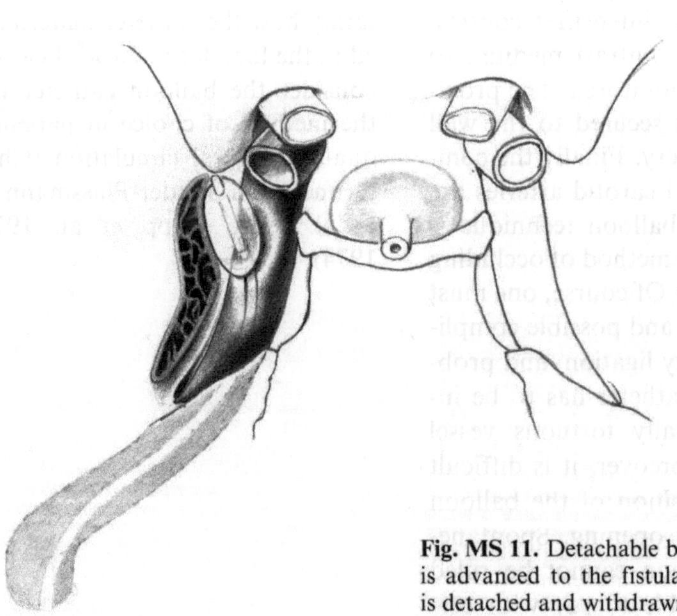

Fig. MS 11. Detachable balloon technique. The balloon is advanced to the fistula with a microcatheter, which is detached and withdrawn sures that would increase the risk of mortality, hemiplegia, or aphasia. These considerations led Mullan to reject traditional techniques of internal carotid artery occlusion.

Detailed study of patients with carotid-cavernous fistulae has shown that each case is unique in terms of the shape and location of the arteriovenous communication, making it necessary to apply a variety or combination of approaches and occlusive methods. The materials used for thrombogenesis include copper-clad steel needles, phosphor bronze wires (0.005 mm in diameter), occlusive balloons, and conventional materials like Gelfoam, oxidized cellulose, and cotton. Thrombosis of the cavernous sinus may be done through any of four approaches. The anterior, lateral, and posterior approaches require a frontotemporal osteoplastic craniotomy, while the fourth approach involves the percutaneous, transjugular introduction of thrombogenic material.

Various types of carotid-cavernous fistula are encountered, and specific techniques of thrombosis are preferred for each:

1) *Radiologically visible fistulous connections.* These are relatively favorable and can be occluded by stereotaxic or direct insertion of copper-clad steel needles into the fistula using the lateral approach.
2) *Fistulae that drain exclusively anteriorly into the ophthalmic vein* direct their entire force into the orbit and produce severe ophthalmologic complications. They are most easily treated through an anterior approach. The junction between the ophthalmic vein and sinus is entered, and the sinus is thrombosed with conventional material. If the cavernous sinus component of the fistula is small, copper needle insertion may be adequate.
3) *Fistulae that drain exclusively posteriorly.* The posterior approach to these lesions is difficult. Oculomotor nerve palsy is a potential complication. Various techniques may be used in these cases: (a) Direct insertion of wires or needles below and behind the oculomotor nerve, using intraoperative angiography to avoid internal carotid injury; (b) direct insertion of thrombogenic material into the superior petrosal sinus a few millimeters before its entry into the cavernous sinus, provided the superior petrosal sinus has an adequate lumen; and (c) percutaneous retrograde insertion of an occlusive balloon via the internal jugular vein in cases where the inferior petrosal sinus is adequately developed.
4) *Large long-standing fistulae* are relatively easy to manage. They are approached laterally. Because the internal carotid artery cannot be visualized by intraoperative angiography in such cases, wire is first inserted into the relatively safe anterior inferior portion of the cavernous sinus. When this corner is occluded, the internal carotid artery begins to show up on the angiogram, and further wire insertion can be done close to the artery. Up to 24 m of 0.005-mm phosphor bronze wire may be needed to occlude the entire fistula.
5) *Smaller, recent fistulae draining in all directions* usually require a combination of approaches and often are difficult to occlude.
6) *Bilateral fistulae* are treated in the same way as unilateral fistulae. They are approached one at a time, making an effort to occlude each side completely.
7) *Fistulae that are intolerant to carotid compression* because of insufficient collateral flow. These can result in bilateral cases where the contralateral fistula has been treated by carotid occlusion, or in cases where the collateral circulation is already anatomically deficient. Care must be taken to avoid vasospasm by irritation of the internal carotid artery; this is especially likely to occur when copper needles are used. One should either use a different material or insert the needle a few millimeters distant from the artery, even if a small residual pouch persists.

Two main problems have been encountered in this type of treatment:

1) Occlusion of the posterior exit from the cavernous sinus before the anterior outlet is thrombosed can lead to acute orbital symptoms requiring immediate treatment.

2) Occlusion of the anterior and posterior portions of the sinus without obliterating the middle can result in a central aneurysm with transient cranial neuropathies. This, too, requires further treatment once the condition is diagnosed.

To avoid these problems, an attempt should be made to thrombose one side completely in one session if at all possible. To date, 24 patients have been treated by this technique. There was one case of transient abducens nerve palsy, and one other patient developed a temporary aneurysm. A partial ophthalmoplegia became complete for a time and later resolved. There were no deaths and no evidence of hemispheric blood flow deficiency in any patient.

Direct Operations on the Cavernous Sinus

Parkinson (1965, 1967, 1982) performed the first selective closure of a fistulous opening in the cavernous sinus, doing this first in a patient with an unsuccessfully treated carotid-cavernous fistula and later in patients not previously treated, since it was found that the transcavernous approach made it possible to preserve the patency of the internal carotid artery.

The operation is performed under deep hypothermia and circulatory arrest. Parkinson used a transfrontotemporal approach and exposed the fistula through an incision in the lateral wall of the cavernous sinus, which is traversed, from above downward, by cranial nerves III, IV, V, and VI. The edges of the incision are separated to expose the cavernous segment of the internal carotid artery with its branches, and the fistula and smaller involved vessels are repaired by angioplasty. Carotid patency can be saved with this operation, although it has resulted in deaths and complications such as aphasia, meningitis, and obstructive hydrocephalus (Parkinson et al. 1974).

A competition exists at present between the direct approach to the cavernous sinus, practiced by surgeons experienced in microsurgery, and the catheter techniques for fistula occlusion that preserve carotid patency, favored by many neuroradiologists. Further experience is needed in order to establish patient selection criteria for the different techniques.

Given the systemic stress imposed by the direct, open approach to the cavernous sinus, current opinion seems to favor the less invasive detachable balloon technique. The direct approach nevertheless remains a valid alternative in case the balloon technique is unsuccessful.

Transtemporal Extradural Approach to the Anterior Surface of the Petrous Pyramid and Internal Auditory Canal

Introductory Remarks. The development of antibiotics and the introduction of the operating microscope have stimulated renewed interest in the extradural approach to the middle cranial fossa for fenestration of the superior semicircular canal in otosclerosis and chronic otitis media (Wullstein 1951), for facial nerve grafts and repair (Clerc and Batisse 1954), and for vestibular neurectomy and excision of acoustic neurinomas (House 1961, 1966). Fisch (1969, 1970, 1976) in particular has reviewed the potential applications, technical modifications, and advantages of this approach as well as the results of surgery on the internal auditory canal (Harker and McCabe 1984). The transtemporal extradural approach to the anterior surface of the pyramid and internal auditory canal has gained an established place in the traumatology of the lateral skull base (Unterberger 1959). The principal indications for this approach are persistent cerebrospinal fluid leaks and irreversible facial paralysis associated with longitudinal and transverse fractures of the petrous pyramid. The basic principles of the treatment of cerebrospinal fluid leaks following laterobasal fractures were discussed previously (p. 234). The decision whether to perform duraplasty by the transtemporal or transmastoid route is influenced both by the extent of the fracture and by auditory function. In extensive fractures that are not associated with damage to hearing, we favor the transtemporal route because it avoids the necessity of enlarging the traumatic bone defect, with risk of dural herniation, and it avoids further irritation of the acoustic organ. Duraplasty over the roof of the antrum and mastoid often can be performed more simply through the transmastoid approach from below. However, cerebrospinal fluid leak through the roof of the tympanic cavity can be repaired through the transtemporal route with no difficulties in terms of sparing the tympanic membrane-ossicular apparatus and perhaps reconstructing it at the time duraplasty is performed. If a transverse fracture has caused irreversible damage to the inner ear, even fractures situated far medially can be explored from below when a cerebrospinal fluid leak exists, and necessary duraplasty can be performed and combined with facial nerve exploration and repair as far as the cerebellopontine angle from below through the translabyrinthine approach. The presence of facial paralysis, discussed later in detail, can also influence the choice of surgical approach to the pyramid. In rare cases one may consider transtemporal exposure of the internal auditory canal for vestibular nerve or cochlear nerve section in patients with posttraumatic disturbances of vestibulolochlear function (e.g., patients with deficient central compensation for vestibular nerve injury or with a disabling noise in the ear) (Geyer and Helms 1983; Helms 1985).

Operative Technique
(Fig. MS 12a–n)

The patient is positioned supine with the body tilted slightly toward the affected side and the head turned to the side and slightly extended. The vertical skin incision starts just above the temporal muscle, extends down to the root of

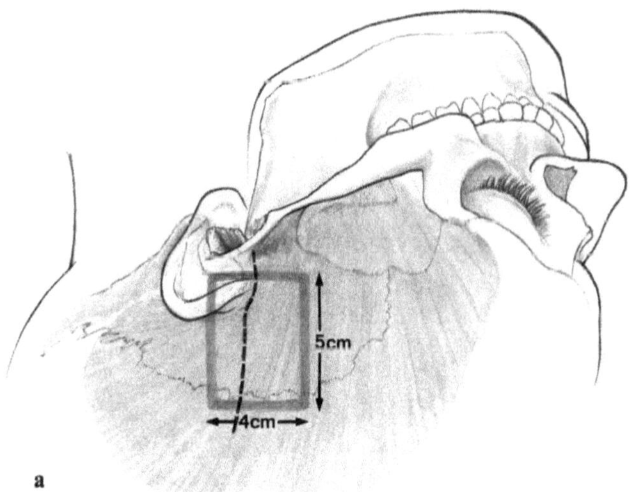

a

Fig. MS 12a–n. The transtemporal extradural approach to the anterior surface of the petrous pyramid and internal auditory canal.
a The skin incision (---) and extent of the osteoplastic craniotomy are indicated.
b The bone flap is outlined with the cutting burr.
c Here the craniotomy is made using burr holes and an osteotome.
d The craniotomy is extended basally with a rongeur

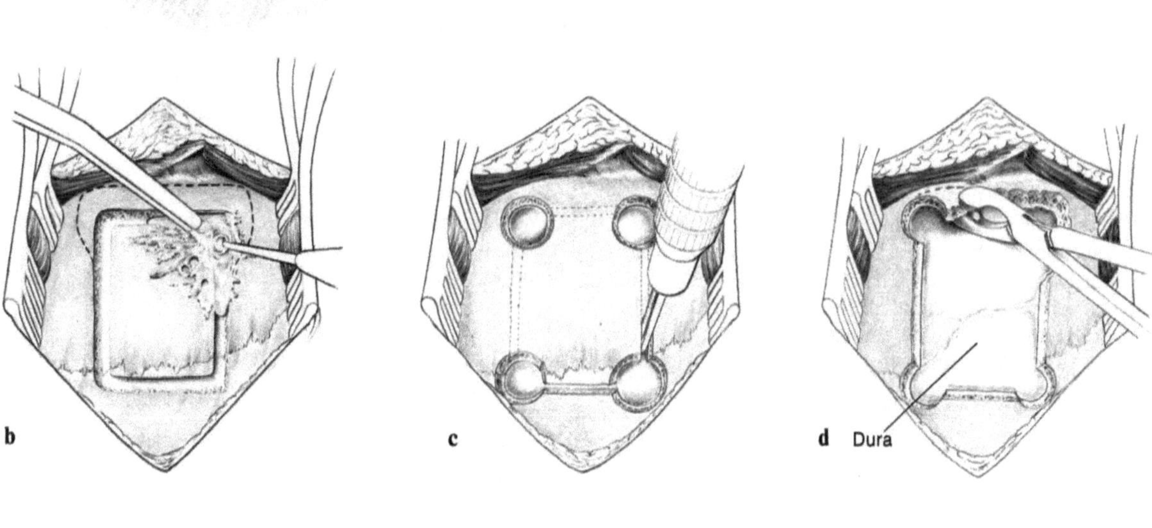

b c d

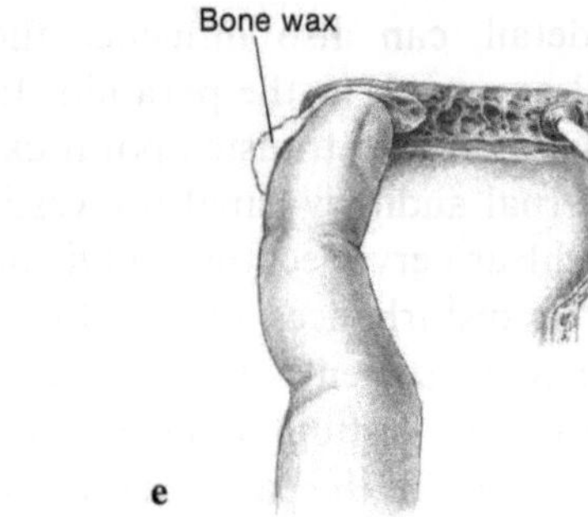

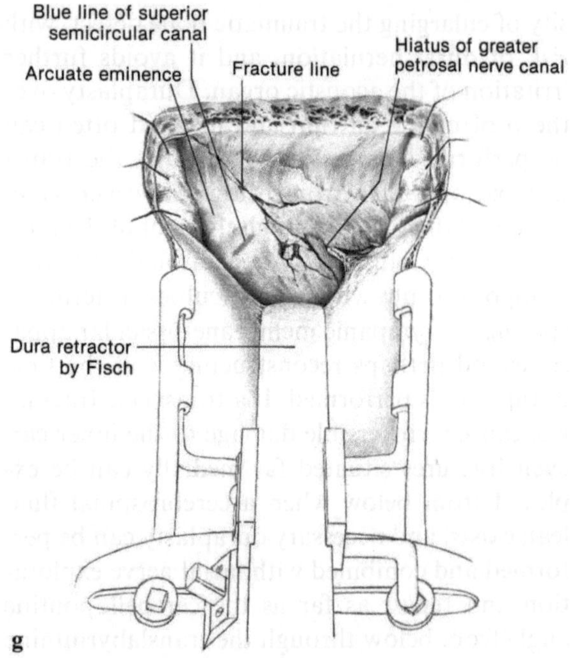

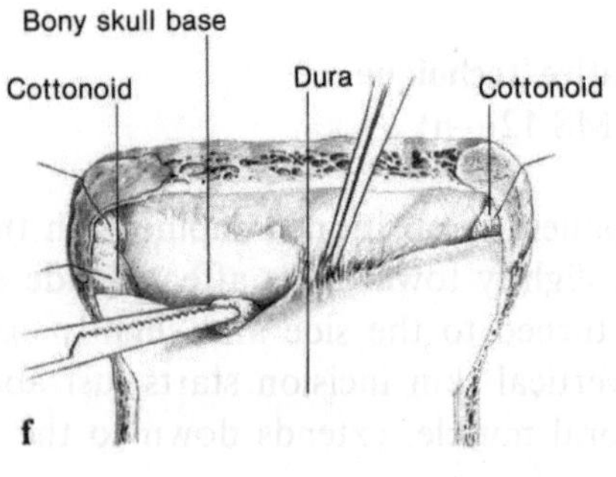

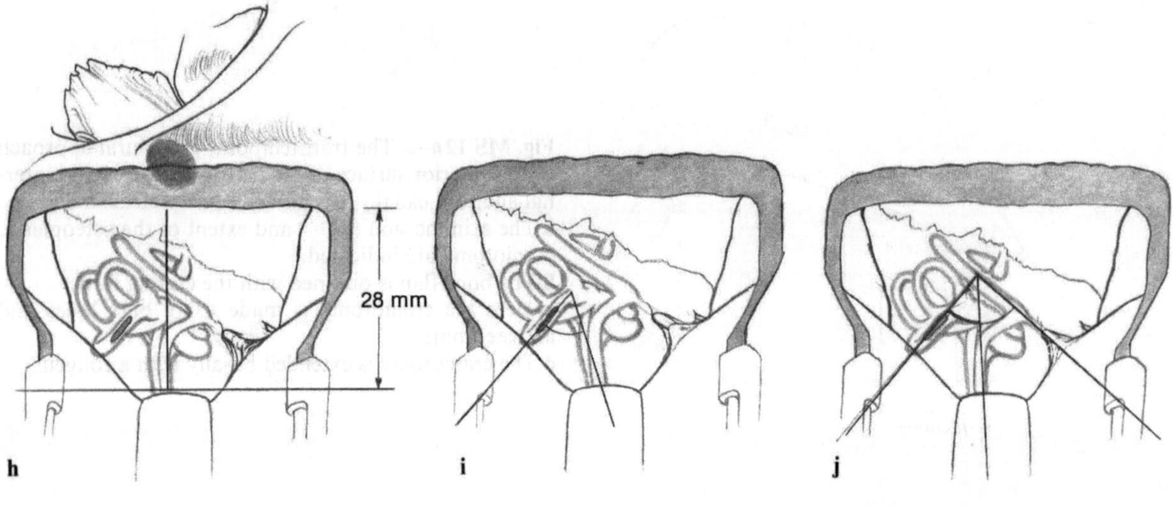

Fig. MS 12e–j.
e The bone edges are smoothed with the diamond burr, and bleeding is controlled with bone wax.
f The dura is elevated, and dural vessels are coagulated. The anterior edge of the wound (middle meningeal artery) and the posterior edge (venous vessels) are protected with cotton paddies.
g The anterior surface of the petrous bone is exposed, revealing the fracture line. Dural retraction is maintained using a Fisch retractor. The "blue line" of the superior semicircular canal presents somewhat medial and anterior to the arcuate eminence; the petrosal nerve is visible at its site of emergence, the hiatus of the greater petrosal nerve canal.
h–j Methods of identifying the internal auditory canal (IAC). **h** Portman et al. use an imaginary line drawn 28 mm from the occipital squama and parallel to it. The IAC is located by drilling superficially in the area where this line intersects the perpendicular O line. **i** Fish subtends an angle of 60° from the blue line of the superior semicircular canal as a means of locating the IAC. **j** Wigand bisects the obtuse angle between the greater petrosal nerve and the blue line of the superior semicircular canal to find the axis of the IAC

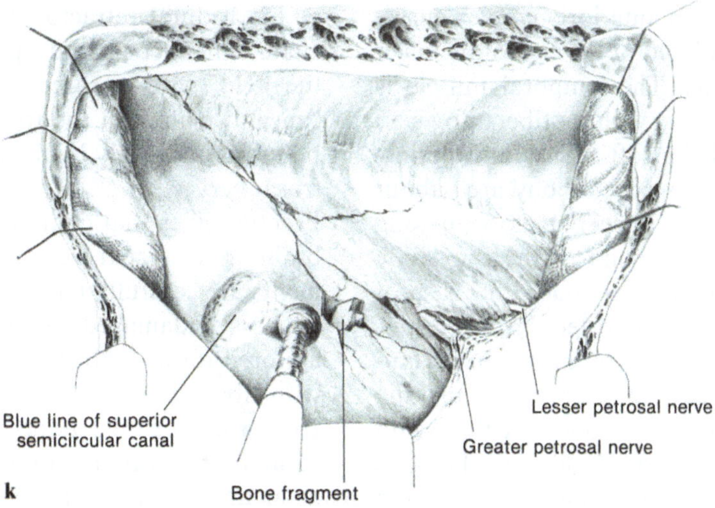

k

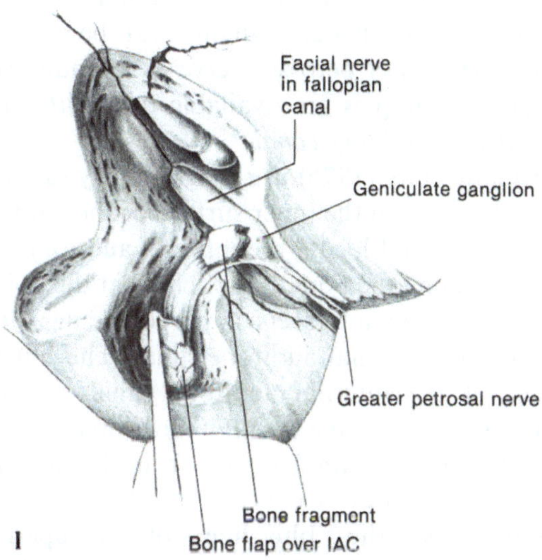

l

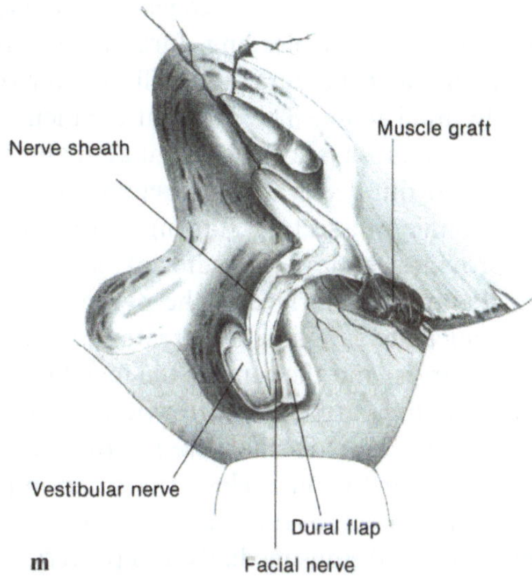

m

Fig. MS 12k–n.
k The roof of the IAC is progressively thinned by drilling superficially in front of the superior semicircular canal. With significant pneumatization, the operator will first encounter supralabyrinthine cells before reaching the yellow, compact labyrinthine bone.
l The roof of the IAC is pried upward as a bone flap. A bone fragment is seen impinging on the facial nerve at the inlet of the fallopian canal.
m An anteriorly based dural flap is raised in trap-door fashion to enter the IAC. The bone fragment impinging on the facial nerve is removed to decompress the nerve.
n At the end of the procedure the IAC is covered with a piece of muscle or fascia secured with fibrin glue, and the entire fracture area is covered with a larger piece of lyophilized dura

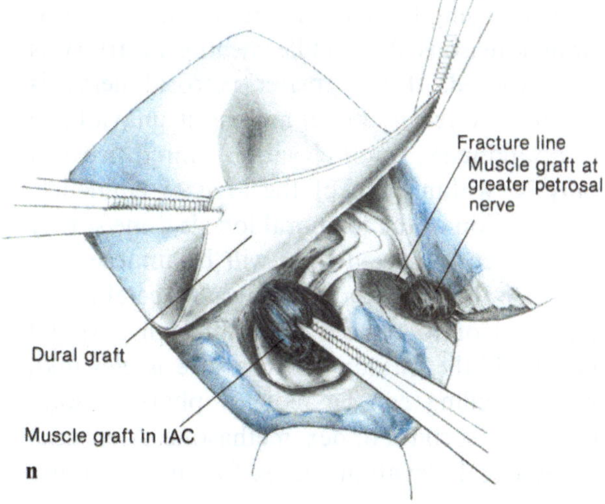

n

the auricle, forming an anteriorly convex curve, and passes down in front of the ear to the lower border of the tragus. The temporal muscle is incised vertically in line with its fibers down to the squamosa, and the soft tissues and periosteum are reflected to expose a bony area about 7 × 10 cm in size. The bone flap is 5 cm long and 4 cm wide; the midpoint of the short side of the rectangle should just touch the base of the zygomatic arch. The osteoplastic craniotomy may be performed by outlining the rectangular flap with a cutting burr or by making corner burr holes and interconnecting them with a pneumatic osteotome or Gigli saw. The bone flap is carefully separated from the dura and removed, whereupon the basal part of the craniotomy is extended with a rongeur or cutting burr. Bleeding from the bone edges is controlled with bone wax, and bleeding dural vessels are coagulated. Next the dura is mobilized over the middle cranial fossa. The dural attachment in the petrosquamosal suture is coagulated and divided. Then dural elevation is begun with the aid of a microdissector, starting posteriorly. This provides better exposure of structures about the anterior surface of the pyramid such as the geniculate ganglion, the greater and lesser petrosal nerves, and the genu of the facial nerve. These structures are exposed to view in about 10% of cases even in the absence of a bony injury (Fisch 1976). Dural elevation is continued to the foramen spinosum anteriorly and to the superior petrosal sinus medially and posteriorly. The dura is not mobilized over the facial hiatus, as this might cause bleeding from numerous veins coursing between the dura and bone. For similar reasons the middle meningeal artery is not exposed. If the greater petrosal nerve is largely covered by bone, making it unavailable as a landmark, dural elevation should proceed only to within 2 cm of the arcuate eminence. If retraction of the temporal lobe is done slowly and patiently, it generally will be unnecessary to incise the dura for withdrawal of cerebrospinal fluid or to remove fluid through a spinal needle. If the intracranial pressure is elevated, brain swelling can be reduced pharmacologically with sorbitol or dexamethasone. After adequate dural elevation, the self-retaining House or Fisch dural retractor is introduced. The arcuate eminance should appear at the center of the field, with an area which Fisch calls the "meatal plane" in the foreground. The field is bounded anteriorly by the lesser and greater petrosal nerves.

Fracture lines that contain entrapped dura and brain are dissected free, and smaller bone fragments are carefully removed. If the facial nerve appears undamaged, the dura is repaired with a stored dural graft attached to the skull base with fibrin glue, retraction is released from the temporal lobe, the bone flap is replaced and secured, the temporal muscle is reapproximated, a suction drain is inserted, and the scalp is closed with all-layer sutures.

If facial paralysis exists, it is necessary to explore the fallopian canal and internal auditory meatus. The geniculate ganglion can be located using the greater petrosal nerve as a landmark. Several techniques are available for *identifying the internal auditory canal:*

Portmann et al. (1975) use an imaginary sagittal line 28 mm from the inner surface of the temporal squama and locate the internal auditory canal by drilling the bone superficially at the point where the line intersects a perpendicular line joining the external auditory canal. The bluish luster of the internal auditory canal and its borders will be visible through the thinned bone. The roof of the canal ranges from 4–7 mm in thickness and may be covered by apical air cells. Fisch exposes the "blue line" of the superior semicircular canal with a diamond burr and locates the internal auditory canal by subtending a 60° angle anteriorly from the blue line. Wigand (1979) bisects the obtuse angle formed by the greater petrosal nerve and the blue line of the semicircular canal. When attempting to locate the internal auditory canal, it should be noted that the highest elevation of the arcuate eminence does not necessarily correspond to the course of the superior semicircular canal. Especially when there is extensive apical pneumatization, it can be difficult to identify the yellowish, compact labyrinthine bone. Just anterior to the fundus of the internal auditory canal and labyrinthine portion of the fallopian canal, attention must be given to the basal turn of the cochlea. The internal auditory canal is exposed by superficial drilling with the diamond burr under constant irrigation. When the bone has been adequately thinned, the roof of the internal auditory canal is raised as a flap, and the canal is entered by coagulating and incising the dura in the area of the posterior wall of the internal auditory canal. The facial nerve is encountered in the anterior superior portion of the internal auditory canal, the superior part of the vestibular ganglion lies posterosuperiorly, the inferior part lies posteroinferiorly, and the cochlear division of the vestibulocochlear nerve is located caudally and posterior to the facial nerve.

The "transverse crest" divides the fundus of the internal auditory canal into an upper and a lower compartment. The upper compartment contains the facial nerve anteriorly and the superior part of the vestibular ganglion posteriorly. The lower compartment houses the cochlear division of the vestibulocochlear nerve anteriorly and the inferior part of the vestibular ganglion posteriorly. In the upper compartment of the fundus, the facial nerve is separated from the superior part of the vestibular ganglion by a vertical bony crest known as "Bill's bar." This bar is an important landmark for identifying the facial nerve, especially in the translabyrinthine approach to the internal auditory canal (see p. 258). It must be decided whether and what kind of measures need to be performed on the facial nerve, such as incision of the sheath. At the end of the operation we cover the internal auditory canal and any opened air cells with a dural graft. The graft may be attached with fibrin glue. To prevent constricting scars, Wigand applies a sheet of silicone film covered by a myoperiosteal graft attached with tissue adhesive.

The Transmastoid Translabyrinthine Approach

Introductory Remarks. Exploration of the traumatized lateral, middle, *and* posterior skull base from the caudal aspect is accomplished through a transmastoid approach. The indications for this approach in the presence of a cerebrospinal fluid leak were discussed previously. In cases where hearing has been lost, even fractures located far medially can be explored and treated from below through this approach, performing labyrinthectomy as required, and the facial nerve can be exposed as far as the cerebellopontine angle. If hearing is intact, this approach is contraindicated for exploration of the internal auditory canal or for exposing medially situated fractures, because it results in loss of hearing and peripheral balance dysfunction. A major advantage is the ability to expose the middle and posterior basal portions of the petrous pyramid concurrently. The translabyrinthine approach to the internal auditory canal was first described by the otologist Panse (1904), and in 1911 Quix was the first to attempt the removal of an acoustic neurinoma via this route. The method later fell into disfavor because of technical problems relating mainly to the lack of suitable optical magnification. It was not until 1966 that House and Hitselberger, using microsurgical technique, successfully reintroduced the approach into otoneurosurgical practice (Brackmann 1984).

Operative Technique
(Fig. MS 13a–e)

The mastoid plane and temporal squama are widely exposed through a postauricular skin incision, which may be S-shaped or C-shaped depending on the trauma to the cranial vault, and the fracture lines are sought along the middle and posterior skull base and posterior meatal wall through a wide mastoidectomy. The dura behind the fracture lines is exposed with the diamond burr and examined for injuries. Dural injuries, when present, must be completely exposed with a surrounding margin of intact dura. Necrotic portions of brain are removed. The defect is closed with autogenous or xenogenous material inserted between the bony skull base and dural margins. If labyrinthectomy is necessary to expose a fracture line that extends far medially, the mastoid portion of the bony fallopian canal is first identified below the lateral

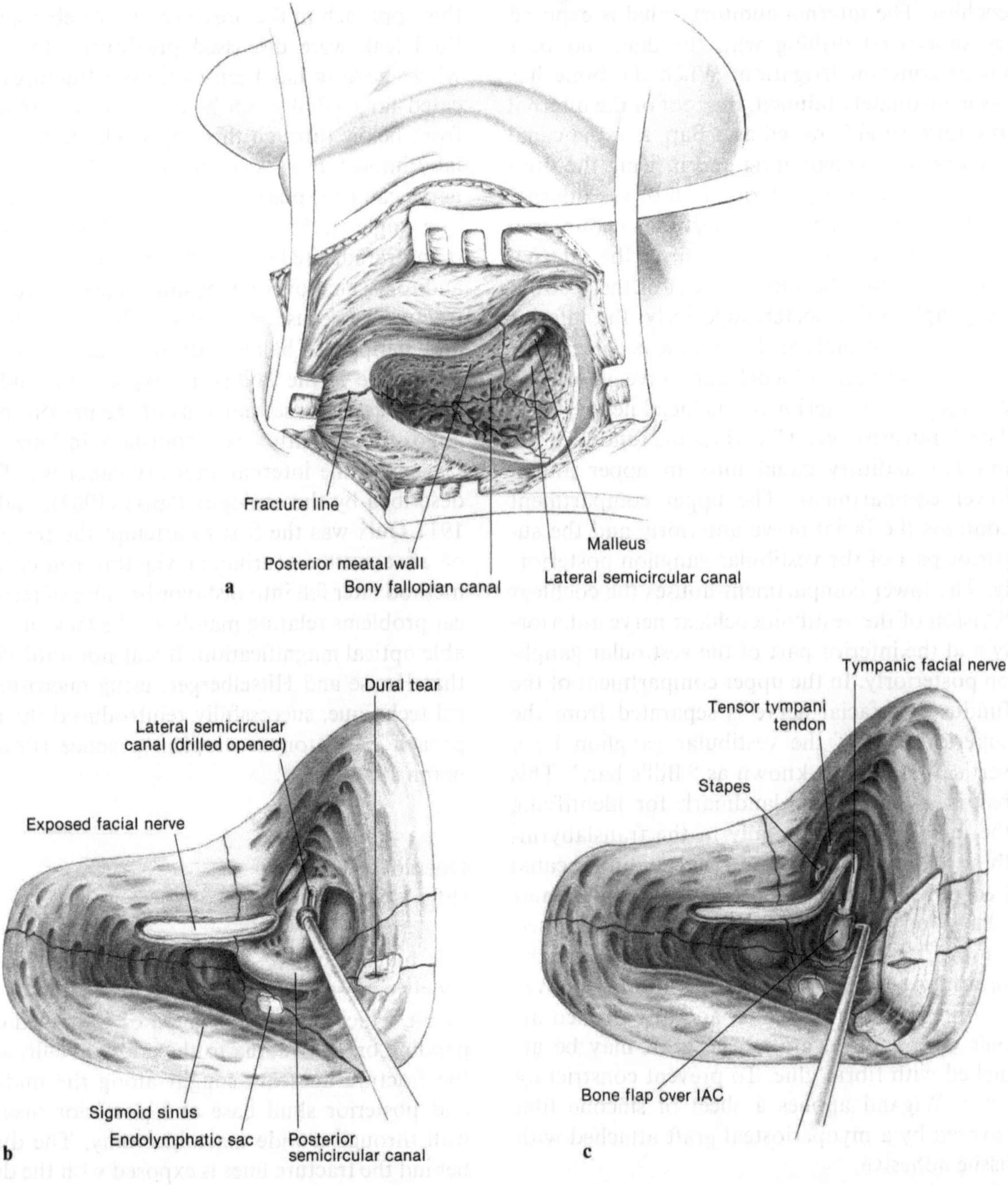

Fig. MS 13a–e. The transmastoid-translabyrinthine approach to the IAC, illustrated for a laterobasal fracture with exposure of the facial nerve.

a Mastoidectomy with preservation of the posterior meatal wall has been performed. The bony mastoidal fallopian canal, the lateral semicircular canal, the epitympanic recess with the body of the anvil, and the fracture lines are visible.

b The fracture lines are traced farther with exposure of the facial nerve. The labyrinthine system is opened and removed, and the dura of the posterior and middle fossae is exposed along with the endolymphatic sac.

c The facial nerve is exposed up to its entrance into the IAC. The ossicular chain is dismantled to expose its tympanic portion. A defect in the middle fossa dura is visible. A bone flap is outlined with the cutting burr in the posterior wall of the internal meatus.

d The IAC is entered, and the dural defect is covered with a dural graft. The horizontal bony ridge of Bill's bar is visible between the vestibular nerve and the emergence of the facial nerve from the IAC.

e The procedure is concluded by covering cranial bone defects with lyophilized dura and fibrin glue. The mastoid is obliterated with pieces of fat

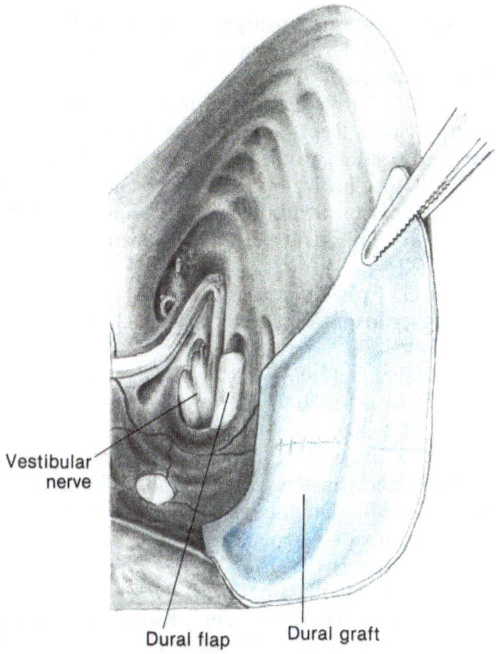

d

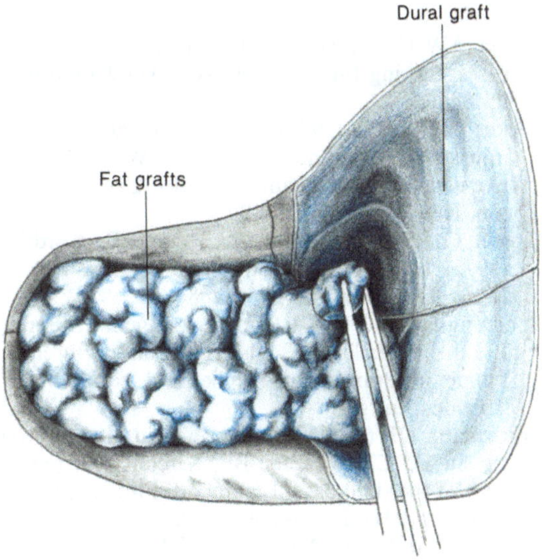

e

semicircular canal so that it will remain in view when the semicircular canal is removed. If the mastoid part of the fallopian canal is fractured, the nerve must be exposed at that site and its sheath incised. Next the retrolabyrinthine cells and posterior semicircular canal are removed along the posterior skull base, and the superior semicircular canal along the middle skull base. The subarcuate artery is generally encountered below the superior semicircular canal; it can be occluded with the diamond burr by stopping the irrigation briefly. The posterior wall of the internal auditory canal is identified and is marked cranial to the anterior and lateral ampullary nerve and caudal to the posterior ampullary nerve. Additional labyrinthine bone is removed to expose the posterior wall of the internal auditory canal as far as the posterior lip of the porus acusticus. Any small fracture fragments that are encountered are removed. In a patient with irreversible facial paralysis, the VII cranial nerve can be explored through this approach over its entire course including the cerebellopontine angle segment. We recommend removing the incus and the head of the malleus. The dura of the posterior cranial fossa must be widely exposed. Next the posterior wall of the internal auditory canal is thinned down until the blue luster of the canal is visible through the bone. A rectangular bone flap is outlined with the burr and is carefully elevated from the dura. Before opening the dura, the surgeon should identify Bill's bar at the junction of the fallopian canal and the fundus of the internal auditory canal to make sure that the facial nerve is localized. The dura of the internal auditory canal is then opened close to the floor to avoid hazard to the facial nerve. It should be noted that the labyrinthine artery and anterior inferior cerebellar artery may wind into the fundus of the internal meatus and are vulnerable during opening of the dura or section of the vestibular nerve.

If the central stump of the facial nerve cannot be located in the internal auditory canal, the dura of the posterior fossa is coagulated and incised between the sigmoid sinus and posterior lip of the porus, the cerebellopontine cistern is opened, cerebrospinal fluid is withdrawn, the cerebellum is protected with cotton paddies, and an attempt is made to locate the central portion of the facial nerve. After the ablative part of the surgery has been completed, the dural openings are covered with stored dura attached with adhesive, and the mastoid is obliterated with autogenous pieces of abdominal fat removed earlier. Finally the wound is closed in layers.

References

Adson AW (1942) Surgical treatment of vascular diseases altering functions of eyes. Am J Ophthalmol 25:824

Becker DP, Ward J (1982) Surgical management of head injuries. In: Schmideck HH, Sweet WH (eds) Operative neurosurgical techniques, vol 1. Grune and Stratton, New York, pp 175–190

Besson G, Guy G, Bedon G, Becume B, Kerdiles Y (1975) Les fistules carotido-caverneuses. Rev Oto-Neuro-Ophthalmol 47:259–268

Boenninghaus HG (1979) Ohrverletzungen. In: Berendes J, Link R, Zöllner F (eds) Hals-Nasen-Ohren Heilkunde in Praxis und Klinik, 2nd edn. Ohr I/20. Thieme, Stuttgart

Brackmann DE (1984) The translabyrinthine approach. In: Sasaki CT, McCabe BF, Kirchner JA (ed) Surgery of the skull base. Lippincott, Philadelphia

Brooks B (1931) Discussion: Noland L, Taylor AS: Trans South Surg Ass 43:176–177

Bushe KA (1973) Unabweisbare neurochirurgische Akutsituationen im allgemeinen Krankenhaus. Langenbecks Arch Chir 334, 336

Chowdhary UM (1978) Treatment of carotid-cavernous fistula using a ballon-tipped intra-arterial catheter. J Neurol Neurosurg Psychiatr 41:996–1000

Clerc PR, Batisse R (1954) Abord des organes intrapetreux par voie endo-cranienne (greffe du nerf facial). Ann Otolaryng 71:20–38

Cophignon J, Djindjian R, Rey A (1974) Treatment of carotid-cavernosus fistulae. Ann Radiol 17:275–277

Dandy WE (1935) The treatment of carotid cavernosus aneurysms. Ann Surg 102:916–920

Dandy WE (1937) Carotid cavernous aneurysms (pulsating exophthalmos) 2 bl Neurochir 2:77–206

Debrun G (1982) Treatment of certain intracerebral vascular lesions with balloon catheters. In: Schmideck HH, Sweet WH (ed): Operative neurosurgical techniques, vol 2. Grune & Stratton, New York, London, pp 789–811

Debrun G, Lacour P, Caron JP, Hurth M, Comoy J, Keravel Y (1975) Experimental approach of treatment of carotid-cavernosus sinus fistulaes with an inflatable and isolated balloon. Neuroradiology 9:9–12

Debrun G, Lacour P, Vinuela FV, Fox AJ, Drake Ch, Caron JP (1981) Treatment of 54 traumatic carotic cavernosus fistulaes. In: J Neurosurg 55:678–692

Dietrich U (1981) Karotis-Sinus Cavernosus Fisteln. Dissertation, University of Mainz

Djindjian R (1974) Superselective arteriographic embolization by the femoral route in neuroradiology. Neuroradiology 6:143–152

Echols DM, Jackson JD (1959) Carotid cavernosus fistula. A perplexing surgical problem. J Neurosurg 16:619–628

Escher F (1973) Das Schädelbasistrauma in otorhinologischer Sicht. HNO 21:129

Fisch U (1969) Oto-neurosurgical operation. In: Yasargil MG (ed) Microsurgery applied to neurosurgery. Thieme, Stuttgart

Fisch U (1970) Transtemporal surgery of the internal auditory canal. Report of 92 cases, technique, indications and results. Adv. Otorhinolaryngol 17:203

Fisch U (1976) Chirurgie am inneren Gehörgang und an benachbarten Strukturen. In: Naumann HH (ed) Kopf und Halschirurgie, vol 3. Thieme, Stuttgart, pp 457–543

Friedmann G, Frowein RA, Luster G (1970) Karotis-Sinus-cavernosus-Aneurysmen. Fortschr Neurol Psychiatr 38:57–79

Geyer G, Helms J (1983) Wertigkeit der Neurektomie bei cochleovestibulären Störungen. Laryngol Rhilon Otol 62:302–305

Gillingham FJ, Shaw JF, Fraser J, Hitchcock ER, Harris P (1971) Head Injuries. Livingstone, Edinburgh

Goldhahn G (1967) Diagnose und Therapie der Karotis-Sinus-cavernosus-Aneurysmen. Psychiatr Neurol Psychol (Leipzig) 19:218–229

Grunert V, Sunder-Plassmann M (1971) Beitrag zur chirurgischen Therapie der Karotis-Kavernosus Fisteln. Acta Neurochir 25:109–114

Guleke N (1950) Die Eingriffe am Gehirnschädel, Gehirn, an der Wirbelsäule und am Rückenmark. Springer, Berlin Göttingen Heidelberg, chaps 2, 3, 9, 10, 17

Hamby WB (1964) Carotid cavernous fistula. Report of 32 surgically treated cases and suggestions for definitive operation. J Neurosurg 21:859–867

Hamby WB (1966) Carotid-Cavernous Fistulae. Charles C Thomas, Springfield, Illinois

Hamby WB, Gardner WS (1933) Treatment of pulsating exophthalmos with report of 2 cases. Arch Surg (Chicago) 27:676–685

Harker LA, McCabe BF (1984) Middle cranial fossas approach to skull base surgery. In: Sasaki CT, McCabe BF, Kirchner JA (ed) Surgery of the Skull Base. Lippincott, Philadelphia

Helms J (1985) Die chirurgische Therapie des M. Meniere. Arch Otorhinolaryngol Suppl 1985/I p 68–118

Hermann HD, Fischer D, Loew F (1975) Experiences with intraluminal occlusion with the Fogarty catheter in the treatment of carotid-cavernous sinus fistulaes and other lesions at the base of the skull. Acta Neurochir 32:35–54

House WF (1961) Surgical exposure of the internal auditory canal and its contents through the middle cranial fossa. Laryngoscope 71:1363–1385

House WF, Hitselberger WE (1966) Surgical approaches to acoustic tumors. Arch otolaryngol 84/3:286–291

Isamat F, Salleras V, Miranda AM (1970) Artificial embolisation of carotid-cavernous fistula with postoperative potency of internal carotid artery. J Neurol Neurosurg Psychiat 33:674–678

Isfort A (1967) Probleme der chirurgischen Behandlung von Carotis-Cavernosus-Fisteln. Zbl Chir II:1519–1524

Jaeger R (1942) Intracranial aneurysms. South Surg 15:205–217

Kessel FK, Guttmann L, Maurer G (1969) Neuro-Traumatologie mit Einschluß der Grenzgebiete. Urban & Schwarzenberg, München
Kley W (1968) Die Unfallchirurgie der Schädelbasis und der pneumatischen Räume. Arch Ohr Nas Kehlk Heilk 191:1
Kley W (1976) Operationen bei Verletzungen der Ohrregion. In: Naumann HH (ed) Kopf- und Halschirurgie, vol 3: Ohrregion. Thieme, Stuttgart, p 259–294
Krayenbühl W (1967) Treatment of carotid-cavernous fistula consisting of a one-stage operation by muscle embolization of the fistulous segment. In: Donaghy and Yasargil (eds) Microvascular surgery. Thieme, Stuttgart
Krayenbühl H, Yasargil MG (1965) Die zerebrale Angiographie. Thieme, Stuttgart
Land ER, Bucy PL (1965) Treatment of carotid-cavernous fistula by muscle embolisation alone: The Brooks method. J Neurosurg 22:387–392
Lang J (1979) In: von Lanz T, Wachsmuth W (eds) Praktische Anatomie, vol 1, part 1. Springer, Berlin
Lang J, Schäfer K (1976) Über Ursprung und Versorgungsgebiete der intracavernösen Strecke der A. carotis interna. Gegenbauers Morphol Jahrb 122:182
Lanksch W, Grumme Th, Kazner E (1978) Schädelhirnverletzungen im Computertomogramm. Springer, Berlin
Larson SJ, Worman LW (1968) Internal carotid artery flow rate during craniotomy and muscle embolisation for carotid-cavernous fistula; report of four cases. J Neurosurg 29:60–64
McCormick WF, Kelly PJ, Sarwar M (1976) Fatal paradoxical muscle embolisation in traumatic carotid-cavernous fistula repair: case report. J Neurosurg 44:513–516
Metzel E (1973) Dringende diagnostische und therapeutische Maßnahmen bei Schädelhirnverletzungen. Z Allgemeinmed 49:271–276
Metzel E (1980) Pathologische Prozesse der Schädelbasis. Diagnostik und Therapie aus neurochirurgischer Sicht. In: Berendes J, Link R, Zöllner F (eds) Hals Nasen Ohren Heilkunde in Praxis und Klinik, 2nd edn, vol 6, Ohr II. Thieme, Stuttgart 36, p 1–42
Michailow SS (1964) Makro- und mikroskopische Untersuchungen des Baues des Sinus cavernosus. Anat Anz 115:233
Moniz I (1934) L'angiographie cerebrale. Paris, Masson
Moringlane JR, Samii M (1981) Beitrag zur Behandlung des chronischen subduralen Hämatoms und Hygroms des Erwachsenen. Neurochirurgie 24:158–162
Mullan JF (1982) Techniques of thrombosis of carotid cavernosus fistulae. In: Schmideck HH, Sweet WH (ed) Operative neurosurgical techniques Vol 2, p 813–818, Grune and Stratton, New York
Mullan S (1974) Experiences with surgical thromboses of intracranial berry aneurysms and carotic cavernous fistulas. Neurosurg 41:657–670
Nau HE, Bork WJ, Brkic J (1977) Klinische und elektroencephalographische Befunde bei Carotis-Sinus-Cavernosus Fisteln. 32 EEG-EMG 8:65–69
Noordenbos W (1968) Traumatic carotis-cavernous fistula. Psychiatr Neurol Neurochir 71:93–98, Amsterdam
Obrador S, Gomez-Bueno J, Silvela J (1974) Spontaneous carotid-cavernous fistula produced by ruptured aneurysm of the meningohypophyseal branch of the internal carotid artery: case report. J Neurosurg 40:539–543
Ohta T, Nishimura S, Kikuchi H (1973) Closure of carotid-cavernous fistula by polyurethone foam embolus (technical note) J Neurosurg 40:539–543
Panse R (1904) Ein Gliom des Akustikus. Arch Ohrenheilk 61:251
Parkinson D (1965) A surgical approach to the cavernous portion of the carotic artery. J Neurosurg 23:477–483
Parkinson D (1967) Transcavernous repair of carotid cavernous fistula: case report. J Neurosurg 26:420–424
Parkinson D (1982) Surgical management of internal carotid artery aneurysms within the cavernous sinus. In: Schmideck HH, Sweet WH (ed) Operative neurosurgical techniques Vol 2, Grune & Stratton, New York London, p 819–828
Parkinson D, Downs AR, Whytehead LL (1974) Carotid cavernous fistula: direct repair with preservation of carotid. Surgery 76:882–889
Pieritz UR, Schmidseder A (1981) Central dislocation of the Jaw-joint into the middle cranial fossa. Case report. J Max Fac Surg 9:61–63
Pool JL, Poots DG (1965) Aneurysms and arteriovenous anomalies of the brain: diagnosis and treatment. Harper and Row, New York
Portmann M, Sterkess JM, Charachon R, Chouard CH (1975) The internal auditory meatus. Anatomy, pathology and surgery. Churchill Livingstone, Edinburgh
Prolo DJ, Hanbery JW (1971) Intraluminal occlusion of a carotid cavernous sinus fistula with a balloon catheter: Technical note. J Neurosurg 35:237–242
Quix F (1911) Ein Akustikustumor. Arch Ohrenheilk 84:252
Reulen HJ, Faupel G (1980) Behandlung des traumatischen Hirnödems mit hochdosiertem Dexamethason. In: Wieck HH (ed) Neurotraumatologie. Thieme, Stuttgart, pp 185–192
Rey A, Cophignon J, Thurel C, Thiehaut JB (1975) Treatment of Traumatic Cavernous Fistulae. In: Krayenbühl H (ed) Advances and technical standards in neurosurgery. Springer, New York
Rougerie J, Guilmet D, Bamberger-Bopo C (1973) Anevrysme carotid-caverneux. A propos d'une orientation therapeutique nouvelle. Neurochirurgie 19:649–654
Rupp N, Piger A, Ultsch B (1975) Karotis-Cavernosus-Fistel: Behandlung mit einem Ballon-Katheter. Fortschr Geb Röntgenstr Nuklearmed 122:215–217
Samii M (1972) Autologe Nerventransplantation im Trigeminusbereich. Med Mittlg (Melsungen) 46:189
Samii M, Brihaye J (1983) Traumatology of the Skullbase. Springer, Berlin Heidelberg New York Tokio

Sedzimir CB, Occleshaw J (1967) Experience with 2 cases of muscle embolisation of carotid-cavernous fistula. J Neurol Neurosurg Psychiatr 30:586

Serbinenko FA (1971) Balloon occlusion of cavernous portion of the carotid artery as a method of treating carotid-cavernous fistulae. In: Vopr Neirokhir 6:3–9

Serbinenko FA (1972) Reconstruction of cavernous part of carotid artery in case of carotid-cavernous fistulae. In: Vopr Neirokhir 36:3–9

Serbinenko FA (1974) Balloon catheterization on occlusion of major cerebral vessels. In: J Neurosurg 41:125–145

Stern WE, Brown WD, Alksne JF (1967) The surgical challenge of carotid cavernous fistula: the critical role of intracranial circulatory dynamics. J Neurosurg 27:298–308

Unterberger S (1959) Neuzeitliche Behandlung von Schädelverletzungen mit Beteiligung der fronto- und laterobasalen pneumatischen Räume. Laryng Rhinol 38:441

Wigand ME (1979) Transtemporal extradural surgery of the internal auditory canal. In: Samii M, Draf W (Org) Course on surgery of the Skullbase, Hannover

Wullstein HL (1951) Die extratympanale endocranielle Fensterung bei chirurgischer Otitis media and Labyr. Z Laryng Rhinol 30:203–216

Wullstein HL (1972) Hat Terminologie zur Definition unseres Faches eine praktische Bedeutung? HNO (Berl) 20:259–261

Surgery of Inflammatory Disorders of the Middle Skull Base

Introductory Remarks. The close proximity of the external, middle, and inner ear and associated air spaces to the adjacent temporal portion of the cranial cavity creates conditions favorable for the extension of inflammatory processes of this region into the middle and posterior cranial fossae. These complications of inflammatory diseases of the external and especially the middle ear can invade the cranial cavity directly through the middle and posterior skull base as well as through the complex soft and hard structures of the petrous pyramid. Sinus thrombosis, labyrinthitis, suppuration of the petrous apex, epidural and subdural abscess formation with empyema, brain abscess, and otogenic meningitis and encephalitis have become rare complications of acute or chronic otitis media since the advent of antibiotics. But for that very reason, they present a special diagnostic and therapeutic challenge (see recent literature in Alford 1973, Beck 1979, Bluestone and Klein 1983, Ganz 1979, Kornmesser 1979, Kressner 1979, Paparella and Capps 1973).

Cholesteatoma continues to be a major factor in the development of intracranial inflammatory complications. The "true" cholesteatoma of embryologic origin is a benign mass that can attain considerable size in the petrous bone and cerebellopontine angle region before symptoms such as hearing loss, vestibular nerve deficit, facial paralysis, or tinnitus cause the patient to seek medical attention. This entity differs from "false" cholesteatoma, which is a primary or secondary lesion occurring in association with chronic otitis media. "Primary cholesteatoma" develops from an epitympanic invagination of the initially intact tympanic membrane, whereas "secondary cholesteatoma" results from the entry of squamous epithelium into the middle ear cavity through a perforated tympanic membrane. The false cholesteatomas of the otosurgeon can also result from the traumatic introduction of meatal epithelium into the middle ear. Through expansive growth and pressure atrophy, these false cholesteatomas can erode through the bony skull base, invade the internal auditory canal through the labyrinth, and grow from there (or directly) into the cerebellopontine angle. These possibilities should be considered when evaluating the extent of cholesteatomas on axial and coronal tomograms and CT scans, especially if previous operations have been performed on the ear for cholesteatoma removal. The pioneers of modern ablative and reconstructive microsurgery of the middle ear (Heermann and Heermann 1964; Kley 1957 a, b, 1976; Plester 1959, 1961; Plester and Zöllner 1979; Shambaugh 1967; Wullstein 1952a, b, 1968; Zöllner 1954, 1955, 1957) formulated these goals for the treatment of cholesteatoma:

1) Complete removal with maximum preservation of function.
2) Reconstruction of the tympanic membrane-ossicular chain.

The primary emphasis is placed on excision of the pathological process. Very extensive cholesteatomas that have grown into the internal auditory canal and cerebellopontine angle causing damage to the facial nerve in that area may require surgery on the internal auditory canal through the transmastoid-translabyrinthine approach with exploration of the cerebellopontine angle (pp. 257–259), or the transtemporal extradural approach (pp. 252–257), or a combination of both. The techniques of facial nerve dissection and reconstruction developed for the surgery of trauma and acoustic neurinoma (see p. 392) can be applied with great advantage to the skull base surgery of inflammatory ear diseases. For epidermoids of the petrous bone and cerebellopontine angle and in other special cases, cooperation between otosurgeons and neurosurgeons can contribute greatly to a successful diagnosis and operative treatment. This is discussed further in connection with the surgery of tumors of the posterior skull base and cerebellopontine angle.

Principles of Cholesteatoma Removal
(Fig. MS 14a–c)

The middle ear cavity is exposed through the auditory canal or through a postauricular approach, the posterior meatal wall is partially or completely removed, and the cholesteatoma sac is dissected free. Some authors reconstruct the posterior meatal wall with autogenous material or with a plastic implant. The cholesteatoma wall (matrix) must be progressively dissected from underlying tissues in its entirety. If the matrix involves the bones, the bone must be ablated with the diamond burr to destroy any residual epithelial cells that might lead to a recurrence.

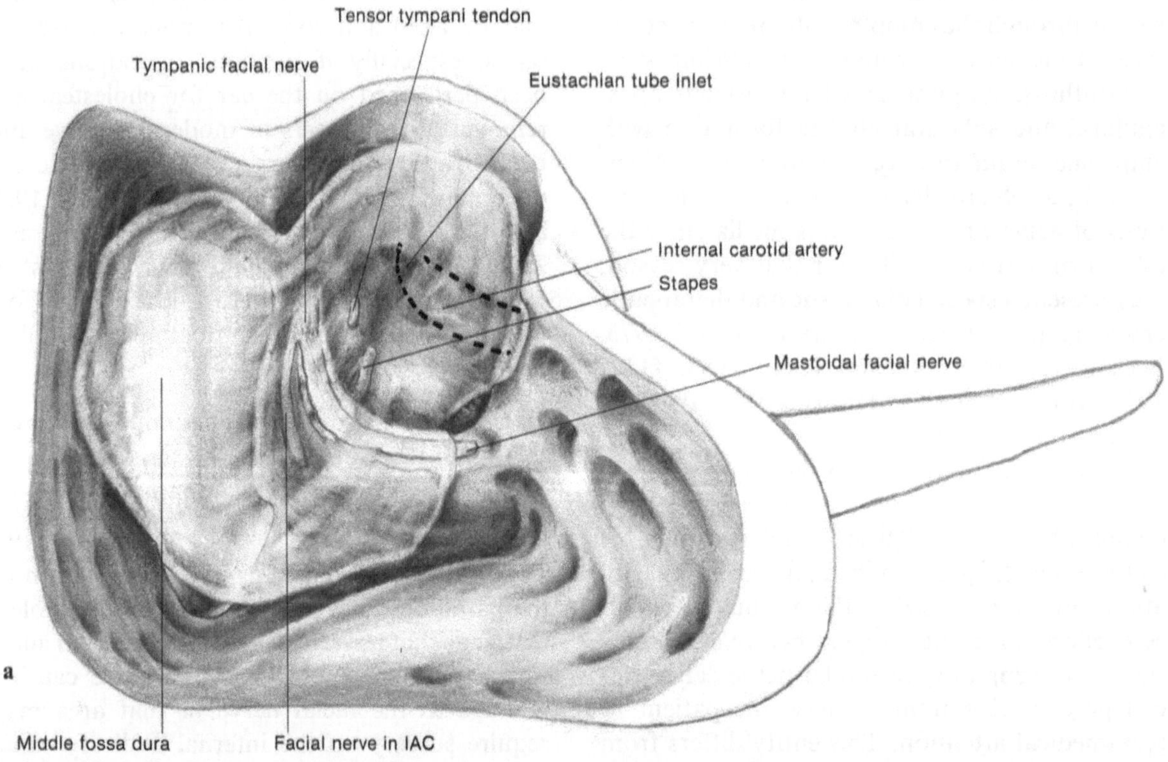

Fig. MS 14a–c. Principle of cholesteatoma removal, illustrated for an extensive cholesteatoma with destruction of the roof of the IAC and bony carotid canal in the transverse portion of the internal carotid artery.
a Removal of the posterior meatal wall exposes the cholesteatomatous lining of the mastoid and tympanic cavity. Destruction of the ossicular chain, bony fallopian canal, and middle skull base is apparent. Cholesteatoma has overgrown the inlet to the eustachian tube. The posterior meatal wall was removed. The internal carotid artery is indicated by a *dashed line*, and a "transparent" view is given of the cholesteatoma.
b Further exposure reveals that the cholesteatoma has grown anterolaterally over the roof of the IAC and has invaded the labyrinth.
c The bony internal carotid canal is seen following removal of the eustachian tube orifice

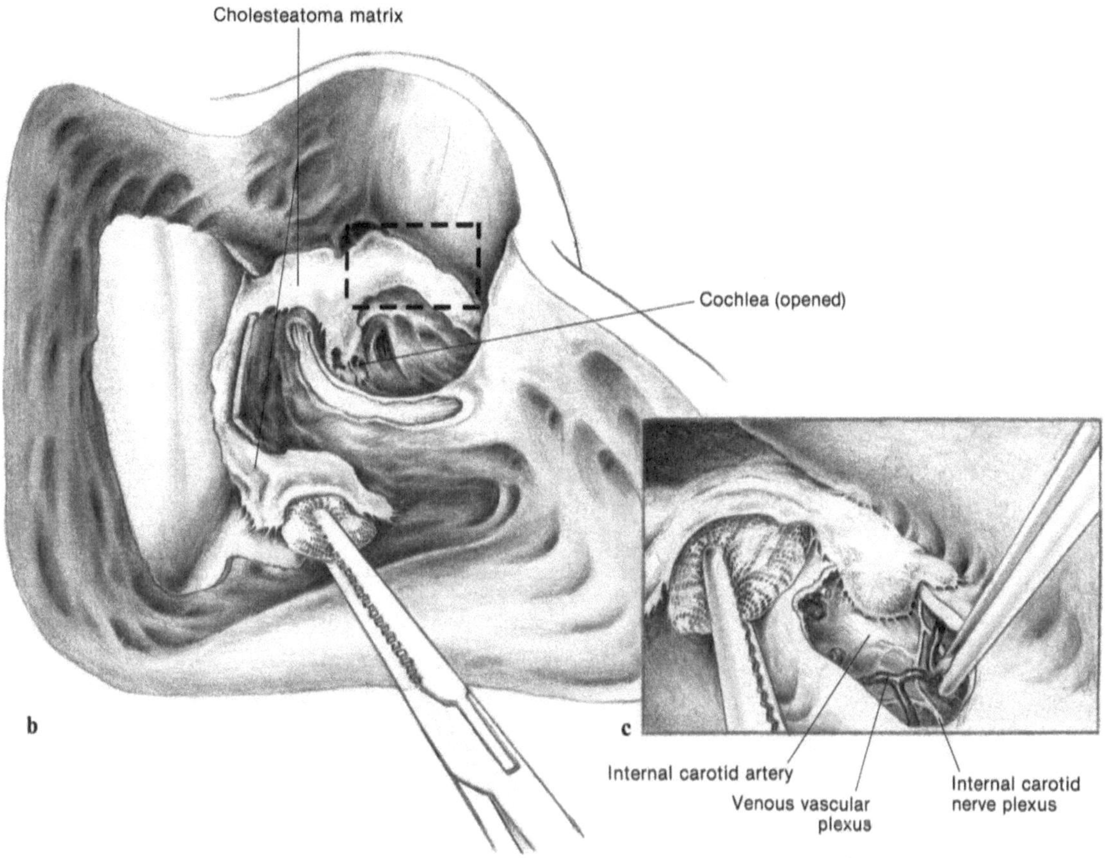

If the cholesteatoma is adherent to soft structures such as nerves (e.g., the facial nerve) or blood vessels, it is separated from those structures microsurgically using sickle knives, straight or angled dissectors, and careful traction. We advise against removing the matrix from different sites in small pieces, as this virtually guarantees that epithelial remains will be left in hidden corners of the labyrinth or at the upper or lower margins of the petrous bone. Once the dura is exposed, it must be determined whether matrix has grown epidurally between the dural surface and bony skull base or has invaded the labyrinth. It is imperative that these epithelial extensions be removed completely with a portion of the skull base or by performing a labyrinthectomy. This is necessary to prevent intracranial recurrences, which are difficult to diagnose and fraught with complications. Details on operative strategy in the middle ear and mastoid region may be found in the specialized literature.

Surgical Treatment of Otogenic Jugular Vein-Sigmoid Sinus-Transverse Sinus Thrombosis

Introductory Remarks. The basic principles of the surgical treatment of these otogenic, intracranial complications as stated by Grunert (1894) and Voss (1904) are still valid today. Grunert's operation on the jugular bulb forms an important basis of modern skull base surgery. We are indebted to Denecke (1953), Fleischer (1976), and Theissing and Theissing (1975) for their excellent illustrations on the surgery of sigmoid sinus complications. The development of antibiotics has brought changes in the frequency and indications for operative intervention. If a perisinus abscess is found during the course of an ablative procedure in a patient who does not show clinical signs of septic thrombosis, it is appropriate to expose the sigmoid sinus and use needle aspiration to confirm or exclude a thrombosis.

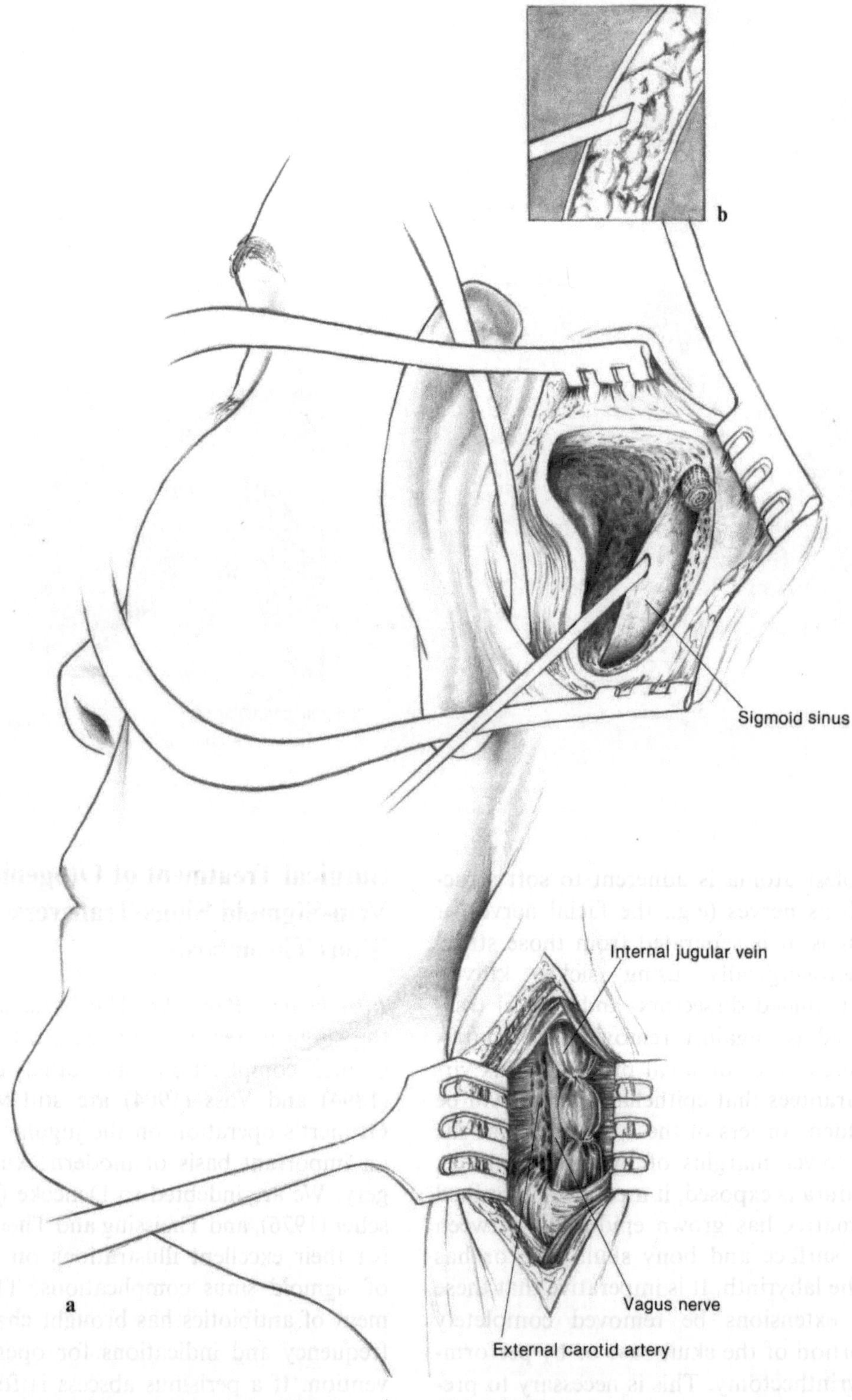

Fig. MS 15a–d. The surgical treatment of otogenic jugular vein-sigmoid sinus-transverse sinus thrombosis.
a The sigmoid sinus is exposed superiorly to its junction with the transverse sinus and inferiorly to the jugular bulb. The sinus is aspirated with a flat-bevel needle to check for thrombosis. If thrombosis is confirmed, an absorbable cellulose gauze roll is packed up into the sinus to create a tamponade. At the neck, the vascular package is exposed just above the carotid bifurcation, and the internal jugular vein is doubly ligated after isolating the vagus nerve.
b Cross-sectional view of the aspirating needle in the sigmoid sinus

In the absence of septic signs it is appropriate to keep the patient under clinical observation, even when thrombosis exists. If sepsis is apparent, treatment consists of cervical ligation of the internal jugular vein and occlusion of the sigmoid or transverse sinus at the intracranial end of the thrombosis before incising the venous sinus and removing the thrombus.

Operative Technique
(Fig. MS 15a–d)

When there is clinical suspicion of sinus thrombosis, the sigmoid sinus is exposed cephalically to its junction with the transverse sinus and caudally to the jugular bulb (Fig. MS 9a). The sinus is aspirated with a relatively flat-beveled needle of medium caliber, avoiding injury to the medial sinus wall (Fig. MS 9b). Failure to obtain blood with several trial aspirations confirms that thrombosis exists. The exposure may have to be continued as far proximally as the sinus confluence. The sinus will tend to appear bluish in its nonthrombosed portion, while it

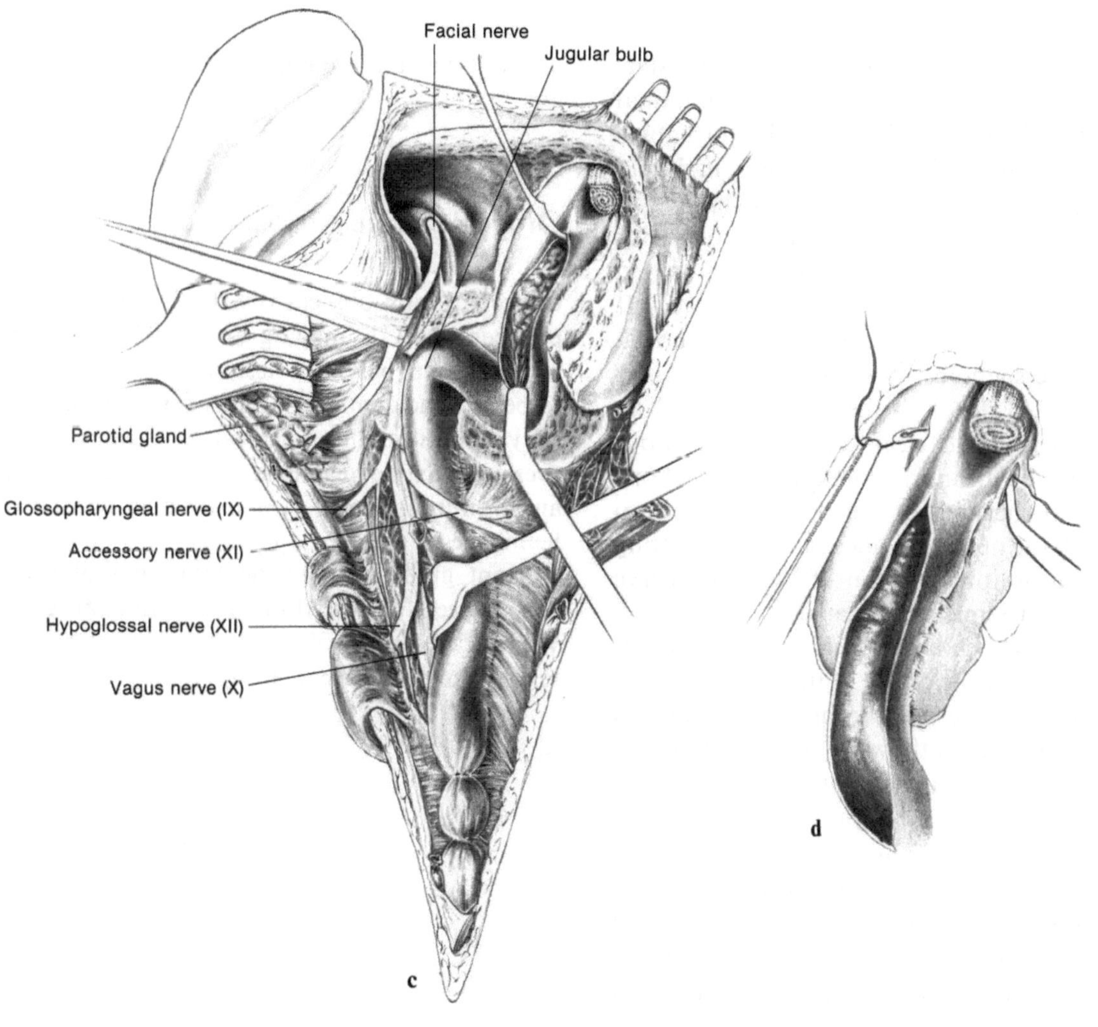

c

d

Fig. MS 15c, d.
c With extensive thrombosis the internal jugular vein, jugular bulb, and sigmoid sinus are exposed, preserving the cranial nerves emerging from the jugular foramen, the vessel is opened, and the thrombosis is evacuated.
d If packing is not sufficient, it is necessary to ligate the sigmoid sinus after bilateral incision of the dura

will appear yellowish and indurated about the thrombosis. To aid orientation, the surgeon can recall that the course of the transverse sinus is roughly on a line between the meatal roof and the external occipital protuberance. Small gauze rolls are prepared in advance, before the sigmoid sinus is incised, so that the sinus can be tamponaded quickly (Draf 1976). We have had excellent results with cellulose gauze, which is absorbable and may be left in place. After incision of the sinus, the thrombus is progressively removed proximally until bleeding is elicited. This is controlled by compression with the prepared gauze rolls. The distal portion of the clot is evacuated in the same way. If it appears that the thrombus extends past the jugular bulb, the jugular vein should be isolated through a skin incision along the anterior border of the sternocleidomastoid muscle before attempting final removal of the proximal part of the thrombus. During dissection of the jugular vein, it should be noted that the accessory nerve often crosses the vein directly at the level of the posterior belly of the digastric muscle. The vein is snared with a tape so that it can be easily ligated. If the thrombus cannot be completely removed through the sigmoid sinus, the internal jugular vein is ligated distal to the thrombus, and an attempt is made to clear the septic thrombus from below by means of irrigation. During bone removal in the area of the bulb, it is best to work with the operating microscope and cutting burr to ensure preservation of the facial nerve and posterior semicircular canal.

Occasionally it can be difficult to control bleeding from the upper portion of the sinus by external tamponade. It then becomes necessary to occlude the sinus outflow by suture ligation or by applying metal clips. In both cases it is necessary to make a small dural incision on both sides of the sinus. For ligation, two threads on a Dechamps needle are wound around the sinus and tightened, avoiding injury to underlying brain and vascular structures. This procedure may tear a thin sinus wall, requiring additional ligating sutures for repair.

In sinus occlusion with metal clips, the dural incision should be sufficient to permit visual inspection of the medial sinus surface, as it is common for "bridging veins" to communicate with that aspect of the sinus. These venous openings are electrocoagulated if possible before clips are applied. If bleeding from the intracranial cavity is noted after the sinus has been clipped, the sinus must be divided after placing a second metal clip, and the cerebral cortex is carefully explored to exclude a subdural hemorrhage. Because the metal clips produce artifacts that interfere with postoperative CT imaging, preference should be given to suture ligation whenever possible. At the end of the sinus procedure, the dural incisions are closed with simple interrupted sutures. With a thrombus that extends almost to the sinus confluence, the dissection must be done with extreme care to avoid endangering the critically important cerebral venous outflow through the contralateral transverse sinus.

Otogenic Brain Abscess

Otogenic brain abscess is entirely accessible to preoperative CT imaging and MRI, and there is no reason why this lesion should continue to be an "incidental" finding at operation. *Early symptoms* relating to elevation of intracranial pressure include headache, somnolence, nausea, and vomiting. *Local symptoms* may consist of hemiparesis, aphasia, and visual field defects.

Current guidelines for the treatment of brain abscess were discussed previously in connection with the treatment of brain abscesses of the anterior skull base (see p. 155).

Surgical Treatment of Skull Base Osteomyelitis Associated with Necrotizing Otitis Externa

(Fig. MS 16a–d)

Until about 10 years ago (Draf and Scheifele 1974, Krumpholz 1979, Manolidis et al. 1973, Neveling et al. 1962, Ungerecht 1974), progressive necrotizing otitis externa (Cohn 1974) was virtually unknown in the German otorhinolaryngologic literature. The otologist Chandler (1968) published a comprehensive report on this rare disease, calling it "malignant otitis externa" because of its high mortality. In advanced cases and even in some relatively early cases, it is wise to seek neurologic diagnostic consultation in instances where involvement of the neural foramina in the skull base has caused cranial neuropathies to supervene on the local process in the ear or to develop after the otologic process has resolved (Dinapoli and Thomas 1971, Draf and Regli 1975, Schwarz et al. 1971). A triad of symptoms is characteristic of progressive necrotizing otitis externa: a granulating destructive process in the auditory canal, severe pain, and a yellowish-green ear discharge from which *Pseudomonas* can be cultured. Generally a lowered systemic resistance to infection (diabetes mellitus, advanced age) in an individual infected with *Pseudomonas aeroginosa* is responsible for causing a circumscribed otitis externa to take a fulminating course. The neurologic symptoms can include isolated facial paralysis, multiple cranial neuropathies, cervical root lesions, and meningoencephalitis. The diagnosis is established by clinical findings, tomograms of the petrous bone, high-resolution CT scans,

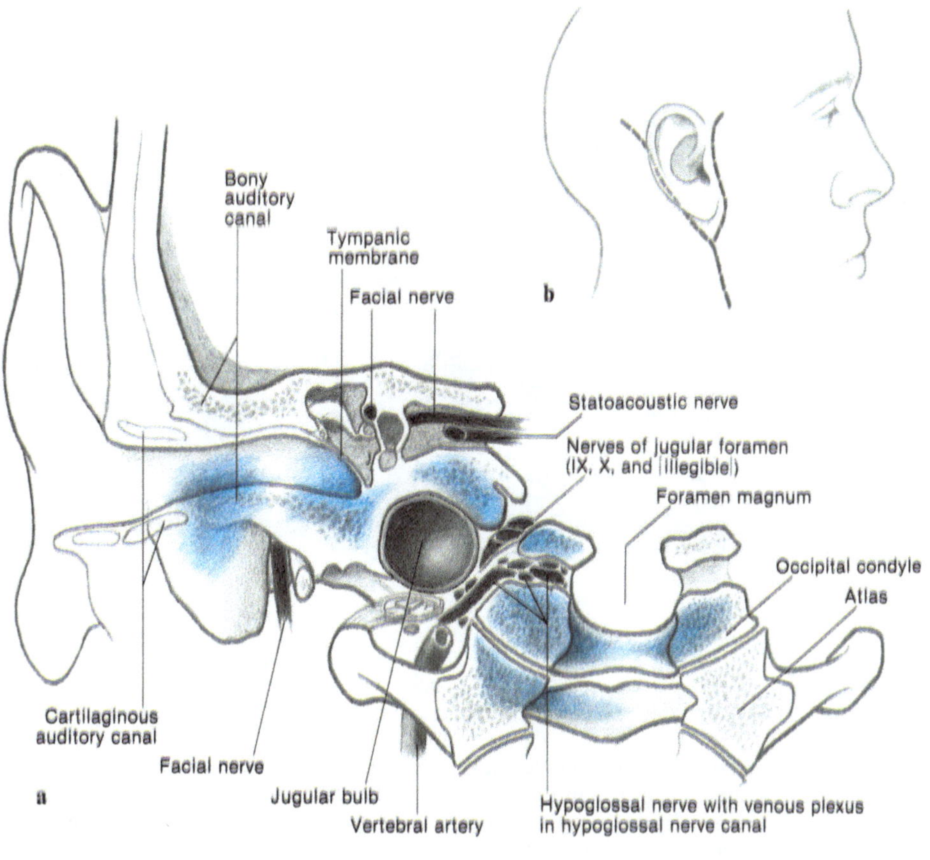

Fig. MS 16a–d. The surgical treatment of necrotizing otitis externa.
a Possible pathways for extension of skull base osteomyelitis.
b Y-shaped incision for exposure of the lateral middle skull base

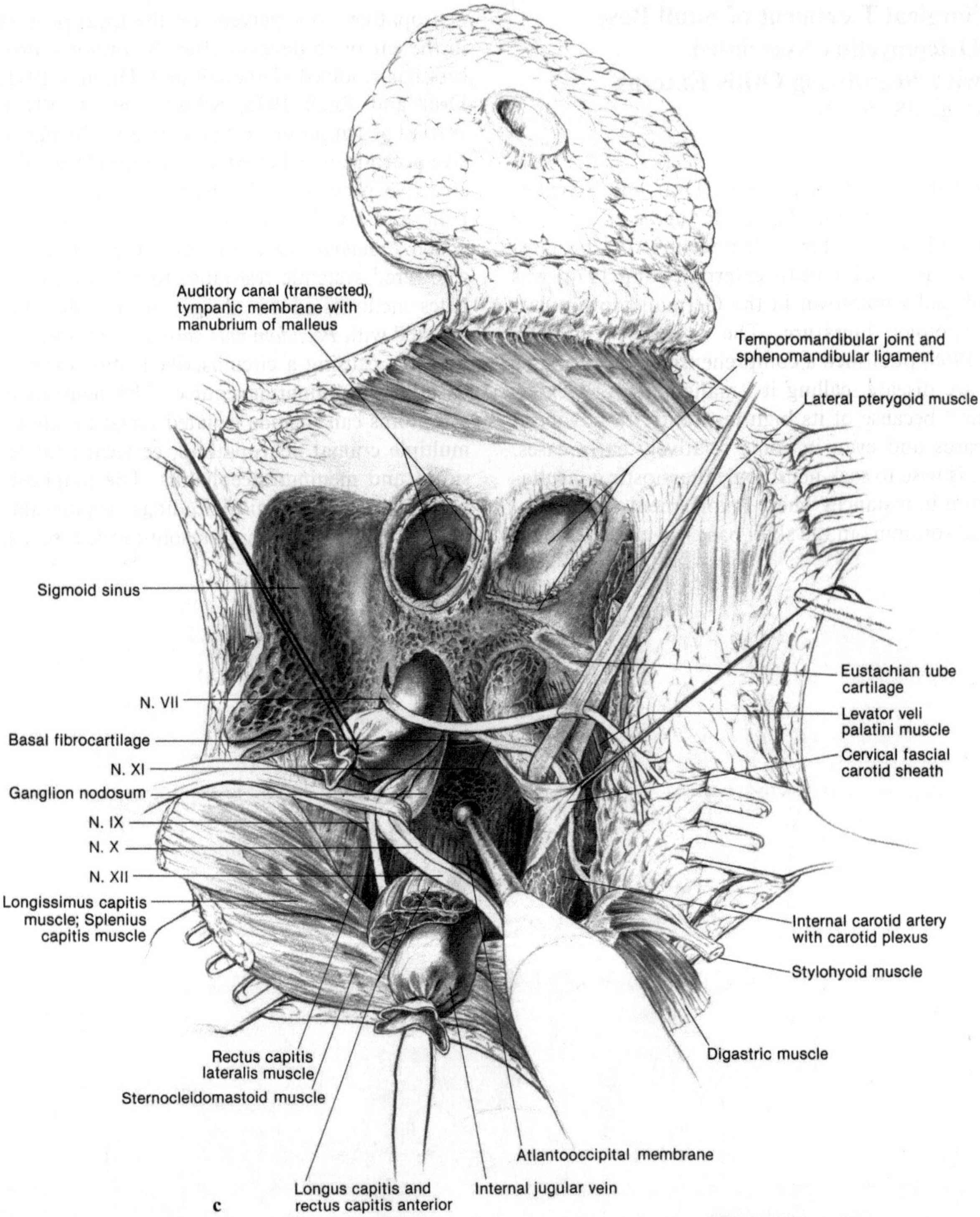

Fig. MS 16. c The facial nerve and cranial nerves transversing the jugular foramen are identified and retracted, and the internal jugular vein is ligated. Parotidectomy also may be required. Starting from the auditory canal, the pathological bone is progressively drilled away. The start of the transverse portion of the internal carotid artery is visible after removal of the mandibular condyle. It may be necessary to continue the bone removal as far as the clivus

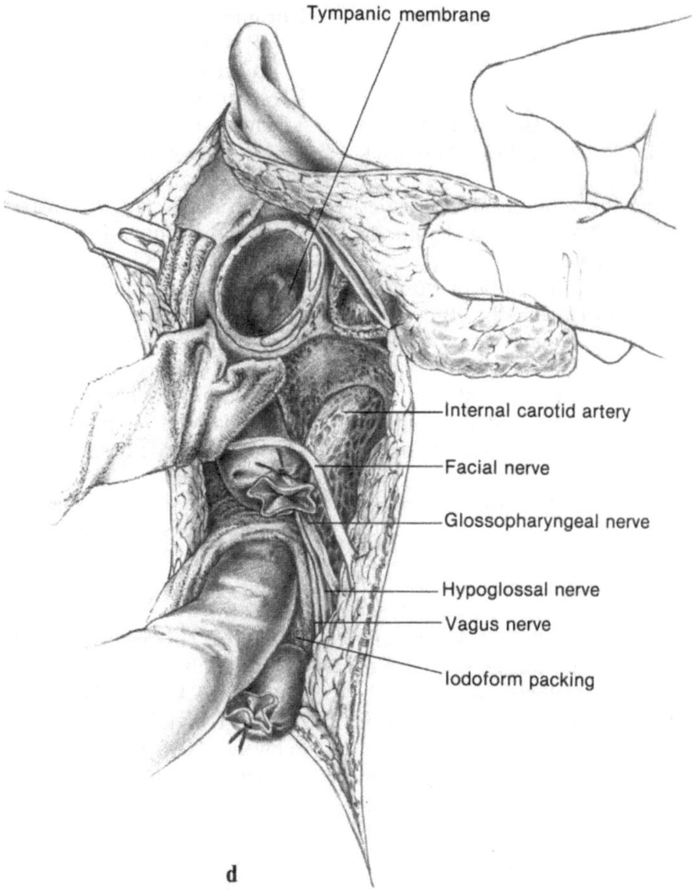

Fig. MS 16. d At the end of the procedure the surgical cavities are packed with iodoform strips, several holding sutures are placed in the upper part of the incision, and the cavity is treated in open fashion

and especially by cranial isotope scans. The latter can provide diagnostic clues before destructive changes become visible on X-rays and can make it easier to monitor treatment response.

When diagnosed early, the disease can be controlled with large doses of a broad-spectrum antibiotic that is absorbed by bone. In doubtful cases, however, there is no alternative to early surgical exposure and removal of all bone showing inflammatory changes. Parotidectomy may be necessary if the process has penetrated the anterior wall of the auditory canal. If the pars nervosa of the jugular foramen is involved, the incision should be extended along the anterior border of the sternocleidomastoid muscle to expose the internal jugular vein, external and internal carotid arteries, and cranial nerves IX, X, XI and XII from below. After resection of the mastoid process, the sigmoid sinus and internal jugular vein can be ligated if necessary and, after the facial nerve is identified, portions of the bony skull base involved by osteitis can be removed as far as the rim of the foramen magnum (Fig. MS 10b, c).

After bone removal is completed, the surgical cavity is packed with iodoform strips and left open for secondary healing (Ungerecht 1974). In severe cases we recommend maintaining high-dosage antibiotic therapy for several months, using isotope scans to evaluate response. The osteomyelitic process in the skull base can spread across the midline to the opposite side or may lead to an abscess with destruction of the cervical vertebrae (Draf and Regli 1975; further references in Krumpholz 1979).

References

Alford BR (1973) Complications of suppurative otitis media and mastoditis. In: Paparella MM, Shumrick DA Otolaryngology Vol 2, p 153–160

Beck Ch (1979) Otogene Sinusthrombosen. In: Berendes JR, Link W, Zöllner F, Hals Nasen Ohren Heilkunde in Praxis und Klinik, Bd V. Thieme, Stuttgart

Bluestone ChD, Klein JO (1983) Intratemporal complications and sequelae of otitis media. In: Bluestone ChC, Stool SE (ed) Pediatric Otolaryngology Vol 1. Saunders, p 513–564

Bluestone ChD, Klein JO (1983) Intracranial suppurative complications of Otitis media and mastoiditis. In: Bluestone ChD, Stool SE (ed) Pediatric Otolaryngology Vol 1, p 565–576

Chandler JR (1968) Malignant external otitis. Laryngoscope 78:1257

Cohn AM (1974) Progressive necrotizing otitis. Malignant external otitis. Arch otolaryng 99:136–139

Denecke HJ (1953) Die otorhinolaryngologischen Operationen. In: Gulecke N, Zenker R (ed) Allgemeine und spezielle chirurgische Operationslehre 2nd Ed. Springer, Berlin Göttingen Heidelberg, Vol 5

Dinapoli RP, Thomas JR (1971) Neurologic aspects of malignant external otitis. Mayo clin Proc 46:339–344

Draf W (1976) Personal communication quoted from Kley W. Operationen bei Verletzungen der Ohrregion. In: Naumann HH (Hrsg) Kopf- und Halschirurgie. Vol 3 Ohrregion. Thieme, Stuttgart, p 278

Draf W, Regli F (1975) Zur Differentialdiagnose von Hirnnervenausfällen: Die progressive, nekrotisierende Otitis externa. J Neurol 210:2119–2226

Draf W, Scheifele J (1974) Die nekrotisierende Otitis externa. Ein Beitrag zur Klinik und Therapie. HNO (Berl) 22:365–367

Fleischer K (1976) Chirurgische Behandlung der otogenen endokraniellen Komplikationen. In: Naumann HH (Hrsg) Kopf- und Halschirurgie. Vol 3. Ohrregion. Thieme, Stuttgart, p 295–319

Ganz H (1979) Otogener Hirnabszeß. In: Berendes JR, Link W, Zöllner F Hals Nasen Ohren Heilkunde in Praxis und Klinik BD VI. Thieme, Stuttgart, p 39

Grunert KA (1894) Die operative Ausräumung des Bulbus venae jugularis (Bulbusoperation) Arch Ohrenheilk 36:71

Heermann H, Heermann J (1964) Endaurale Chirurgie. Urban & Schwarzenberg, München Berlin

Kley W (1957a) Probleme der Tympanoplastik. 4. Mitt.: Die Resorption der Schrammtamponade im Tierversuch. Z Laryng Rhinol 36:277

Kley W (1957b) Über die Nachbehandlung nach hörverbessernden Operationen. Z Laryng Rhinol 36:495

Kley W (1976) Operationen bei Verletzungen der Ohrregion. In: Naumann HH Kopf und Halschirurgie Bd III. Thieme, Stuttgart, 259–294

Kley W (1976) Operative Behandlung der chronischen Otitis media und ihrer unmittelbaren Folgezustände. In: Naumann HH Kopf und Halschirurgie Bd III, Thieme, Stuttgart: 171–258

Kornmesser HJ (1979) Otogene Meningitis. In: Berendes JR, Link W, Zöllner F, Hals Nasen Ohren Heilkunde in Praxis und Klinik. Bd VI. Thieme, Stuttgart: 28

Kressner A (1979) Tympanogene Labyrinthitis. In: Berendes JR, Link W, Zöllner F, Hals Nasen Ohren Heilkunde in Praxis und Klinik Bd VI, Thieme, Stuttgart:29

Krumpholz K (1979) Unspezifische Entzündungen des äußeren Ohres. In: Hals Nasen Ohren Heilkunde in Praxis und Klinik. Bd V. Thieme, Stuttgart:23

Manolidis L, Daniilidis J, Kouloulas A (1973) Bösartige Otitis externa. Z Laryng Rhinol 52:788–792

Neveling R, Nysten H (1962) Die chronische nektrosierende Gehörgangsentzündung und ihre operative Behandlung. Laryngol Rhinol Otol 41:216–224

Paparella MM, Capps MJ (1973) Labyrinthitis. In: Paparella MM, Shumrick DA. Otolaryngology Vol 2, p 338–356

Plester D (1959) Die Gehörverbesserung durch Tympanoplastik bei verschlossener Tube. HNO (Berl) 7:277

Plester D (1961) Problems of Tympanoplasty. J Laryng 75:879

Plester D, Zöllner F (1979) Behandlung der chronischen Mittelohrentzündungen. In: Berendes JR, Link W, Zöllner F Hals Nasen Ohren Heilkunde in Praxis und Klinik Bd VI Thieme, Stuttgart:28

Schwarz GA, Blumenkrantz MJ, Sundmaker WLH (1971) Neurologic Complications of malignant external otitis. Neurology (Minneap) 21:1077–1084

Shambaugh GE (1967) Surgery of the ear. Su Ed Saunders

Theissing G, Theissing J (1975) Kurze HNO-Operationslehre für Ärzte und Studierende. Bd 2 Eingriffe am Ohr. Thieme, Stuttgart

Ungerecht K (1974) Progrediente Otitis externa des Diabetikers durch Pyocyaneusinfektion. Arch Oto Rhino Laryng 207:537–539

Voss O (1904) Zur operativen Freilegung des Bulbus venae jugularis. Z Ohrenheilk 48:265

Wullstein HL (1952a) Funktionelle Operationen im Mittelohr mit Hilfe des freien Spaltlappen-Transplantates. Arch Ohr Kehlk Heilk 161:422

Wullstein HL (1952b) Die Eingriffe zur Gehörverbesserung. In: Uffenorde W Anzeige und Ausführung der Eingriffe an Ohr, Nase und Hals. 2. Aufl Thieme, Stuttgart

Wullstein HL (1968) Operationen zur Verbesserung des Gehörs. Grundlagen und Methoden. Thieme, Stuttgart

Zöllner F (1954) Die Schalleitungsplastiken. I. Teil Acta Oto Laryng (Stockh) 45:370

Zöllner F (1955) Die Schalleitungsplastiken. II. Teil Acta Oto Laryng (Stockh) 45:168

Zöllner F (Kongreßber 1957) Hörverbessernde Operationen bei entzündlich bedingten Mittelohrveränderungen. Arch Ohr Nas Kehlk Heilk 171:1

Surgery of Space-Occupying Lesions of the Middle Skull Base

Surgery of Space-Occupying Lesions of the Sellar Region

Introductory Remarks. Operative exposure of the sellar region is most commonly indicated for the treatment of pituitary neoplasms; for the excision of other tumors such as tuberculum sellae meningiomas (see p. 210), craniopharyngiomas, and optic nerve gliomas (see p. 184); and for the surgical treatment of circle of Willis aneurysms.

Because of its anatomic location, the sella can be approached either transcranially or transsphenoidally through the ethmoid bone, maxillary sinus, or nasal septum (Denker 1921). Horsley (1906) approached a pituitary neoplasm transcranially by way of the middle cranial fossa, while Krause (1905) described an approach through the anterior fossa. Schloffer, in 1907, was the first surgeon to perform a hypophysectomy in a living patient, exposing the pituitary by reflecting the nose laterally and opening the frontal sinus, maxillary sinus, and sphenoid sinus. Later this procedure was greatly simplified by von Eiselsberg (1907, 1912). While Halstead used a sublabial incision for the transnasal approach (1910), Hirsch was the first, in 1909, to enter the sella transsphenoidally through an intranasal mucosal incision. Hirsch was the first rhinologist to remove a pituitary tumor surgically. Cushing, in 1912, combined Halstead's sublabial incision with the submucosal septal resection employed by Hirsch, and in the same year Chiari described the paranasal transethmoidal approach to the pituitary. Angell (1969), and Bateman (1962) combined the transethmoidal approach with the transnasal or transseptal technique. They gained exposure through the ethmoid bone and passed instruments transnasally into the sphenoid sinus. On the other hand, the transpalatal approach recommended by König in 1900 did not gain wide acceptance, although König was the first to attempt to reach the pituitary by way of the sphenoid sinus. Modifications of the transpalatal-transsphenoidal technique by Fein (1910), Löwe (1905), Preysing (1913), and Tiefenthal (1920) have fallen into disuse (Guleke 1950).

The introduction of the operating microscope and special microinstruments reawakened the discussion among neurosurgeons and otorhinolaryngologists as to the most suitable route of surgical access. Many authors have discussed the microsurgery of pituitary tumors – most notably Bateman (1962), Burian (1961, 1969, 1970), Escher (1965), Hamburger et al. (1961), Hamburger and Hammer (1964), and Nager (1940) on the otorhinolaryngologic side, and Fahlbusch (1978), Guiot (1958, 1967, 1973, 1976), Hardy (1969, 1973, 1975), Lüdecke (1982, 1983, 1985), and Nicola (1972) on the neurosurgical side.

The *choice of surgical approach* to the sellar region depends on the results of neuroradiologic studies. Plain radiographs should include special sellar views and tomograms in the lateral and AP projections, giving particular attention to the anatomic relationship of the sphenoid sinus and sella, the degree of pneumatization of the sphenoid sinus, and to any irregularities and asymmetries. CT and MRI scans on multiple planes have superseded encephalotomography for evaluating the suprasellar extent of the tumor. Carotid angiography provides information on the direction of tumor growth and permits differentiation of suprasellar tumors from circle of Willis aneurysms. The latter can cause destructive changes about the sella and invade the sphenoid sinus, mimicking the appearance of a pituitary neoplasm.

There is diversity of opinion concerning the most suitable route of approach for exposure of the sella. There is no general agreement on the tumor extent that would favor a transsphenoidal versus a transcranial procedure. We prefer the transsphenoidal approach for tumors that are located within the sella or whose suprasellar extent does not go beyond the optic chiasm. There is no question that the transsphenoidal approach involves fewer risks and is more easily tolerated than the transcranial. Therefore that approach would be favored in the high-risk patient, even for fairly extensive tumors. The decision becomes easier when extensive bony destruction of the skull base by the tumor precludes surgical exposure from below. It may well be possible to resect tumors with suprasellar and parasellar extension by systematic enucleation through the transsphenoidal route, but removal of parasellar extensions cannot always be satisfactorily accomplished through this approach.

Because the transsphenoidal routes involve the nose and paranasal sinuses, close teamwork between the neurosurgeon and the ENT surgeon is advised. This is very helpful in preventing postoperative complications arising from the paranasal sinuses and in preserving the nasal mucosa, thereby reducing the danger of atrophic rhinopathy with septal perforation and troublesome crusting.

General Operative Techniques

Transsphenoidal Approach to the Pituitary

This approach is best for sellar tumors that have widely invaded a well-pneumatized sphenoid sinus.

In the *transmaxillary-transethmoidosphenoidal hypophysectomy* preferred by Hamburger and Hammer (1964), the sphenoid sinus is opened using the Caldwell-Luc method and the bony medial wall of the sinus is removed. The lateral nasal wall with the inferior and middle turbinates is dislocated medially, and the ethmoid is exenterated. Then, aided by partial removal of the posterior septum, the anterior wall of the sphenoid sinus is removed with a rongeur and cutting burr, and the sphenoid septum is ablated. At this point the operating microscope is brought into the field. The anterior inferior bony wall of the sella is removed, and the sellar dura is coagulated with a bipolar cautery and incised. The distance from the anterior portion of the sphenoid sinus to the pituitary is approximately 9 cm.

The sphenoid sinus also may be approached by performing a *fronto-orbital external ethmoidectomy* through a paranasal incision. After reflection of the soft tissues and periosteum, exposing the trochlea and lacrimal sac, the floor of the frontal sinus is opened, and the ethmoid cells are progressively exenterated along the skull base between the lamina papyracea and lateral nasal wall, establishing a wide communication with the nose. The mucosal flap technique of Uffenorde (1923) is recommended for epithelializing the connection between the frontal sinus and nose. Using the operating microscope, the skull base is smoothened with the cutting burr. After stripping the nasal mucosa from the anterior wall of the sphenoid sinus and creating a medially based mucosal-septal flap, the anterior wall of the sphenoid sinus on the affected side is opened, and the intersphenoid septum is removed. If a laterally based flap of sphenoid mucosa can be mobilized, it may be used later to help seal the opening into the sella (Lehnhardt 1979). The vomer of the bony nasal septum provides a reliable landmark for opening the sella exactly on the midline. The sphenoid septum, on the other hand, is variable in its position and is useful for orientation only if CT scans are consulted.

In both the transmaxillary-transethmoidosphenoidal and the ethmoidosphenoidal approaches, the sella is approached more from the lateral side than anteriorly. This is disadvantageous, because unfavorable pneumatization of the sinus can make it difficult to identify the midline, and the slightly oblique route may come dangerously close to critical structures like the internal carotid artery, cavernous sinus, and cranial nerves II–VI.

For these reasons, we and many other rhinosurgeons and neurosurgeons have come to prefer

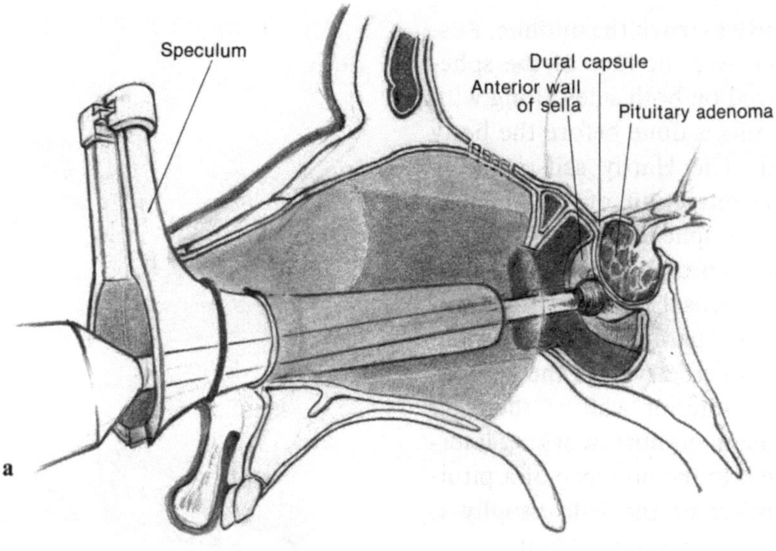

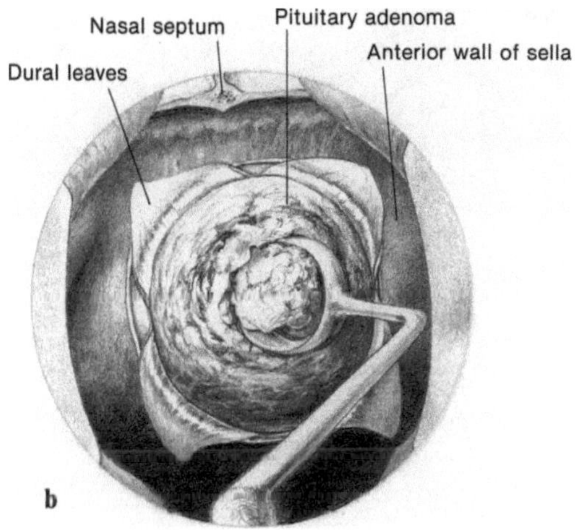

Fig. MS 17a, b. Transseptosphenoidal approach to the pituitary.
a Sagittal section: The cartilaginous septum is swung aside, the anterior wall of the sphenoid sinus is removed, and the Hardy self-retaining speculum is introduced. The anterior wall of the sella can be removed with a diamond burr and micropunch.
b After removal of the anterior wall and floor of the sella, the dura is exposed and opened in cruciate fashion so that the pituitary tumor can be removed piecemeal with a curette using microscopic aid. We recommend leaving part of the bony septum attached to the sphenoid face to provide a landmark for the midline

the *transseptosphenoidal approach* with use of the operating microscope (Fig. MS 17a, b). Because this is a strictly midline approach, the risk of bleeding is decreased, and a greater safety margin is maintained with respect to the structures bordering on the sphenoid sinus and sella. However, care must be taken to spare the mucosa when dissecting about the septum so that an effective septoplasty can be performed. This goal is readily accomplished through teamwork between the rhinosurgeon and neurosurgeon. Failure in this regard can result in an atrophic rhinitis with troublesome intranasal crusting for life.

The *nasal septum* can be approached sublabially through a mucosal incison in the oral vestibule, or intranasally through a "hemitransfixion" incision of the type often used for septoplasty. The incision is placed about 1 mm behind the anterior border of the septum and extends from the attachment of the lateral cartilage to the nasal floor. Elevation of the septal mucosa on one side is done on the side opposite the hemitransfixion incision with a straight nasal septum, and on the concave side if the septum is deviated. A vertical submucous incision is made at the junction of the cartilaginous and bony septa, and the septal cartilage is dislocated from the nasal crest of the maxilla and swung aside, sparing the contralateral mucosa. This is followed by submucous resection of the posterior bony septum. A portion of the vomer should be preserved inferiorly to mark the midline. Posteriorly, the mucosa over the face of the sphenoid sinus is mobilized on both sides along with the septal mucosa; this is done before the bony septum is removed. The Hardy self-retaining speculum maintains retraction of the mucosa from the surface of the sphenoid sinus. The latter is opened with a cutting burr and micropunch, sparing the mucosal lining of the sinus cavity. The mucosa is separated from the sphenoid septum with a microelevator, the septum is removed, and the anterior wall of the sella is opened with the diamond burr, working laterally from the midline. In the presence of a pituitary tumor, the surface of the sella usually is markedly thinned due to pressure atrophy.

The dural capsule is coagulated and opened with a cruciate incision, and the tumor is enucleated piecemeal with a curette. High magnification is used to differentiate tumor from healthy pituitary tissue by its consistency and color (Fig. MS 17b). Not infrequently, the tumor is so soft that it "spills out" through the opening in the pituitary capsule and can be removed with suction. In these cases it is no problem to preserve the considerably firmer, healthy pituitary tissue, which is usually lighter in color than the tumor. If the diaphragma sellae is not breached during tumor removal, cerebrospinal fluid leak will not occur, and it is sufficient to pack the sella with fibrin sponges. If cerebrospinal fluid leak does occur after tumor removal, it is necessary to seal the sella with a myofascial graft. The hemitransfixion incision is closed with mucosal sutures. To avoid submucous septal hematoma, it is recommended that nasal packing be inserted before the transfixion sutures are applied. Septal hematoma represents a potentially dangerous source of infection.

Transcranial Intradural Approach to the Pituitary

(Dandy 1938, Krause 1905, Fig. MS 18a–e)

We recommend the transfrontal approach for tumors that have reached the floor of the third ventricle or have caused its displacement. The transcranial, transfrontal approach begins with

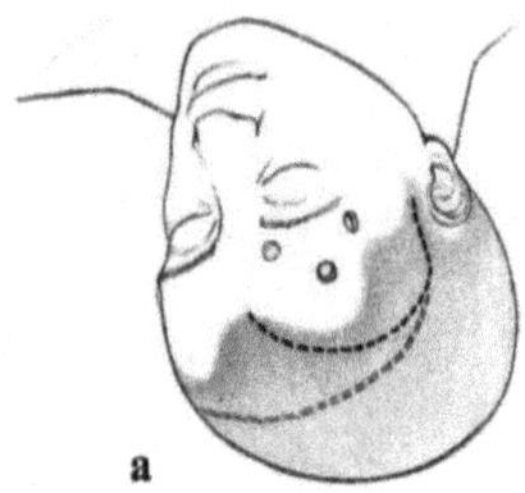

a

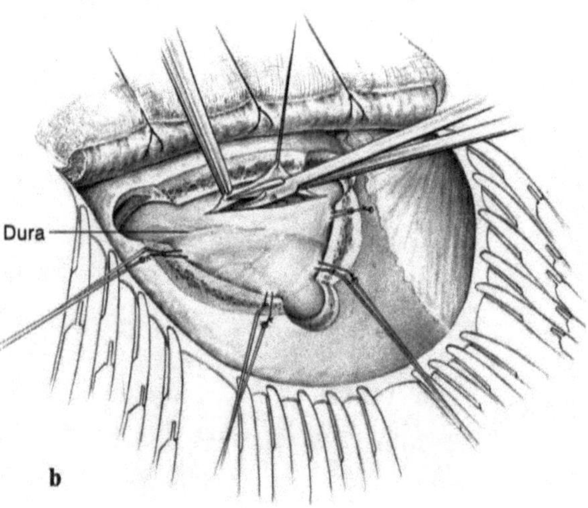

b

Fig. MS 18a–e. Transcranial intradural approach to the pituitary.
a Scalp incisions for unilateral and bilateral craniotomy and burr-hole placement for unilateral craniotomy.
b Unilateral right frontal craniotomy. The osteoplastic bone flap has been removed, and the dura is opened frontobasally with scissors. The dural tack-up sutures are in place. The temporal muscle is preserved.
c After retraction of the right frontal lobe, the suprasellar tumor capsule is identified in the anterior angle of the optic chiasm and opened. The tumor is enucleated piecemeal with a curette and suction tip.
d Surgical cavity following tumor removal. The pituitary stalk is intact.
e Microanatomy as viewed through the anterior angle of the optic chiasm after tumor removal

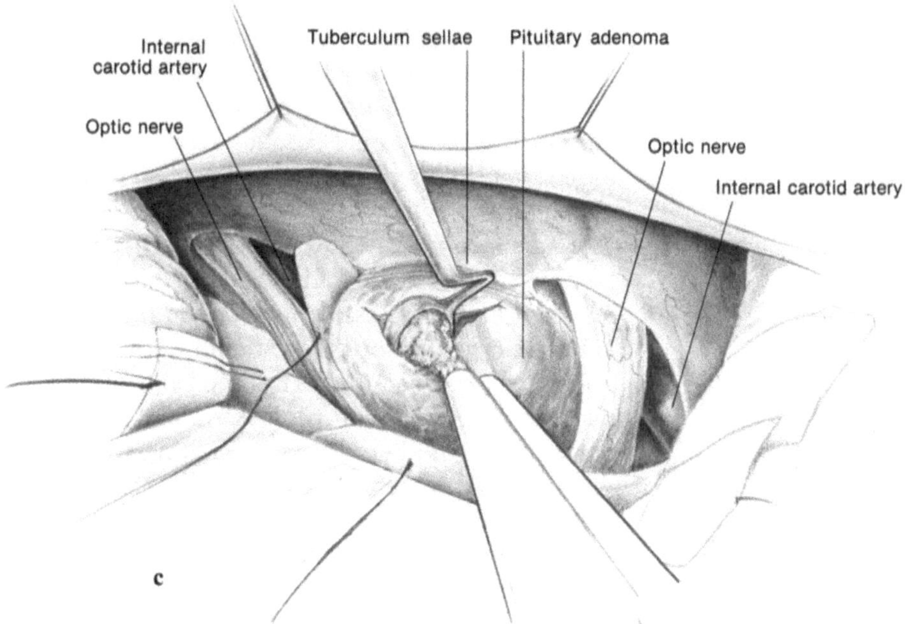
Internal
carotid artery
Tuberculum sellae
Pituitary adenoma
Optic nerve
Optic nerve
Internal carotid artery

c

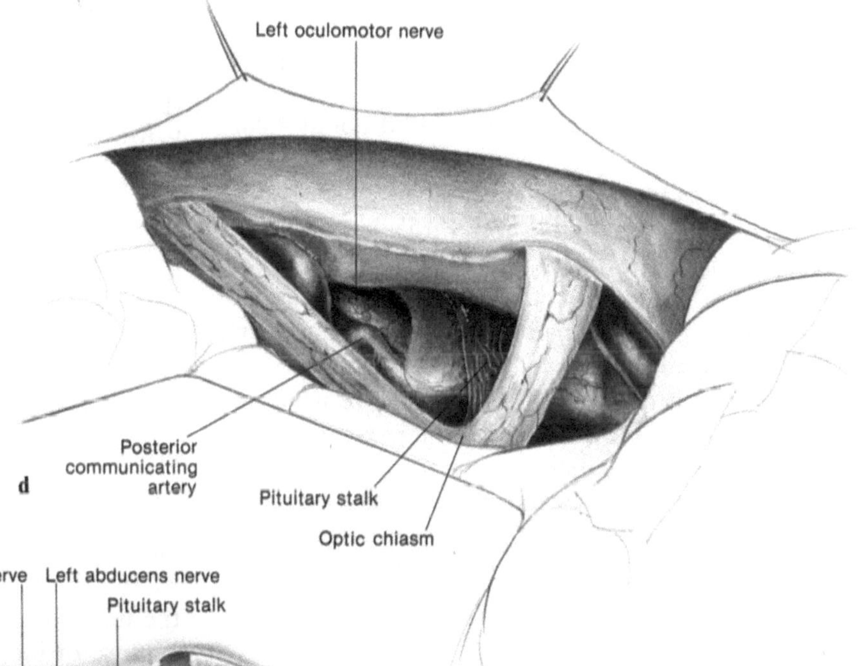
Left oculomotor nerve
Posterior
communicating
artery
Pituitary stalk
Optic chiasm

d

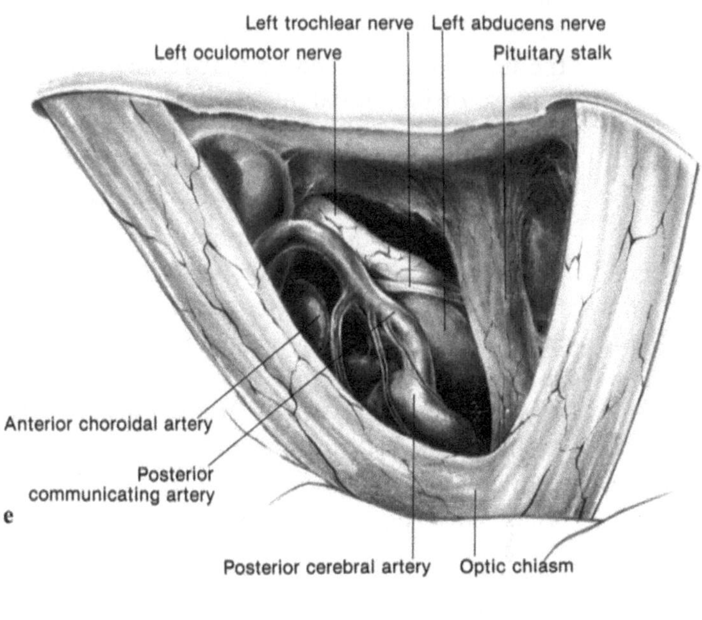
Left trochlear nerve
Left abducens nerve
Left oculomotor nerve
Pituitary stalk
Anterior choroidal artery
Posterior
communicating artery
Posterior cerebral artery
Optic chiasm

e

a bitemporal coronal incision. For cosmetic reasons we prefer this to a circumscribed flap incision on the forehead. Generally three burr holes are sufficient for the craniotomy:

1) The *lateral burr hole* is placed at the root of the zygomatic process of the frontal bone, which forms a palpable ledge at its junction with the infratemporal fossa. The hole should be placed about 1 to 1 1/2 cm above the frontozygomatic suture. A small slit can be made in the aponeurosis of the temporal muscle to expose the bony ledge at the temporal fossa. The burr hole is placed directly on that ridge. As the hole is drilled, care is taken that the burr does not enter the bony orbit, which would injure Tenon's capsule, and that the hole is as close as possible to the floor of the anterior cranial fossa. This will avoid a troublesome bony overlapping later on.
2) The *medial burr hole* is situated about 4 cm from the lateral hole. We try to place the hole as low as possible and close to the midline. This is possible even with a large frontal sinus that extends far superiorly. When the frontal sinus is reached, its mucosal lining is stripped downward so that the burr can be advanced through the posterior sinus wall without damaging the mucosa. We mention this detail in the interest of preventing the spread of pathogenic organisms from the paranasal sinuses into the cranial cavity and obviating the need for tube drainage of the frontal sinus into the nasal cavity.
3) The *superior burr hole* is placed about 3 cm above, and midway between, the lateral and medial perforations.

The interconnecting Gigli saw cuts should be kept as low as possible without damaging the paranasal sinus mucosa. The dura is opened with a frontobasal incision. Intradural exposure of the anterior fossa is carried out in standard fashion, facilitating frontal lobe retraction by progressively opening the arachnoid and withdrawing cerebrospinal fluid. It has proved useful to expose the anterior skull base more from the lateral side, using the lesser sphenoid wing as a landmark. Additional room is gained by microsurgical dissection, aided if necessary by division of the ipsilateral olfactory bulb and further retraction of the frontal lobe. The right optic nerve and underlying internal carotid artery are visualized first, followed by the left optic nerve and optic chiasm.

The next step is to debulk the tumor after coagulating and then opening its capsule. This makes it easier to dissect the capsule from the left optic nerve, following the tumor to the optic chiasm or hypothalamus. This step calls for meticulous dissection with progressive bipolar coagulation of the blood vessels entering the tumor. Working carefully, the surgeon should be able to mobilize the tumor in stages and effect a complete removal. Forcible extraction can cause uncontrolled tearing of blood vessels in the area of the hypothalamus, posing a serious hazard to the patient. In doubtful cases we feel that tumor in contact with the hypothalamus should be left alone in case an adhesion exists between the hypothalamus and tumor capsule that cannot be cleared. Through progressive microsurgical dissection, it is possible to identify the pituitary stalk at the hypothalamus, follow it toward the sella, and separate any uninvolved pituitary tissue from the neoplasm. This avoids undesired traction on the hypothalamus via the pituitary stalk, which can lead to severe postoperative endocrinological and metabolic disorders. Increasingly the use of the operating microscope is expanding our knowledge of the microtopography of this region, enabling us to identify microvessels around the tumor that supply the brain stem. We are convinced that the uncontrolled bleeding that results from the rupture of individual vessels in the area of the hypothalamus inflicts greater tissue damage than the controlled coagulation of individual microvessels that cannot be spared. It is our impression that the interruption of a few "perforating vessels" does not necessarily cause a functionally significant decline of hypothalamic blood flow owing to the abundant collateral connections in this area.

Retrosellar tumors and tumors with *parasellar* extension toward the tentorial incisure are generally approached through a standard, wide *frontotemporal craniotomy* allowing access to

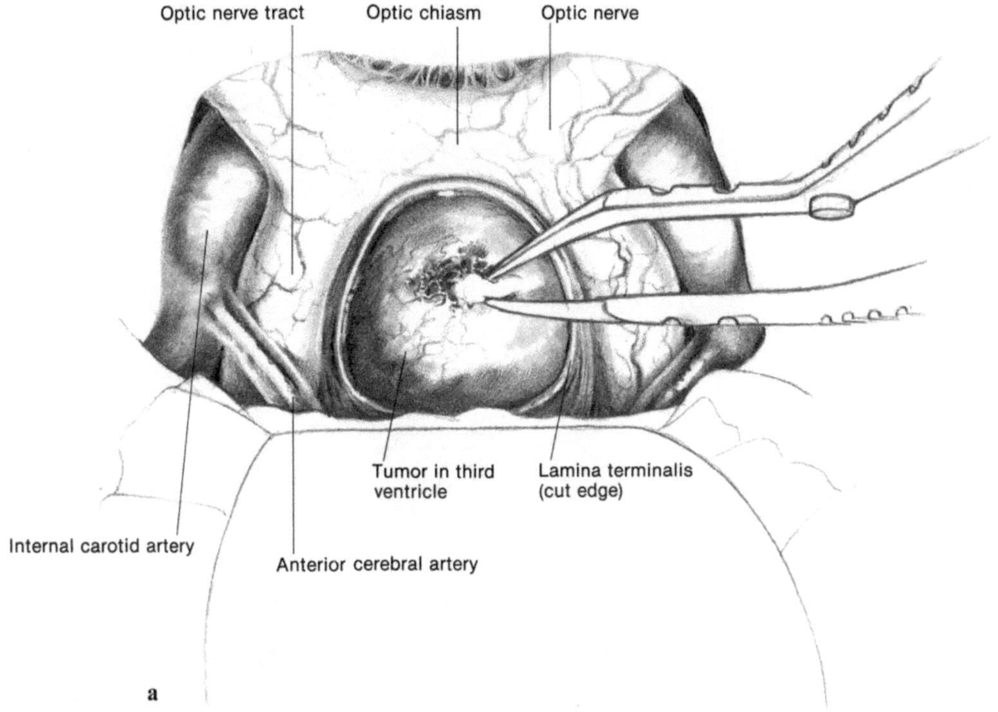

a

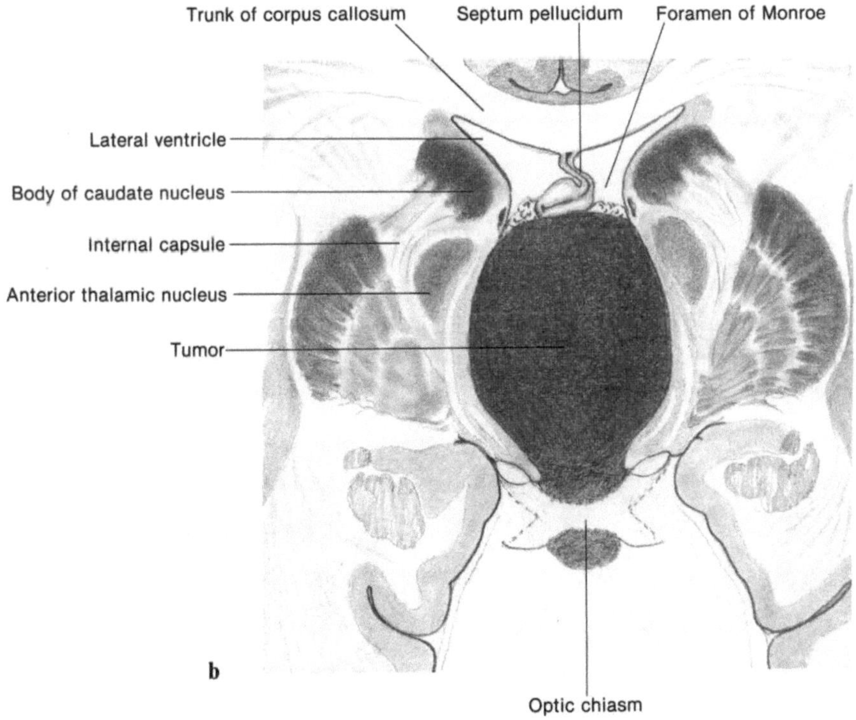

b

Fig. MS 19a–d. Bifrontal, transcranial, intradural approach for removing a tumor with extensive supra- and parasellar growth. With an anteriorly displaced (prefixed) optic chiasm, it is necessary to open the lamina terminalis to remove the suprasellar part of the neoplasm.

a Retrochiasmatic exposure of the tumor after opening the lamina terminalis with a prefixed chiasm.
b Frontal section through the tumor showing its relation to the basal ganglia. To aid orientation, the optic chiasm is shown rotated onto the transverse plane

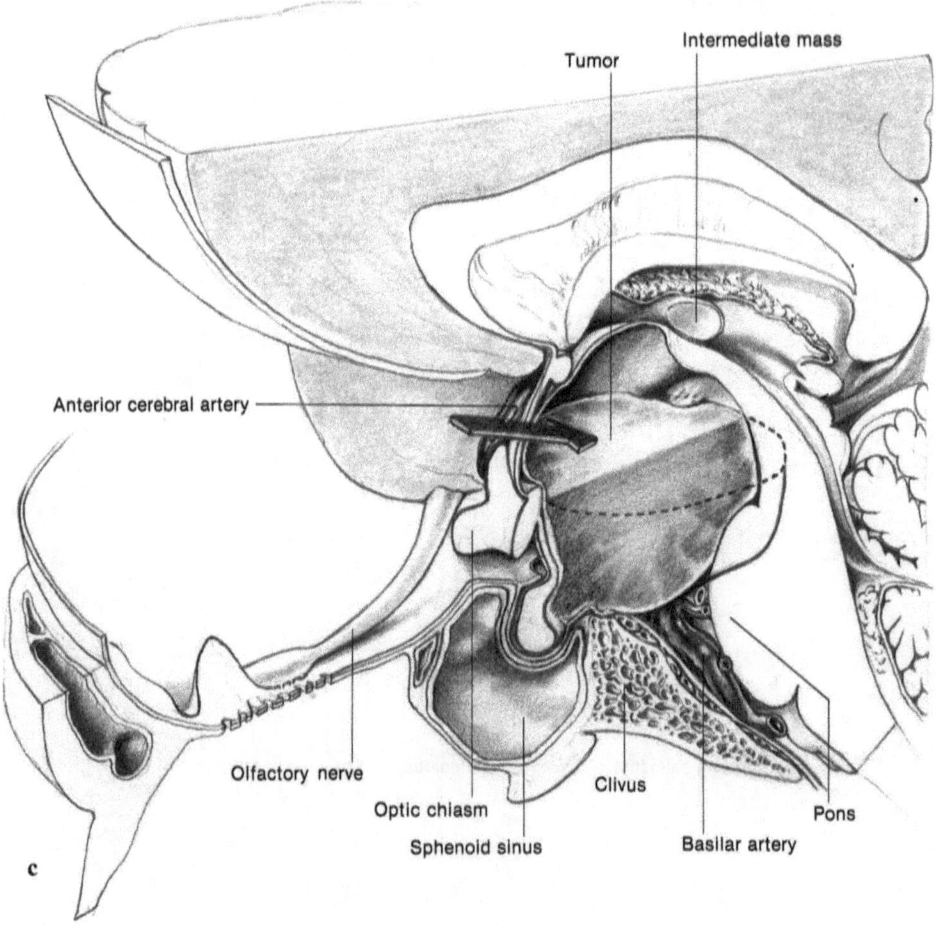

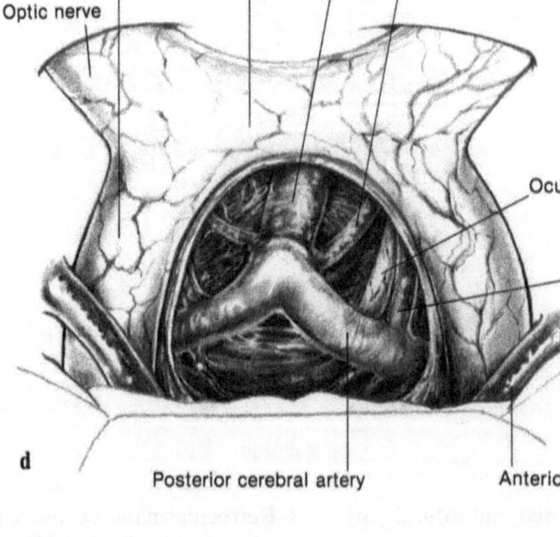

Fig. MS 19c, d.

c Three-dimensional representation of the tumor extent on the transverse and sagittal planes and of the route of surgical access. Both olfactory nerves can be microsurgically dissected and preserved.

d View into the prepontine space showing the microsurgical anatomy following tumor removal the anterior and middle fossae. The sphenoid wing can be exposed as far as the clinoid process by retraction of the temporal lobe, and the edge of the tentorial notch can be identified posterior to the internal carotid artery, making use of available landmarks around the tentorial incisure. The posterior communicating artery, anterior choroidal artery, and oculomotor nerve are always displaced laterally or posteriorly by the tumor. If the tumor extends far posteriorly, it may even displace the trochlear nerve. In our experience, tumors with substantial parasellar and suprasellar extension are approached more simply and less traumatically by the subfrontal route, dissecting obliquely beneath the optic chiasm from the opposite side, because of the uplifted condition of the chiasm and the splaying of its anterior angle (see Figs. MS 22a–c and MS 23a–c; Figs. MS 18a–e, MS 19a–d).

With large pituitary adenomas that have caused extensive bony destruction of the anterior and middle skull base, the goal of surgery is to de-

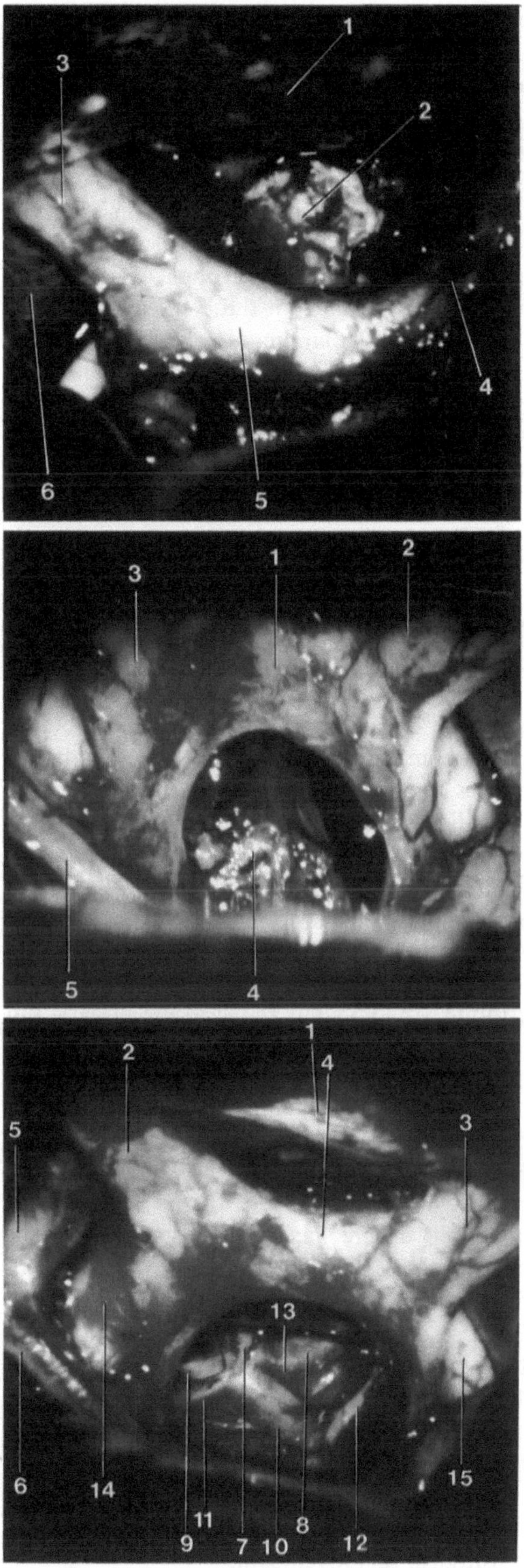

Fig. MS 20a–c. Extirpation of a partially calcified suprasellar craniopharyngioma.
a After bifrontal craniotomy and bilateral retraction of the frontal lobes, the calcified anterior tumor pole is identified in the anterior angle of the optic chiasm.
b To reach all of the tumor, it is necessary to open the lamina terminalis (elevated by the tumor) and expose the posterior angle of the chiasm. Here the lamina has been split, providing a view through the posterior angle of the chiasm into the third ventricle, which contains the posterior part of the tumor.
c With all tumor removed, we can look through the posterior angle of the chiasm and see the prepontine space with the basilar artery and its branches and also the right oculomotor nerve.
a: (*1*) Tuberculum sellae, (*2*) anterior pole tumor, (*3*) left optic nerve, (*4*) right optic nerve, (*5*) optic chiasm, (*6*) left internal carotid artery. **b:** (*1*) Optic chiasm, (*2*) right optic nerve, (*3*) left optic nerve, (*4*) tumor in third ventricle, (*5*) left anterior cerebral artery. **c:** (*1*) Tuberculum sellae, (*2*) left optic nerve, (*3*) right optic nerve, (*4*) optic chiasm, (*5*) left internal carotid artery, (*6*) left anterior cerebral artery, (*7*) basilar artery, (*8*) right superior cerebellar artery, (*9*) left superior cerebellar artery, (*10*) right posterior cerebral artery, (*11*) left posterior cerebral artery, (*12*) right posterior communicating branch, (*13*) right oculomotor nerve, (*14*) left optic tract, (*15*) right optic tract

bulk the tumor to effect decompression of surrounding structure, most notably the optic nerve and chiasm, the oculomotor nerves, and the internal carotid artery and its branches.

Pituitary adenomas and craniopharyngiomas that have invaded the third ventricle, causing obstructive hydrocephalus from occlusion of the third ventricle and the foramen of Monro, cannot be totally removed through a subfrontal, subchiasmatic route. In these cases it is necessary to incise the lamina terminalis to gain access to the intraventricular part of the tumor behind the chiasm (Figs. MS 19a–d and MS 20a–c).

Special Operative Techniques

Introductory Remarks. With advances in endocrinological diagnosis, it has become possible to detect small pituitary tumors at an early stage and refer them for operative treatment before they are manifested clinically by visual disturbances or other cranial neuropathies and radiologically by expansion of the sella. A prime example is the prolactinoma, whose endocrine effects include disturbances of potency and libido and secondary amenorrhea.

At one time it was believed that the pharmacologic treatment of prolactinomas with bromocriptine would obviate the need for surgery, but long-term observations have been disappointing in this regard. It is true that this therapy can lower prolactin levels and produce demonstrable shrinkage of some pituitary adenomas. However, this effect is of but short duration, even with continuation of therapy, and so far a definitive cure has not been achieved. The drug can be given preoperatively, however, to facilitate tumor removal.

Because of the hazards associated with radiotherapy (Atkinson et al. 1979, Lawrence et al. 1971, Pieterse et al. 1982, Raskind 1977), we consider this modality only postoperatively in two situations: 1) when optimum surgical tumor removal has not been effected, and 2) when a recurrence develops shortly after meticulous microsurgical tumor removal.

The *transseptosphenoidal approach* is particularly suitable for small adenomas (Fig. MS 21a–c). The goal of the microsurgical procedure is selective tumor removal, preserving healthy portions of the pituitary to ensure normal postoperative hormone secretion. It is not uncommon for previously infertile women to achieve a normal pregnancy following this type of procedure.

The *transfrontal intradural approach* is the method of choice for larger supra- and parasellar pituitary neoplasms. We feel that the decision whether to perform a right or left frontal craniotomy or a bifrontal craniotomy should depend on the side to which the supra- and parasellar portion of the tumor can be localized.

A midline suprasellar tumor, even when extensive, is operable through a small right frontal craniotomy. This has the advantage of avoiding exposure of the usually dominant left hemisphere. Even large, left-sided parasellar tumor extensions can be removed through this approach (Fig. MS 22a, b).

A tumor that has expanded toward the right side beneath the optic nerve and internal carotid artery to the tentorial margin is not exposed well through a right-sided approach. In these cases we prefer to gain an oblique view of the tumor site through a left-sided exposure.

If the tumor has equivalent parasellar extents on both sides, the bifrontal craniotomy makes it possible to remove the tumor from both the right and left sides under favorable vision. This also satisfies the prerequisite of Suzuki (1981) that both olfactory nerves be visualized and spared if possible (Fig. MS 23a–c).

Pituitary adenomas occasionally expand behind the sella into the prepontine area and impinge upon the basilar artery and its branches. Such tumors can be attacked bifrontally in cases where a coexisting suprasellar portion of the tumor has elevated the optic chiasm and widened its anterior angle (Fig. MS 24a, b).

Sudden visual deterioration signifies enlargement of the tumor mass due to spontaneous hemorrhage. This condition demands immediate surgical intervention (Fig. MS 25a–d).

True skull base problems are posed by mass lesions of the sellar region having both intracranial and extracranial extension.

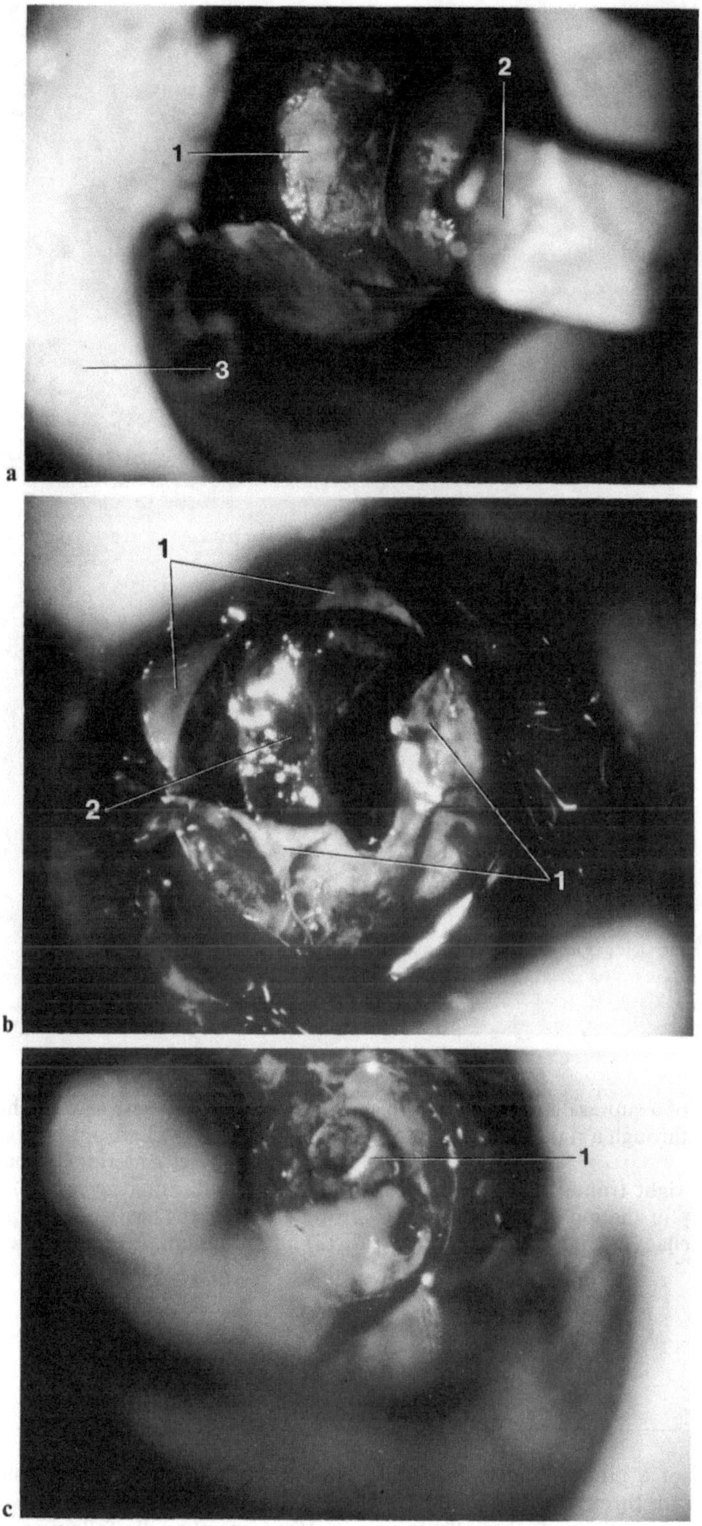

Fig. MS 21 a–c. Transseptosphenoidal removal of a pituitary adenoma.
a The anterior wall of the sphenoid sinus is removed, exposing the anterior wall and floor of the sella turcica. (*1*) Anterior wall of sella, (*2*) speculum, (*3*) ala nasae.
b The dura lining the anterior wall and floor of the sella is opened with a cruciate incision, and the tumor capsule is opened. (*1*) Dural leaves, (*2*) tumor.
c The tumor is removed with a curette (1)

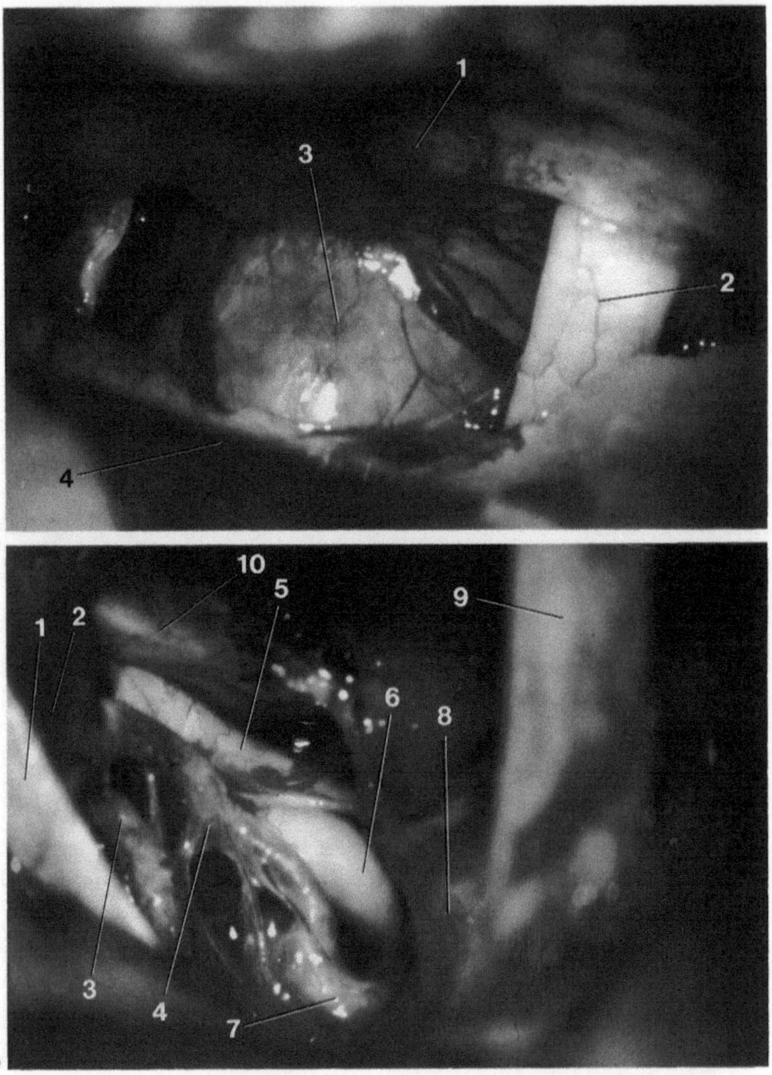

a

b

Fig. MS 22 a, b. Removal of a suprasellar adenoma with a left parasellar extension through a right frontal craniotomy.
a After retraction of the right frontal lobe, the tumor is exposed microsurgically in the anterior angle of the chiasm. (*1*) Tuberculum sellae, (*2*) right optic nerve, (*3*) tumor, (*4*) spatula.
b Subchiasmatic view toward the left side following tumor removal. (*1*) Left optic nerve, (*2*) left internal carotid artery, (*3*) left anterior choroidal artery, (*4*) left posterior communicating artery, (*5*) left oculomotor nerve, (*6*) left abducens nerve, (*7*) left posterior cerebral artery, (*8*) infundibulum, (*9*) right optic nerve, (*10*) dorsum sellae

Fig. MS 23 a–c. Removal of a pituitary adenoma with supra- and parasellar growth through the bifrontal approach with bilateral preservation of the olfactory tracts.
a Both frontal poles have been retracted to expose the tumor. (*1*) Left optic nerve, (*2*) left frontal pole, (*3*) left olfactory tract, (*4*) tuberculum sellae, (*5*) right optic nerve, (*6*) right olfactory tract, (*7*) right frontal pole.
b The tumor capsule is opened with microscissors. (*1*) Tumor, (*2*) microscissors.
c View into the sella following tumor removal. (*1*) Left optic nerve, (*2*) left olfactory tract, (*3*) tuberculum sellae, (*4*) dorsum sellae, (*5*) pituitary stalk, (*6*) pontine cistern, (*7*) right olfactory tract, (*8*) right optic nerve

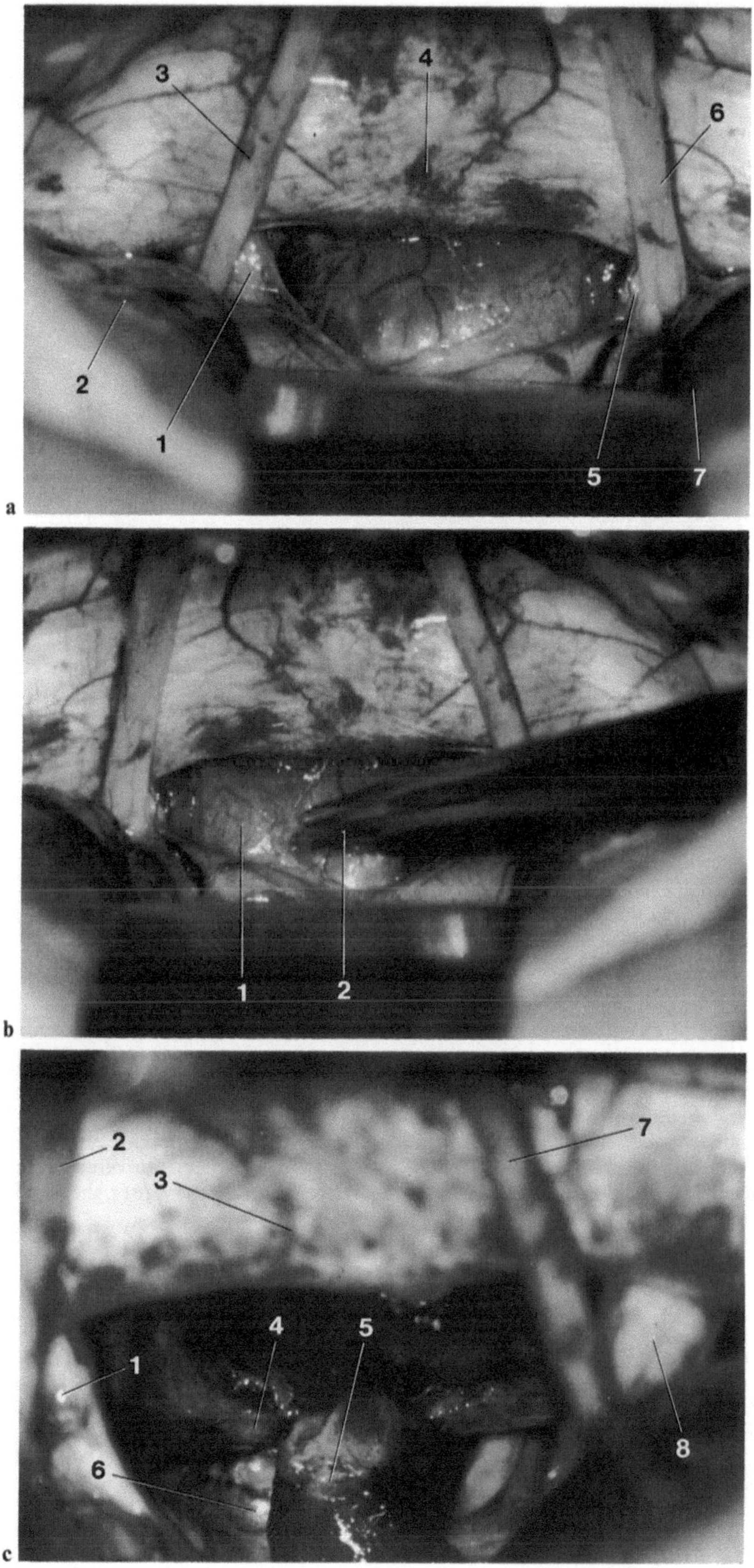

a

b

c

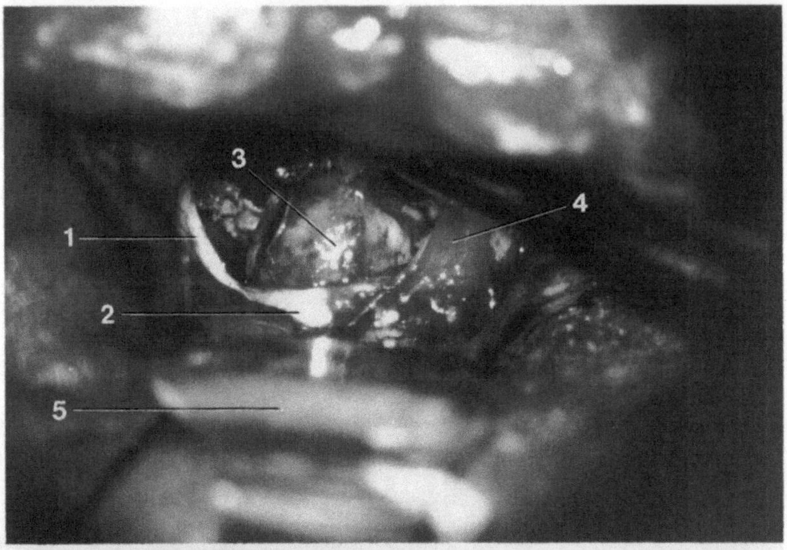

a

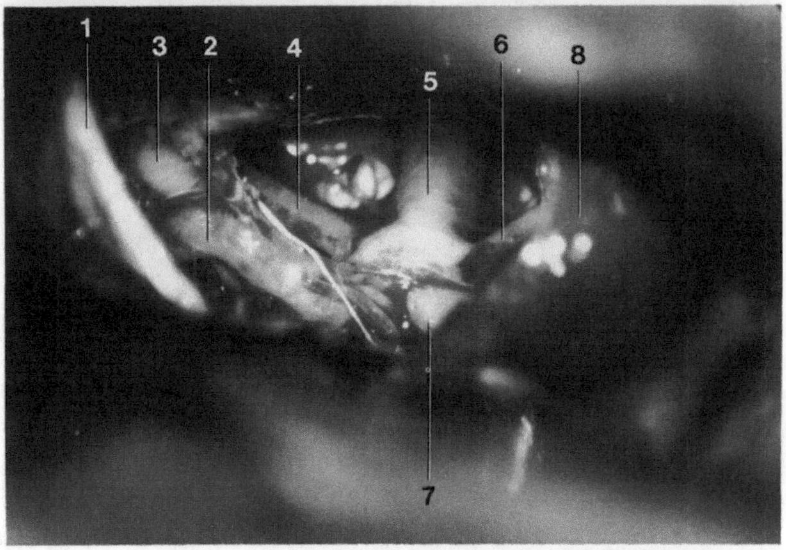

b

Fig. MS 24a, b. Pituitary adenoma with supra- and retrosellar extension.
a The suprasellar part of the tumor has been removed. The retrosellar extension is mobilized anteriorly through the splayed anterior angle of the chiasm. (*1*) Left optic nerve, (*2*) optic chiasm, (*3*) tumor extension, (*4*) right optic nerve, (*5*) spatula.
b Subchiasmatic view of the microanatomy of the prepontine space following tumor removal. (*1*) Left optic nerve, (*2*) left posterior cerebral artery, (*3*) left oculomotor nerve, (*4*) left superior cerebellar artery, (*5*) basilar artery, (*6*) right superior cerebellar artery, (*7*) right posterior cerebral artery, (*8*) right optic nerve

Fig. MS 25a–d. Eosinophilic adenoma of the pituitary in a 17-year-old girl who experienced sudden, left-sided blindness secondary to a tumor hemorrhage.
a Right frontal craniotomy exposing the tumor in the anterior angle of the chiasm. A hematoma is seen below the chiasm and lateral to the left optic nerve. (*1*) Left optic nerve with hematoma, (*2*) tuberculum sellae, (*3*) subchiasmatic hematoma with tumor, (*4*) right optic nerve.
b Evacuation of the hematoma lateral to the left optic nerve. (*1*) Left optic nerve, (*2*) right optic nerve, (*3*) hematoma.
c Preoperative (*1, 2*) and postoperative (*3, 4*) CT scans.
d Visual field maps before and immediately after surgery and at 7 months postoperatively

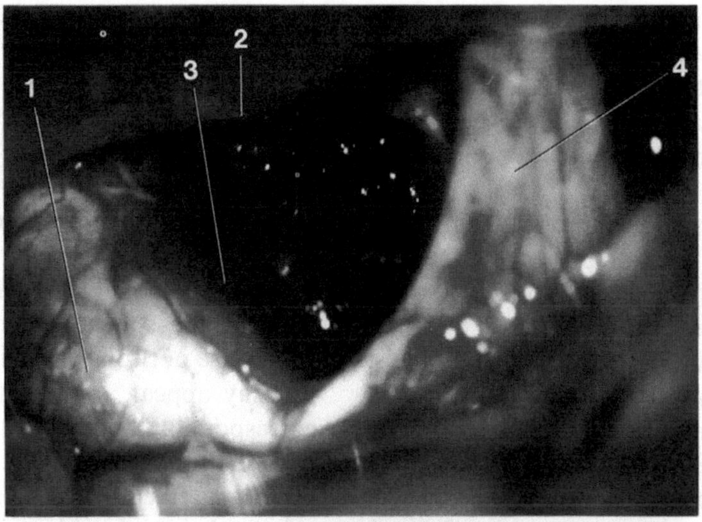
1
2
3
4
a

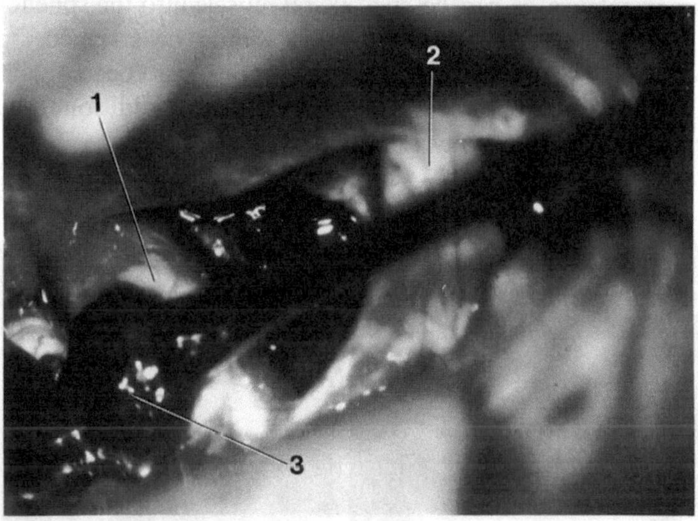
1
2
3
b

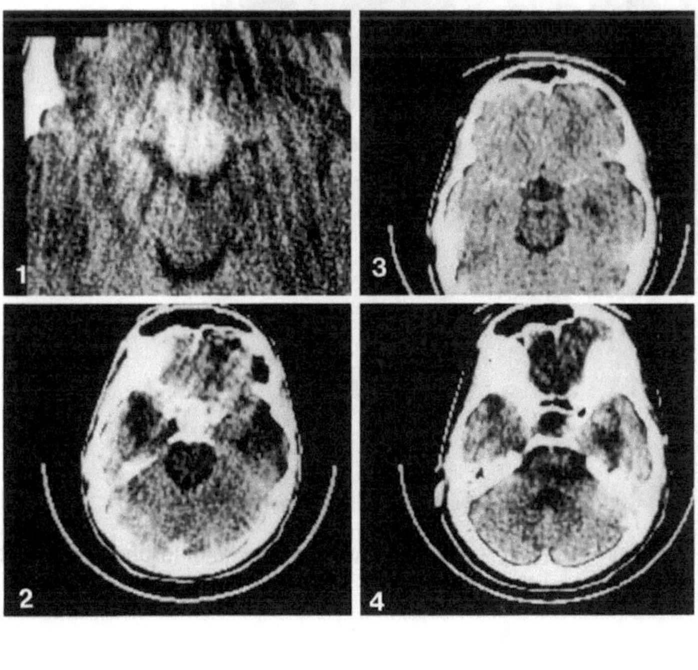
1
2
3
4
c

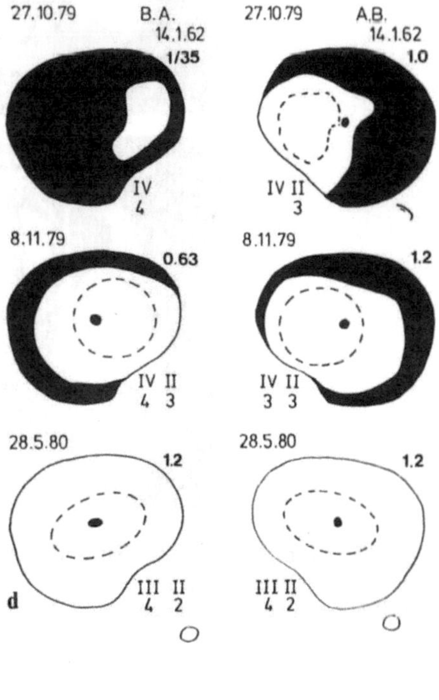
27.10.79
B.A.
14.1.62
1/35
IV
4
27.10.79
A.B.
14.1.62
1.0
IV II
3
8.11.79
0.63
IV II
4 3
8.11.79
1.2
IV II
3 3
28.5.80
1.2
III II
4 2
28.5.80
1.2
III II
4 2
d

Joint work by neurosurgeons and ENT surgeons has shown that a large percentage of these very extensive pituitary adenomas with destruction of the skull base can be attacked by the transethmoidosphenoidal route as well as the transcranial route.

In these extreme cases, the approach from below permits exposure of the skull base from the posterior wall of the frontal sinus over the roofs of the ethmoid and sphenoid sinuses to the anterior wall of the sella and down to the clivus. Laterally, the exposure can extend over the wall of the cavernous sinus, caudal to the optic nerve, as far as the petrous apex and carotid canal.

After this wide approach has been established, even intracranial tumor extensions can be successfully removed after further incision of the dura (Fig. MS 26a–d).

The dural defect is sealed with a piece of fascia lata, which is inserted between the bony skull base and dural margins and supported from below with an iodoform ointment pack for 14 days.

If the transcranial approach is used, it is necessary to enlarge the access to the paranasal sinus system at the anterior angle of the optic chiasm by removing the tuberculum sellae and portions of the planum sphenoidale (Fig. MS 27a–e). In this way it is possible to gain access to the clivus through the sphenoid sinus (see p. 432). The transverse portions of the internal carotid arteries may appear at the sides of the field when corresponding bone destruction is present.

Before the cranial cavity is closed basally by inserting a free myofascial graft from the temporal muscle into the sphenoid sinus, all the mucosa should be stripped from the sinus so that the graft can become firmly adherent to the bony walls. Additional fixation with fibrin glue is recommended.

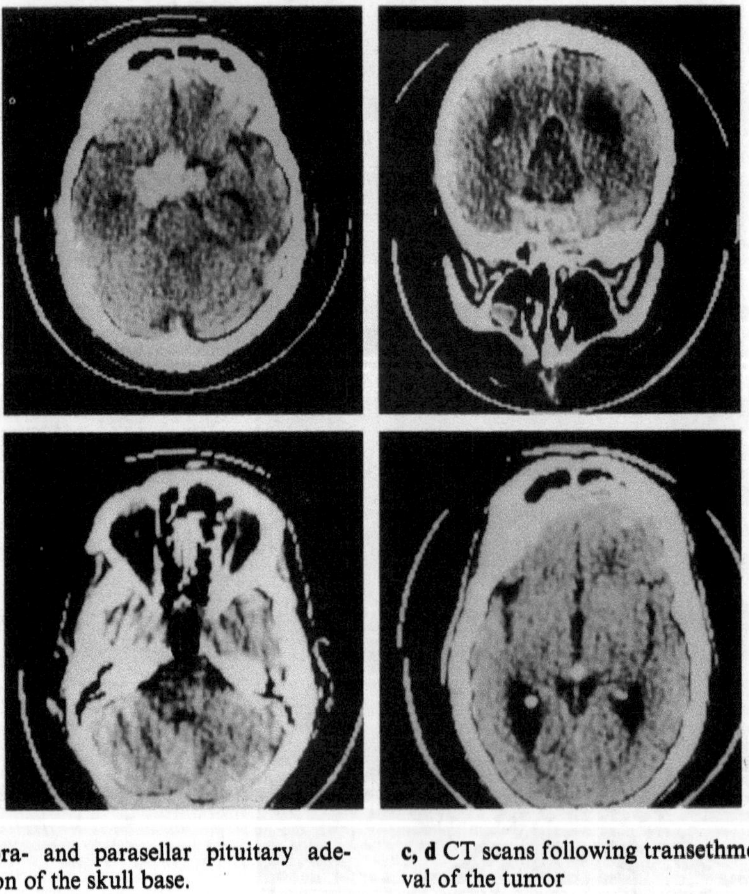

a b c d

Fig. MS 26a–d. Supra- and parasellar pituitary adenoma with destruction of the skull base.
a, b Preoperative axial and coronal CT scans.
c, d CT scans following transethmoidosphenoidal removal of the tumor

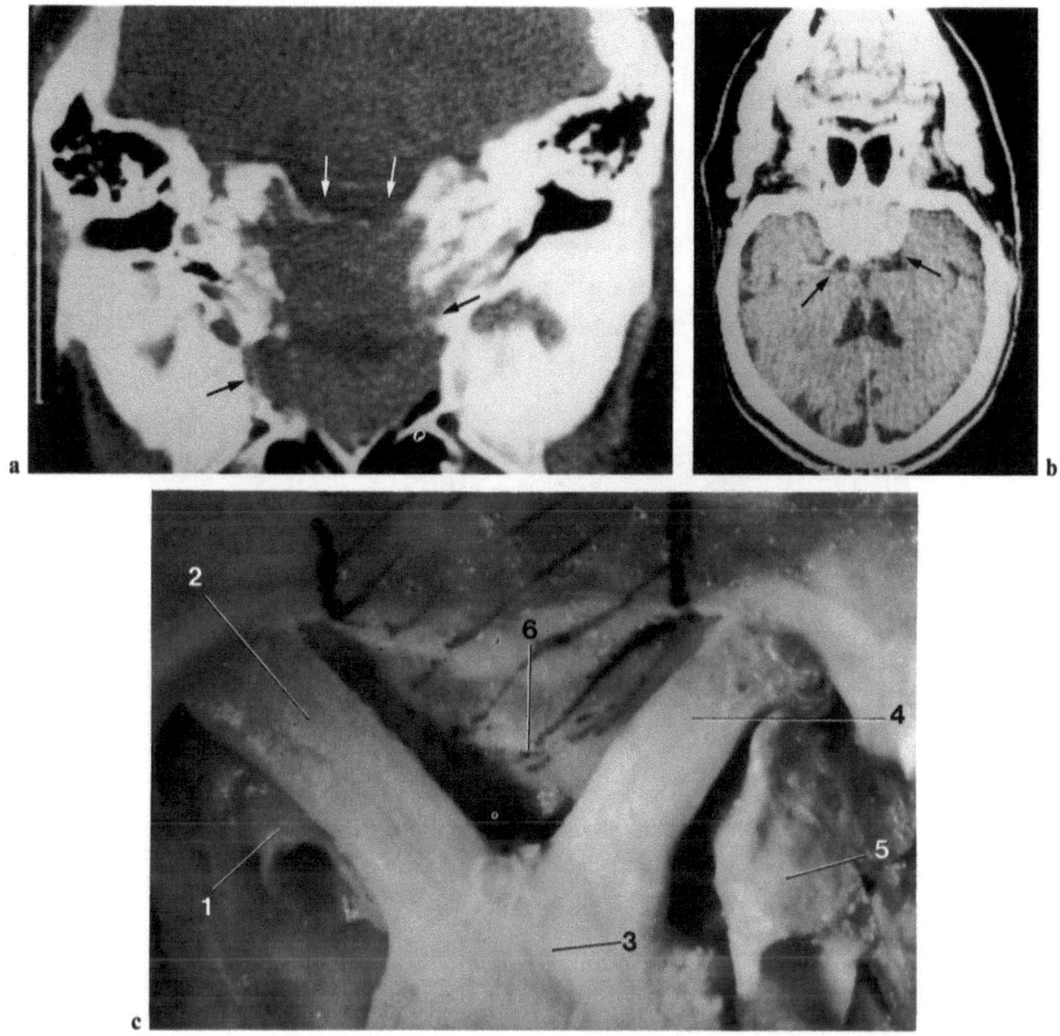

Fig. MS 27 a–e. Pituitary adenoma with extensive skull base destruction in the region of the clivus and petrous apices.
a, b Preoperative CT scans (*arrows*).
c Extent of bone resection for the transcranial approach to the sphenoid sinus and clivus, shown on an anatomic specimen. (*1*) Left internal carotid artery, (*2*) left optic nerve, (*3*) optic chiasm, (*4*) right optic nerve, (*5*) right internal carotid artery, (*6*) tuberculum sellae

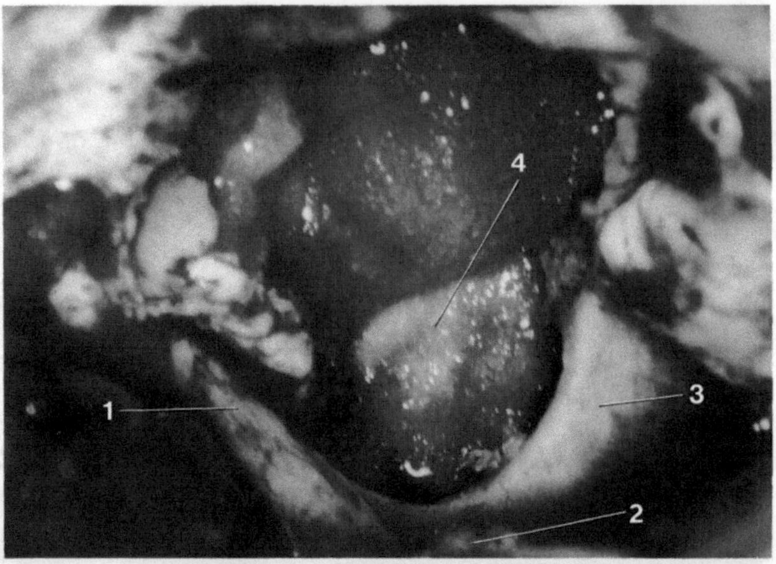

d

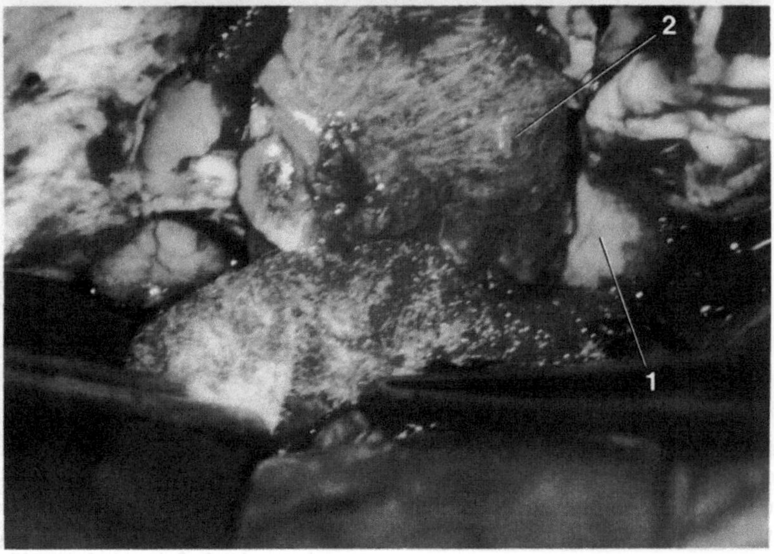

e

Fig. MS 27 d, e.
d Status following transcranial-transsphenoidal tumor removal. (*1*) Left optic nerve, (*2*) optic chiasm, (*3*) right optic nerve. (*4*) former tumor cavity packed with fibrin sponge.

e The cranial cavity is sealed with a free muscle-fascia graft. (*1*) Right optic nerve, (*2*) myofascial graft

Case Report. Large pituitary adenoma with very extensive intracranial growth (Fig. MS 28 a–g). A 69-year-old woman with obesity, diabetes mellitus, hypertension, and congestive heart failure had about a 3-year history of increasingly severe headaches and had noticed bilateral visual deterioration for several months. On admission she was awake and responsive to questions, but she appeared disoriented and apathetic. Examination disclosed decreased visual acuity in both eyes (especially the left), bitemporal hemianopsia, and bilateral papilledema.
CT scans showed a large mass lesion of the sellar region with extreme suprasellar extension, more pronounced on the right side than on the left, and invasion of the frontal horn of the right lateral ventricle. The angiogram showed a hypovascular tumor causing bilateral compression of

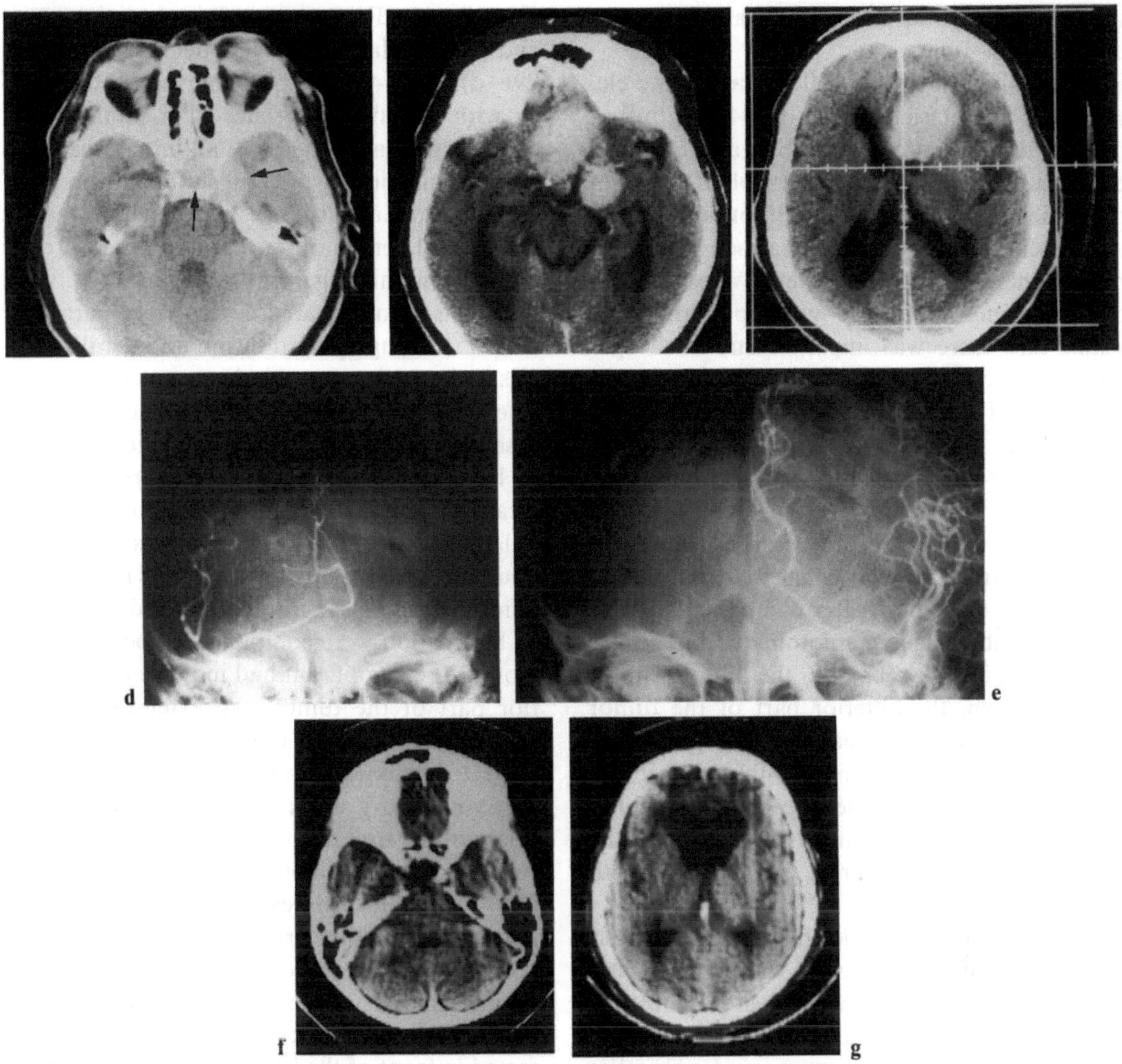

Fig. MS 28a–g. Large intra- and parasellar pituitary adenoma with unusual suprasellar and right frontal extension and invasion of the anterior horn of the right lateral ventricle.
a Axial CT scan at the level of the sella, demonstrating the intrasellar and right parasellar portion of the neoplasm (*arrows*).
b Axial CT scan of the suprasellar region shows extension of the tumor into the frontal and temporal lobes and its relation to the right anterior and middle cerebral arteries.
c Axial CT scan at the level of the lateral ventricle shows the adenoma occupying the anterior horn of the right lateral ventricle.
d, e Right and left carotid angiograms in the AP projection show marked bilateral elevation of the transverse portions of the anterior cerebral arteries, especially on the left, and displacement of the vertical limbs of both anterior cerebral arteries toward the left side.
f Postoperative axial CT scan at the level of the sella.
g Postoperative axial CT scan at the level of the anterior horns

the internal carotid arteries and anterior cerebral arteries.

Endocrinological tests revealed a moderate elevation of the plasma prolactin (34.1 ng/ml), a marked depression of basal FSH, and a significant depression of plasma cortisol. Because of the patient's poor general condition and the tumor extent, a trial course of treatment with bromocriptine was initiated. After 6 weeks of this therapy, tumor shrinkage was apparent on CT scans, and there was improvement in the patient's general condition and of vision in the right eye. The therapy was continued, but 4 weeks later CT showed reenlargement of the mass, and it was decided that surgery could not be delayed further despite the increased risk. Meanwhile the tumor had acquired intracerebral and intraventricular extensions in addition to its supra- and parasellar components. After bifrontal osteoplastic craniotomy and exposure of the anterior fossa back to the anterior angle of the chiasm, the anterior part of the tumor was identified and enucleated after bipolar cautery. At that point it was possible to free the tumor capsule from the left optic nerve and left internal carotid artery and then to follow the tumor-encased left anterior cerebral artery to the midline.

On the right side, the major blood vessels (internal carotid, anterior cerebral and middle cerebral arteries) and optic nerve were completely surrounded and obscured by tumor. After progressive removal of the supra- and parasellar parts of the neoplasm, these structures could be identified and freed of tumor. After further dissection it was possible to separate the tumor capsule from the hypothalamus and follow the nodular projection into the right lateral ventricle and remove it. Evacuation of the intrasellar and right parasellar portions of the tumor at the tentorial margin completed the ablative part of the procedure. The skull base dura was intact, so grafting was unnecessary. The patient tolerated this major operation well and was moved to a rehabilitation center for further medical treatment.

Case Report. Recurrence of an extensive para- and suprasellar pituitary adenoma (Fig. MS 29a–d). A 56-year-old woman was referred to us with a giant recurrence of a pituitary adenoma. She had undergone an initial operation six years previously but still suffered from bilateral dyskinesia, pituitary hypofunction, and a bitemporal hemianopsia that had not improved after the initial surgery.

CT scans demonstrated a very large parasellar mass extending upward into both lateral ventricles and compressing the third ventricle.

The angiogram showed displacement and encasement of the right internal carotid artery and its bifurcation. The tumor was approached surgically through a bifrontal craniotomy. The parasellar part of the lesion compressed the cavernous sinus and right optic nerve. The supraclinoid portion of the internal carotid artery and its bifurcation were completely embedded in tumor, as the angiogram had indicated. The superior part of the tumor had extended through the frontal lobe into both lateral ventricles. It projected backward to the third ventricle.

To avoid injury to surrounding structures, the origin of the supraclinoid portion of the internal carotid artery was identified as a landmark and followed while progressively removing tumor. After exposing the carotid bifurcation, we were able to resect the tumor surrounding the anterior and middle cerebral arteries while sparing the perforating arteries. Next the tumor was resected in front of the lamina terminalis, entering the third ventricle. Finally the nodular extensions into the lateral ventricles were removed. Postoperative course was uncomplicated, and the patient no longer manifested neurologic symptoms. Postoperative CT scans confirmed total removal of the adenoma.

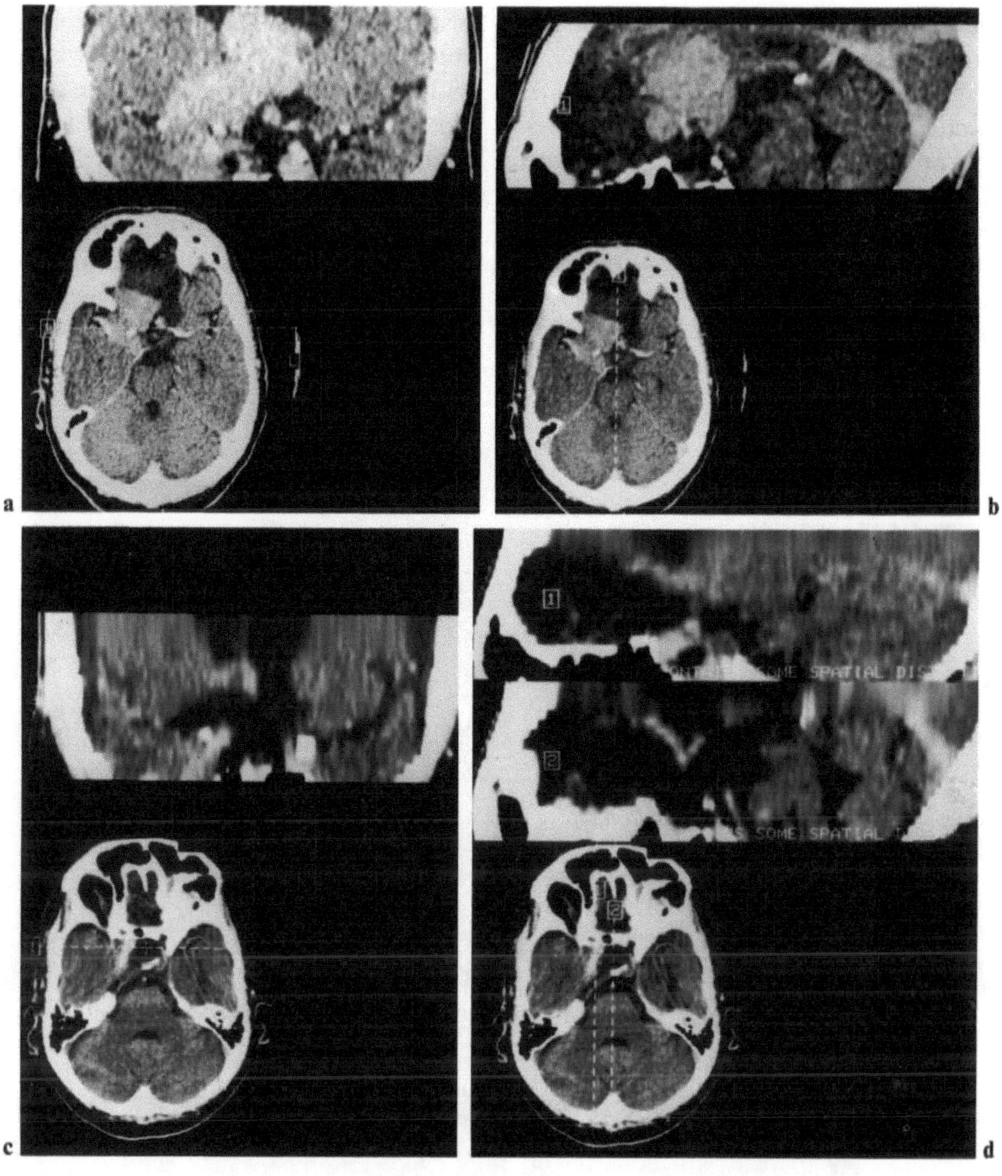

Fig. MS 29a–d. Extensive para- and suprasellar adenoma of the pituitary with invasion of both lateral ventricles and compression of the third ventricle, before and after operation.

a, b Axial CT scans in coronal and sagittal reconstruction, showing considerable para- and suprasellar tumor extension, bilateral invasion of the lateral ventricles, and compression of the third ventricle.
c, d Postoperative CT scans after complete tumor removal

Comments: The unusual feature of this extremely large recurrence of a pituitary adenoma was that the tumor had spread transfrontally into the lateral ventricles and had enveloped the neurovascular structures without displacing them. The surgical strategy in these cases is to locate all involved neurovascular structures in an area where they are not obscured by tumor. From that point dissection is continued along the structures while the tumor is progressively removed.

Case Report. Craniopharyngioma with invasion of the third ventricle and obstructive hydrocephalus (Fig. MS 30a–e). A 9-year-old girl with headache and diminished visual acuity was referred for ophthalmologic evaluation, which disclosed a central scotoma of the left eye. Acuity in the right eye was considerably decreased, only light perception was possible. Examination of the fundus disclosed bilateral optic atrophy. CT scans showed a large, suprasellar, cystic mass with a smaller solid component, which, considering the patient's age, was consistent with a craniopharyngioma. The tumor completely filled the third ventricle and had produced hydrocephalus by obstruction of the foramen of Monro. A ventriculoatrial shunt was inserted to relieve the hydrocephalus, and the patient's level of consciousness improved. Two weeks later operative removal was performed through a bifrontal osteoplastic craniotomy.

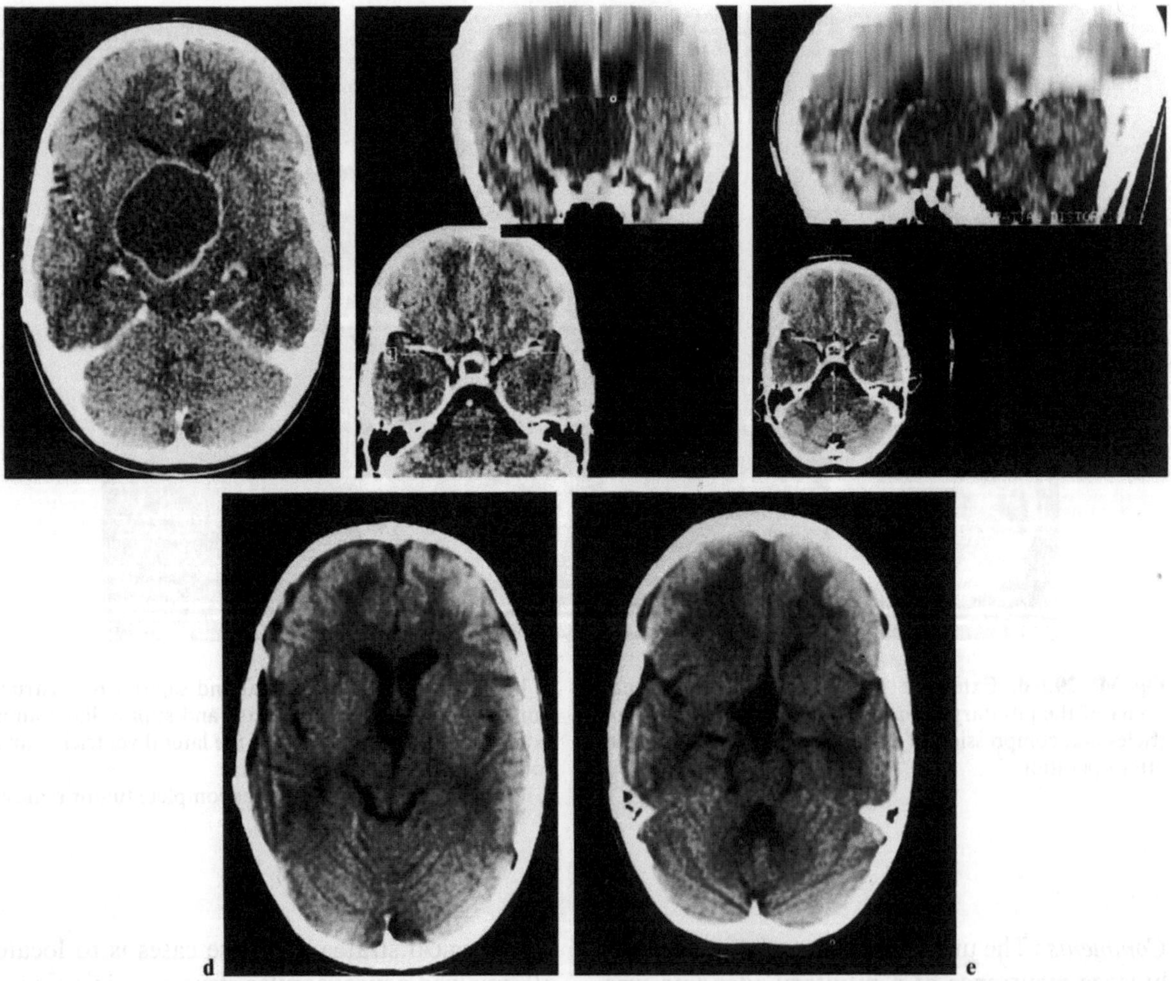

a, b c d e

Fig. MS 30a–e. Large suprasellar craniopharyngioma with invasion of the third ventricle and obstructive hydrocephalus, before and after operation.
a–c Axial CT scans in coronal and sagittal reconstruction following a shunt procedure for obstructive hydrocephalus show the giant tumor and its relations to the third ventricle, lateral ventricles, interpeduncular fossa, and pons. The tumor compresses the temporal lobes laterally on both sides.
d, e Postoperative CT scans confirm complete tumor removal

The anterior pole of the tumor was exposed, tapped, and cystic fluid was aspirated. Then the tumor capsule was progressively separated from both optic nerves and the internal carotid arteries. The bulk of the capsule and tumor could be removed below the optic chiasm. Pathological tissue still remained behind the chiasm and third ventricle, so the ventricle was entered through the lamina terminalis, and the last vestige of tumor was removed. At the end of the procedure we had a clear view of the pons and interpeduncular fossa and of the basilar artery and its branches. Transient symptoms of diabetes mellitus and diabetes insipidus developed in the early postoperative period, and the patient remained somnolent for three days. By five weeks her general condition was very good and she was discharged home, although her visual acuity did not improve. Postoperative CT scans confirmed total removal.

References

Angell J (1969) Transsphenoidal hypophysectomy. In: Hamburger CA, Wersäll J (Ed) Disorders of the skullbase region Almquist & Wiksell, Stockholm, p 163–169

Atkinson AB, Allen IV, Gordon DS, Hadden DR, Maguire CJF, Trimble ER, Lyons AR (1979) Progressive visual failure in acromegaly following external pituitary irradiation. Clinical Endocrinology 10:469–479

Bateman GH (1962) Transsphenoidal hypophysectomy. J Laryng 76:442

Burian K (1969) Die Hypophysektomie aus der Sicht des Rhinologen. HNO 17:193

Burian K, Beringer A, Ellegast H, Frischauf H (1961) Technik, Indikation und Erfahrungen bei partieller Hypophysen-Ausschaltung. Laryng Rhinol Otol (Stuttg) 40:186

Burian K, Pendl G, Salah S (1970) Über die Rezidivhäufigkeit von Hypophysenadenomen nach transfrontaler, transsphenoidaler oder zweizeitig kombinierter Operation. Wie Med Wochenschr 120:833–836

Chiari O (1912) Über eine Modifikation der Schlofferschen Operation von Tumoren der Hypophyse. Klin Wschr Wien 25:5

Cushing H (1912) The pituitary body and its disorders. Lippicott, Philadelphia London

Dandy WE (1938) Hirnchirurgie. Barth, Leipzig

Denker A (1921) Drei Fälle (von Hypophysentumoren) operiert nach transmaxillärer Methode. Int Zbl Laryng 37:225

von Eiselsberg A (1907) Über operative Freilegung der Tumoren in der Hypophysengegend. Neurol Zbl 26:994

von Eiselsberg A (1912) Zur Operation der Hypophysisgeschwülste Langenbecks. Arch Klin Chir 100:8

Escher F (1965) Resultate und Erfahrungen mit der Hypophysenausschaltung. Fortschr Hals Nas Ohrenheilk 12:129–160

Fahlbusch R, Rjosk HK, Werder KV (1978) Operative Treatment of Prolactin-Producing Adenoms. In: Fahlbusch R, Werder KV (Ed) Treatment of pituitary Adenomas. Georg Thieme, Stuttgart 225–237

Fein J (1910) Zur Operation der Hypophyse Wien Klin Wschr 23:1035

Guiot G (1958) Adenom hypophysaires. Masson, Paris

Guiot G (1973) Transphenoidal approach in surgical treatment of pituitary adenomas: general principles and inolisations in non functioning andemonas – Excerpta Medica. International Congress Series No 303, p 159–178

Guiot G, Derome P (1976) Surgical problems of Pituitary Adenoms. In: Advances and Technical Standards in Neurosurgery Vol III. Springer, Wien New York

Guiot G, Bouche J, Oppotu A (1967) Les indicationes de l'ahord transsphenoidal des adenoms hypophysaires. Press med 75:1563

Guleke N (1950) Die Eingriffe am Gehirnschädel, Gehirn, an der Wirbelsäule und am Rückenmark. 2. Aufl Springer, Berlin Göttingen Heidelberg, p 335

Halstead AE (1910) Remarks on the operative treatment of tumors of the hypophysis. Report of two cases operated only an oronasal method. Surg Gynec Obstet 10:494–502

Hamburger CA, Hammer G (1964) Der transnasale Weg der Hypophysektomie. In: Berendes J, Link R, Zöllner F Hals Nasen Ohren Heilkunde 1. Aufl Bd I Thieme S 795–818

Hamburger CA, Hammer G, Noorlen G, Sjogren B (1961) Transsphenoidal hypophysertony. Arch Otolaringol 74:2–8

Hardy J (1969) Transsphenoidal microsurgery of the normal and pathologic pituitary. Clin Neurosurg 16:185

Hardy J (1973) Transsphenoidal surgery of hypersecreting pituitary tumors. ed by Kohler PO, Ross GT Excerpta Med Amsterdam American Elsevier New York

Hardy J (1975) Transsphenoidal microsurgical removal of pituitary micro-adenoma. In: Progr neurol Surg Karger Basel 6:200

Hirsch O (1909) Eine neue Methode der endonasalen Operation von Hypophysentumoren. Wie med Wschr 636

Horsley V (1906) On the technique of operation on the central nervous system. Brit med J II:411–423

König F (1900) quoted from Guleke (1950) Die Eingriffe am Gehirnschädel, Gehirn, an der Wirbelsäule und am Rückenmark. In: Guleke N, Zenker R (Hrsg) Allgemeine und spezielle chirurgische Operationslehre. 2nd Ed. Vol 2 p 335. Springer, Berlin Göttingen Heidelberg

Krause T (1905) Hirnchirurgie (Freilegung der Hypophyse). Dtsch Klin 8:1004–1012

Lawrence AM, Pinsky SM, Goldfine ED (1971) Conventional radiation therapy in acromegaly Arch Intern Med 128:369–377

Lehnhardt E (1979) Septum-Schleimhautplastik zur Dauerdrainage der Keilbeinhöhle. Arch Otolaryngol 222:43–46

Löwe L (1905) quoted from Guleke (1950) Die Eingriffe am Gehirnschädel, Gehirn, an der Wirbelsäule und am Rückenmark. In: Guleke N, Zenker R (Hrsg) Allgemeine und spezielle chirurgische Operationslehre 2nd. Ed. Vol 2, p 335. Springer, Berlin Göttingen Heidelberg

Lüdecke DK, Niedworok G (1985) Results of Microsurgery in Cushing's Disease and Effect on Hypertension. Cardiology 72 (Suppl 1):91–94

Lüdecke DK, Brenstedt HJ, Brömswig J (1982) Evaluation of surgically treated Nelson's Syndrome. Acta Neurochirurgica 65:3–13

Lüdecke DK, Herrmann HD, Hörmann K (1983) Comparison of effects of Dopamine Agonist and microsurgeries in GH and PRL serreting adenomas. In: Cain DB (Ed) Liseride and other Dopamine Agonists. Raven Press, New York, pp 271–289

Nager FR (1940) The paranasal approach to intrasellar tumors. Semon Lecture 1939 J Laryng 55:361

Nicola G (1972) Transsphenoidal surgery for pituitary adenomas with extrasellar extension. In: Progress in Neurological Surgery Vol VI. Karger, Basel

Pieterse ST, Dinning TAR, Blumbergs PC (1982) Postirradiation sarcomatous transformation of a pituitary adenoma: a combined pituitary tumor J Neurosurg 56:783–787

Preysing (1913) Beiträge zur Operation der Hypophyse. Verh dtsch Laryng 20:51

Raskind R (1977) Central nervous system damage after radiation therapy. International Surgery 48:430–441

Schloffer H (1907) Zur Frage der Operation an der Hypophyse. Beitr Klin Chir 50:767

Suzuki S, Yashimoto T, Mizoi K (1981) Preservation of the olfactory tract following operation on anterior communicating artery aneurysm using bifrontal craniotomy and its functional prognosiș. In: Samii M, Jannetta PJ (Ed) The cranial nerves. 59–65 Springer, Berlin Heidelberg New York

Tiefenthal (1920) Technik der Hypophysenoperation. Münch Med Wschr 67:794

Uffenorde W (1923) Orbitale Stirnhöhlenoperation. Z Hals-Nas-Ohren-Heilk 6:117

Surgery of Space-Occupying Lesions of the Lateral Middle Skull Base

Introductory Remarks. Whereas the inside of the skull base is very clearly divided into the anterior, middle, and posterior fossae by the lesser sphenoid wing and anterior border of the petrous pyramid, this subdivision is not so apparent when the skull base is viewed from below. It is fairly common for tumors of the middle skull base to spread to involve the anterior as well as the posterior skull base. This fact must be kept in mind when determining the extent of these neoplasms by clinical and radiologic investigations.

Malignant or benign tumors of the middle skull base, infratemporal fossa, and petrous pyramid can attain considerable size before producing *clinical* manifestations. If the bulk of the tumor is in the infratemporal fossa and pterygoid fossa, it can produce fullness on one side of the face, chewing difficulties due to infiltration of the masticatory muscles, headache due to trigeminal nerve irritation, and orbital symptoms. With involvement of the maxillary sinus, X-rays will show a more or less pronounced opacity: the tumor may extend into the nasopharynx and oropharynx, creating the impression of a tumor primarily originating.

If the tumor is localized farther posteriorly in the region of the petrous pyramid, the symptoms depend largely on the involvement of the cranial nerves located there. With involvement of the jugular foramen, vocal cord paralysis may occur as the initial symptom. Thus, when recurrent laryngeal nerve palsy is noted, the course of the vagus nerve should be checked not only in the mediastinum and thyroid gland but also in the region of the skull base. Swallowing difficulties can result from irritation of the glossopharyngeal nerve and vagus nerve. Tumor infiltration of the accessory nerve is manifested by limitation of shoulder motion. Hearing loss, tinnitus, and vertigo are symptoms of a vestibulocochlear nerve lesion, or they may signify tumor involvement of the cochlea and semicircular canals, internal auditory canal, or cerebellopontine angle. Facial paralysis is uncommon but can occur in association with malignancies of the parotid gland and tumors of the facial nerve itself or of its surrounding structures, especially the pyramidal portion of the bony fallopian canal.

If the bulk of the skull base tumor is intracranial, it may produce a mass lesion in the temporal lobe with corresponding neurologic deficits. With medial tumor growth toward the tentorial incisure, the following clinical signs can occur: visual field defect from compression of the optic nerve, oculomotor palsy (nerves III, IV, VI), trigeminal nerve irritation with areas of facial hypo- or anesthesia, and facial pain. If the tumor penetrates the surface of the petrous pyramid or invades the infratentorial space through the tentorial incisure, cranial nerves VII and VIII may additionally be affected. If further tumor growth produces compression of the brain stem, contralateral pyramidal tract disturbances can arise with signs of hemiparesis. Compressive occlusion of the internal carotid artery develops gradually over a period of years and usually remains clinically silent. In our experience, a general rise of intracranial pressure with papilledema and obstructive hydrocephalus is rarely if ever observed even in connection with very large tumors of this region.

Besides conventional radiologic imaging procedures such as survey films, tomography, angiography, and cranial isotope scans, computed tomography (CT) and magnetic resonance imaging (MRI) have greatly enhanced our ability to determine the extent of space-occupying lesions in this region. These modalities have largely eliminated the need for invasive diagnostic procedures such as pneumoencephalography (Samii 1974) and ventriculography. But despite success in determining the extent of lesions, it usually is not possible to establish the presence and extent of dural infiltration with techniques currently available. Preoperatively, then, it is usually unclear how much of the dura will have to be resected. Cases of this kind should be discussed jointly by the neurosurgeon and ENT surgeon so that they can properly assist and support each other during the operation.

Benign tumors are removed at the earliest opportunity, using either a transcranial intradural approach or a primary extradural approach depending on the principal site of the tumor. Because the use of microsurgical techniques has greatly reduced the frequency and severity of iatrogenic injuries, it is unwise to wait for an initially small lesion to attain a greater size. The functional results of the operation are best when the lesion has caused minimal destruction. Also, cranial neuropathies that develop with further tumor growth have less chance of functional regression, even if the nervous structures can be preserved at operation (Neely 1979).

The surgical resection of *malignancies* is appropriate only if a complete removal seems feasible. We are against mutilating resections that not only are pointless from an oncologic viewpoint but also introduce risks of complications (Fig. MS 31).

The *operative strategy* depends on the nature of the tumor. A preoperative histologic diagnosis should be obtained if at all possible. With a deeply situated intracranial neoplasm, stereotaxic needle biopsy can be used to establish the histology of the lesion. The combination of macrosurgical and microsurgical techniques has proven an effective means of preserving important structures such as the internal carotid artery, the cranial nerves, and the inner ear.

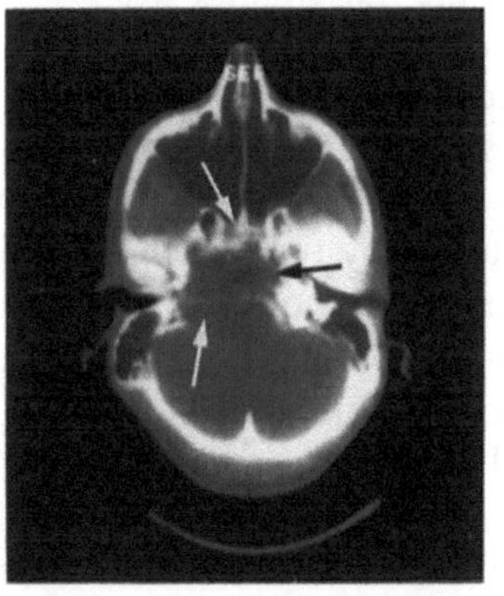

Fig. MS 31. Very extensive, predominantly left-sided chordoma of the middle skull base with extension across the midline (*arrows*) in a 23-year-old man. The disease is too extensive for surgical resection

General Operative Techniques

Extracranial Lateral Approach to the Middle Skull Base (Temporal and Infratemporal Fossae)

Introductory Remarks. Wide access to the lateral aspect of the middle skull base can be gained through this approach following removal of the zygomatic arch and, if necessary, partial mandibulectomy (Attenborough 1980; Braeucker, quoted in Guleke 1959; Denecke 1970; Zehm 1970). The maxillofacial surgeon Obwegeser (1985) uses this approach for the removal of lesions of the temporomandibular joint, the orbit, and the retromaxillary space. We agree with him that this technique 1) provides excellent exposure with a minimal scar and 2) allows optimum preservation of the temporomandibular joint. It is indicated for tumors that encroach upon the middle skull base from below, where the main tumor mass is located in the temporal or infratemporal fossa.

Operative Technique
(Fig. MS 32a, b)

The skin incision is shown in Fig. AS 32a. The coronal incision across the midline starts horizontally along the frontal hairline and curves downward behind the temporal hairline, passing in front of the auricle and around the lobule of the ear down to the anterior border of the sternocleidomastoid muscle.

When the skin flap is developed, the temporal muscle may be left attached to it if the muscle is not infiltrated by tumor. This avoids trauma to the frontal branch of the facial nerve. Otherwise the temporal muscle is included in the en-bloc tumor resection. The zygomatic arch is osteotomized at its root and is turned downward, leaving it attached to the masseter muscle, which is released from the lateral aspect of the vertical ramus of the mandible. Once the vertical ramus has been adequately exposed, it may be marginally resected behind the coronoid process, removing only the condyle, or it may suffice to perform a temporary mandibulotomy. The parotid gland with the facial nerve branches may be retracted posteriorly, leaving it on the lobule, or if necessary it is completely removed while preserving the facial nerve branches. This approach gives exposure of the lateral plate of the pterygoid process, the maxillary artery, and the lateral wall of the maxillary sinus. The skull base may be exposed to the lateral wall of the nasopharynx or even as far as the clivus if necessary, providing wide exposure of the lesion.

The surgeon can now proceed with the tumor resection at the bony skull base, removing the dura as required and repairing the defect by duraplasty. Wound closure and reconstruction are performed from within outward. The mandible, if temporarily osteotomized, is reapproximated and fixed with a wire or plate. Before the skin flap is replaced, the zygomatic arch also may be wired back into position to achieve an optimum cosmetic result. The wound is closed in layers over a suction drain.

Fig. MS 32a, b. The lateral extracranial approach to the lateral middle skull base (temporal and infratemporal fossae).
a Possibilities for resection or osteotomy of the vertical ramus of the mandible. Resection of the mandibular condyle (*dark*), wide marginal mandibulectomy including the condyle (*dark* and *light gray*), fenestration of the posterior border of the vertical ramus (...), and temporary transverse osteotomy (— — —).
b The scalp and facial soft-tissue flap is prepared, and the temporal muscle is temporarily released from its insertion. Marginal mandibulectomy is performed with inclusion of the condyle. The parotid gland is removed, exposing the facial nerve in the lower part of the wound. The zygomatic arch is turned downward on the masseter muscle. At this stage there is free access to the infratemporal fossa and pterygoid fossa. Important landmarks are the mandibular nerve and the lateral plate of the pterygoid process. Bone is removed from the anterior border of the clivus with the cutting burr, partially exposing the dura of the medio-lateral skull base. The lateral pharyngeal wall is visible anterior to the clivus. At the end of the procedure the zygomatic arch is wired back into place, and the facial soft tissues are restored (see Fig. AS 23g)

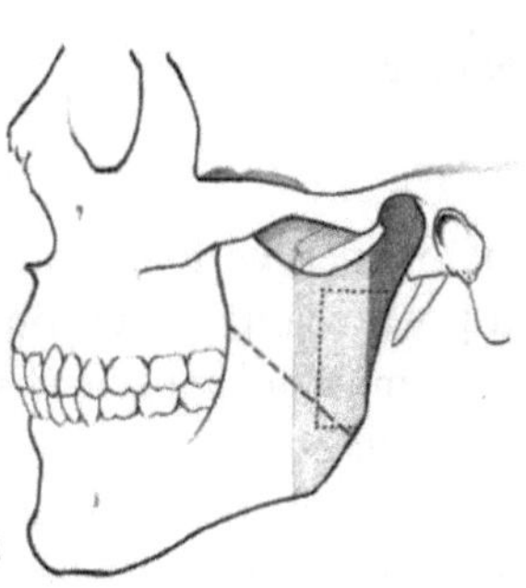

a

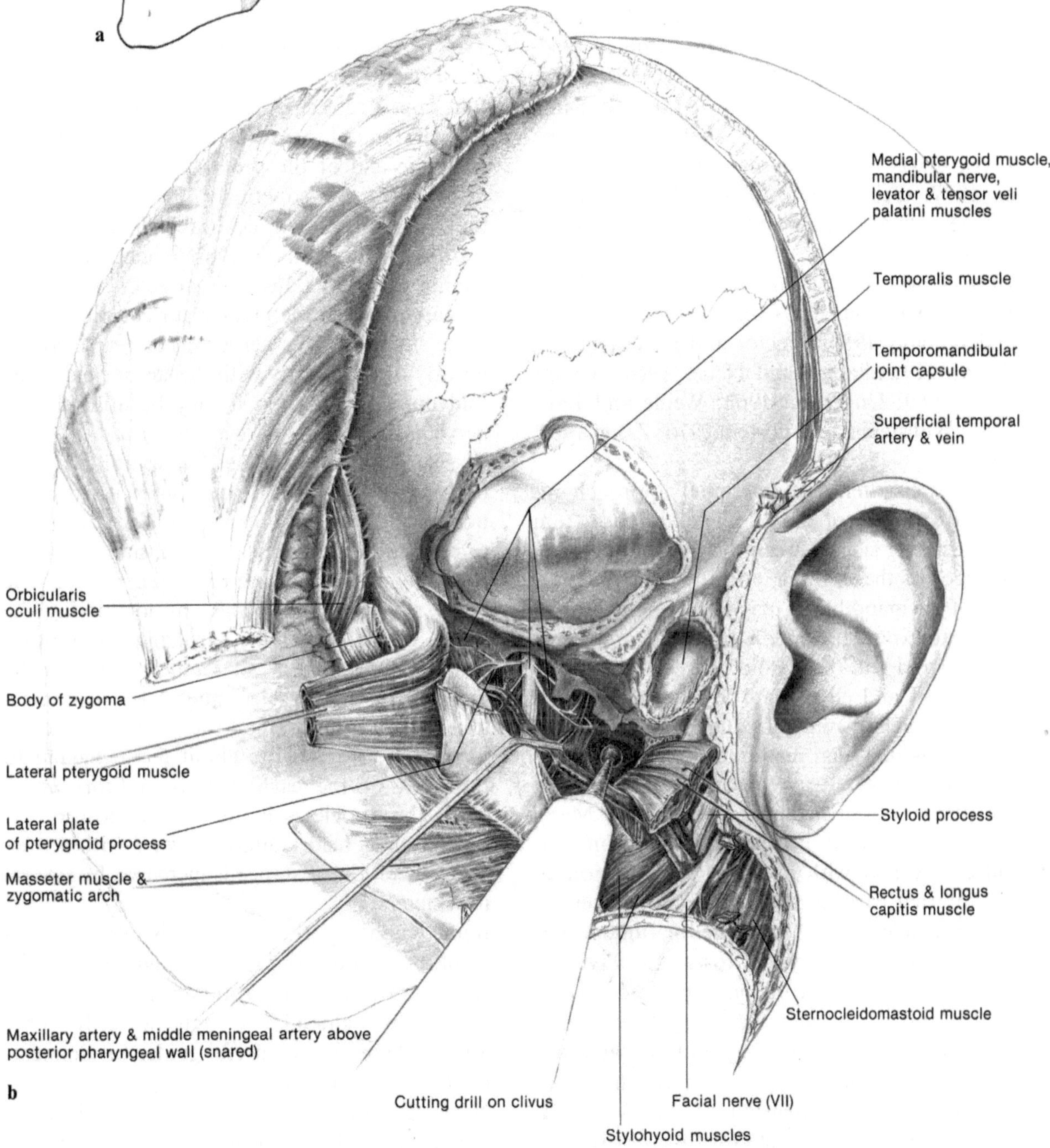
Medial pterygoid muscle, mandibular nerve, levator & tensor veli palatini muscles
Temporalis muscle
Temporomandibular joint capsule
Superficial temporal artery & vein
Orbicularis oculi muscle
Body of zygoma
Lateral pterygoid muscle
Lateral plate of pterygnoid process
Masseter muscle & zygomatic arch
Styloid process
Rectus & longus capitis muscle
Sternocleidomastoid muscle
Maxillary artery & middle meningeal artery above posterior pharyngeal wall (snared)
Cutting drill on clivus
Facial nerve (VII)
Stylohyoid muscles

b

Extracranial Posteroinferior Approach to the Middle Skull Base (Carotid Canal, Jugular Foramen)

Introductory Remarks. Extracranial approaches to the posterior portion of the middle skull base have been described in numerous publications (Arena 1974, 1976; Champy et al. 1964; Coleman 1966; Columella et al. 1957; Conley 1964; Conley and Novack 1960; Denecke 1959/1960, 1966, 1969 a/b, 1970, 1978; Draf and Samii 1977, 1982; Fisch 1977 a/b, 1979, 1983; Gacek 1976; Gacek and Goodman 1977; Gardner et al. 1977; Gejrot 1965; Glasscock et al. 1974; Grunert 1894; Hilding and Selker 1969; Hilding and Greenberg 1971; Hunt 1961; Kempe et al. 1971; Lewis et al. 1966; Meacham and Capps 1960; Michelson and Conolly 1962; Mischke and Balbany 1980; Proctor and Lindsay 1947; Rehn 1919; Shapiro and Neues 1964; Thoms et al. 1960; Ungerecht 1963; Weille and Lane 1951; Wullstein and Wullstein 1976; Zehm 1969, 1970).

The posteroinferior extracranial approach involves exposure of the middle skull base from the posterior side between the mastoid process, the root of the zygoma, and the condylar process of the mandible. It may additionally be necessary to expose the middle ear cavity and resect the mastoid and the styloid process. The pterygoid fossa and clivus can be reached through this approach by removing the mandibular condyle or by marginal mandibulectomy. This approach is indicated for tumors in the region of the jugular foramen and carotid canal. Many of these lesions can be reached without mandibulectomy and with excellent visualization of the internal carotid artery and cranial nerves. The principle of this technique for tumors that spread from the pterygoid fossa and clivus to involve the auditory canal and mastoid process is also applied in extensive benign and malignant tumors of the parotid gland and auditory canal. An advantage of this approach is that it readily permits extension of the skull base resection back to the posterior fossa for tumors occurring at the junction of the middle and posterior fossae.

Operative Technique
(Fig. MS 33a–h)

The skin may be opened with an anteriorly concave, C-shaped postauricular incision extending to the sternocleidomastoid muscle (Fisch 1983). Alternatively, a Y-shaped incision with pre- and postauricular limbs may be employed (Conley 1964; Wullstein and Wullstein 1976). The latter incision creates a superiorly based auricular flap that can be retracted upward. If portions of the temporal muscle are to be used as filling material at the end of the procedure, the incision is extended farther superiorly. The lower limb of the Y incision extends a variable distance downward, depending on the tumor extent. When dissecting the skin flaps, the surgeon should try at least to spare the greater auricular nerve. In some situations this nerve can be retracted anteriorly or posteriorly with the sternocleidomastoid muscle; in others it may be utilized as a nerve graft.

The surgeon now isolates the anterior border of the sternocleidomastoid muscle with its insertion on the mastoid tip and mobilizes the inferior pole of the parotid gland, exposing the posterior belly of the digastric (biventer) muscle. The facial nerve can be located by identifying the sharp, medial tip of the cartilaginous auditory canal (the "pointer" of Conley 1975) at the junction of the digastric and sternocleidomastoid muscle insertions on the mastoid. The stylomastoid foramen lies about 5 mm medial to the apex of the cartilaginous auditory canal when the auricle is in its normal position. If the auricle is held laterally upward with a traction suture, this distance is increased by several millimeters.

Immediately *before* the tumor is exposed, it is helpful to expose the internal jugular vein, the common or internal carotid artery, and the accessory, hypoglossal, and vagus nerves from below, as these provide useful guides for delineating the tumor inferiorly.

Next the sternocleidomastoid and digastric muscles are released from the mastoid and the mastoid tip is resected, depending on the posterior and medial extents of the neoplasm. The digastric muscle is reflected anteriorly down-

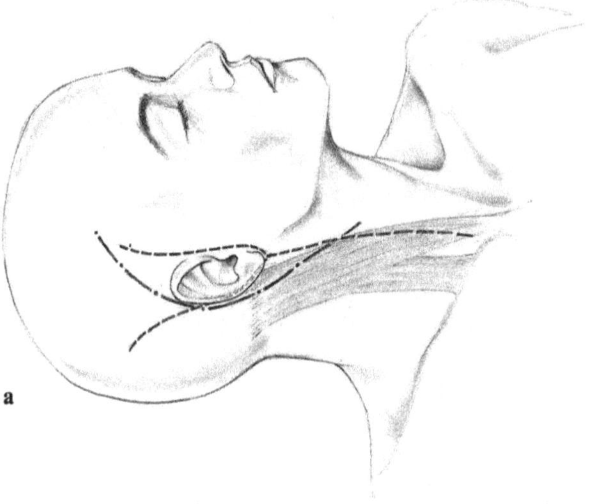

a

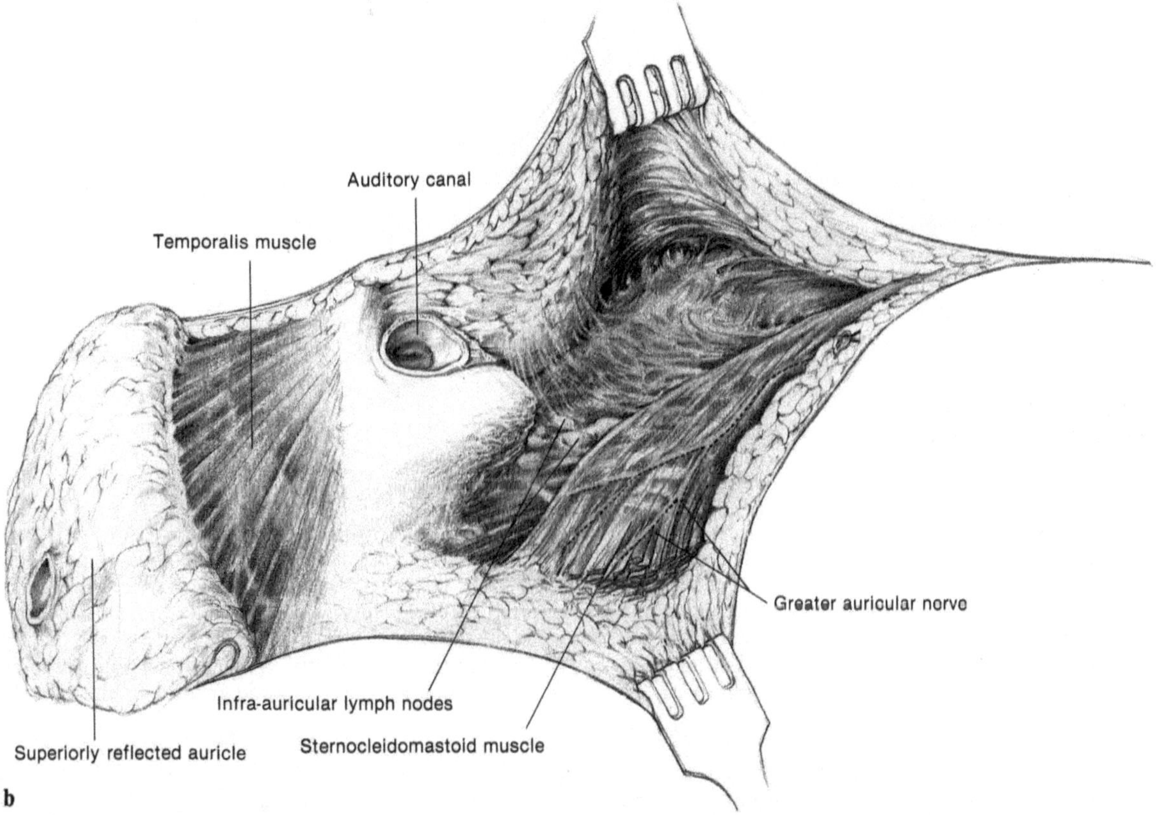

b

Fig. MS 33a–h. The extracranial posteroinferior approach to the posterior part of the lateral middle skull base.
a Possible skin incisions: Y-shaped incision (– – –), C-shaped incision of Fisch (*dots and dashes*).
b With the Y incision, the auricle is reflected upward to expose the mastoid plane and mastoid tip, the anterior sternocleidomastoid border, and the inferior part of the parotid gland. Here the sternocleidomastoid muscle has been released from the mastoid tip and turned inferiorly, preserving its cutaneous attachment. A transparent view is given of the greater auricular nerve and its branches. Where necessary, the greater auricular may be utilized as a nerve graft

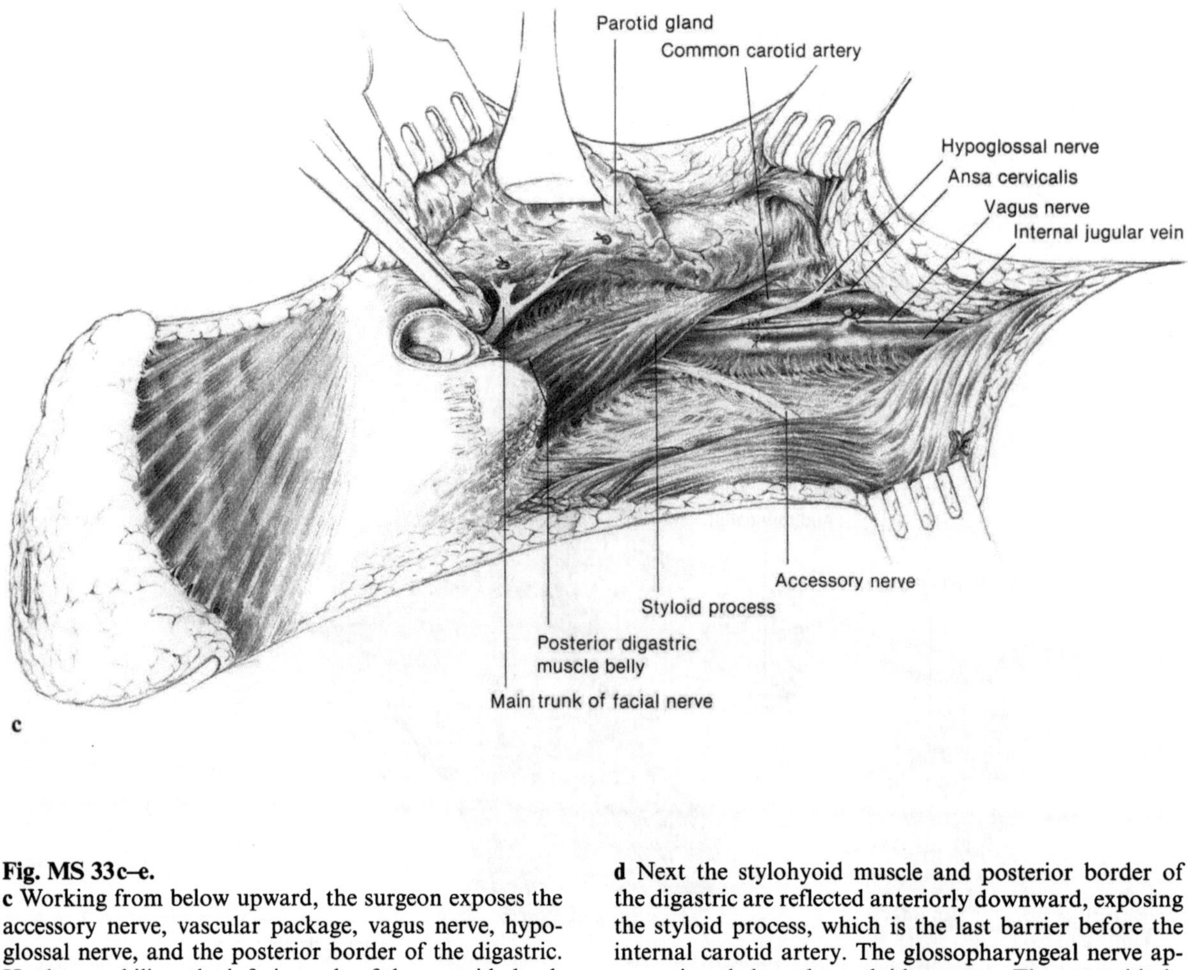

Fig. MS 33c–e.
c Working from below upward, the surgeon exposes the accessory nerve, vascular package, vagus nerve, hypoglossal nerve, and the posterior border of the digastric. He then mobilizes the inferior pole of the parotid gland. The medial point of the cartilaginous external auditory canal and the anterior border of the insertion of the sternocleidomastoid and posterior digastric muscle border serve as landmarks for locating the facial nerve. The stylomastoid foramen lies about 5 mm medial to the cartilaginous point of the auditory canal when the auricle is in its normal position. The connective tissue fibers between the cartilaginous ear canal and the parotid capsule are cleared over a wide area. The final warning sign before reaching the facial nerve is bleeding from a large arterial vessel that passes just lateral to the nerve.
d Next the stylohyoid muscle and posterior border of the digastric are reflected anteriorly downward, exposing the styloid process, which is the last barrier before the internal carotid artery. The glossopharyngeal nerve appears just below the styloid process. The mastoid tip is osteotomized at this time. The stylomastoid foramen is located slightly posterior and medial to the base of the styloid process.
e Possibilities for extension of the posteroinferior approach by removal of the mastoid and styloid process and marginal mandibulectomy (*shaded areas* and *dashed line*).

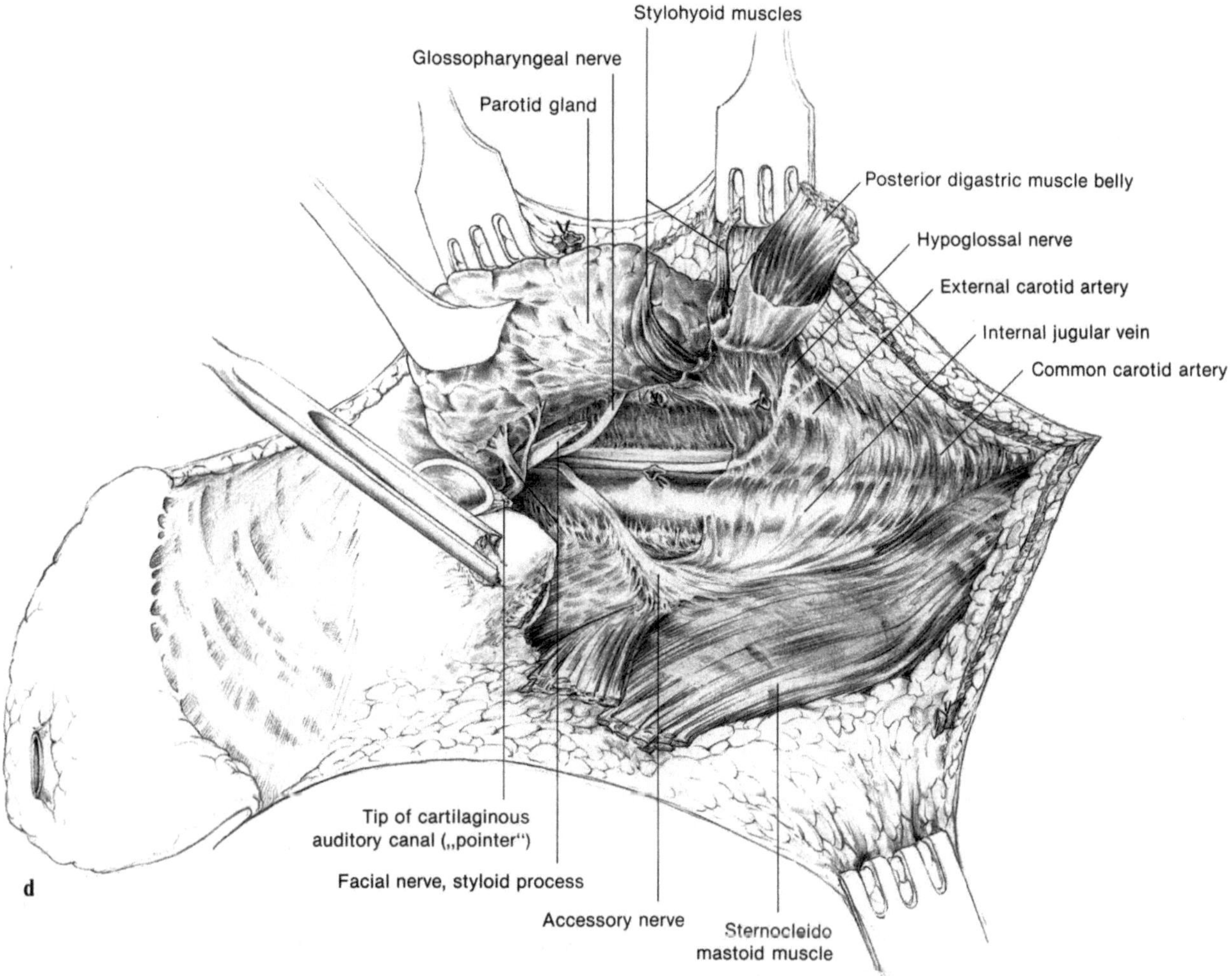
Stylohyoid muscles
Glossopharyngeal nerve
Parotid gland
Posterior digastric muscle belly
Hypoglossal nerve
External carotid artery
Internal jugular vein
Common carotid artery
Tip of cartilaginous auditory canal („pointer")
Facial nerve, styloid process
Accessory nerve
Sternocleido mastoid muscle

d

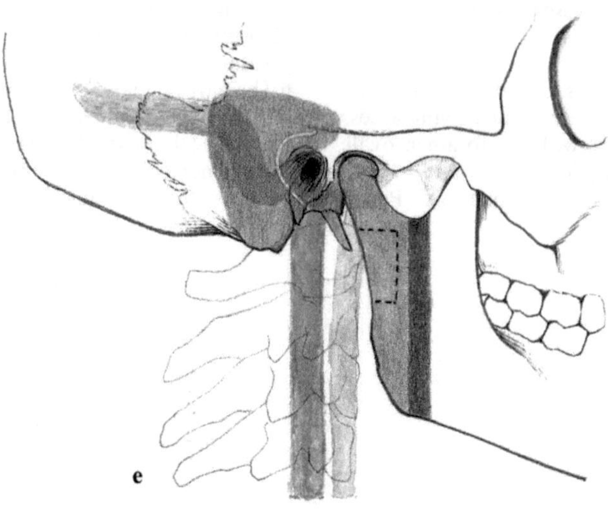

e

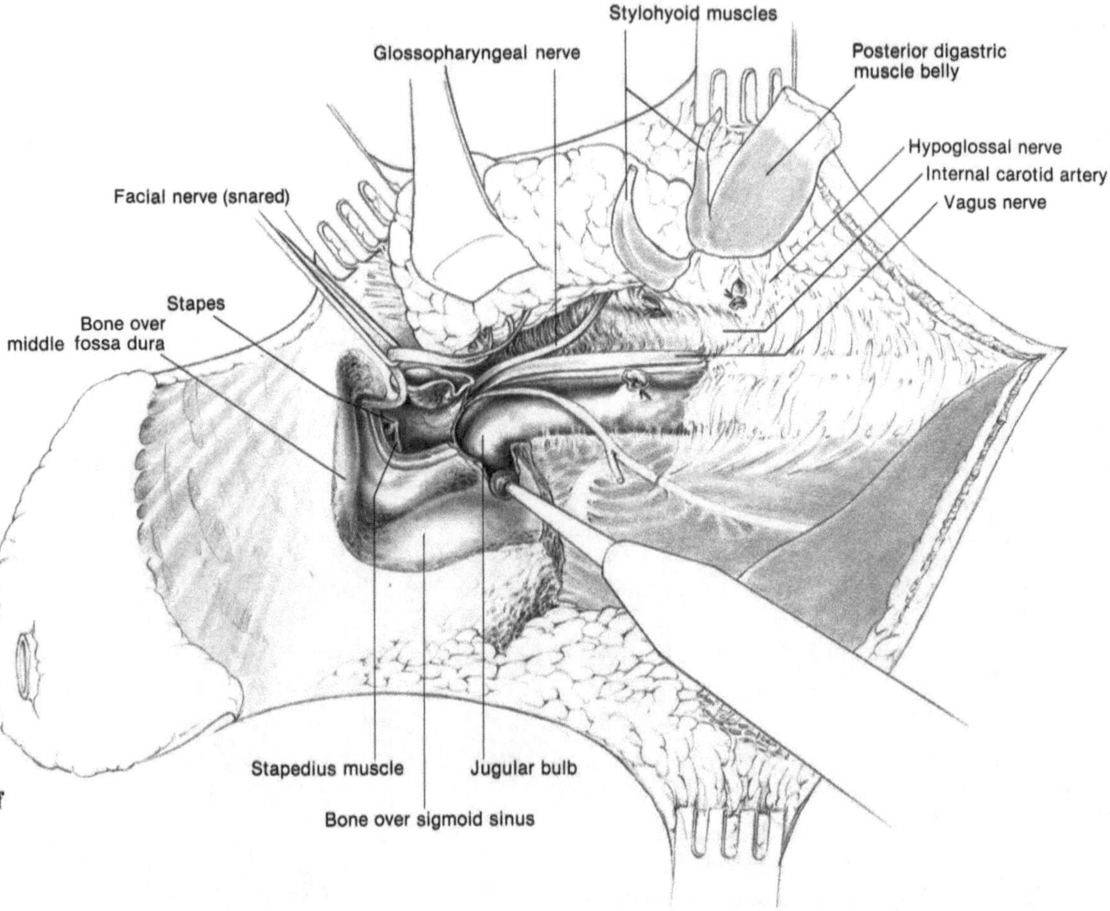

f

Fig. MS 33f–h.

f Most of the mastoid has been removed to expose the jugular bulb and posterior wall of the auditory canal. The tympanic and mastoid portion of the facial nerve has been mobilized from its bony canal and retracted anteriorly (Fisch). The jugular bulb is further exposed with the cutting burr. The accessory nerve branch to the sternocleidomastoid muscle is sectioned, preserving the branch to the trapezius.

g The posteroinferior approach is extended by marginal resection of the vertical mandibular ramus, giving access to the lateral middle skull base with the foramen ovale and lateral plate of the pterygoid process, and also to the lateral pharyngeal wall and nasopharynx. Posteriorly, intracranial access can be gained by removing the dura of the posterior and middle fossae. The sigmoid sinus and internal jugular vein are ligated. The defect in the dura is repaired with a dural graft. The petrous bone is partially resected including the medial wall of the tympanic cavity, leaving the petrous apex intact. The opening of the eustachian tube is occluded with the incus after inverting the mucosa, and the stump of the external carotid artery is ligated.

h The parotid gland is restored to its bed, and a temporal muscle flap is rotated into the field to partially restore the surgical cavity. This is done when distal release of the sternocleidomastoid muscle from the sternum and clavicle is not available for cavity ablation

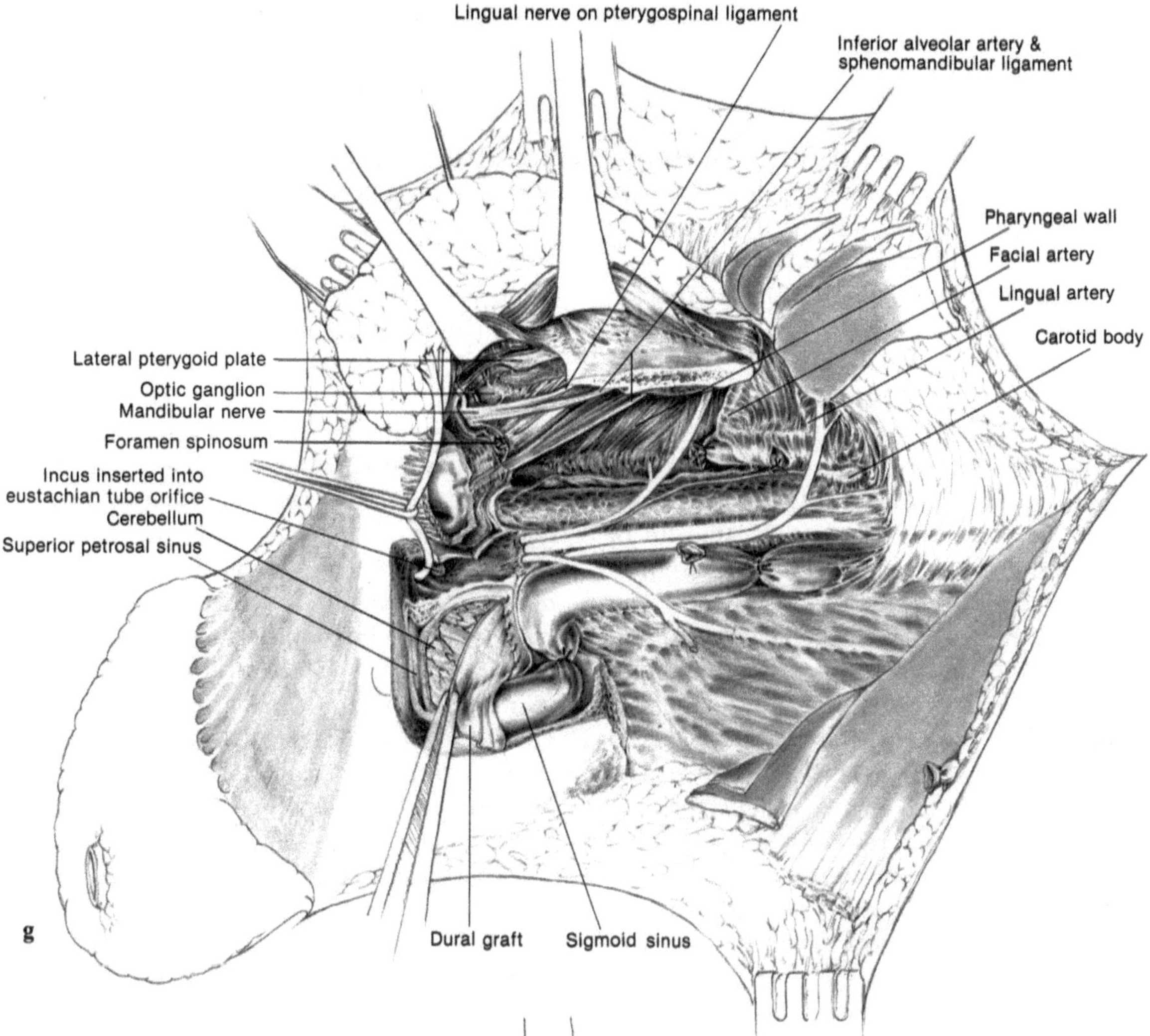

Lingual nerve on pterygospinal ligament
Inferior alveolar artery & sphenomandibular ligament
Pharyngeal wall
Facial artery
Lingual artery
Carotid body
Lateral pterygoid plate
Optic ganglion
Mandibular nerve
Foramen spinosum
Incus inserted into eustachian tube orifice
Cerebellum
Superior petrosal sinus
Dural graft
Sigmoid sinus

g

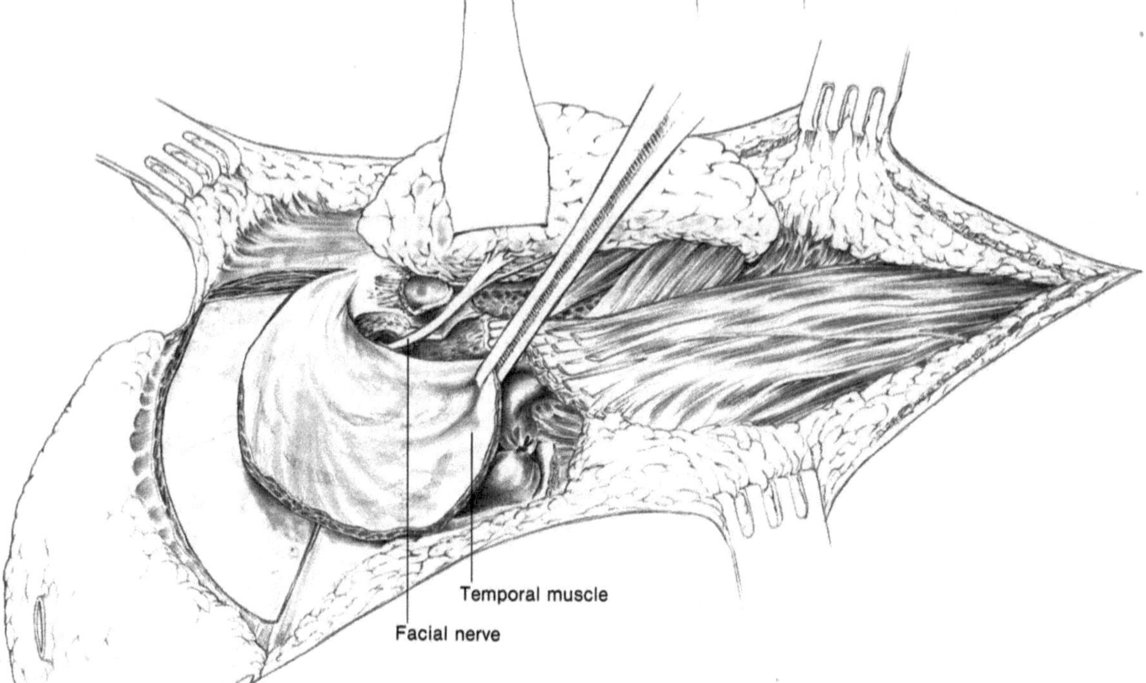

Temporal muscle
Facial nerve

h

ward, while the sternocleidomastoid muscle is retracted posteriorly, preserving its cutaneous attachment. Following the removal of extensive tumors, the sternocleidomastoid can be utilized as a superiorly based muscle flap, following a suggestion of Denecke (1966), for surgical cavity obliteration (see Fig. MS 42a–d). The temporal muscle can be similarly transposed following a neck dissection with resection of the sternocleidomastoid.

This approach can be extended medially by removing the styloid process after releasing and mobilizing the stylohyoid muscles (Fig. MS 33e).

If necessary, the approach to the jugular foramen can be facilitated by removing the tip of the mastoid process. Following a standard mastoidectomy with exposure of the bony fallopian canal, it can be determined whether and to what extent a middle skull base tumor has spread to involve the petrous pyramid. If the neoplasm has penetrated the petrous bone and reached the dura, the tumor is encompassed by exposing the sigmoid sinus and jugular bulb, including adjacent dura in the resection as necessary. Opening the inner ear, whether this is done through the mastoid or from the tympanic cavity, means functional loss of the ear and labyrinthine system and establishes a communication with the subarachnoid space. This should be done, therefore, only if necessary to ensure completeness of tumor removal.

The jugular vein and sigmoid sinus are ligated if more medial tumor extension is found in the infratemporal area or in the petrous bone itself. First it must be confirmed by angiography that adequate venous drainage exists on the contralateral side. Fisch (1977a) and ourselves prefer to apply silk ligatures after anterior and posterior incision of the dura. Following jugular vein ligation, the jugular bulb can be removed to expose cranial nerves IX to XI. Usually at this stage there is bleeding from the inferior petrosal sinus, which communicates with the jugular bulb, and this is controlled by packing the sinus with cellulose. Next the tumor is dissected away from the caudal cranial nerves using microsurgical technique. Even in patients with marked preoperative facial paralysis, satisfactory functional recovery is possible if the nerve was only compressed by the tumor and has been preserved. On the other hand, we have found that vocal cord paralysis related to a preexisting recurrent nerve palsy does not regress, even if vagus nerve continuity has been maintained.

The facial nerve can be transposed anteriorly by completely freeing the nerve from its bony canal as far as its entry into the internal auditory canal (Fisch 1977a; Fig. MS 33f). This enables the surgeon to spare the facial nerve while following tumor extensions along the internal carotid artery into the carotid canal as far as the carotid-cavernous sinus junction and removing them. The result is a subtotal petrosectomy with complete or partial resection of the bony eustachian tube. To avoid wound infection with the danger of meningitis, the eustachian tube should be occluded with bone paste, an ossicle, or a myofascial graft. The parotid gland is returned to its bed, and the surgical cavity is partially ablated with a temporal muscle rotation flap in cases where this cannot be done with a sternocleidomastoid flap detached from the sternum and clavicle.

The posteroinferior approach is extended by marginal resection of the *vertical ramus of the mandible* to gain access to tumor extending toward the infratemporal fossa. Following release of the masseter muscle, the posterior border of the vertical ramus is identified, and a window is cut into the bone beneath the condylar process with a burr or rongeur, sparing the mandibular nerve. If this measure is insufficient, the condylar process may be resected without serious compromise of masticatory function.

In our experience, it is often possible to expose the middle skull base up to the lateral pharyngeal wall and clivus without performing a mandibulectomy or mandibulotomy. A temporarily osteotomized mandible is subsequently repaired by internal fixation with a wire or plate.

Intracranial Extradural Approach to the Middle Skull Base

Introductory Remarks. Lesions of the middle skull base that are predominantly intracranial but have not penetrated the dura may be approached through a frontotemporal or temporal craniotomy or craniectomy. In this approach the middle skull base can be exposed epidurally from the lesser sphenoid wing to the posterior border of the pyramid. The transtemporal, extradural exposure of the anterior surface of the pyramid to gain access to the internal auditory canal represents a limited extradural exposure of the middle skull base.

Operative Technique
(Fig. MS 34a–d)

The craniotomy is oriented more anteriorly when the lesion is located below the lesser sphenoid wing in the area of the superior orbital fissure or in proximity to the anterior clinoid process. In this case the dura of the anterior and middle fossa is elevated from the margin of the lesser sphenoid wing. Following retraction of the frontal and temporal lobes, the lesser wing can be removed as far as the clinoid process and internal carotid artery, affording a superolateral view of the bony optic canal and lateral orbital wall.

In the anterior part of the middle fossa, dural elevation is limited in the anterior-to-posterior direction by the superior orbital fissure, the foramen rotundum, the foramen ovale, and the foramen spinosum if the structures traversing these openings are to be preserved. If necessary, the surgeon can elevate the dura as far as the internal carotid artery after dividing the maxillary and mandibular nerves and coagulating the middle meningeal artery. When dissecting along the anterior surface of the pyramid, it must be remembered that the greater petrosal nerve and geniculate ganglion may course immediately below the dura without bony protection. The gasserian ganglion is completely ensheathed by dura. As a rule, the extradural exposure is not carried beyond the superior petrosal sinus. After removal of the tumor, the craniotomy flap is replaced. Craniectomy defects are repaired with methylmethacrylate.

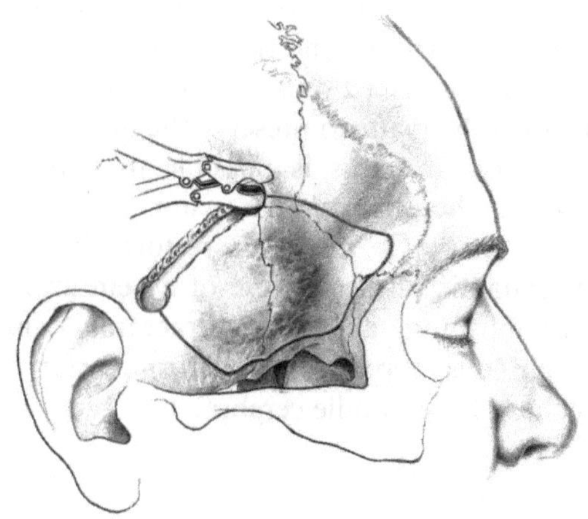
a

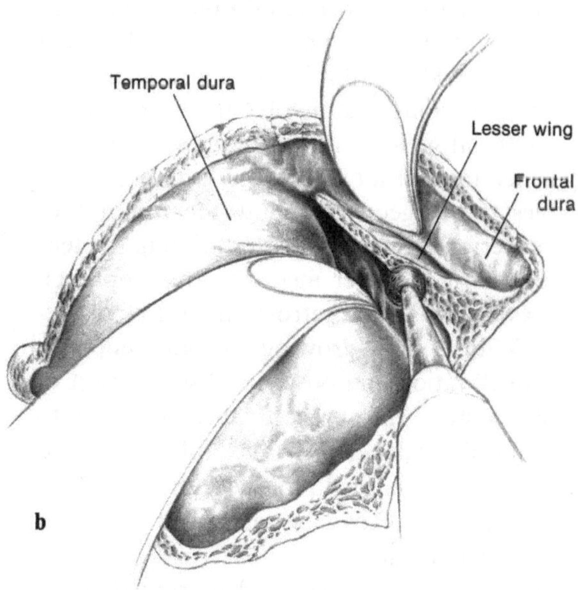

b

Fig. MS 34 a–d. The intracranial, extradural approach to the lateral middle skull base. With involvement of the temporal squama (e.g., by osteoma), the skull is opened by craniectomy.
a Outline of the temporal craniectomy, which is traversed obliquely by the squamous suture. The craniectomy is performed in healthy bone following the placement of burr holes.
b The frontal lobe is retracted anteriorly upward, the temporal lobe is retracted posteriorly, and the dura is progressively elevated to give access to the minor sphenoid wing, which is ablated.

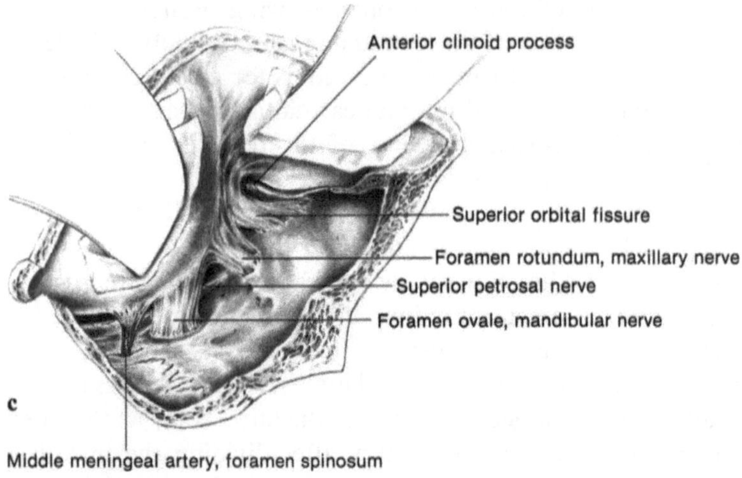

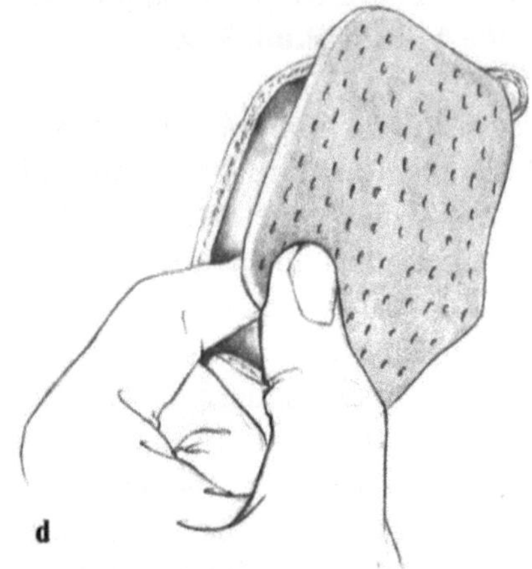

Fig. MS 34c, d.
c The superior orbital fissure, the foramen rotundum, the foramen ovale, and the foramen spinosum must be left intact in the anterior part of the middle skull base if the structures transversing these openings are to be spared.
d The craniectomy defect is repaired with a methylmethacrylate implant

Temporal Intracranial Intradural Approach to the Middle Skull Base and Tentorial Incisure (Pterional Approach)

Introductory Remarks. This approach is used for tumors with considerable intracranial extent that presumably have infiltrated a large area of the dura. Lesions that involve the structures of the tentorial incisure at the brain stem are approached intradurally along the skull base. This enables the surgeon to follow the tumor into the posterior cranial fossa after incising the tentorial margin. Farther medially, this approach permits access to the retrosellar and clivus region. With a slow-growing benign neoplasm causing elevation and posterior displacement of the brain stem, the surgeon can gain access to the contralateral petrous apex following enucleation of the tumor. In this case the structures of the brain stem can be visualized as far as the foramen magnum.

With a lesion at the tentorial margin that extends posteriorly to the cerebellopontine angle and also inferomedially to the clivus, we have been able to extend the approach considerably by coagulating the superior petrosal sinus and drilling away the petrous apex. In dissections around the cavernous sinus, the extent of resection of benign tumors is guided by preoperative ocular motility and vision. Under no circumstances should intact ocular motor nerves (especially cranial nerve III) be sacrificed with the cavernous sinus to ensure a complete tumor removal. With preexisting amaurosis, the decison whether to include the motor nerves in the resection will depend on how much esthetic importance is placed on ocular motility. An effort should be made to preserve the internal carotid artery, and this is possible in many instances. If there is tumor invasion into the artery, an effort is made to restore favorable hemodynamics either by use of a vein graft or by establishing an extra-intracranial shunt through the superficial temporal artery to branches of the middle cerebral.

Operative Technique
(Fig. MS 35a–h)

The lesion is exposed through a temporal craniotomy, which may be placed frontotemporally if required. The dura is secured up to the bone margins and opened basally. The temporal or

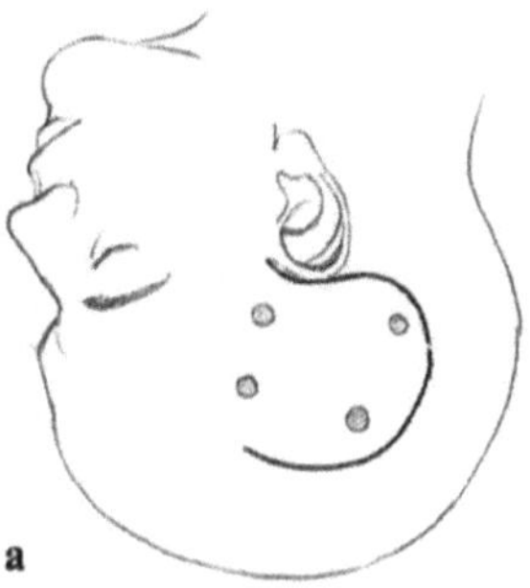

a

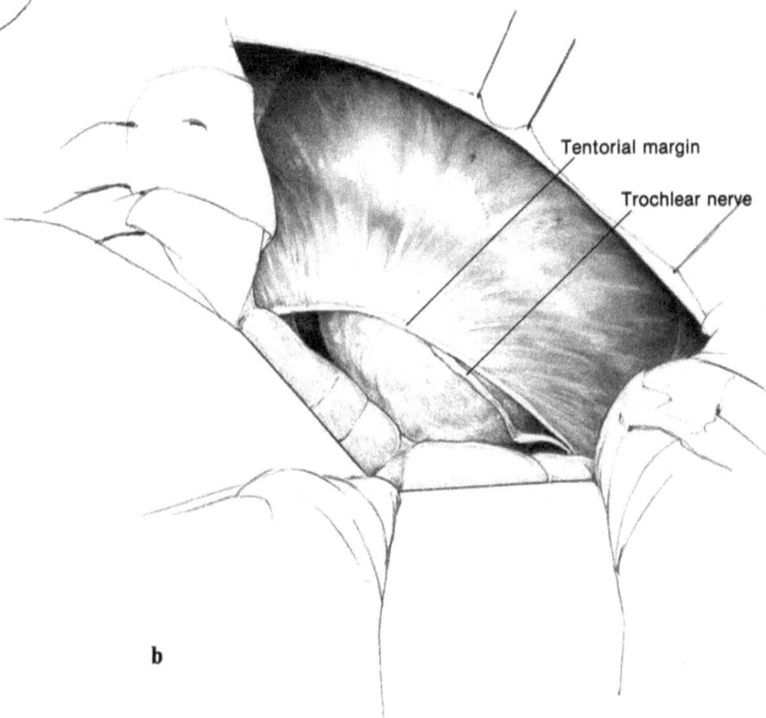

b

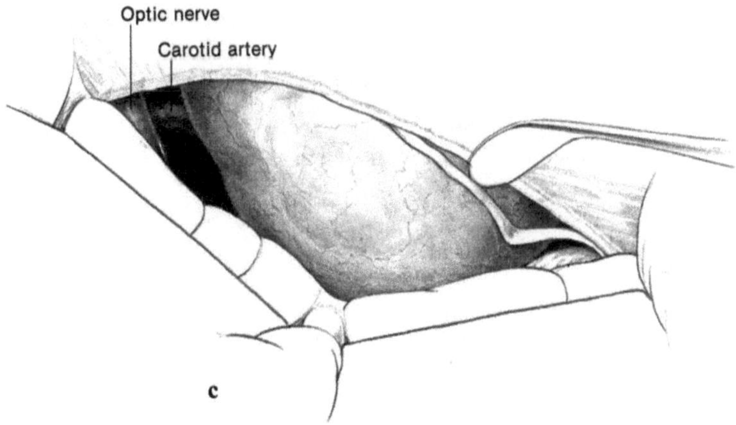

c

Fig. MS 35a–h. Temporal, intracranial, intradural approach to the middle skull base and tentorial incisure (pterional approach).
a Scalp incision and burr holes.
b After incision of the dura, the frontal lobe is retracted anteriorly and the temporal lobe posteromedially to expose the tumor in the tentorial incisure. The trochlear nerve passes over the tumor surface.
c Further brain retraction uncovers the internal carotid artery and optic nerve anteriorly. The trochlear nerve is very carefully mobilized from the tumor capsule.

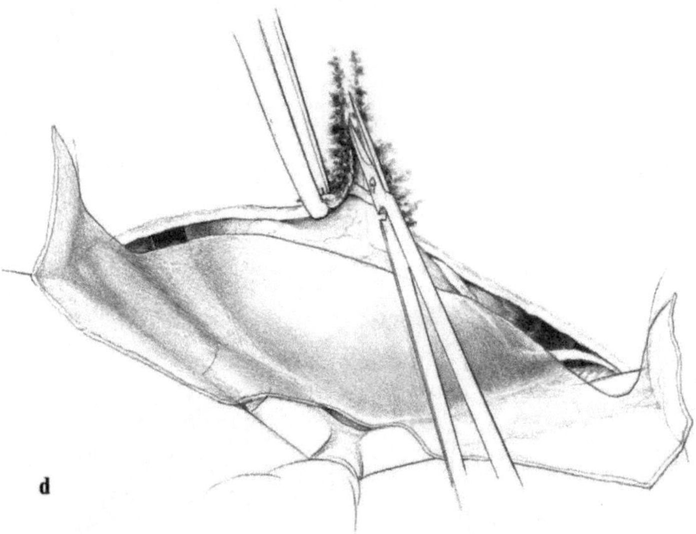

d

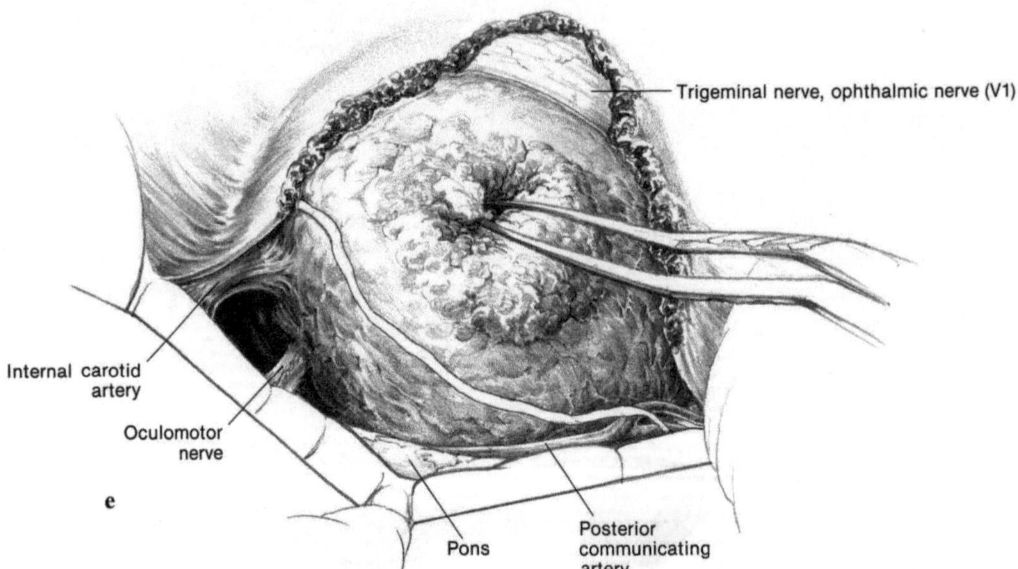

e

Fig. MS 35 d–h.
d Further tumor exposure can be gained by cutting across the tentorial margin after bipolar coagulation. Care is taken not to damage the subjacent trochlear nerve.
e Piecemeal enucleation of the tumor follows. The oculomotor nerve is visible deep in the field.
f As tumor removal is carried farther posteriorly, the trigeminal nerve comes into view.
g The view into the cerebellopontine angle is facilitated by drilling away the medial part of the petrous apex. This is done after coagulating and dividing the superior petrosal sinus and resecting the dura of the pyramidal surface. The posterior limit of bone removal is defined by the anterior wall of the IAC, and the lateral limit by the medial wall of the carotid canal. The anterior limit is the dura of Meckel's cave. The medial portion of the petrous apex also may be removed through an extradural, transtemporal approach (see p. 379).
h Appearance of the surgical cavity at the end of the procedure. Brain and neurovascular structures have been preserved

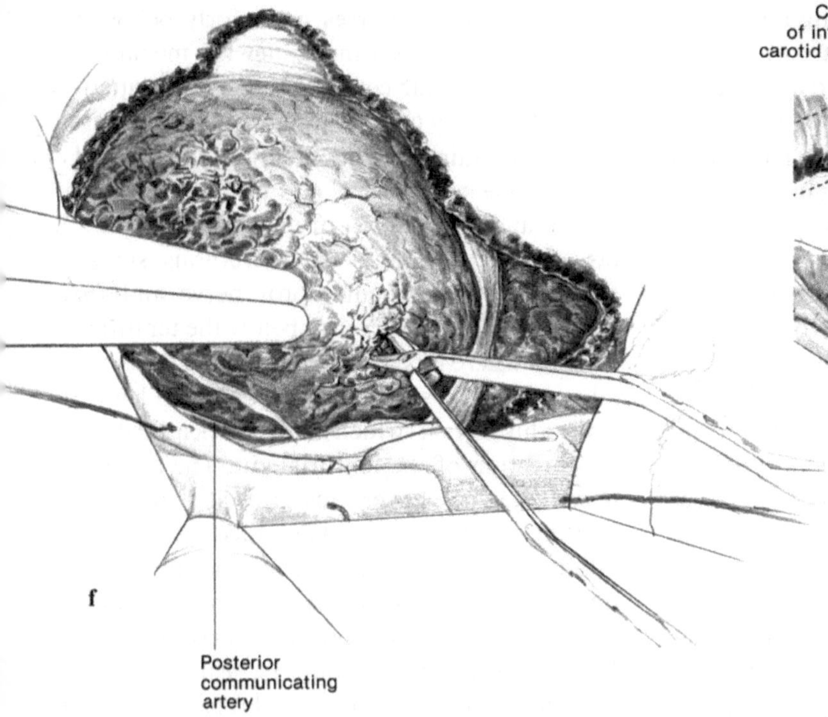
Posterior
communicating
artery

f

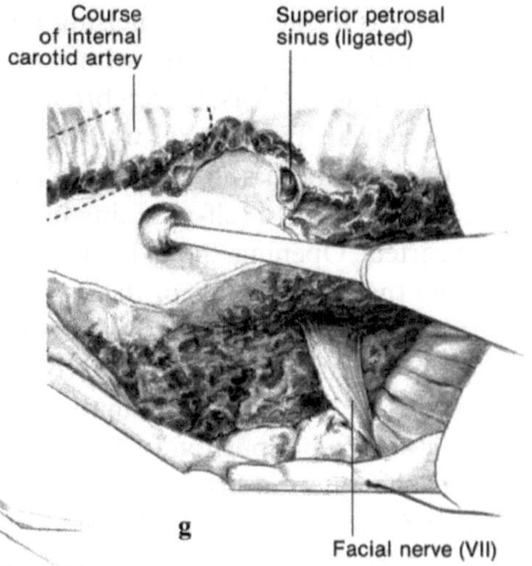
Course
of internal
carotid artery
Superior petrosal
sinus (ligated)
Facial nerve (VII)

g

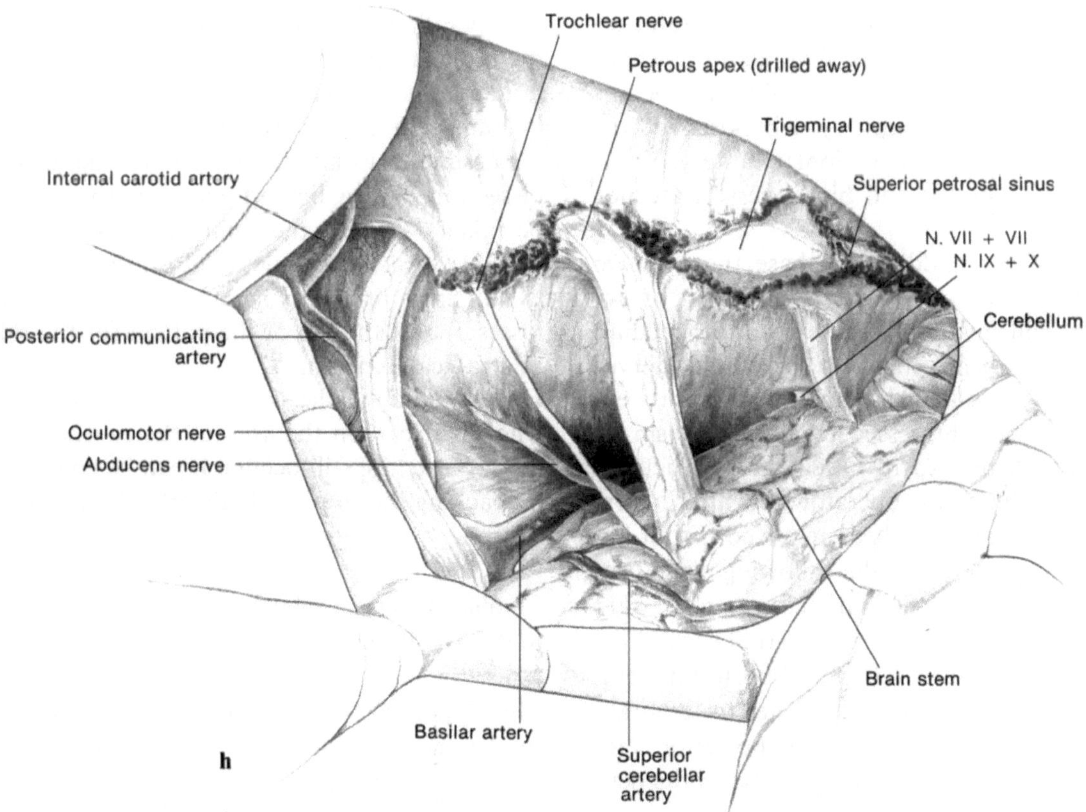
Trochlear nerve
Petrous apex (drilled away)
Trigeminal nerve
Superior petrosal sinus
N. VII + VII
N. IX + X
Cerebellum
Internal carotid artery
Posterior communicating
artery
Oculomotor nerve
Abducens nerve
Brain stem
Basilar artery
Superior
cerebellar
artery

h

frontal lobe is retracted after incising the arachnoid and protecting the brain with cotton paddies while slowly releasing cerebrospinal fluid from the sylvian fissure (Yasargil et al. 1976). When the skull base and the tumor have been adequately exposed, a self-retaining brain spatula is inserted. Opening the sylvian fissure and retracting the anterior pole of the temporal lobe posteromedially, with earliest possible exposure of the optic nerve and internal carotid artery, has proven an especially atraumatic means for exposing the medial portion of the middle skull base and the anterior structures of the tentorial incisure (Yasargil et al. 1976). The temporal lobe is elevated from laterally to medially to uncover the anterior and posterior parts of the tentorial incisure. This involves somewhat greater pressure on the temporal lobe than the pterional approach. Congestive phenomena have occasionally resulted from the partial coagulation and division of basal veins coursing at right angles to the direction of this dissection. This tends to occur when the veins are of relatively large caliber and thus contribute to venous drainage. Laterally situated tumors that do not extend into the tentorial incisure usually can be removed without difficulty by debulking the tumor piecemeal and using bipolar cautery. Vitally important nerves and blood vessels are not violated.

Tumors of the middle skull base that involve the tentorial incisure, either primarily or by extension, will invariably cause anterior, medial, or posterior displacement of the cranial nerves and blood vessels in that area. The brain stem itself may be compressed by the neoplasm or may be adherent to it. Often these structures become visible to the operator only after a portion of the tumor has been removed. From anteriorly to posteriorly, the following structures are present in the tentorial incisure and should be watched for: optic nerve, internal carotid artery, anterior choroidal artery, posterior communicating artery and its branches to the brain stem, the basilar artery, and the posterior cerebral and superior cerebellar arteries. Of the ocular motor nerves, one initially encounters cranial nerve III (the oculomotor nerve) close to the tentorial margin where it enters the cavernous sinus. The nerve courses posteriorly below the tentorium before passing somewhat medially to cross the posterior cerebral artery; the superior cerebellar artery courses inferior to it. The nerve leaves the brain stem between these two vessels. The trochlear nerve has a considerably smaller caliber and may consist of one or more separate fascicles. Posterior to the cavernous sinus it passes below the oculomotor nerve and then takes a more lateral course below the tentorium. In cases where it is necessary to incise the tentorial margin, the surgeon must be careful not to sever this nerve, which runs perpendicular to the direction of the tentorial cut. The abducens nerve enters the cavernous sinus at a rather low level at the clivus and then runs lateral to the internal carotid artery, entering the superior orbital fissure. Occasionally it is not visualized when dissecting in the tentorial incisure.

Even extensive benign tumors, usually well encapsulated, can be completely removed with preservation of the above structures by meticulous microsurgical dissection. Even when using the operating microscope, the surgeon may face the limit of operability with tumors that manifest a plaquelike type of growth, like some meningiomas. In these cases it can be difficult or impossible to isolate the involved structures by dissection, and a limited-goals approach must be taken – reduce the tumor size as much as possible to achieve functional improvement. It is not appropriate to accept major functional losses or risk the life of the patient for the sake of a radical excision.

Understandably, the tumor must be mobilized with great care in the area of the cavernous sinus. If bleeding still occurs, it can be controlled by packing the sinus with absorbable sponge.

Combined Extracranial-Intracranial Approach to the Middle Skull Base

This approach to the middle skull base for the total removal of tumors with intracranial and extracranial components is analogous to the combined craniofacial approach for tumors of the anterior skull base (see p. 169). With very extensive osseous tumors such as fibrous dysplasia or meningeoma, it will occasionally be necessary to limit surgery to a palliative resection. It may be advisable in such cases to perform the extra- and intracranial parts of the operation in separate stages. On the other hand a combined extirpation in one session offers a means of achieving a complete resection even in difficult cases.

Special Operative Techniques

The principles of the surgery of space-occupying lesions of the anterior skull base apply with equal validity to the middle skull base region.

Surgery of Benign Space-Occupying Lesions of the Middle Skull Base with Predominantly Extradural Growth

Lymphangioma

Tumorous affections of the lymphatic system include lymphangiectasis, lymphangioma, and lymphangiosarcoma (Batsakis 1980). The malignant form is extremely rare and is practically unknown in the head and neck region. Lymphangiomas of the neck region usually occur in the posterior cervical triangle or below the sternocleidomastoid muscle. They can extend upward to the parotid gland and skull base, and very extensive tumors can produce tracheal compression. Of the three types of lymphangioma, lymphangioma simplex, cavernous lymphangioma, and cystic lymphangioma (Landing and Tarber 1956), the cavernous lymphangioma exhibits a more aggressive type of growth than the cystic. Characteristically, this tumor does not grow along predefined pathways, but sends fingerlike projections into tissue spaces. Because of the tendency of this tumor to recur, an effort should be made to effect a complete removal.
The preservation of functionally important structures can pose difficulties, especially in small children. If the thin-walled tumor extends from the parotid gland to the skull base, it is microsurgically dissected medial to the facial nerve to permit a total removal.

Case Report. Large lymphangioma of the right side of the neck, extending to the skull base (Fig. MS 36a–d). An 18-month-old child was brought to us with a lump in the area of the right posterior quadrant of the neck that had attained considerable size over a period of months. We found a soft, nontender, nonpitting mass that caused a mild limitation of neck motion. The decision for surgery was based on the rapid increase in the size of the mass. Swelling was noted behind the auricle and in the parotid area, extending upward past the auditory canal.
The tumor was prepared from below upward, exposing the vascular sheath, accessory nerve, vagus nerve, and hypoglossal nerve, and carefully dissecting away tumor that had grown between these structures. Care is taken in cases of this type not to injure the tumor, because it collapses easily and becomes more difficult to dissect. After exposure of the posterior belly of the digastric, the facial nerve trunk was identified, its peripheral branches isolated, and the lateral portion of the parotid gland resected en bloc with the tumor, excising it from the skull base at the level of the foramen jugulare. Postoperatively the patient manifested no functional disturbances.

Comments: A benign, fast-growing, extracranial lymphangioma extending to the middle skull base in a small child was removed via the posteroinferior approach to the middle skull base.

Von Recklinghausen's Neurofibromatosis

Von Recklinghausen's neurofibromatosis is an inherited disease that may be associated with pigmented patches or "café au lait" stains on the skin, multiple neurofibromatous vegetations (mostly cutaneous), and central nervous system tumors (Holt 1978; Hommerich 1977). This systemic disease is included in the class of "hamartoses." Its prevalence is 1 in 2500–3300 births

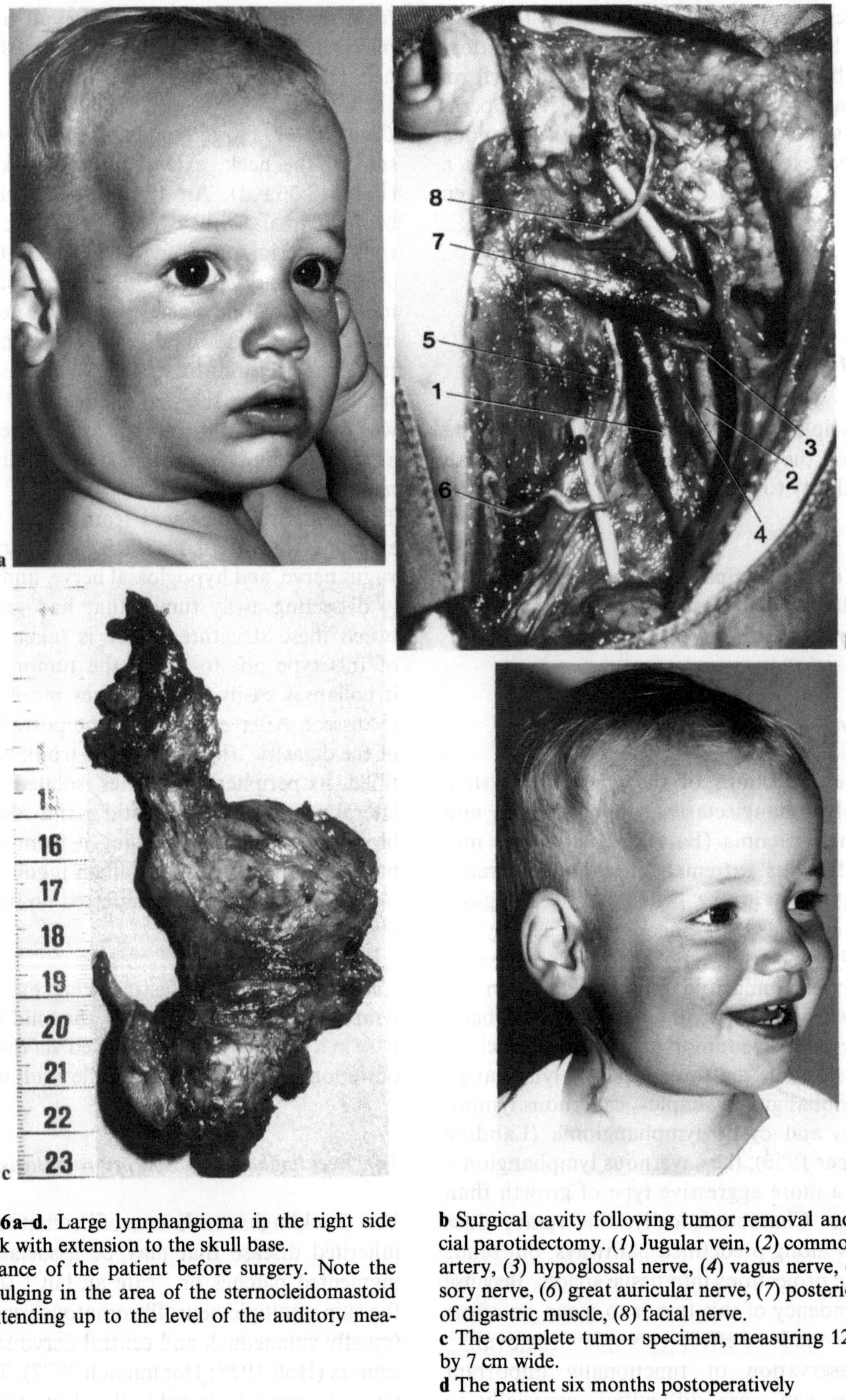

Fig. MS 36a–d. Large lymphangioma in the right side of the neck with extension to the skull base.
a Appearance of the patient before surgery. Note the marked bulging in the area of the sternocleidomastoid muscle extending up to the level of the auditory meatus.
b Surgical cavity following tumor removal and superficial parotidectomy. (*1*) Jugular vein, (*2*) common carotid artery, (*3*) hypoglossal nerve, (*4*) vagus nerve, (*5*) accessory nerve, (*6*) great auricular nerve, (*7*) posterior border of digastric muscle, (*8*) facial nerve.
c The complete tumor specimen, measuring 12 cm long by 7 cm wide.
d The patient six months postoperatively

(Feinmann and Yakovac 1970). The characteristic café-au-lait spots are an important diagnostic criterion in patients with subcutaneous tumors. The disease is often combined with other neurologic abnormalities or developmental anomalies such as gliomas, meningeomas, acoustic neurinomas, and spina bifida. Neurofibromatous lesions can also develop in the skeleton and lead to asymmetries, especially when the facial bones are involved (Draf 1974; Heard 1962; Ungerecht 1966). Data on the incidence of sarcomatous transformation or coexisting neurogenic sarcoma range from 5.5% (Holt and Wright 1948) to 16% (Martin and Kleinsasser 1981; Preston et al. 1952). Very rarely, the tumors can develop in the cervical region and infiltrate the skull base. Problems in the dissection of these tumors relate to the fact that they can arise from various nerves, can become very firmly adherent to the nerves and adjacent vessels, and can acquire a luxuriant blood supply. The tumors grow in a manner that can make them almost impossible to distinguish from healthy tissue.

Case Report. Extensive neurofibromatosis of the left side of the neck with invasion of the skull base (Fig. MS 37a–i). A 7-year-old boy presented with an extensive neurofibromatous tumor compressing the larynx and trachea, causing increasing interference with respiration. Facial asymmetry, especially around the orbits, and corresponding clinical signs made possible a diagnosis of von Recklinghausen's neurofibromatosis.

Involvement of the left petrous pyramid and jugular foramen had produced a gradual paralysis of cranial nerves VIII, IX, X, and XI. An operation attempted 4 years earlier had been discontinued because the tumor could not be dissected free from the carotid artery. Radiologic studies showed considerable destruction of the left pyramid and posterior displacement of the internal carotid artery. The maxillary artery was the only external carotid branch that could be visualized. The tumor, which was extensively adherent to the carotid vessels, was progressively isolated from the inferior aspect. It was necessary to dissect the tumor sharply from the internal carotid artery and at the same time remove the adventitia. The hypoglossal nerve had been severed in the previous operation. The facial nerve was identified at the stylomastoid foramen, and it was possible to spare the main trunk and its peripheral branches as the operation progressed. The mastoid was partially resected, and the sigmoid sinus was ligated. Then the tumor was removed from the petrous bone; this necessitated removal of the bony eustachian tube, but the inner ear structures were preserved. The patient recovered from the surgery well and had no further difficulties with swallowing or respiration. Facial nerve function was intact. The only postoperative sequela was a moderate conductive hearing loss on the left side.

Comments: Extensive neurofibromatosis of the left side of the neck and middle skull base was managed surgically following unsuccessful operative treatment 4 years earlier. The decision for surgery was due to respiratory difficulty and increasing infiltration of the petrous pyramid. The tumor was completely removed through a posteroinferior approach. The increased risk of malignant degeneration following multiple operations (Kern 1977; Miehlke 1977) emphasizes the importance of achieving a radical removal during initial surgery. In the present case there was no evidence of malignancy at the second operation, 9 years later.

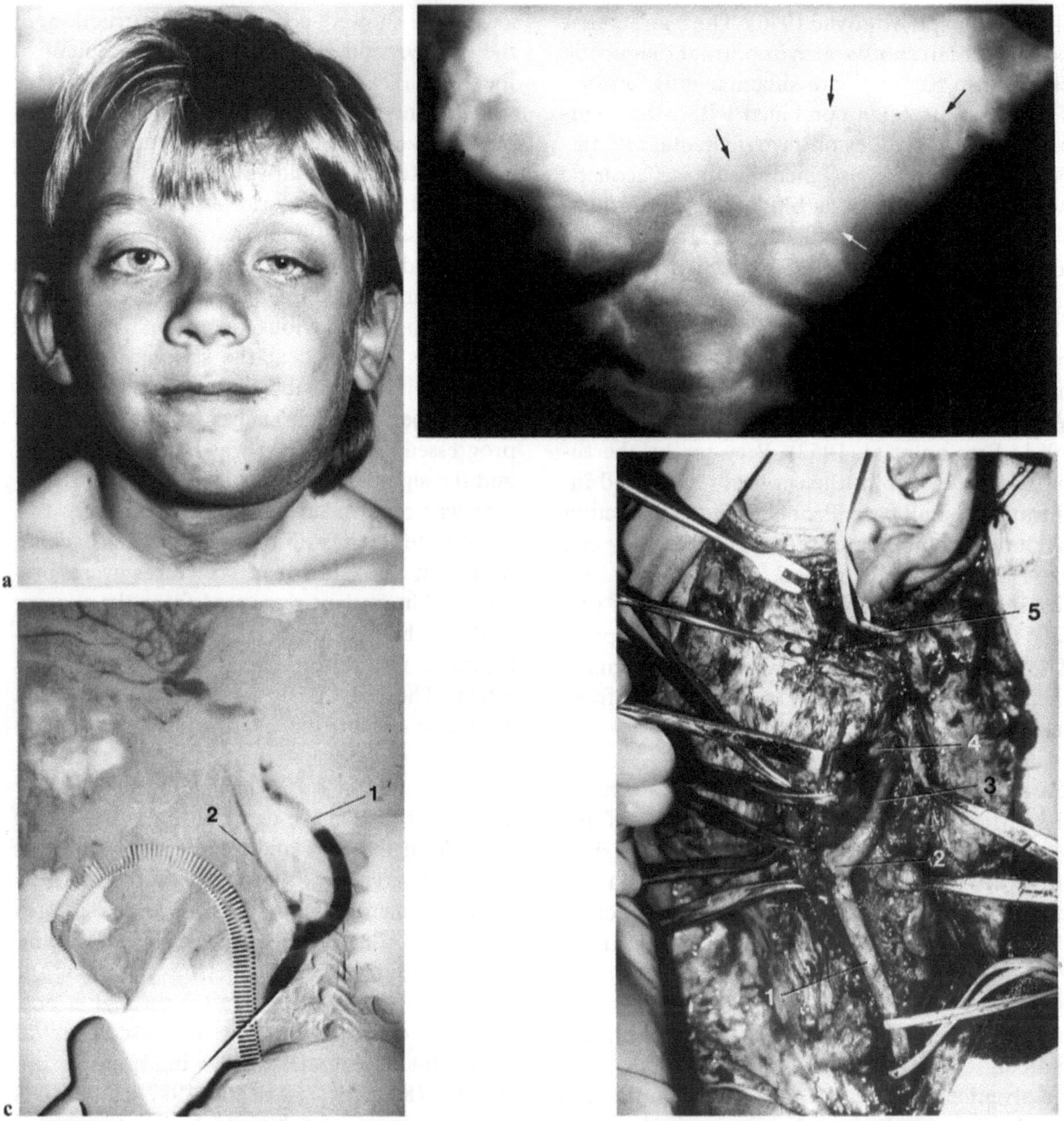

Fig. MS 37a–i. Von Recklinghausen's neurofibromatosis with a tumor in the left side of the neck invading the skull base.

a Facial asymmetry is pronounced, especially in the area of the orbits. The patient had other skeletal asymmetries and cafe-au-lait spots.

b AP tomogram of the skull base shows destruction of the pyramid and of the medial skull base as far as the arch of the atlas (*arrows*).

c Carotid angiogram shows posterior displacement of the internal carotid artery by the tumor. The maxillary artery is the only external carotid branch that is visualized. (*1*) Internal carotid artery, (*2*) maxillary artery.

d Here the common carotid artery is completely exposed, and the internal carotid artery is partially exposed. The external carotid branches were ligated in a previous operation. The hypoglossal nerve, lesioned in previous surgery, is seen as it crosses over the internal carotid artery; the facial nerve is visible at the stylomastoid foramen. (*1*) Common carotid artery, (*2*) carotid bifurcation, (*3*) internal carotid artery, (*4*) hypoglossal nerve, (*5*) facial nerve

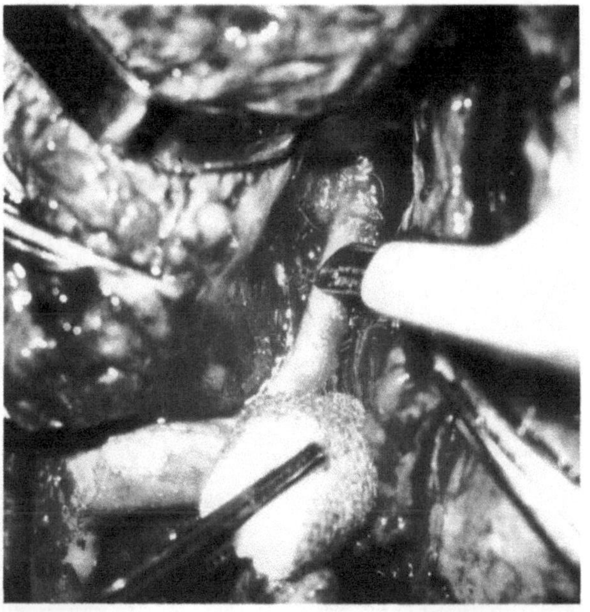

e

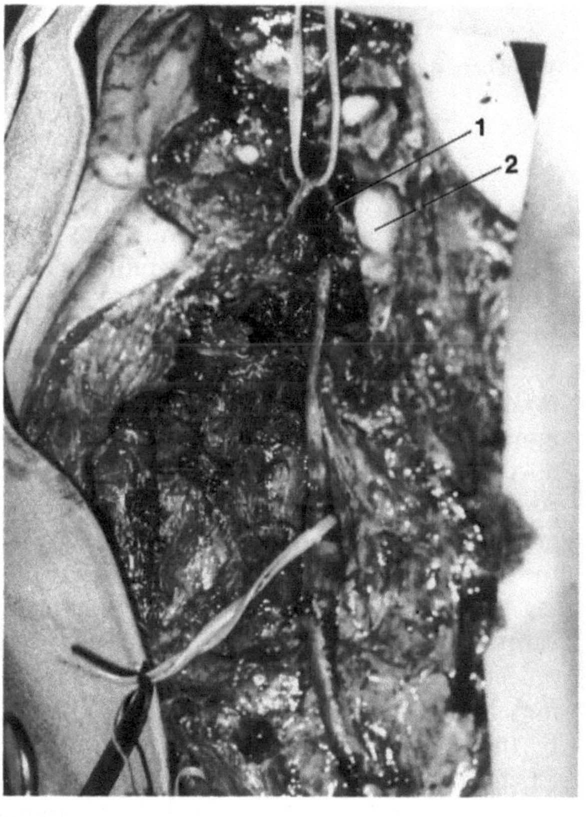

f

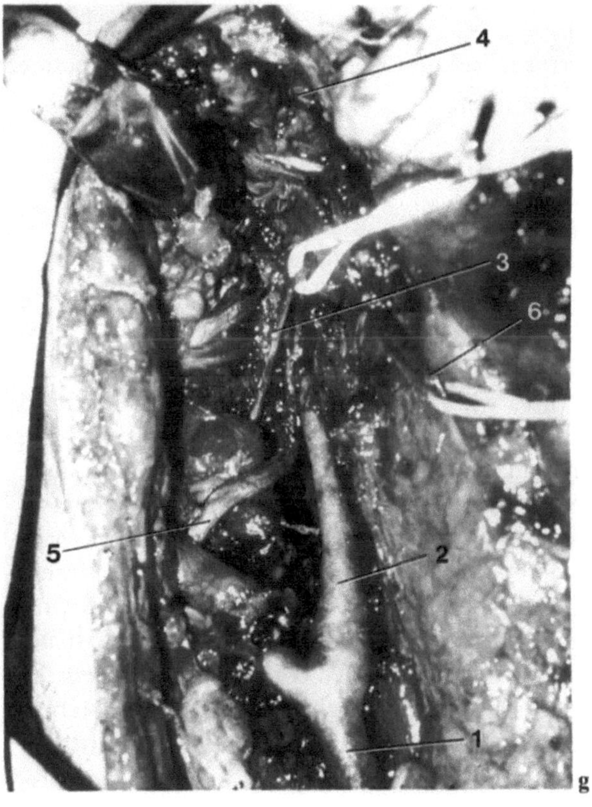

g

Fig. MS 37e–g.

e The tumor had to be sharply separated from the carotid artery with concurrent removal of the adventitia.

f After partial mastoidectomy, the lesion was removed from the petrous bone with preservation of inner ear structures; the bony eustachian tube was also removed. The sigmoid sinus was underrun and ligated. (*1*) Facial nerve, (*2*) middle fossa dura.

g Appearance of the field at the end of the operation. (*1*) Common carotid artery, (*2*) internal carotid artery, (*3*) facial nerve, (*4*) posterior cut edge of mastoid, (*5*) N. hypoglossus (*6*) accessory nerve.

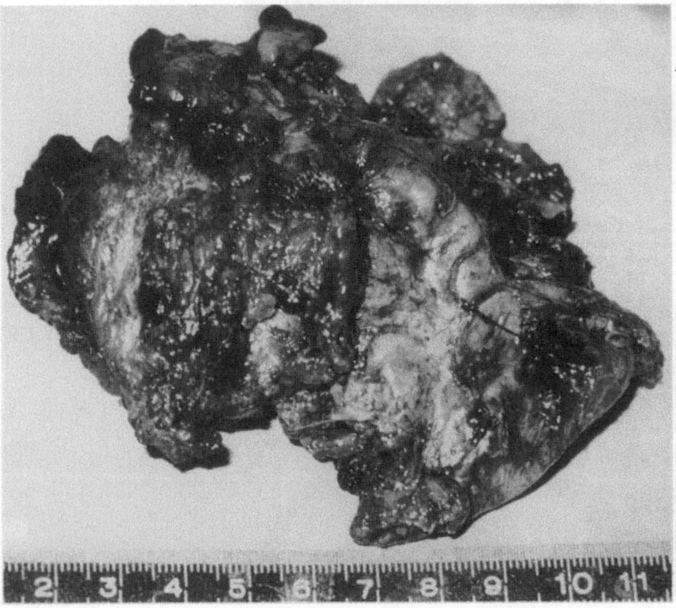

h

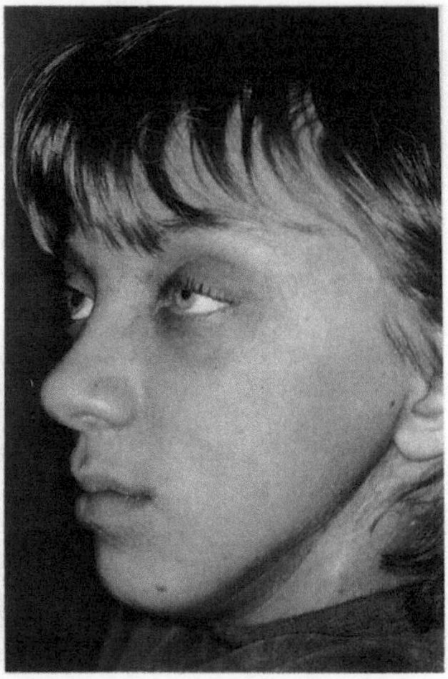

i

Fig. MS 37h, i.
h The surgical specimen. **i** The patient nine years postoperatively. There is no evidence of tumor recurrence

Fibromyxoma

Myxomas are exceedingly rare neoplasms in the head and neck region (Hommerich 1977). Ungerecht in 1966 reported on 20 cases in the literature, while Dechaume et al. (1968) reported on 10 personal cases, 5 of which involved the maxilla. The rate of tumor growth is slow. Schwab observed a myxoma of the paranasal sinuses that had penetrated the skull base (1951). The recommended treatment for these usually benign tumors is surgical removal with preservation of functionally important structures. Opinions differ concerning the need for radiotherapy. The high recurrence rates after incomplete removal have led some authors to question the benignancy of these lesions (Eckert-Möbius 1929; Lewin 1966; Tesarik 1959; Tesarik and Hubacek 1968).

Case Report. Extensive fibromyxoma of the left temporal fossa, infratemporal fossa, and pterygoid fossa (Fig. MS 38a–h). A 38-year-old man had had two previous operations in the two years before the present hospitalization, one involving a "face lift." For several months the patient had noticed an increasing fullness in the left temporal area with headaches, which he attributed in part to an injury.

Excisional biopsy identified the lesion as a fibromyxoma. CT scans clearly demonstrated the tumor mass in the left temporal region. There was no evidence of middle fossa bone destruction. As the tumor appeared highly vascular on angiograms, we began the operation by exposing the left carotid bifurcation and selectively ligating the tumor-feeding branches of the external carotid. The scalp and facial soft tissues were reflected anteriorly downward. The temporal muscle was found to be extensively infiltrated by tumor. The zygoma was osteotomized with a Gigli saw. The tumor was then separated from the bony middle skull base, which the tumor had reached but had not grossly infiltrated. The fibromyxoma extended into the pterygoid fossa. The facial nerve trunk was identified at the beginning of the procedure, and the main branches were preserved initially during tumor dissection and parotidectomy. Because of a nodular tumor extension medial to the vertical ramus of the

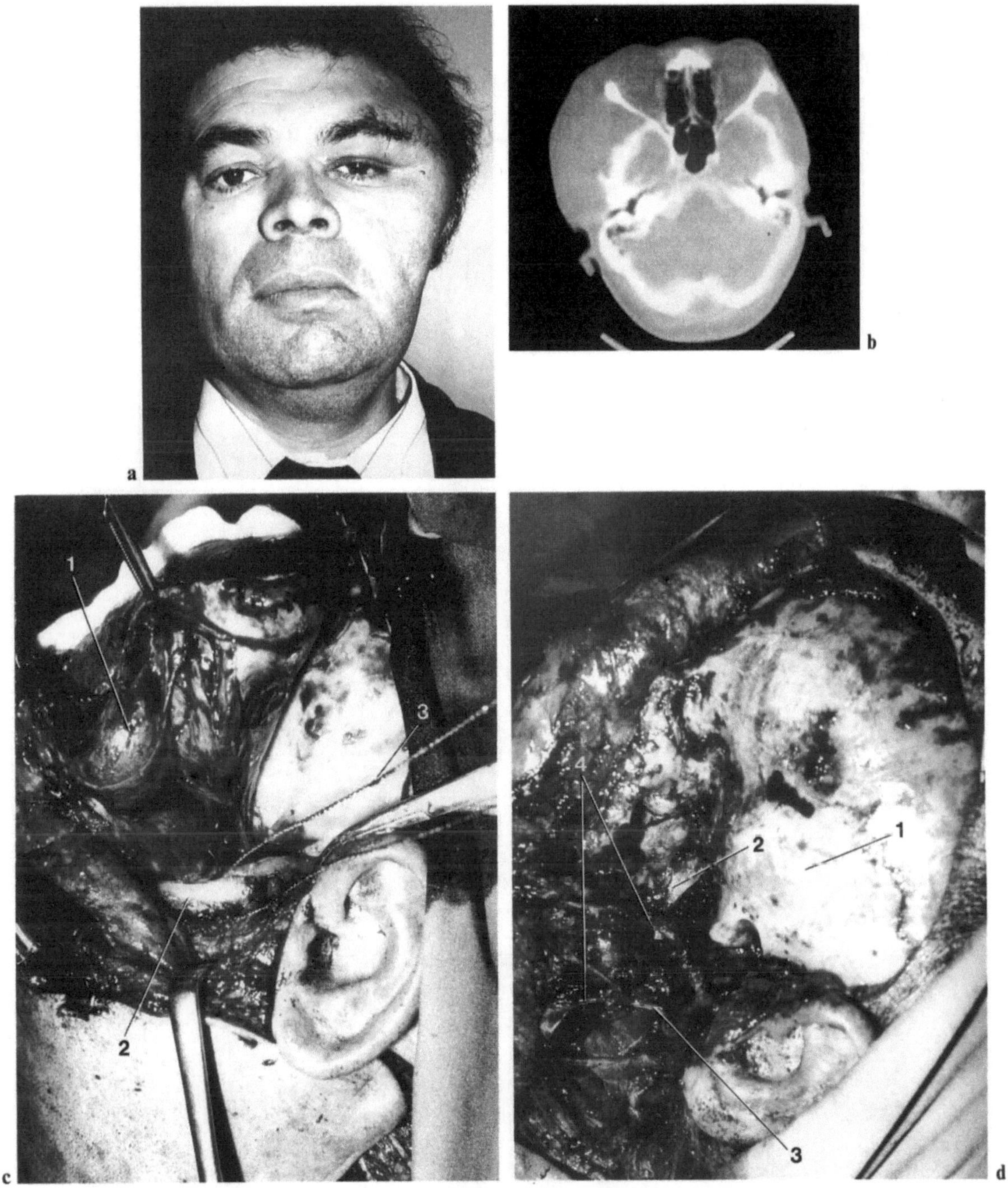

Fig. MS 38a–h. Extensive fibromyxoma of the left temporal, infratemporal, and pterygoid fossae with broad involvement of the middle skull base but no gross evidence of bone destruction.
a Firm swelling in the left temporal region; excisional biopsy was previously done in the area of the left eyebrow.
b Axial CT scan demonstrates the soft-tissue mass in the left temporal area.
c The tumor is partially separated from the temporal squama. The zygomatic arch is osteotomized with a Gigli saw. (*1*) Tumor, (*2*) zygomatic arch, (*3*) wire saw.
d Portions of the temporal bone in contact with the tumor were drilled down to the inner cortex. The lateral plate of the pterygoid process is visible deep in the field. The facial nerve and its major branches were spared initially. The left facial skin showed tumor involvement on frozen-section examination, so most of it had to be resected. (*1*) Temporal bone, (*2*) lateral plate of pterygoid process, (*3*) main trunk of facial nerve, (*4*) facial nerve branches

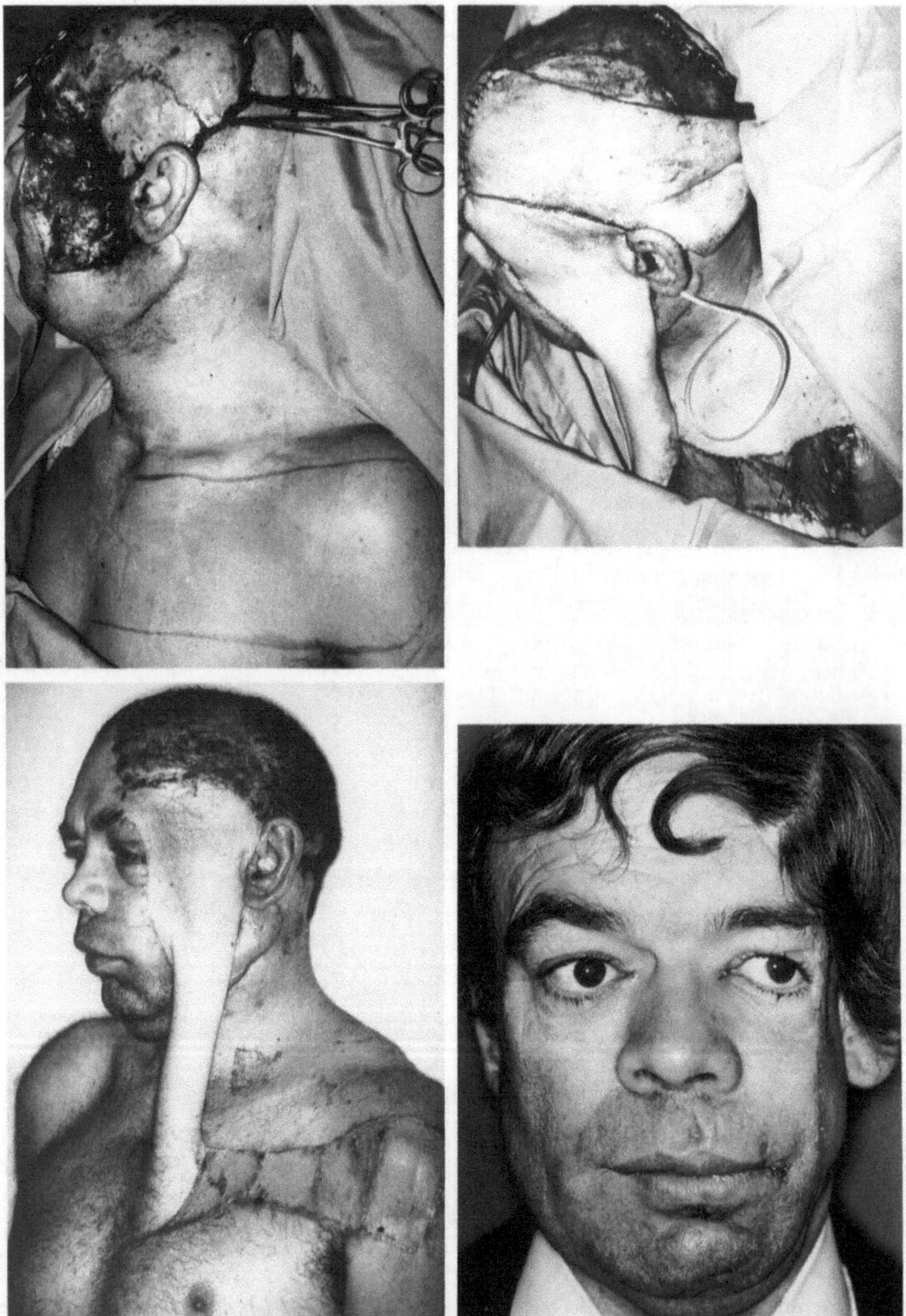

e f g h

Fig. MS 38e–h.
e Status following wide resection of the tumor and involved facial skin. The deltopectoral flap has been outlined with a marker.
f After transfer of the deltopectoral flap, the anterolateral scalp was resurfaced with a posteriorly based parietal rotation flap. The donor site was covered with split-thickness skin.
g Both regional flap transfers healed well.
h The patient five years postoperatively. The pedicle of the deltopectoral flap was deepithelialized and used to fill out the left infratemporal contour. Hair growth partially conceals the facial deformity on the left side

mandible, the latter was transversely osteotomized at the mandibular angle and disarticulated at the temporomandibular joint. Histologic examination of the facial skin at several sites showed that the tumor had infiltrated the skin over a wide area, making it necessary to resect most of the facial skin on the left side and portions of the temporal scalp, also sacrificing the facial nerve branches. All surgical margins were negative at the end of the operation. The large facial soft-tissue and scalp defect was covered inferiorly with a deltopectoral flap and superiorly with a posteriorly based scalp flap rotated from the parietal area. The donor site for the scalp flap was resurfaced with split-thickness skin. The advanced scalp flap was hair-bearing, and this helped to conceal the disfigurement of the left facial half. Both flaps healed completely without complications. The pedicle of the deltopectoral flap was deepithelialized and used to fill the deep facial depression.

Five years postoperatively the patient is doing well and is free of the agonizing headaches that he had experienced previously. His appearance was improved secondarily by raising the left corner of the mouth and the outer canthus of the left eye.

Comments: An extensive fibromyxoma of the left side of the face extending to the middle skull base was completely removed by facial soft-tissue resection including the facial nerve, partial mandibulectomy, and exposure of the middle skull base through the lateral extracranial approach.

Recurrence of a Pleomorphic Adenoma of the Parotid Gland with Intracranial Extension

Pleomorphic adenoma, a frequently benign salivary gland tumor, is characterized histologically by a diverse mixture of epithelial and mesenchymal elements. Most authors assume a purely epidermal histogenesis for both the epithelial and mesenchymal components of the lesion (literature in Eneroth 1976; Kleinsasser 1975). Pleomorphic adenoma accounts for 70%–80% of all parotid neoplasms. The incidence of malignancy is estimated to be 1%–3%. Conley (1975) states that two types of malignancy occur. One involves a malignant focus in a mixed tumor, which probably arises from the mixed lesion (Kleinsasser and Klein 1968). In the second type the malignant component is predominant, and very little of the tumor shows the typical features of pleomorphic adenoma, suggesting the possibility of a primary carcinoma. The danger of malignant transformation of a pleomorphic adenoma increases with age. Rarely, a tumor may grow between the mandible and mastoid process into the parapharyngeal space, causing a medial bulge of the lateral pharyngeal wall. In the series of Eneroth (1969), fewer than 1% of pleomorphic adenomas of the parotid gland extended to the pharynx. Denecke (1959) and others have seen a very few cases where such tumors reached the skull base and spine, causing compression of the internal carotid artery. The term "iceberg tumor" has been applied to this deep type of growth. Even with very large tumors, facial paralysis is rarely seen as long as the tumor is benign.

These neoplasms are not radiosensitive, so the treatment of choice is surgical extirpation. If the tumor occurs in the superficial part of the parotid gland, this portion is excised with preservation of the facial nerve. If the deep part of the gland is involved, the entire gland must be removed. Great care should be taken at operation not to open the tumor capsule, but to remove it en bloc with the surrounding tissues. That is the only way to prevent a recurrence due to cell dissemination. Also, the site of the intraoperative frozen section biopsy should be closed with sutures to prevent tumor spread. With very large neoplasms, it can be quite difficult to preserve the tumor capsule.

Case Report (Fig. MS 39 a–d). A 75-year-old woman had surgery elsewhere 9 years earlier for removal of an extremely large pleomorphic adenoma of the right parotid gland. The tumor was fused to the internal carotid artery where the genu of the artery joins its transverse segment in the petrous bone, causing hemorrhage from that portion of the vessel.

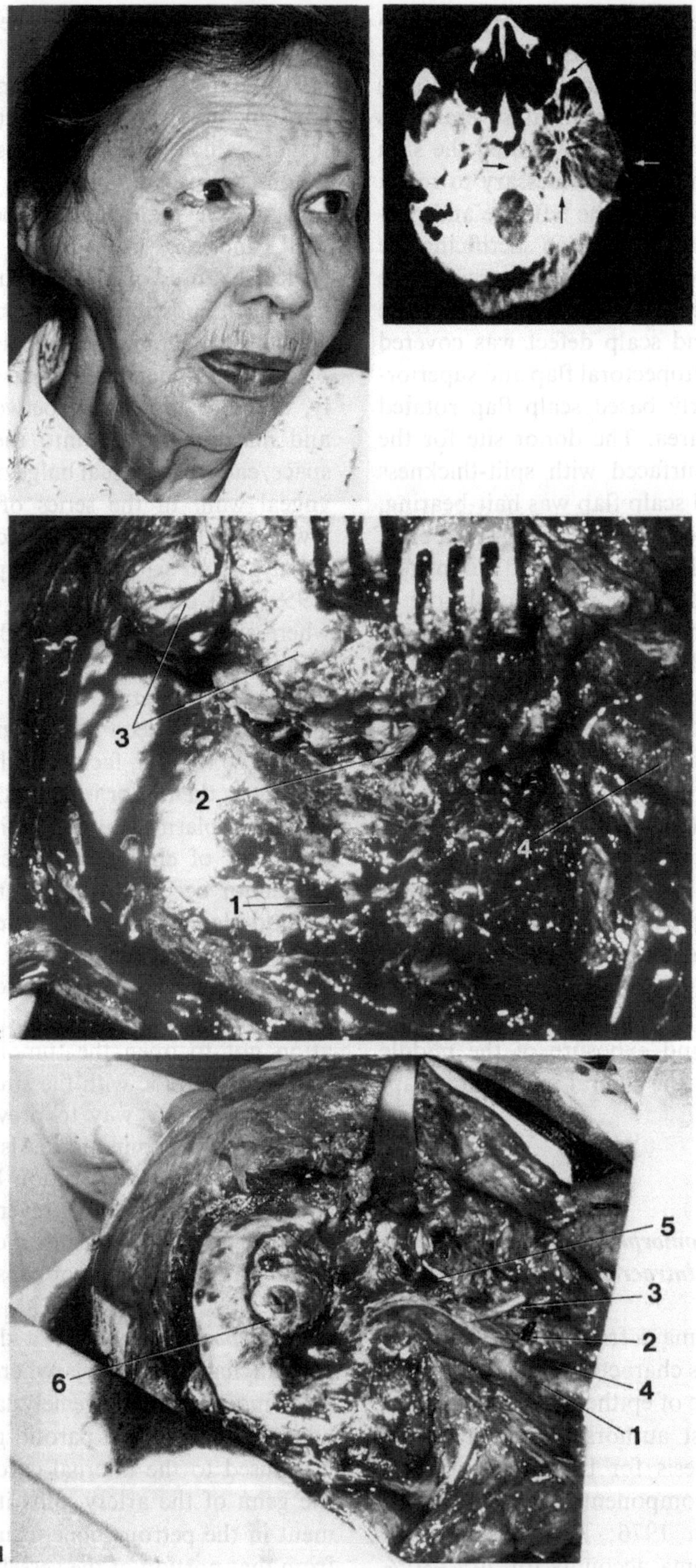
a
b
3
2
4
1
c
5
3
2
6
4
1
d

A clinical recurrence gradually developed, and when we first saw the patient approximately six years after her first operation, CT scans revealed destruction of the temporal skull base. Angiograms showed that the tumor was heavily vascularized. The patient's general condition was compromised by cardiac symptoms and other problems, so when she urgently requested radiotherapy as a means of relieving her severe headaches, we complied and initiated treatment with an exposure of 20 gray. This had no effect on tumor size or clinical symptoms. Because the pain was reaching an intolerable level, we decided to perform surgery despite the high risk. At operation the tumor and involved skin were resected with a wide margin of healthy tissue. The peripheral facial nerve branches were isolated, divided, and marked with threads to leave open the option for subsequent reconstruction of the facial nerve, which could not be spared.
The tumor had invaded the mastoid process, most of which had to be resected. The facial nerve was identified below the semicircular canal and resected. The vertical ramus of the mandible had already been removed in the previous operation. A strong bleeding tendency made the dissection difficult. The tumor was adherent to the right temporal lobe dura over an area of 6 × 5 cm, had displaced the dura upward, and in one place had greatly thinned it.

Fig. MS 39 a–d. Recurrence of a pleomorphic adenoma of the parotid gland with intracranial extension.
a Tumor recurrence in the right parotid area of a 75-year-old woman suffering severe headaches.
b CT scan shows tumor growth in the infratemporal fossa and parapharyngeal area and intracranial extension toward the temporal lobe (*arrows*).
c The tumor was encompassed posteriorly with resection of the mastoid, which the tumor had invaded and partially destroyed. The facial nerve trunk is visible. (*1*) Sigmoid sinus, (*2*) facial nerve, (*3*) tumor extension into mastoid, (*4*) internal jugular vein.
d The tumor has been completely removed in a combined extracranial-intracranial extradural operation with craniectomy and pharyngotomy. (*1*) Internal jugular vein, (*2*) internal carotid artery, (*3*) hypoglossal nerve, (*4*) vagus nerve, (*5*) opened pharynx with feeding tube, (*6*) exposed dura

It was necessary at this point to extend the operation intracranially through a craniectomy so that the tumor could be totally encompassed. We were able to separate the tumor progressively from the first bend of the carotid artery and from its transverse portion, finding no evidence of infiltration of the carotid wall or dura. The lateral superior pharyngeal wall on the right side was resected along with the last parapharyngeal tumor extension to decrease the risk of recurrence. The internal jugular vein, jugular bulb, sigmoid sinus, and all caudal cranial nerves had been identified at the beginning of the operation, and all were preserved. Following the ablative phase of the procedure, the pharyngeal defect was repaired with preserved dura, and the temporal lobe dura was similarly reinforced with stored dura to prevent cerebrospinal fluid leak. The wound was closed in layers and healed well. After six weeks the patient was discharged home in good condition and suffered no further headaches. In this case the anesthetic risk was considered too high to reconstruct the facial nerve in the same sitting. The patient has been free of disease for six years.

Comments: A recurrence of a radioresistant pleomorphic adenoma of the right parotid gland with intracranial and parapharyngeal extension was removed in a combined extra/intracranial extradural operation with a craniectomy.

Benign Chondroblastoma

(Jaffe and Lichtenstein 1942)

Zülch (1956) places *chondromas* in the class of rare brain tumors (cf. literature in Zülch 1956). They originate from the dura, which, as an internal periosteum, has cartilage-forming properties. Chondromas occur in the plexus, usually of the lateral ventricles, and on the dura of the convexity, the frontal falx, and skull base, most commonly in the middle cranial fossa near the foramen lacerum.
Klingler (1951) states that the following groups of chondromas are frequently encountered:

1) Chondromas originating in the nose and paranasal sinuses and invading the cranial cavity in the area of the sella.
2) Chondromas of the petrous apex with extension toward the posterior fossa, sella, and greater sphenoid wing.
3) Chondromas arising from the dura of the convexity or falx.

Hommerich (1977) stresses the distinction between *benign chondroblastoma* [Jaffe and Lichtenstein; synonyms: chondro-osteoblastoma, Codman's tumor (Codman 1931), epiphyseal chondroblastoma] and differentiated chondroma. Von Albertini (1974) defines the neoplasm as a pleomorphic, highly cellular, and definitely benign tumor arising from cartilage-forming matrix. Chondroblastomas of the cranial region are extremely rare (Jaffe and Lichtenstein 1942).

With chondromas and chondroblastomas of the skull base, attention should be given not only to the intracranial extent of the lesion but also to the possibility of tumor spread below the skull base. Chondromas have the appearance of cartilage, and most are globular in shape and have a knobby or lobulated surface. (Chondroblastoma has more of a connective-tissue structure.) They grow slowly and tend to have "pushing" margins, although infiltration is occasionally seen. They erode through the skull base by pressure. Many are made radiopaque by the presence of calcium or bone. Recurrence is avoided by completely encompassing the tumor and surrounding dura.

Case Report (Fig. MS 40 a–h). A 48-years-old man noticed a slowly increasing swelling above the left zygomatic arch and in the preauricular area six months before he was hospitalized. CT showed a large mass extending into the middle cranial fossa, reaching the lesser sphenoid wing anteriorly and the sigmoid sinus posteriorly causing extensive destruction of the left temporal bone and petrous bone. Excisional biopsy raised the suspicion of a malignant connective-tissue tumor, such as a malignant fibrous histiocytoma of the bone. A giant cell tumor and osteosarcoma were also considered in the differential diagnosis. The tumor was approached through a combined extra/intracranial intradural operation using the lateral approach to the middle lateral skull base via an anteriorly based frontotemporal scalp flap. First the tumor was encompassed from below. After identifying the vessels, caudal cranial nerves and facial nerve, the parotid gland was resected, sparing the facial nerve branches, and the condylar process of the mandible was removed. Next the tumor was encompassed posteriorly with adequate margins; this involved resection of the mastoid and exposure of the sigmoid sinus. The temporal muscle was found to be widely infiltrated by tumor. Through the craniotomy opening the tumor was removed cranially and anteriorly through extensive temporal bone resection. This was followed by subtotal resection of the petrous pyramid, sparing the area where the intact facial nerve entered the internal auditory canal. Finally the tumor-infiltrated temporal lobe dura was resected in the concluding, intradural phase of the procedure. Examination of the inner surface of the resected dura showed that the tumor had breached only a relatively circumscribed area of the thick dural sheet. The tumor itself was separated from the intracranial structures by a thin fibrous capsule and had not infiltrated the brain. Following removal of the tumor (see Fig. MS 40f) the facial nerve trunk and several of its branches were visible centrally, the internal carotid artery was seen anterior to the facial nerve, and the temporal lobe appeared in the right part of the field. The dural defect was repaired with three grafts attached with simple interrupted sutures and a continuous suture. The surgical cavity was largely obliterated with a superiorly based sternocleidomastoid muscle flap. The cranial vault was repaired with methylmethacrylate, and the skin flaps were turned back into position and sutured.

Postoperative healing was uncomplicated, and two days after surgery the patient could be moved from intensive care. A moderate facial paralysis resolved without treatment.

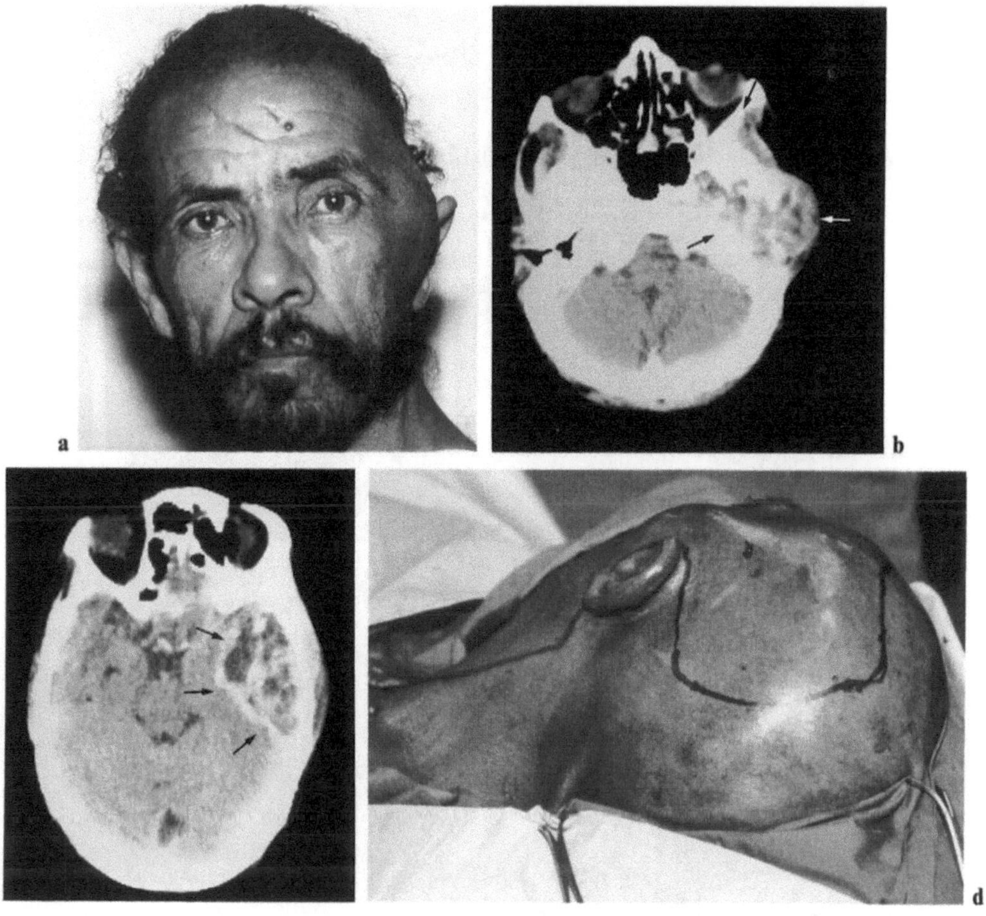

Fig. MS 40a–h. Benign chondroblastoma of the left middle skull base with intracranial extension.
a The patient before surgery, with a tumorous swelling in the left temporal region and temporal/infratemporal fossa.
b, c Preoperative CT scans show destruction of the petrous pyramid, temporal bone, and significant intracranial growth on the left side (*arrows*).
d The incision was placed so as to create an anteriorly based frontotemporal skin flap

Comments: An extra/intracranial tumor of the middle skull base, ultimately classified as a benign chondroblastoma, was removed through a combined extra/intracranial lateral approach to the middle skull base involving subtotal resection of the petrous bone and removal of a large section of dura, with preservation of the facial nerve. The dura was repaired with a graft, and the osseous defect was reconstruced with methylmethacrylate, followed by an uneventful postoperative course.

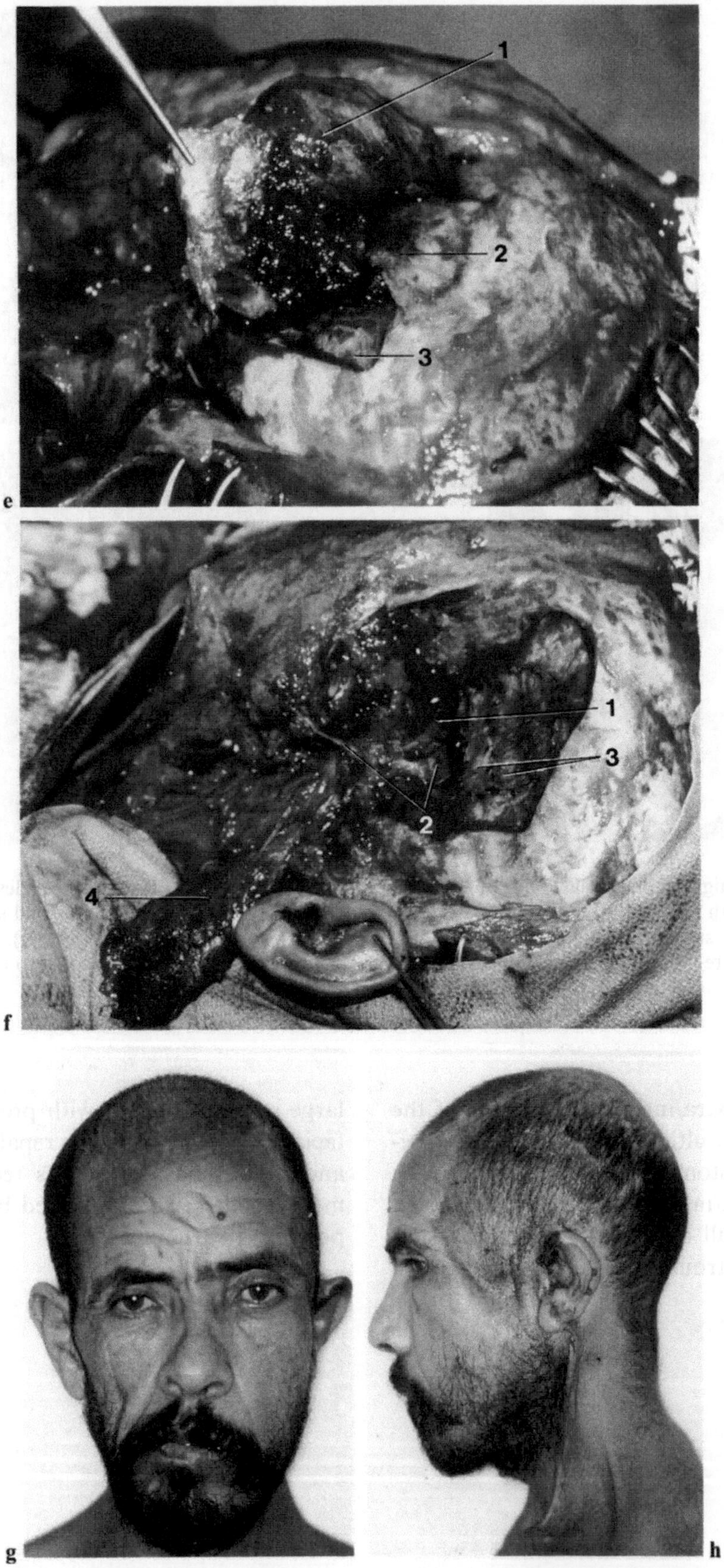
1
2
3
e
1
3
2
4
f
g
h

Extensive Osteoma of the Temporal Bone and Middle Skull Base

Osteomas of the cranial vault are less common than similar lesions of the paranasal sinuses. According to Zülch (1956, see also references in that publication), a few osteomas have a growth tendency comparable to that of autonomous tumors. It is unusual for osteomas of the inner cranial vault to show sufficient growth to cause intracranial displacement.

Case Report. Osteoma of the left temporal squama (Fig. MS 41 a–g). A 40-year-old woman presented with an osteoma of the temporal squama that had spread to the middle skull base. The extent of the neoplasm was evident on plain skull films and CT scan (Fig. MS 41 a–c). The tumor had reached a diameter of 10 cm and was causing headaches.
Because the lesion was entirely intracranial, it was exposed transcranially through a temporal craniectomy.
The tumor was progressively separated from the dura. The midportion of the dura had been greatly thinned by the tumor and had to be resected and resurfaced by duraplasty. The cranial defect was repaired with methylmethacrylate. A temporal muscle was preserved and used to cover the plastic implant.

Fig. MS 40e–h.
e The mastoid was resected and the tumor encompassed from behind. The sigmoid sinus is visible, and there is obvious tumor infiltration of the temporal muscle and squamosa. (*1*) Temporal muscle, (*2*) temporal bone, (*3*) sigmoid sinus.
f Surgical cavity after removal of all tumor and subtotal resection of the petrous bone. The facial nerve is visible in its extratemporal portion and at its entrance into the IAC; anterior to it is the transverse segment of the internal carotid artery. The dural defect has been repaired, and a sternocleidomastoid muscle flap with a superior, retromastoid cutaneous pedicle has been prepared for cavity ablation. (*1*) Internal carotid artery, (*2*) facial nerve, (*3*) dural graft, (*4*) sternocleidomastoid muscle.
g,h The patient several weeks after surgery. The facial weakness on the left side is regressing

Comments: An extensive osteoma of the inner temporal bone with compression of the temporal lobe was removed through a craniectomy. The dura was repaired with a graft, and the bony defect was reconstituted with methylmethacrylate.

Carotid Body Tumor

Batsakis (1980) states that neoplastic diseases are the only kind of pathology known to affect the tissues of the paraganglia. The most common of these are carotid body tumors (chemodectomas). The tumor may originate from the carotid bifurcation and closely envelop the external and internal carotid vessels by infiltrating the adventitia. It is composed of epitheloid-like cells embedded in a highly vascular connective-tissue matrix. The arteriolar vessels feeding the tumor may arise from the carotid bifurcation, but with further growth the tumor may derive blood from the external carotid artery and especially from its ascending pharyngeal branch. Most carotid body tumors are slow-growing and cause a progressive, painless swelling that develops toward the skull base and oropharynx in 5%-10% of cases. In extreme cases the tumor may penetrate the skull base, resulting in a "dumbbell" type of intracranial component. It is not unusual for a carotid body tumor to coexist with a glomus jugulare or glomus tympanicum tumor (see p. 414). Inheritance may play a role in the etiology of carotid body tumors (Resler et al. 1966). According to Batsakis, the question of the malignancy of these lesions is difficult to resolve. He feels that there is no true correlation between the histologic features of the tumor, which may show criteria of malignancy, and its biologic behavior. If we accept metastases as a histologic criterion of malignancy, then fewer than 10% of all paragangliomas are malignant. Generally the lesion can be diagnosed by angiography, which shows the typical expansion of the carotid bifurcation with splaying of the internal and external carotid arteries. The tumor bleeds very strongly when biopsied, so this procedure should be avoided if possible. The diagnosis is established by the

a, b

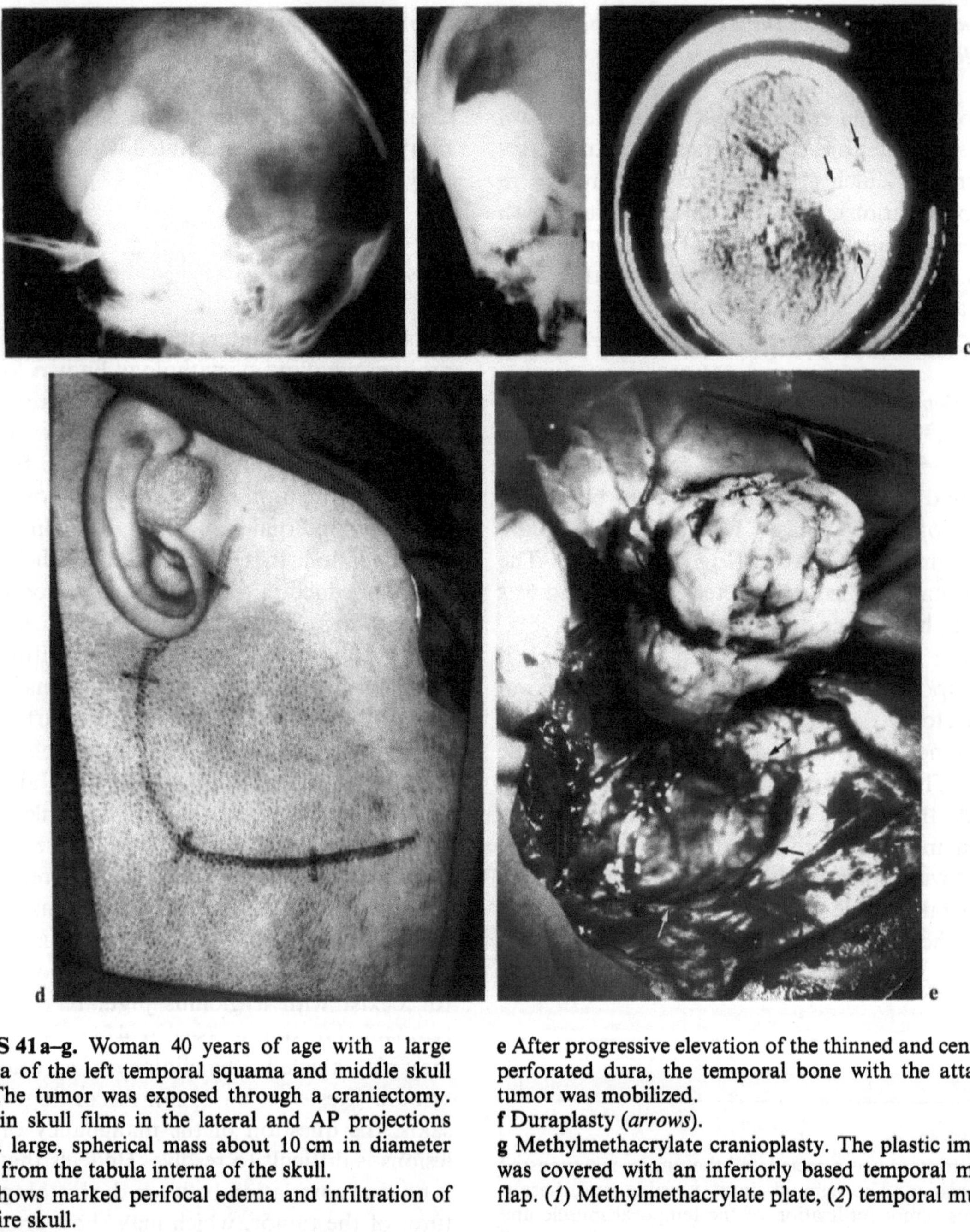

c

d

e

Fig. MS 41 a–g. Woman 40 years of age with a large osteoma of the left temporal squama and middle skull base. The tumor was exposed through a craniectomy.
a,b Plain skull films in the lateral and AP projections show a large, spherical mass about 10 cm in diameter arising from the tabula interna of the skull.
c CT shows marked perifocal edema and infiltration of the entire skull.
d The skin was opened with a temporal scalp flap behind the hairline.
e After progressive elevation of the thinned and centrally perforated dura, the temporal bone with the attached tumor was mobilized.
f Duraplasty (*arrows*).
g Methylmethacrylate cranioplasty. The plastic implant was covered with an inferiorly based temporal muscle flap. (*1*) Methylmethacrylate plate, (*2*) temporal muscle

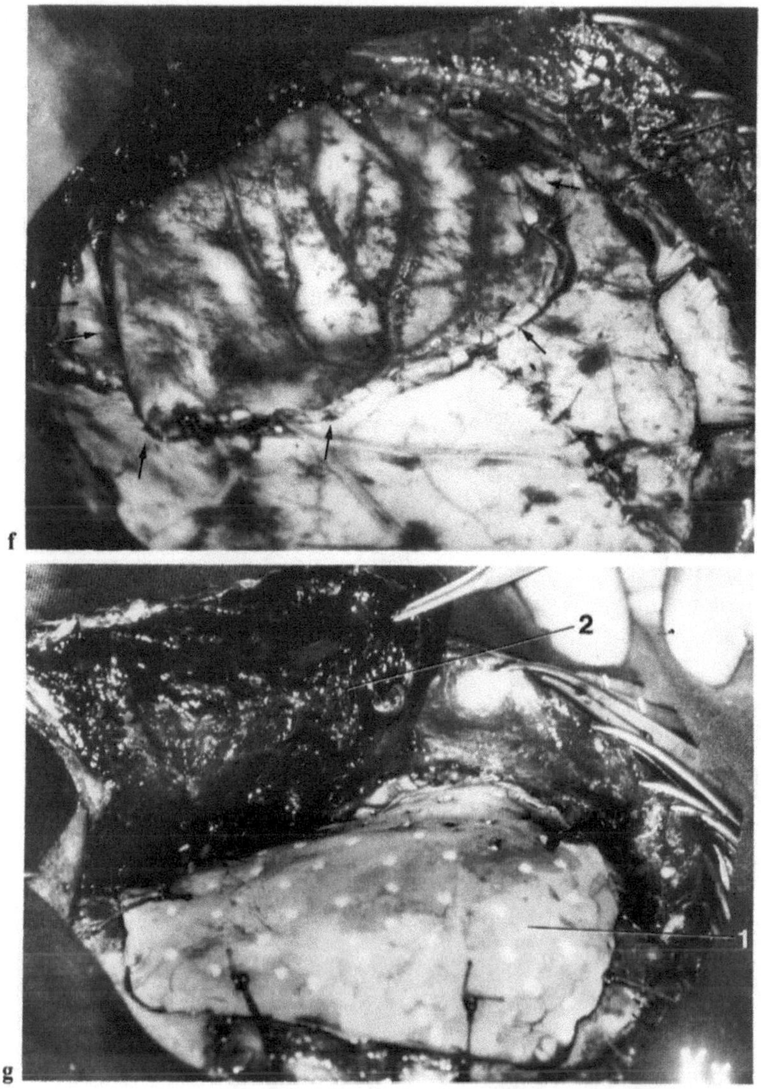

location of the tumor and its angiographic appearance.

If we assume on the one hand that the tumor is very slow-growing, remains asymptomatic for a long period, and metastasizes extremely rarely, and on the other that it may form an intracranial mass lesion and cause multiple cranial nerve deficits, we must weigh carefully the benefits of surgery, especially in elderly patients, and the technical difficulties of separating the tumor from the blood vessels in the neck. The marked bleeding tendency of the lesion and its very close relation to the vessel wall make surgical removal extremely difficult (Conley 1963; Gejrot 1969; Irons et al. 1977; Lack et al. 1977; Vollmar 1975; Voss et al. 1977). Preoperative embolization of the tumor vessels by superselective angiography facilitates removal (Lasjaunias 1980). Prolonged intraoperative occlusion of the internal carotid artery should be avoided, for in the absence of collateral circulation via the circle of Willis, transient or permanent hemiparesis can result even if the vessel is preserved. Elderly patients whose general health is compromised should receive a trial of radiotherapy in an attempt to arrest tumor growth.

Case Report. Left carotid body tumor (Fig. MS 42a–d). A large carotid body tumor of the right side was diagnosed clinically and by carotid angiography in a 62-year-old male. The tumor had caused marked bulging of the oropharynx, hypoglossal and soft-palate weakness, and dysphagia. The neoplasm was approached through the extracranial posteroinferior approach to the middle skull base. First, adjacent structures including the internal jugular vein, vagus nerve, common carotid artery, and accessory nerve were isolated. The sternocleidomastoid muscle was left attached to the skin below the mastoid tip. The tumor was firmly adherent to the common and external carotid arteries and their branches and also to the internal carotid artery and the hypoglossal nerve. We were able to separate the tumor from the vessels by sharp, subadventitial dissection. Bipolar coagulation must be used continuously

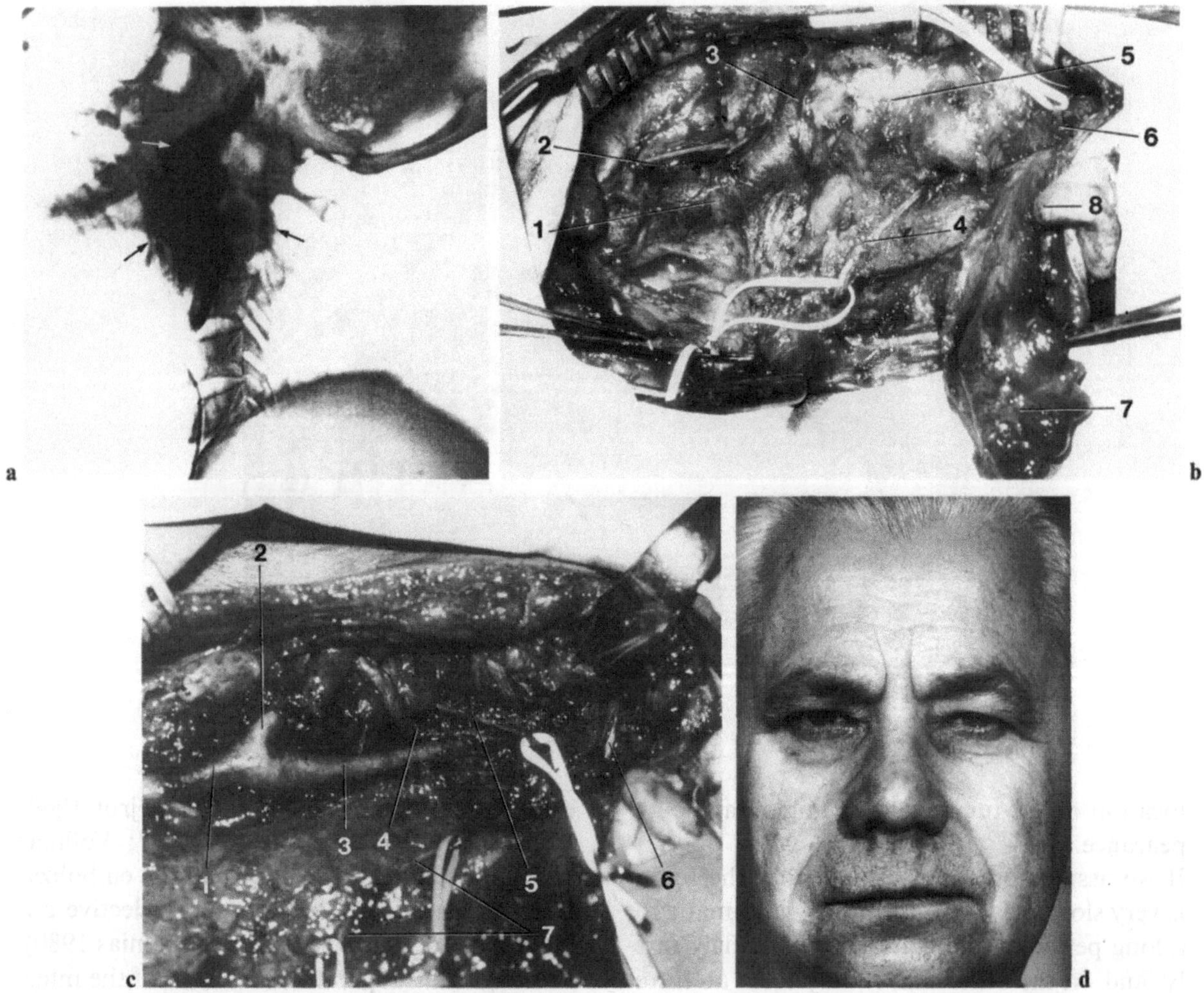

Fig. MS 42 a–d. Large glomus body tumor of the left side.
a Subtraction angiography shows the tumor mass extending to the jugular bulb (*arrows*).
b Operative field before tumor removal. (*1*) Congested internal jugular vein, (*2*) vagus nerve, (*3*) carotid bifurcation, (*4*) accessory nerve, (*5*) tumor, (*6*) facial nerve, (*7*) sternocleidomastoid muscle, (*8*) lobule of ear.
c Operative field after complete tumor removal. (*1*) Common carotid artery, (*2*) stump of external carotid artery, (*3*) internal carotid artery, (*4*) hypoglossal nerve, (*5*) glossopharyngeal nerve, (*6*) facial nerve, (*7*) accessory nerve.
d The patient 1 1/2 years postoperatively

during the dissection of this hypervascularized tumor. The best technique is to cut through the adventitia almost to the vessel wall at one site and from there dissect the tumor from the vessel in cuff-like fashion, staying in the subadventitial plane. Most of the external carotid branches were ligated as the dissection proceeded. The continuity of the hypoglossal nerve was preserved. As the dissection approached the skull base, the facial nerve was identified, and the inferior part of the parotid gland was resected with the mass, preserving the peripheral facial nerve branches. After complete removal of the tumor, the common and internal carotid arteries and the hypoglossal, glossopharyngeal, facial, and accessory nerves could be seen. The initially isolated vagus nerve was lost in the tumor tissue and ultimately could not be spared. At the end of the procedure, the sternocleidomastoid muscle was used for cavity obliteration. A transient facial paralysis regressed completely within a few weeks, and the patient had no significant, permanent postoperative functional impairment.

Comments: A carotid body tumor extending to the skull base was removed through the extracranial posteroinferior approach. Except for the vagus nerve, all cranial nerves and vascular structures were preserved.

Internal Carotid Aneurysm Close to the Skull Base

Aneurysms may be "congenital" or may develop secondary to arteriosclerosis, syphilis, or trauma. An internal carotid aneurysm occurring close to the skull base occasionally leads to medial displacement of tonsillar structures and may be mistaken for a peritonsillar abscess. The palpation of an aneurysmal thrill in these cases avoids the potentially disastrous error of "abscess incision." Angiography should be done to establish the extent and location of the lesion and provide a basis for operative planning. Surgical treatment is indicated for such a lesion that appears suddenly, enlarges rapidly with danger of rupture, and is associated with significant dysphagia or cranial neuropathy. The operation should be performed by an individual experienced in vascular and skull base surgery (Vollmar 1975; Voss et al. 1977).

Case Report. Aneurysm of the right internal carotid artery (Fig. MS 43a–d). A woman 79 years of age experienced increasing dysphagia and respiratory difficulties over a period of several days and was referred with suspicion of a right peritonsillar abscess. On examination, a thrill and pulsations were felt over the entire right pharyngeal wall. Angiography confirmed the suspicion of an internal carotid aneurysm. Because of the rapid enlargement of the aneurysm and the danger of rupture, we decided to operate despite the patient's advanced age.

The skin was incised from the right mastoid tip to the level of the thyroid cartilage, and a second, perpendicular incision was made two fingerwidths below the mandible to expose the cervical vascular structures, the caudal cranial nerves, and the mandible. The mandible was osteotomized at the junction of the angle and horizontal ramus to gain the wide access necessary for dissecting an aneurysmal sac in danger of rupture. The main trunk of the facial nerve was dissected so that the facial nerve could be kept safely under control. After isolating the external carotid artery and ligating its upper branches, we isolated the internal carotid artery immediately above its origin from the carotid bifurcation and also the distal part of the artery beyond the aneurysm up to its entry into the skull base.

There was a pronounced looping of the internal carotid artery toward the lateral pharyngeal wall. The large aneurysm was dissected free on the ascending limb of the vessel, and a smaller calcified aneurysm was dissected free on the distal portion close to the skull base.

Because of the looping of the artery, it was possible to perform an end-to-end anastomosis following excision of the aneurysm and placement of an intraluminal shunt by the vascular surgeon. Although the surgery went well, the patient manifested increasing somnolence and died several days after the operation. Autopsy disclosed high-grade arteriosclerosis distal to the

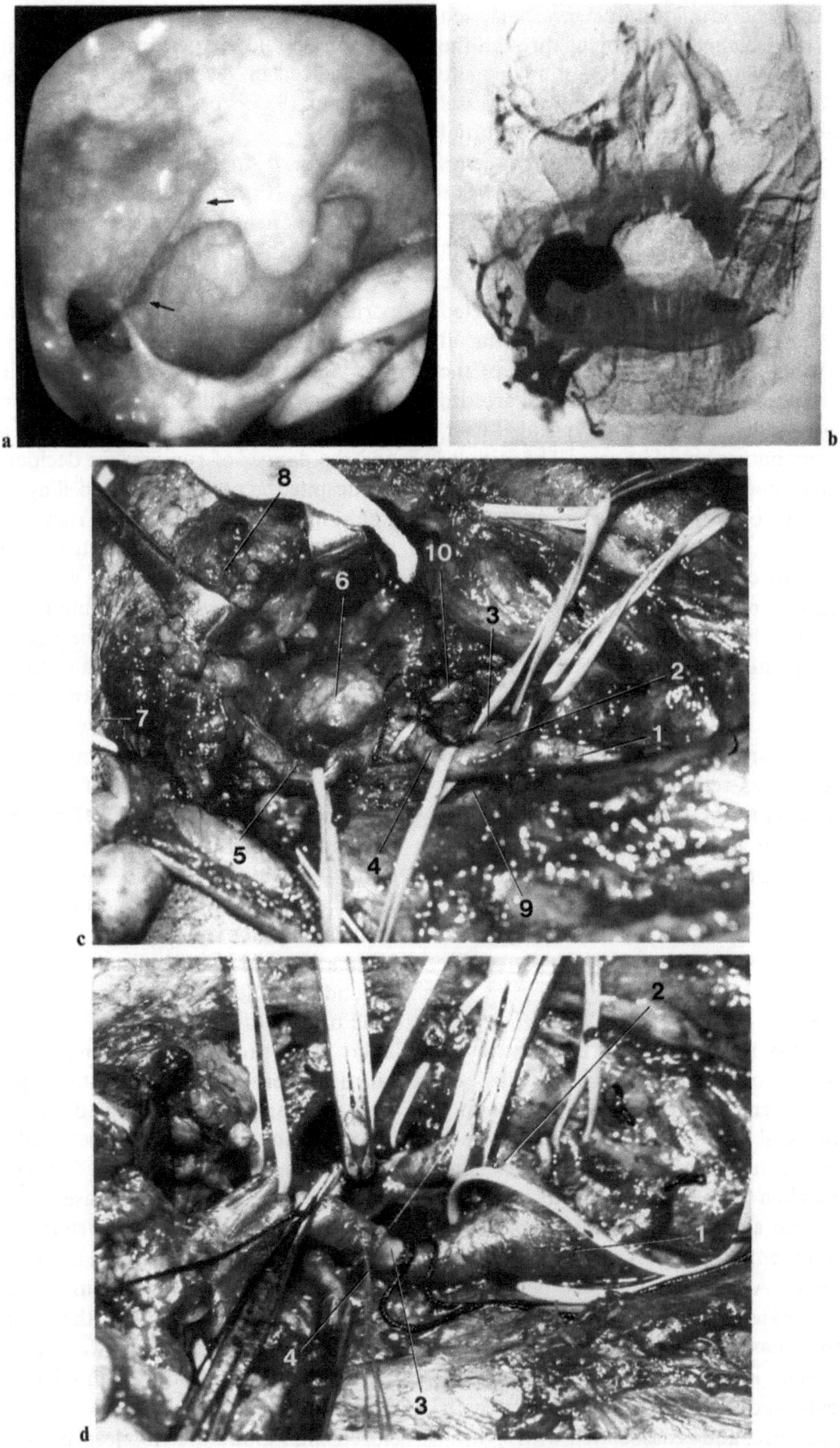
a
b
8
10
6
3
2
7
1
5
4
9
c
2
1
4
3
d

anastomosis with thrombosis accompanied by aplasia of the anterior communicating branch of the circle of Willis.

Comments: An internal carotid aneurysm near the skull base was removed in a patient with severe arteriosclerosis. Because of the location of the aneurysmal sac, the resection and end-to-end anastomosis of the artery were performed with the assistance of a vascular surgeon.

Surgery of Benign Space-Occupying Lesions of the Middle Skull Base with Predominantly Intradural Growth into the Tentorial Incisure

Introductory Remarks. With predominantly intracranial tumors of the middle skull base that are compressing only the temporal lobe and cerebellum, the surgical risk is fairly low. However, when the tumor extends into the tentorial incisure, causing compression of the important vascular and nervous structures located there (including the mesencephalon), it may pose a significant threat to the life of the patient and to the postoperative quality of life, depending on the tumor size and its degree of adherence to surrounding structures. Through microsurgical technique, it has been possible to reduce substantially the mortality and morbidity from operations in this region. It has also been possible to lower the recurrence rate in many cases through the complete and atraumatic removal of these lesions. In addition, use of the operating microscope has expanded our knowledge of the normal microtopographic anatomy of this region, its pathologic anatomy, and the normal variants that are encountered.

We still do not fully understand the function of the individual perforating vessels that arise from the circle of Willis. While a number of authors have noted the importance of the perforating vessels in maintaining the function of brain stem structures, our experience indicates that the plexus-like vascular connections and variants that occur around the brain stem provide this region with a highly adaptable hemodynamic reserve.

In the operative treatment of lesions at the tentorial margin, we are faced with the critical question of whether it is possible to sacrifice these brain stem vessels to effect a complete tumor removal without causing significant functional deficits.

If we examine the variable anatomy of the circle of Willis (Mitterwallner 1955), it becomes clear that large variations must exist in the distributions of the individual vessels. Moreover, in the presence of a highly vascular lesion, the development of new feeding vessels combined with gradual compression of the normal vessels to the point of occlusion can so alter the hemodynamics that the brain stem derives its essential blood supply not from the vessels in the area of the tumor, but largely from the surrounding, normal vascular structures.

With diagnostic techniques currently available, we are unable to measure the preoperative perfusion of deep-lying brain structures accurately enough to provide a basis for planning the operative strategy.

Based on experience to date, we feel strongly that the selective bipolar coagulation of a few of these microvessels has no significant impact on brain stem perfusion. On the other hand, uncontrolled lacerations of the brain stem vessels can be life-threatening, as retraction of the vessel and subsequent intraparenchymal hemorrhage cause profound and irreversible damage to the brain tissue.

Fig. MS 43a–d. Large right internal carotid aneurysm close to the skull base.
a Swelling in the right tonsillar region mimicking a peritonsillar abscess (*arrows*).
b Carotid angiogram shows a large aneurysmal sac in the vertical portion of the internal carotid artery, close to the skull base.
c The mandible has been osteotomized to expose the large cervical vessels, the cranial nerves, and the large aneurysmal sac. (*1*) Common carotid artery, (*2*) carotid bifurcation, (*3*) external carotid artery, (*4*) proximal portion of internal carotid artery, (*5*) distal portion of internal carotid artery, (*6*) aneurysmal sac, (*7*) facial nerve, (*8*) mandible, (*9*) vagus nerve, (*10*) hypoglossal nerve.
d Initial stage of vascular suture. (*1*) Common carotid artery, (*2*) external carotid artery, (*3*) internal carotid artery, (*4*) threads of intraluminal shunt

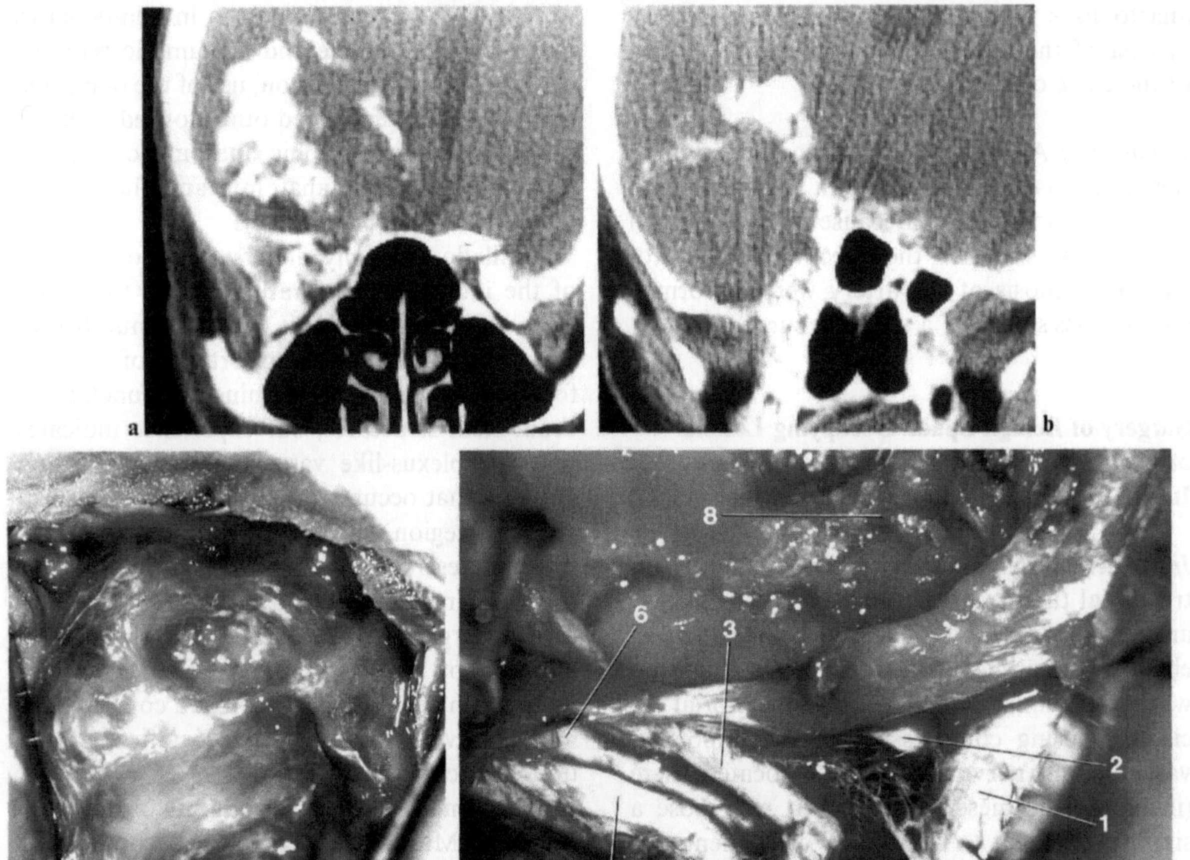

Fig. MS 44 a–f. Chondroma of the right middle cranial fossa with amaurosis and complete ophthalmoplegia.
a, b Preoperative CT scans show extensive calcified foci and destruction of the middle skull base and right clinoid process.
c Exposure of the tumor in the middle fossa.
d The structures in the tentorial incisure are exposed by opening the sylvian fissure and retracting the anterior pole of the temporal lobe. The tumor has already been removed in this area. Remaining tumor is visible at the top of the field. (*1*) Right anterior temporal pole, (*2*) oculomotor nerve, partially covered by tentorial margin, (*3*) internal carotid artery, (*4*) middle cerebral artery, (*5*) anterior cerebral artery, (*6*) optic nerve, (*7*) olfactory tract, (*8*) tumor in area of right middle skull base, (*9*) brain spatula. **e, f** Postoperative CT scans

Chondroma

The pathoanatomic features of this tumor were previously described (see p. 323).

Case Report. Chondroma of the middle cranial fossa with amaurosis and complete ophthalmoplegia (Fig. MS 44a–f). A woman 56 years of age had a 15-year history of right-sided amaurosis and complete ophthalmoplegia. Because of increasing headaches, she was referred for a thorough neurologic and neuroradiologic workup, which disclosed a large space-occupying lesion in the area of the right middle cranial fossa. The lesion had caused significant destruction of the middle skull base as far as the clinoid process. Carotid angiography showed total occlusion of the right internal carotid artery with a well-developed collateral circulation. The lesion was approached through a right frontotemporal craniotomy as used in the standard pterional approach. The sylvian fissure was opened, and the tumor was identified and removed piecemeal, working downward toward the skull base. After posterior retraction of the anterior temporal pole and further separation of the sylvian fissure, we were able to isolate the individual, medially displaced structures in the tentorial incisure. The tumor and surrounding dura were completely removed, whereupon the adjacent bony skull base was drilled down with the diamond burr to obliterate completely the area of tumor attachment. With removal of the tumor, the structures in the tentorial incisure were decompressed without iatrogenic injury. Despite the successful decompression, the longstanding amaurosis and oculomotor paralysis did not improve.
Postoperative CT documented the complete tumor removal.

Comments: An extensive, slow-growing intradural chondroma of the middle skull base with amaurosis, oculomotor paralysis, and internal carotid arterial occlusion was removed microsurgically through a transcranial intradural approach without injury to structures in the tentorial incisure. Preexisting nerve lesions did not improve, underscoring the importance of removing benign tumors as early as possible to avoid permanent functional deficits.

Neurinoma of the Left Trochlear Nerve with Brain Stem Compression

The literature on the biology and pathology of neurinomas was reviewed extensively by Zülch (1956), who described the surgical treatment of cerebellopontine angle neurinomas in some detail. Solitary neurinomas are most common in the cerebellopontine angle, where they usually originate from the vestibulocochlear nerve (cranial nerve VIII). The solitary involvement of other cranial nerves is less common (occasionally V, very rarely III, VII, IX, XI, XII). Zülch does not mention a neurinoma arising from cranial nerve IV (the trochlear nerve), so we may assume that this is exceedingly rare. Specific aspects of the surgical removal of neurinomas are discussed in the section on Cerebellopontine Angle Neurinomas (p. 376).

Case Report. Neurinoma of the left trochlear nerve with brain stem compression and displacement (Fig. MS 45a–d). Mild rightsided hemiparesis and diplopia secondary to oculomotor and trochlear nerve palsies led a 53-year-old woman to seek treatment. CT scans demonstrated a tumor in the tentorial incisure on the left side of the brain stem with associated displacement of the brain stem and basilar artery. An osteoplastic frontotemporal craniotomy was performed, and the lesion was exposed through a left pterional approach. After opening the sylvian fissure and identifying the left internal carotid artery and its branches as well as the left optic nerve, we placed more retraction on the anterior pole of the temporal lobe to expose the anterior part of the tumor. The oculomotor nerve was displaced anteriorly by the tumor and was compressed against the skull base at the posterior clinoid process. The trochlear nerve, from which the tumor arose, was pressed downward against the tentorial margin. During progressive removal and bipolar coagulation, the tumor was found to have considerable extension into the infratentorial space. To aid dissection

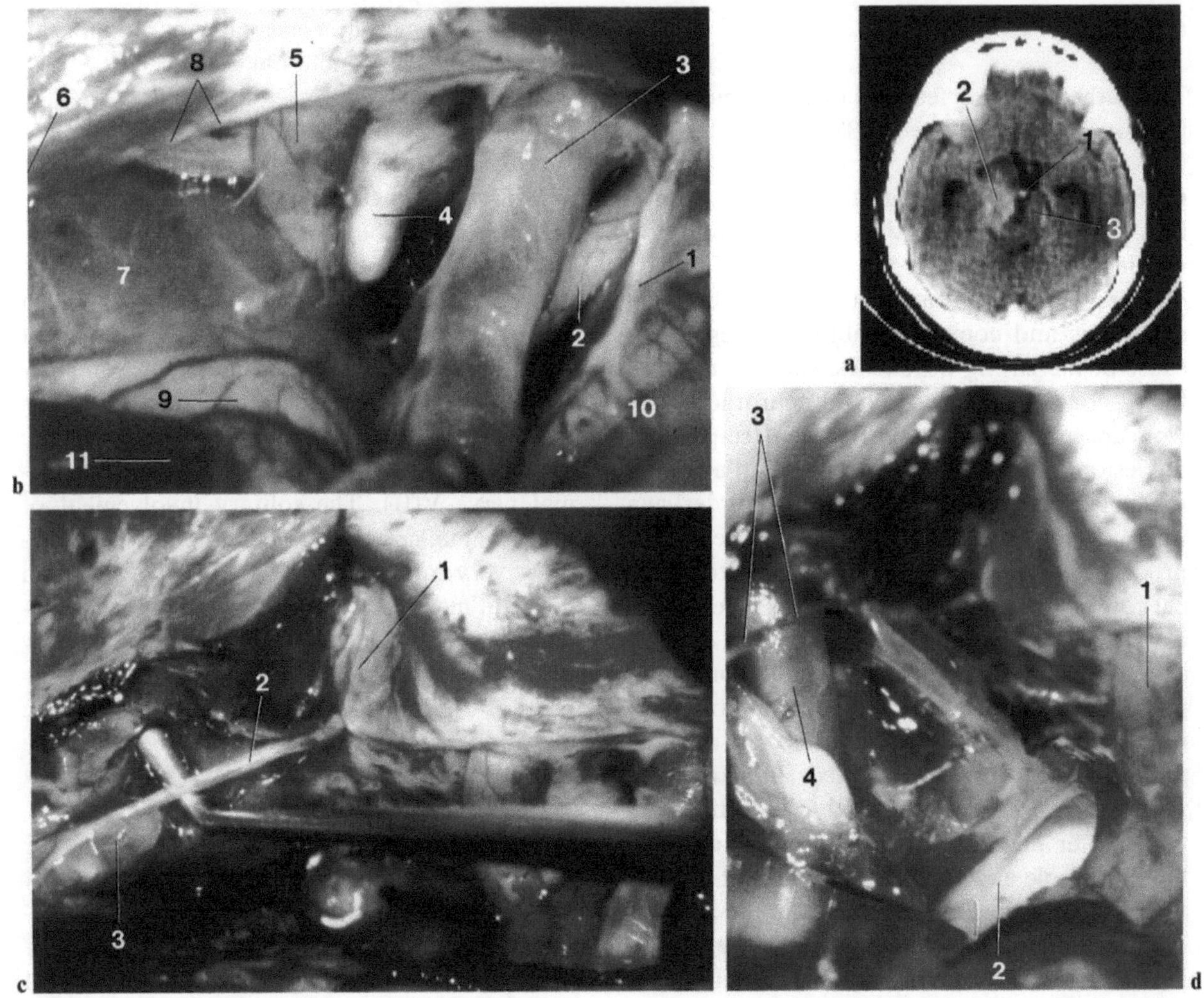

Fig. MS 45 a–d. Extensive neurinoma of the left trochlear nerve with brain stem compression and displacement.

a Axial CT shows displacement of the brain stem by a large mass lesion. The basilar artery is also displaced. (*1*) Basilar artery, (*2*) tumor, (*3*) brain stem.

b The anterior pole of the temporal lobe and posterior frontal lobe have been retracted to expose the internal carotid artery, optic nerve, and the oculomotor and trochlear nerves. (*1*) Olfactory nerve, (*2*) optic nerve, (*3*) internal carotid artery, (*4*) posterior clinoid process, (*5*) oculomotor nerve, (*6*) trochlear nerve, (*7*) tumor, (*8*) tentorial margin, (*9*) anterior pole of temporal lobe, (*10*) frontal lobe, (*11*) brain spatula.

c Here the tumor has been partially removed, and the tentorium has been incised and the flap turned upward. The trochlear nerve has been almost completely freed of tumor (hook). It is still in contact with tumor laterally. (*1*) Tentorial flap, (*2*) trochlear nerve, (*3*) infratentorial part of tumor.

d Operative field following tumor removal. (*1*) Intact oculomotor nerve, (*2*) abducens nerve, (*3*) trochlear nerve, (*4*) basilar artery of the intratentorial part of the tumor, we made an incision behind the site of entry of the trochlear nerve into the cavernous sinus, at right angles to the tentorial margin, and raised the edges of the tentorium with traction sutures. We were then able to expose the trochlear nerve over its entire length and dissect the tumor free from the nerve, including its site of origin, while preserving the continuity of the uninvolved fascicles. The individual anatomic structures were clearly visible and appeared intact following complete removal of the neoplasm. The preexisting trochlear paralysis persisted after surgery, but the mild preoperative weakness of the eye muscles supplied by the oculomotor nerve resolved completely.

Comments: An extremely rare, predominantly infratentorial neurinoma of the trochlear nerve was removed through a left pterional approach. Preoperative oculomotor weakness regressed after the surgery, while paralysis of the trochlear nerve, from which the tumor arose, persisted. The tumor was identified histologically as a neurinoma.

Case Report. Trigeminal neurinoma of the middle skull base (Fig. MS 46a–h). The patient, a 33-year-old woman, had experienced right-sided Migraine attacks"for years. She had a 3-year history of progressive visual deterioration and diplopia with a marked motility disturbance of the right eye.

Axial CT scans showed a large, round, smooth-margined mass lesion with destruction of the petrous apex and the medial two-thirds of the middle skull base. Involvement of the right posterior paranasal sinus system and posterior orbital wall also was apparent. Medially, the tumor extended across the midline to the oppposite side. Magnetic resonance imaging on the coronal plane revealed compression of the right temporal lobe and cerebrum with displacement of the third ventricle. The tumor appeared to be divided into a larger lateral lobe and a smaller medial lobe by the right internal carotid artery. Sagittal MR imaging showed that the tumor had grown obliquely upward from the pterygopalatine fossa, displacing the cerebrum superiorly. Carotid angiography demonstrated medial and posterior displacement of the internal carotid artery by the mass.

A right frontotemporal osteoplastic craniotomy was performed, the dura was opened, and the middle skull base was exposed as far as the tentorial margin. The temporal lobe was retracted to uncover the large tumor. The oculomotor and optic nerve, the internal carotid artery, were microsurgically isolated from the tumor and preserved. Examination of the trigeminal nerve at the brain stem showed that the tumor originated from that nerve and had spread in the area of the bony middle skull base. After bipolar coagulation of the middle fossa dura, the neurinoma was successively removed. The trochlear nerve had to be sacrificed along with the trigeminal nerve to effect a radical removal. After resection of the lateral part of the tumor, the internal carotid artery was progressively exposed in its transverse, petrosal segment. The carotid canal was completely eroded due to pressure from the tumor, and the artery had lost its bony containment. Under high magnification, some of the lateral branches of the internal carotid artery were coagulated and transected so that the vessel could be adequately mobilized. After this had been done, it was possible to remove the remaining, medial portion of the neoplasm. The temporal muscle was used to cover the basal dural defect at the middle skull base, the craniotomy flap was replaced and secured, and the wound was closed over a subgaleal suction drain. Histologic examination identified the tumor as a neurinoma.

Cerebrospinal rhinorrhea was noted about 14 days after the surgery. Erosion of the medial and posterior ethmoid walls by the tumor had allowed the mucosa – intact at operation – to rupture from excessive cerebrospinal fluid pressure. The cerebrospinal fluid leak was repaired transfacially with a fascial graft and packing (Dr. L. Osterwald).

Comments: A large neurinoma of the middle skull base arising from the trigeminal nerve and causing extensive bone destruction was completely removed through a temporal transcranial intradural approach. A postoperative cere-

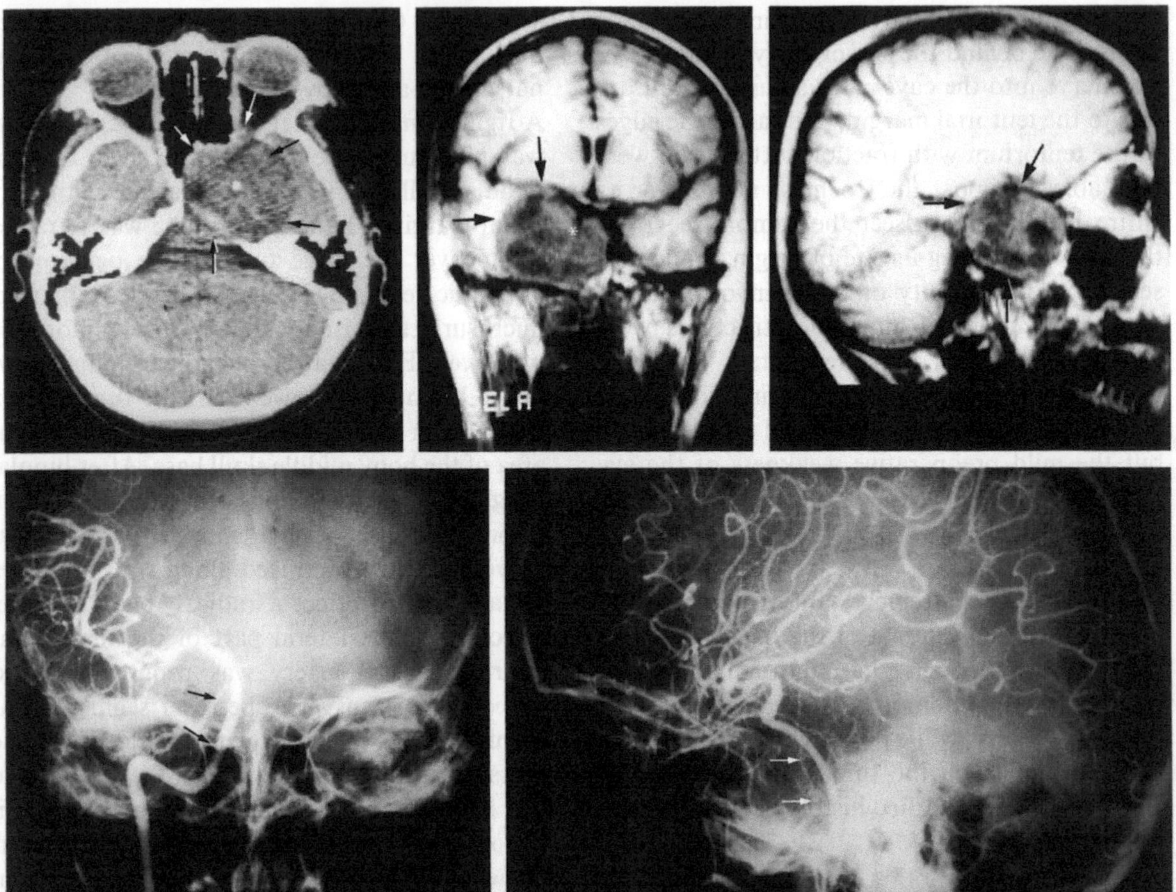

Fig. MS 46a–h. Trigeminal neurinoma of the middle skull base.
a Axial CT scan shows a large mass lesion of the middle skull base extending across the midline to the contralateral side. There is associated destruction of the skull base, the anterior petrous bone, and the posterior walls of the paranasal sinuses.
b, c Magnetic resonance (MR) images in the coronal and sagittal projections. The coronal image (**b**) shows displacement of the temporal lobe to the right and superior displacement of the cerebrum, so that the third ventricle also appears displaced. The internal carotid artery divides the tumor into a medial and a lateral lobe. The sagittal image (**c**) shows the tumor reaching the pterygopalatine fossa and eroding the posterior wall of the maxillary sinus. The cerebrum is displaced superiorly.
d, e Angiograms of the right internal carotid artery show obvious medial and posterior displacement of the vessel.
f Intradural exposure of the tumor by retraction of the frontal and temporal lobes. (*1*) Olfactory tract, (*2*) optic nerve, (*3*) internal carotid artery, (*4*) oculomotor nerve, (*5*) tumor.
g After removing the lateral part of the tumor (*2*), the internal carotid artery (*1*) is isolated in its transverse, petrosal portion.
h Surgical cavity following complete tumor removal. The internal carotid artery now freely traverses the space formerly occupied by the tumor. (*1*) Internal carotid artery (petrosal part), (*2*) internal carotid artery (supraclinoid part), (*3*) destruction of the skull base, (*4*) tentorial margin, (*5*) suction tip

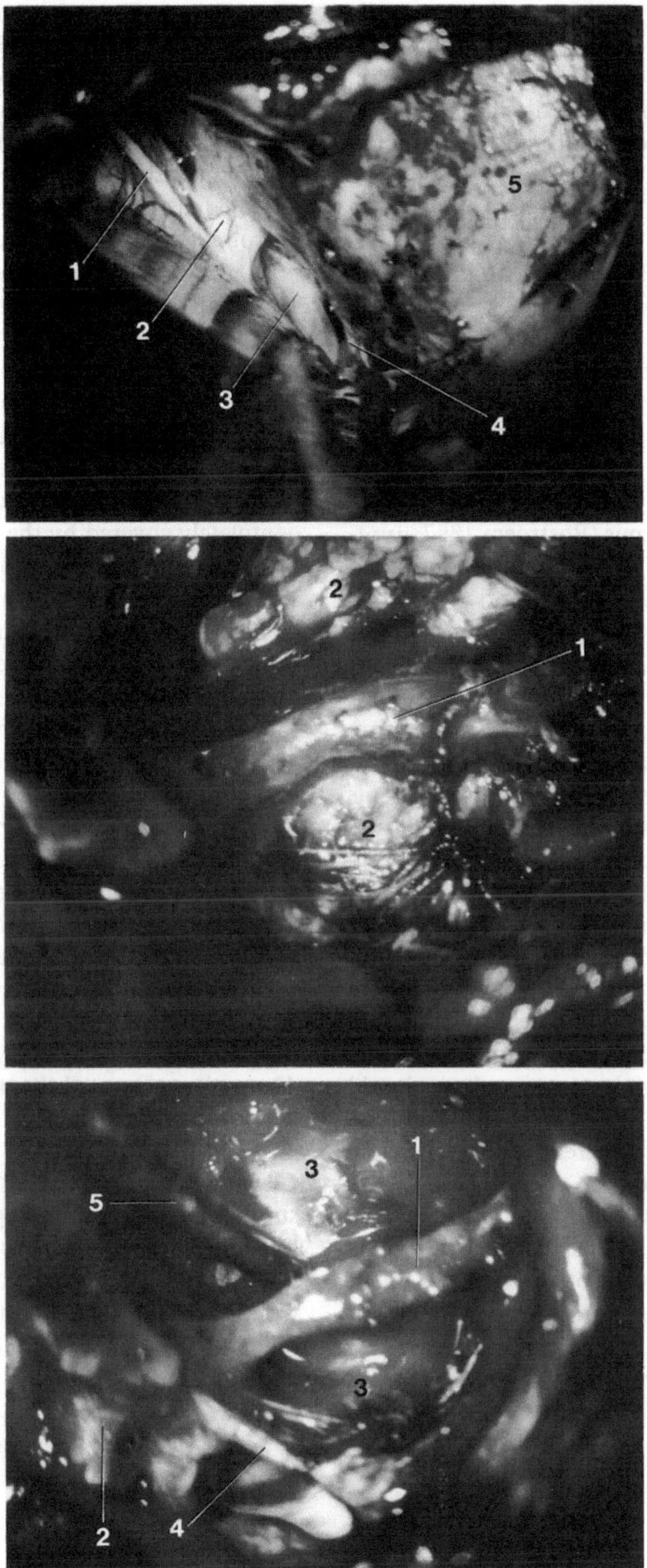

f

g

h

brospinal fluid leak was repaired secondarily with fascia through a transfacial approach. A mild postoperative oculomotor weakness resolved before the patient was discharged. Anesthesia of the right facial half and trochlear paralysis persisted.

Epidermoid of the Medial Middle Skull Base ("True Cholesteatoma")

Some aspects of epidermoids, or cholesteatoma, were discussed earlier in connection with inflammatory disorders of the middle skull base (see p. 264). Epidermoids are tumors that are filled with cholesterol-rich material and whose capsule consists of epidermis (Bostroem 1897, quoted in Zülch 1956). The tumors are considered to be of developmental origin, and reports on the incidence of intracranial occurrence range from 0.6% to 1.8%. Most epidermoids occur in the subarachnoid cisterns, and all are solitary. According to Rand and Reeves (1943), no more than 200 cases were known in the world literature prior to 1943. The behavior of epidermoids and dermoids in relation to surrounding tissues is variable. Epidermoids can damage the brain tissue extensively and can spread along small connective-tissue pathways, even of the central nervous tissue (Zülch 1956). It is important surgically that these tumors are delimited from the brain and surrounding structures by a capsule. Epidermoids attached to the meninges can "blend in" with the pia mater and arachnoid and become fused to the brain. In the skull base region they are often adherent to blood vessels. Extracranial extension is possible along the fissures. The contents of the tumor may undergo autolysis and soften. Recurrence is inevitable with incomplete removal of the capsule, but it is questionable whether transplanted pieces of the capsule can "take" and cause a recurrence (Zülch 1956). Epidermoids generally appear as low-density areas on CT scans.

Case Report. Extensive epidermoid of the medial middle cranial fossa (Fig. MS 47a–f). A 50-year-old man was referred for CT evaluation because of headaches and generalized weakness. Surprisingly, CT scans showed an extensive, predominantly right-sided low-density mass in the medial part of the middle skull base that surrounded and partially compressed the brain stem. Although it appeared that the lesion involved all the ocular motor nerves, ocular motility was clinically normal. A right frontotemporal craniotomy was performed, and the sylvian fissure was opened to reveal, in the tentorial incisure, a tumor comprised of multiple silvery, globular masses surrounded by arachnoid. The internal carotid artery and optic nerve were completely covered by the tumor.
Using microsurgical technique, the tumor and its capsule were removed piecemeal until the optic nerve and posteriorly displaced internal carotid artery were visualized. Through this approach we were able to dissect the tumor from the vessels originating from the internal carotid artery while preserving the oculomotor, trochlear, and abducens nerves. The tumor also had to be removed from the basilar artery and its branches and from the posterior cerebral and superior cerebellar arteries. After complete tumor removal, the "basilar knob or button" with its contralateral posterior cerebral and superior cerebellar arterial branches could be seen. The oculomotor nerve was visible between these two vessels.
The patient tolerated the operation well and experienced no sequelae.

Comments: A large, predominantly right-sided supra- and infratentorial epidermoid in the pontine and interpeduncular cistern was successfully removed microsurgically through a right frontotemporal osteoplastic craniotomy, with bilateral preservation of the ocular motor nerves and vascular structures.

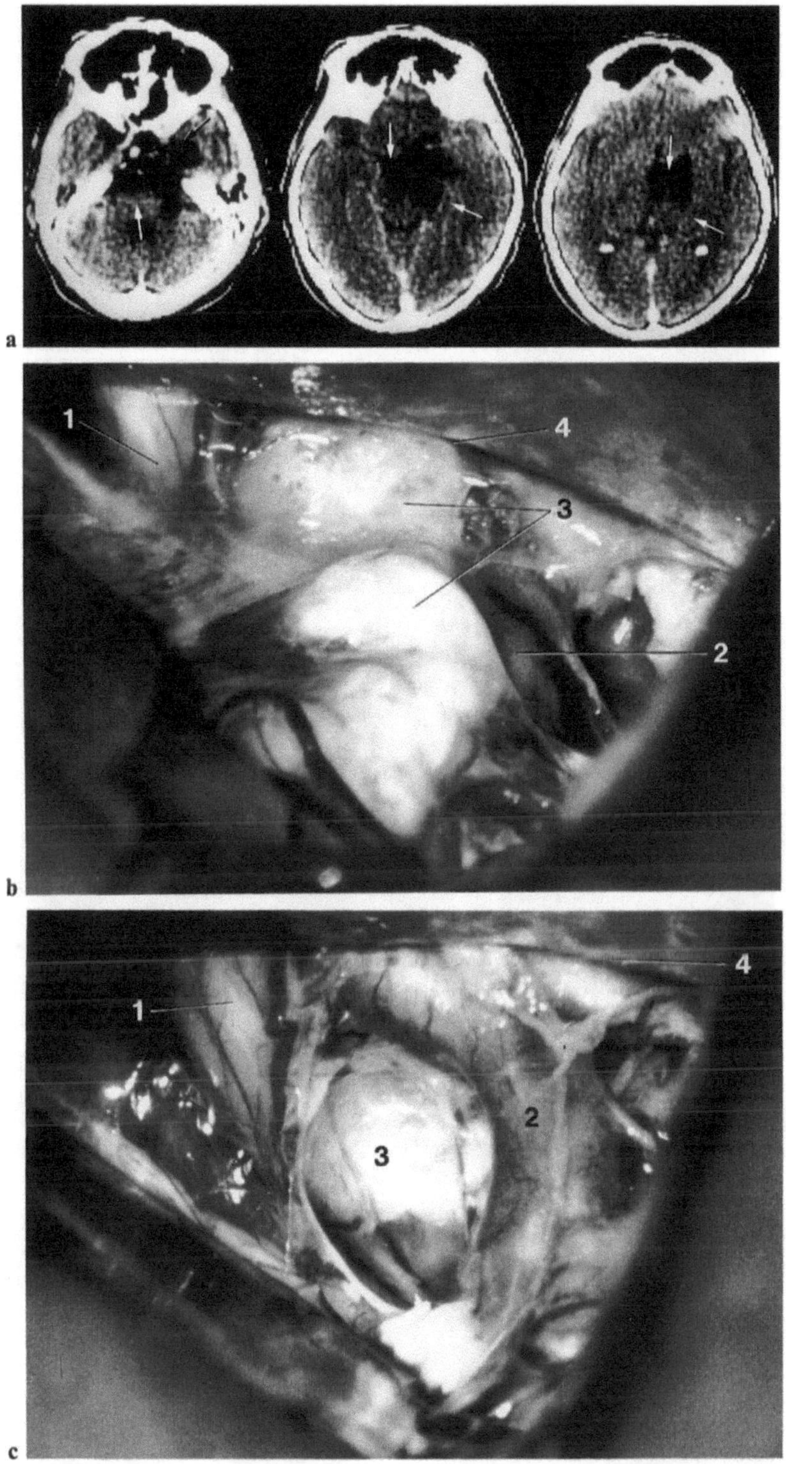

Fig. MS 47a–f. Extensive epidermoid of the medial part of the middle cranial fossa.
a CT scans demonstrate an extensive epidermoid tumor (*arrows*).
b A frontotemporal craniotomy was performed, and the tentorial incisure exposed. The optic nerve and internal carotid artery are largely covered by the silvery, globular tumor masses. (*1*) Optic nerve, (*2*) internal carotid artery, (*3*) tumor, (*4*) tentorial margin.
c The cranial parts of the tumor have been removed, exposing most of the optic nerve and internal carotid artery. (*1*) Optic nerve, (*2*) internal carotid artery (arched), (*3*) tumor, (*4*) tentorial margin

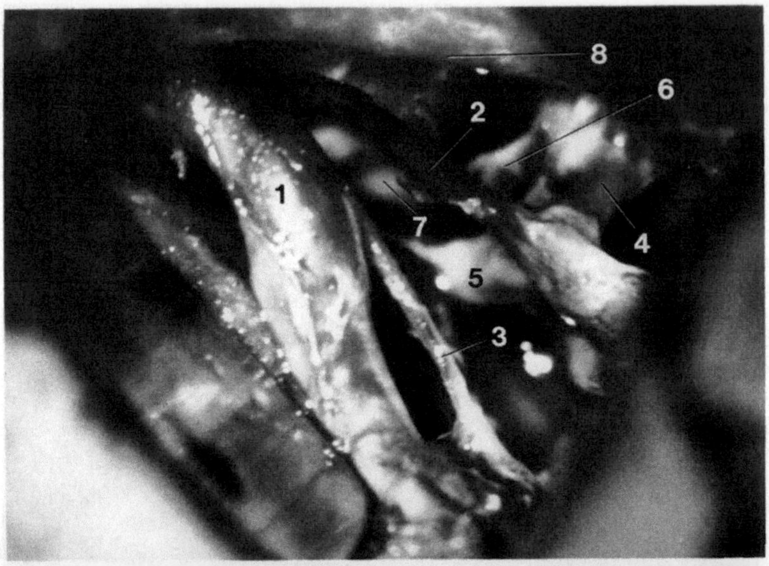

d

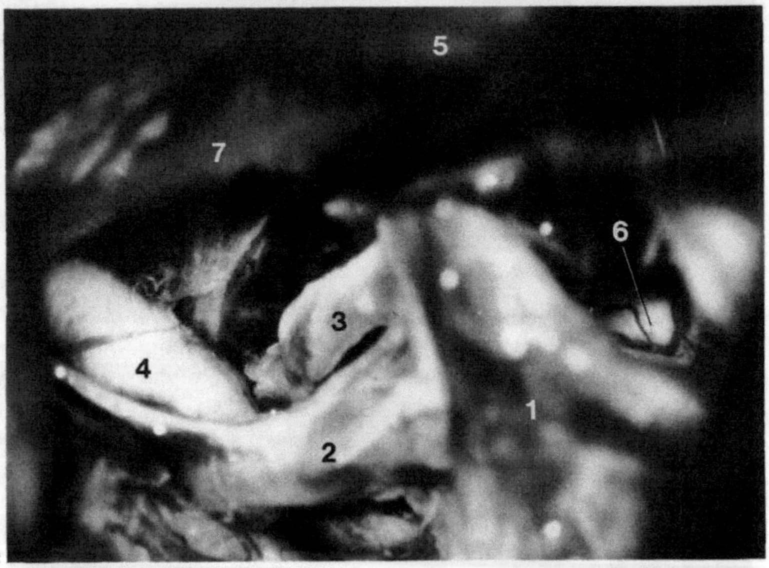

e

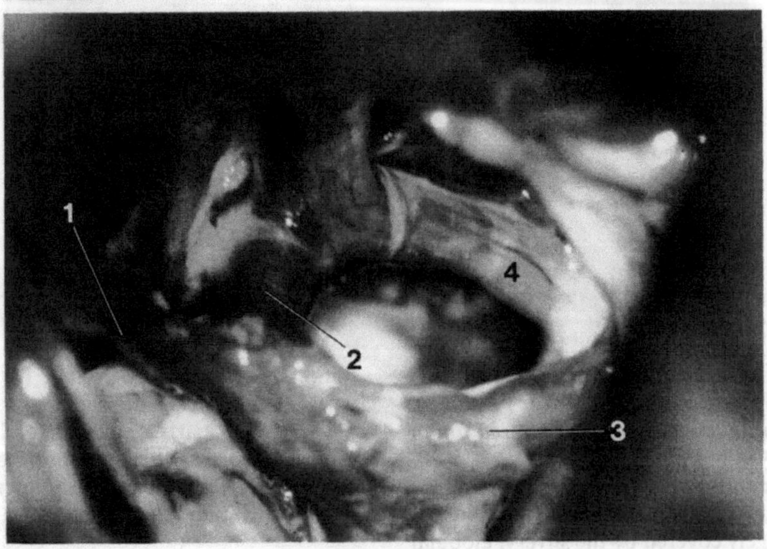

f

Meningiomas of the Middle Cranial Fossa with Extension to the Anterior and Posterior Skull Base

It is significant in terms of otologic diagnosis that the symptom of unilateral secretory otitis media with conductive hearing loss may be secondary to an early-stage meningioma of the middle cranial fossa, prior to the development of mass-lesion symptoms and cranial neuropathies. The middle ear effusion results from compression of the eustachian tube from the medial aspect and an associated disturbance in the aeration of the middle ear.

The classification and biology of meningiomas was discussed previously in connection with anterior skull base tumors (see p. 208). Here we shall focus our attention on the surgical aspects of meningiomas involving the brain stem.

We recognize *two different types* of meningioma from the surgical viewpoint:

1) Globular meningiomas that displace adjacent structures as they enlarge.
2) Enplaque meningiomas that spread over the surfaces of structures and envelop them.

The second type presents greater surgical difficulties, especially at the tentorial incisure, where a number of vitally important structures occur in close proximity to one another. While even large globular meningiomas often can be completely removed by piecemeal extirpation, this is generally not the case with enplaque growths, which are a challenge even to modern microsurgical techniques. The goals of surgery in such cases are three-fold: 1) histologic confirmation of the clinical diagnosis, 2) decompression of important structures, and 3) removal of as much tumor as possible without causing iatrogenic trauma.

The difficulties of dissecting enplaque growths can be formidible, and the surgeon must continually decide the extent to which he can and should continue the tumor removal while avoiding iatrogenic lesions. It is better to leave behind portions of these slow-growing neoplasms than endanger the patient's life or inflict severe, irreversible damage. Removal in several stages should be considered for very extensive, bilateral meningiomas.

Case Report. Petroclival meningioma (Fig. MS 48a–f, see also Fig. MS 35a–h). A 64-year-old woman noticed a sensation of numbness at the inner canthus of the right eye spreading to the right nostril and right upper lip one year prior to operation. Subsequently the patient developed dysarthric speech problems and an increasing unsteadiness of gait, accompanied by general weakness. Neurologic examination disclosed dysesthesia in the first and second trigeminal nerve divisions on the right with an abolished corneal reflex. The patient manifested right-sided bradydiadochokinesia and dysmetria with a tendency to fall to the left side. The gag reflex was diminished. Minimal facial nerve weakness on the right side also was detected. These findings, along with the dysarthric disturbances, suggested an irritation of the caudal cranial nerves. A mild left-sided hemiparesis developed just prior to operation.

CT scans showed a paramedian mass lesion on the right side approximately 5 cm in diameter arising from the tentorial margin and causing very marked displacement of the brain stem and cerebellum.

In view of the tumor location, it was decided to expose the lesion through a transtemporal, transtentorial approach.

◄

Fig. MS 47d–f.
d View into the right tentorial incisure after tumor removal. (*1*) Internal carotid artery, (*2*) posterior communicating artery, (*3*) anterior choroidal artery, (*4*) basilar artery, (*5*) left posterior cerebral artery, (*6*) left superior cerebellar artery, (*7*) oculomotor nerve, (*8*) right tentorial margin.
e Under magnification, the right posterior communicating artery has been retracted toward the tentorial margin with a dissecting forceps, exposing the oculomotor nerve between the left posterior cerebral artery and the left superior cerebellar artery. (*1*) Site of division of the basilar artery, (*2*) left posterior cerebral artery, (*3*) left posterior cerebellar artery, (*4*) oculomotor nerve, (*5*) right tentorial margin, (*6*) pons, (*7*) right posterior communicating artery.
f Here the posterior communicating artery is retracted medially to expose the arched and displaced right oculomotor nerve. (*1*) Posterior communicating artery, (*2*) basilar artery, (*3*) right posterior cerebral artery, (*4*) right oculomotor nerve

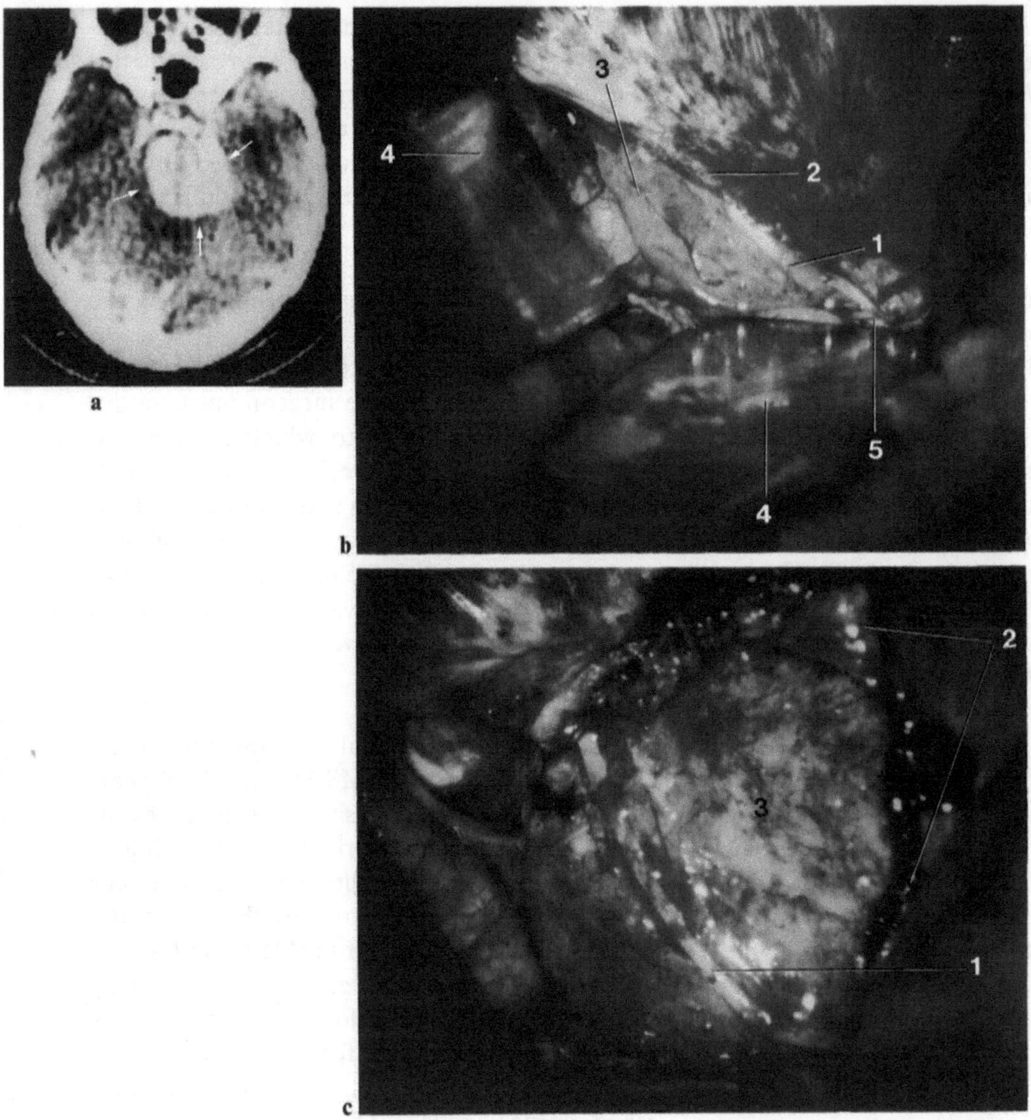

Fig. MS 48 a–f. Transfrontotemporal, transtentorial removal of a petroclival meningioma.
a Axial CT shows a large meningioma arising from the right tentorial margin with marked compression and displacement of the brain stem and cerebellum.
b Transfrontotemporal, intradural approach to the tentorial margin with exposure of the medial tumor pole and trochlear nerve. (*1*) Trochlear nerve, (*2*) tentorial margin, (*3*) tumor, (*4*) spatula, (*5*) trigeminal nerve
c Extended exposure of the tumor by lateral incision of the tentorium. The trochlear nerve passes over the tumor capsule. (*1*) Trochlear nerve, (*2*) tentorial flaps, (*3*) tumor.
d The tumor has been partially removed by combined enucleation and bipolar cautery. The impingement on the brain stem is visible, and the tumor capsule has been partially disengaged at that site. The basilar artery appears medially. (*1*) Trochlear nerve, (*2*) brain stem, (*3*) tumor, (*4*) basilar artery, (*5*) arachnoid.
e Status following complete tumor removal. From left to right we see the oculomotor nerve, which is displaced anteriorly; the trochlear nerve, which is stretched by the tumor; the trigeminal nerve; and the brain stem. (*1*) Trochlear nerve, (*2*) trigeminal nerve, (*3*) oculomotor nerve, (*4*) basilar artery, (*5*) internal carotid artery.
f Status following complete tumor removal, viewing posteroinferiorly toward the cerebellopontine angle. The trigeminal nerve is seen on the left; at the top are the coagulated and divided superior petrosal sinus with the partially resected petrous apex and the facial nerve at its site of entry into the IAC. The structures of the brain stem and cerebellum are readily differentiated. (*1*) Facial nerve, (*2*) trigeminal nerve, (*3*) superior petrosal sinus (coagulated and divided), (*4*) petrous apex (partially removed), (*5*) brain stem, (*6*) cerebellum

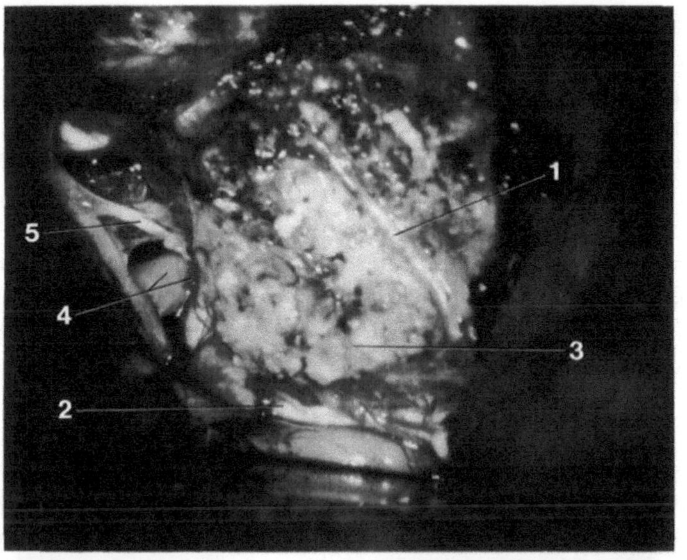

d

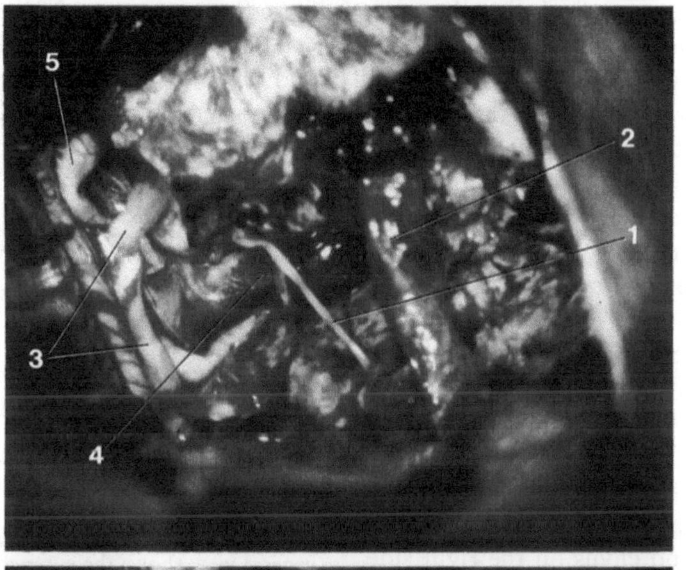

e

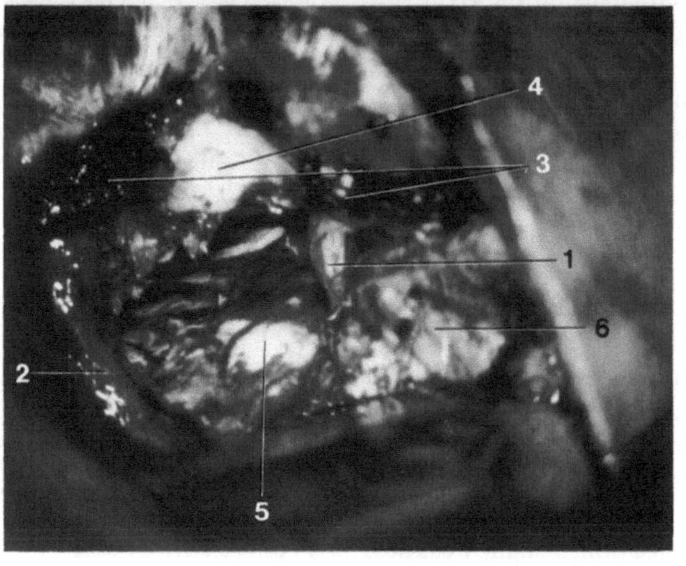

f

A right frontotemporal osteoplastic craniotomy was performed, and the dura was opened temporobasally creating a flap based on the superior sagittal sinus. The middle fossa was exposed, and the tumor was identified in the tentorial incisure. The optic nerve and internal carotid artery were free of tumor, but the trigeminal nerve was greatly compressed by the tumor and displaced anteromedially. The trochlear nerve was displaced upward from below. At this stage the operating microscope was brought into position; the tentorial margin was incised between the trigeminal nerve and trochlear nerve, and the tumor surface was widely exposed. The tentorium was also incised posteriorly over the cerebellum to expose the posterior tumor pole, which was compressing and displacing the cerebellum. The tumor was debulked stepwise, and its capsule was separated from the brain stem. To improve vision for removing the infratentorial tumor extension, the superior petrosal sinus was coagulated and ligated. Then the dura was partly mobilized from the petrous bone, and the petrous apex was removed with the diamond burr. Finally we were able to remove the tumor completely while dissecting free and preserving the basilar artery, the posterior cerebral artery, the facial and vestibulocochlear nerves, and the caudal cranial nerves.

Comments: An extensive meningioma of the skull base involving the tentorial incisure, cerebellopontine angle, and clivus on the right side (petroclival meningioma) was completely removed through a frontotemporal osteoplastic craniotomy with transtentorial exposure of the posterior cranial fossa. A ventriculoperitoneal shunt was inserted.

Case Report. Meningioma of the petrous margin with extension into the middle and posterior fossae on the left side (Fig. MS 49a–f). A 50-year-old woman had a 2-year history of increasing sensory disturbances in the left facial half and experienced disturbances of equilibrium in the months prior to surgery.

On admission the patient had hypalgesia and hyperesthesia of the left facial half, an ipsilateral disturbance of taste sensation, a slight weakness of the oral facial nerve branch, and a paretic nystagmus toward the contralateral side. She also manifested impairment in coordination with a tendency to lose her balance.

Axial and coronal CT scans showed a large mass lesion in the middle and posterior cranial fossae with extension to the cerebellopontine angle and clivus. In the middle fossa the tumor extended to the cavernous sinus.

The tumor was first exposed in the middle fossa through a left frontotemporal osteoplastic trephine opening. The anterior tumor pole had displaced the trochlear and oculomotor nerves upward and anteriorly and extended to the cavernous sinus. The tumor was progressively debulked until its capsule could be dissected free from those nerves and from the cavernous sinus wall. The optic nerve, the internal carotid artery and its branches, the anterior choroidal artery and posterior communicating branch also could be preserved.

Fig. MS 49a–f. Removal of a meningioma at the tentorial margin with extension into the left middle and posterior cranial fossae.

a–c Axial and coronal CT scans demonstrate a large tentorial meningioma with extension into the middle and posterior fossae.

d, e Status following complete tumor removal on the left side through an extended transfrontotemporal, osteoplastic, intradural approach with resection of the tentorium and partial resection of the left pyramid. The general view shows the suprachiasmatic and prepontine region with the following structures: left optic nerve, left internal carotid artery, residual left petrous pyramid with coagulation tracks, and the basilar artery with the origins of the right superior cerebellar and posterior cerebral arteries. Part of the right oculomotor nerve is visible within the arterial bifurcation. (*1*) Left optic nerve, (*2*) left internal carotid artery, (*3*) left oculomotor nerve, (*4*) left petrous bone, (*5*) basilar artery, (*6*) right oculomotor nerve. Panel **(e)** shows a highly magnified view of the basilar artery and its branches, looking into the prepontine space from above and to the left. We clearly recognize the right and left superior cerebellar arteries, the right and left posterior cerebral arteries, and the right oculomotor nerve in the angle between the superior cerebellar and posterior cerebral arteries. (*1*) Basilar artery, (*2*) right superior cerebellar artery, (*3*) right oculomotor nerve, (*4*) right posterior cerebral artery, (*5*) left posterior cerebral artery, (*6*) left superior cerebellar artery.

f Postoperative CT scan

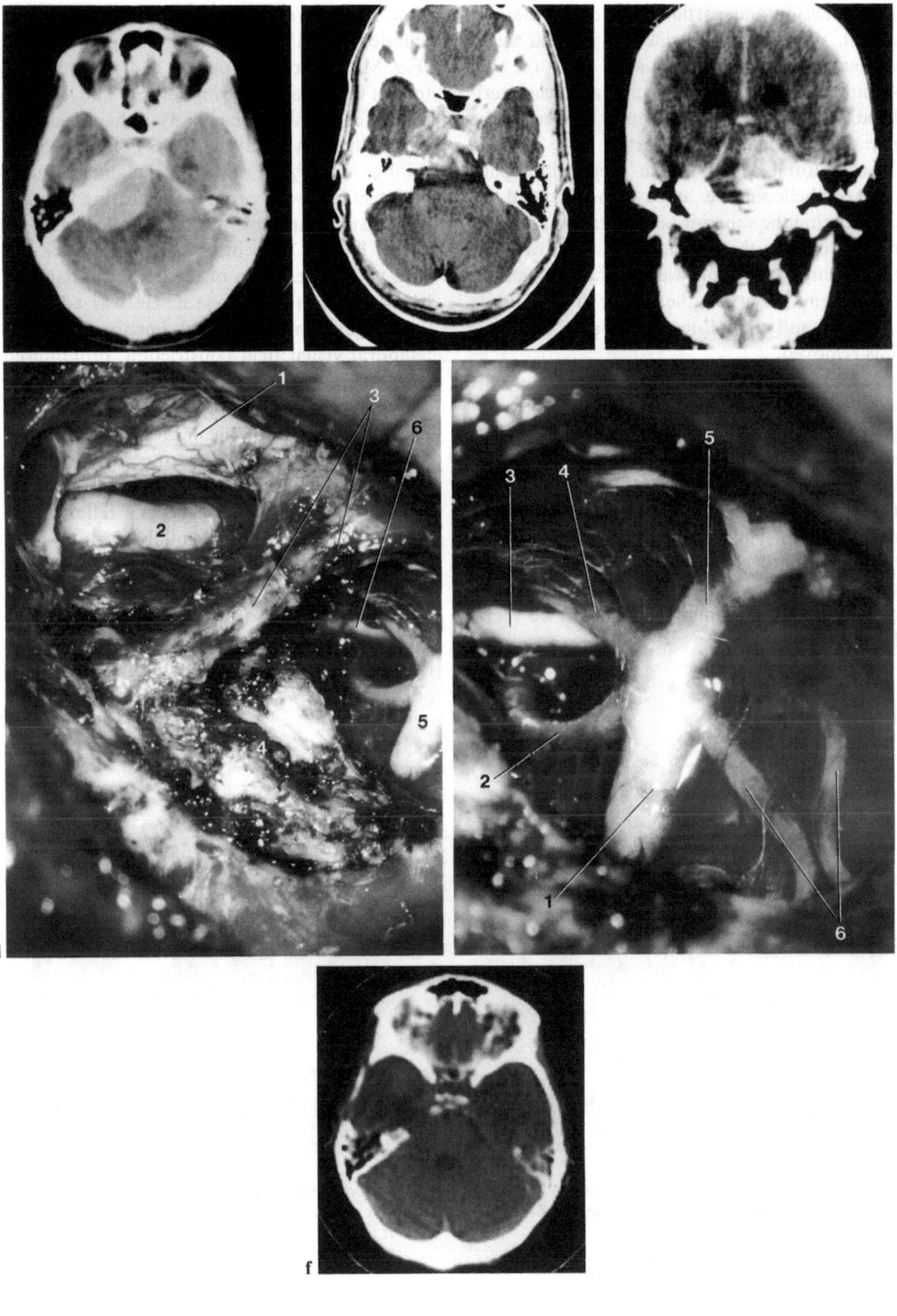

a, b c d e f

After incision and partial resection of the tentorium, the tumor-infiltrated trigeminal nerve was exposed from the brain stem up to the gasserian ganglion and its branches and was sacrificed with the surrounding tumor in view of the preexisting damage to the nerve.
Transtentorial access to the prepontine space and cerebellopontine angle was extended by coagulating the superior petrosal sinus and partially removing the petrous apex. The transtentorial tumor extension was separated from the brain stem, preserving the basilar artery and its branches and cranial nerves VII and VIII, and was removed.

Comments: A meningioma of the tentorial margin extending into the middle and posterior fossae was separated from the cavernous sinus and removed with preservation of functional neurovascular structures, most notably the ocular motor nerves. The extended subtemporal transtentorial approach provides good exposure of the infratentorial region. The trigeminal nerve was infiltrated by tumor and had to be sacrificed.

Case Report. Very extensive meningioma of the anterior, middle, and posterior cranial fossae (Fig. MS 50a–c). The patient had an 8-year history of diplopia of varying severity and a 6-year history of left abducens paralysis, having undergone a tenomyotomy in 1978. For six months prior to surgery the patient complained of noise in the left ear with progressive hearing loss and mild visual impairment. A 2-month history of severe levator palpebrae paralysis on the left side, with hypesthesia of the left facial half and headaches was also present. He was admitted with significant left visual impairment, right temporal visual field constriction, pronounced left oculomotor paresis, and mild left trochlear and abducens paresis. In addition, he had anesthesia and hypoesthesia in all three trigeminal nerve divisions on the left, paresis of the masticatory muscles, slight left facial nerve paresis, a diminished swallowing and gag reflex, slight right hemiparesis, and a mildly positive right Babinski sign with bilateral dysdiadochokinesia. A combined conductive-sensorineural hearing loss in the left ear was also present.
CT scans demonstrated a very extensive mass lesion on the left side extending from the midportion of the anterior cranial fossa across the

a, b

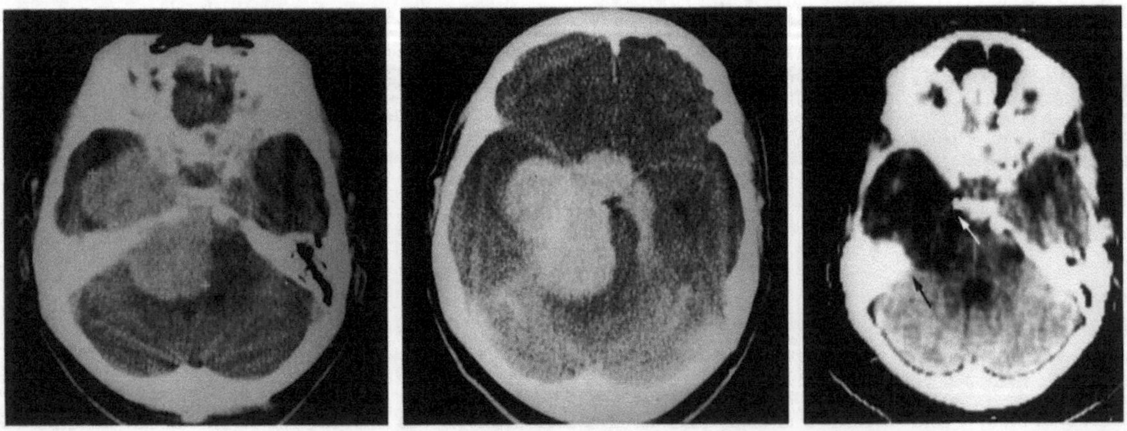

c

Fig. MS 50a–c. Very extensive meningioma involving the anterior, middle, and posterior fossae on both sides, the left side more.
a, b Preoperative CT scans document the displacement of the cerebrum, midbrain, and cerebellum.
c Tumor components are no longer visible on the postoperative CT scan. The surgical defect at the apex of the left petrous pyramid (*arrows*) is apparent

middle fossa into the posterior fossa. The mass had also spread relatively far across the clivus into the middle fossa on the right side. It compressed the brain stem and displaced it to the right and had destroyed the right anterior skull base in the area of the lesser sphenoid wing and orbital roof. Suprasellar extension into the temporal lobe and cerebellum on the left side was also noted. On the right side the tumor had spread posteriorly along the tentorial margin.

Because the tumor involved practically all three parts of the skull base on the left side, more so than on the right, and because the surgical goal was total removal with maximum preservation of important intracranial structures, we elected to perform a multi-stage removal. In an initial operation the main tumor mass in the left middle and posterior fossae was removed through an extended transfrontotemporal osteoplastic intradural approach, starting with exposure and piecemeal debulking of the tumor in the middle fossa. Next, the tumor was removed along the sphenoid wing to the left optic nerve and to the suprasellar space after elevation of the frontal lobe. The tumor encased the left optic nerve, internal carotid artery, and oculomotor and trochlear nerves and had to be progressively dissected from these structures intradurally using microsurgical technique. The cavernous sinus and all the structures transversing it were enveloped by tumor and were so badly damaged that they had to be removed with preservation of the internal carotid artery. The posterior communicating artery, anterior choroidal artery, and the perforating vessels to the brain stem were dissected free of tumor. We were also able to remove piecemeal the tumor extension into the tentorial incisure, which had caused marked displacement of the brain stem, and gained wide access to the infratentorial space and especially the cerebellopontine angle and clivus by resecting a large portion of the tentorium and removing the petrous apex. Through progressive removal, we succeeded in extirpating all infratentorial tumor extension on the left side while preserving the basilar artery and all its branches.

The patient recovered from the surgery quickly and was discharged five weeks after the initial operation. Two months later the tumor was removed from the right tentorial incisure using an analogous approach from the opposite side. Four weeks after that, the patient was again released in good condition. After another four months, during which time the patient experienced increasing visual deterioration, removal of the last, suprasellar part of the tumor was undertaken. Thus a complete tumor removal, confirmed by CT, was accomplished in three separate stages.

Comments: A very extensive, predominantly left-sided meningioma of the anterior, middle, and posterior skull base causing displacement of the cerebrum, midbrain, and cerebellum was removed in multiple stages. The middle fossa involvement in this case was manifested early by a secretory otitis media caused by compression of the eustachian tube from the medial side. This case illustrates the point that very extensive lesions may have to be excised in several stages. Although the severe cranial nerve dysfunction caused by the tumor proved to be irreversible, microsurgical dissection provided a means of avoiding additional deficits that could seriously compromise vital functions. Complete removal of the tumor-involved cavernous sinus was justified, as the nervous structures transversing the sinus were irreversibly damaged by the neoplasm.

Surgery of Malignant Space-Occupying Lesions of the Middle Skull Base

Introductory Remarks. As in the anterior skull base, it is rare for primary intracranial malignancies to penetrate the middle skull base from within. It is much more common for lesions to arise primarily in the posterior paranasal sinuses, nasopharynx (squamous cell carcinoma, adenocarcinoma, lymphoepithelial carcinoma), petrous pyramid, or in the skull base itself (chordoma, chondrosarcoma) and spread from there to the cranial interior. Because treatment is determined largely by the tumor type, a tissue sample should be obtained by the simplest means possible whenever a malignancy is sus-

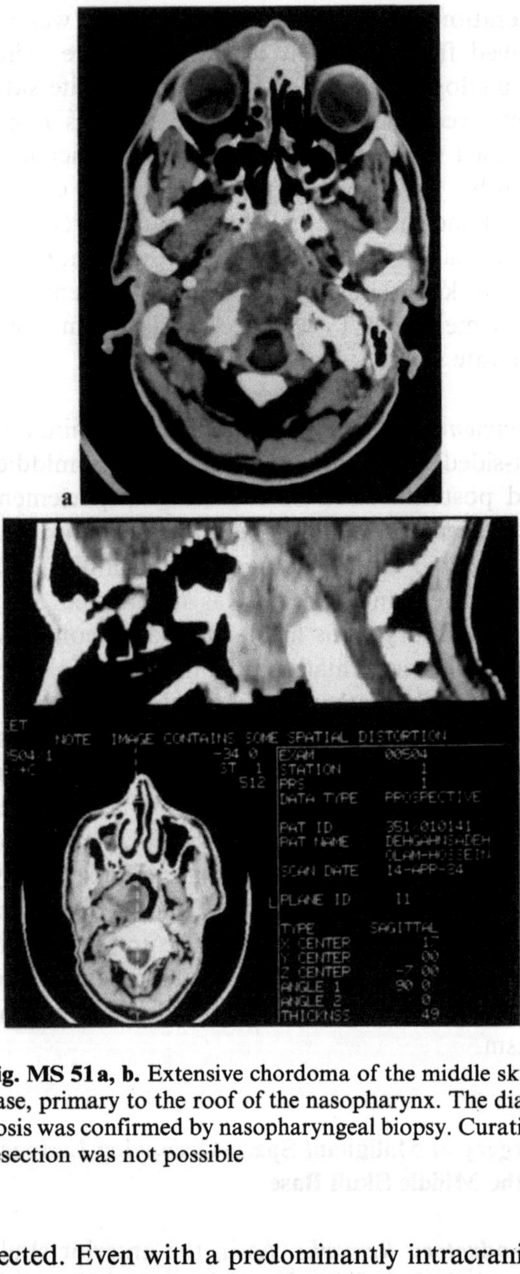

Fig. MS 51 a, b. Extensive chordoma of the middle skull base, primary to the roof of the nasopharynx. The diagnosis was confirmed by nasopharyngeal biopsy. Curative resection was not possible

pected. Even with a predominantly intracranial mass, the initial biopsy should be obtained by endoscopy of the nasal cavity, paranasal sinuses, or nasopharynx or by opening the middle ear space. This is particularly recommended when radiologic studies have confirmed destruction of the skull base. Thus, in a 43-year-old patient with a large intra/extracranial mass lesion of the middle skull base, we were able to identify the lesion as a chordoma by means of a nasopharyngeal biopsy and also debulked the extracranial portion of the tumor (Fig. MS 51 a, b).

If these measures do not supply a diagnosis, intracranial biopsy is required. During preoperative planning one should consider placing the cranial opening so that much of the tumor can be removed following the frozen section examination. Even with malignancies, this can have palliative benefit in terms of delaying neurologic deficits and increasing life expectancy, provided the resection does not significantly compromise the quality of life. This procedure was followed in a child with an extensive mass lesion arising from the left skull base. After transcranial debulking of the tumor mass, a diagnosis of rhabdomyosarcoma was established histologically, and treatment with cytostatics was initiated (Fig. MS 52).

The middle skull base is a difficult area in terms of surgical access, and the radical extirpation of malignancies in that region is most readily accomplished when a tumor has reached the skull base but has not yet penetrated the dura over a significant area. Slow-growing malignancies, even extensive intracranial growths, tend to displace the dura for a long period without infiltrating it. In all cases the mutilating effects of a proposed radical excision should be considered in relation both to the prognosis and to the quality of life. Because tolerance varies greatly from one individual to the next, there are no firm rules concerning patient selection. Rather, the decision for surgery must be based on a detailed consultation with the patient in the presence of his family.

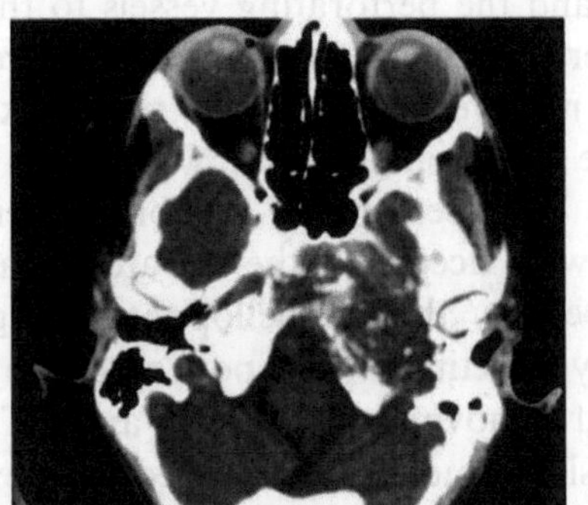

Fig. MS 52. Rhabdomyosarcoma of the left middle skull base. The diagnosis was established and the tumor size palliatively reduced through a temporal osteoplastic craniotomy. Cytostatic therapy was initiated after surgery

Carcinoma of the Auditory Canal

The earlier surgical treatment is undertaken for carcinoma of the ear canal, and the more radical the removal, the better the prognosis. If the bony auditory canal is involved, partial resection of the petrous pyramid is necessary, sacrificing the facial nerve. In the rare cases where the cancer spreads to the middle ear, the prognosis rapidly worsens. The most common cancers of the auditory canal are cornifying squamous cell carcinomas. According to the statistics of Leroux and Ennueyer (1957), 90% of ear cancers are auricular, 7% originate in the middle ear, and only 3% arise in the external auditory canal.

Case Report. Carcinoma of the right auditory canal (Fig. MS 53a–g). A 56-year-old woman presented with a circumscribed carcinoma of the right external auditory canal that involved the bony ear canal. There were no clinically palpable metastases. It appeared that the prognosis would be relatively favorable with radical surgical treatment. Thus the operation was performed as an en bloc resection that included part of the petrous bone, radical parotidectomy, and radical neck dissection on the right side, as well as facial nerve resection and grafting.
A Y-shaped incision was made around the auricle, which was reflected upward, and the cutaneous and cartilaginous auditory canal were circumscribed well into the cavum conchae. The peripheral facial nerve branches were identified and marked at the anterior border of the parotid capsule, and the cervical soft-tissue block was prepared from below upward. Next the dura of the middle and posterior fossae was exposed with the cutting burr, the mastoid was resected, preserving the sigmoid sinus, and the petrous pyramid was included with the surgical specimen on the plane of the jugular bulb and internal carotid artery (Fig. MS 19b). After division of the facial nerve at the geniculate ganglion and removal of the bony labyrinth with the cutting burr, the specimen was removed. The parotid gland and mandibular condyle were included in the specimen. An ossicle was used to occlude the bony eustachian tube.
Facial nerve reconstruction was performed with a cervical plexus graft. One branch of the graft was anastomosed to the temporal branch of the facial nerve, one to the zygomatic branch, and a third to the oral branch. The temporal muscle was swung into the surgical cavity to reduce its size. Finally the auricular flap was turned back into position, and the wound was closed in layers. Good recovery of facial nerve function was achieved within one year. The cosmetic result is acceptable.

Comments: A carcinoma of the right auditory canal was radically removed through an extra/intracranial, extradural approach (subtotal resection of the petrous pyramid, radical neck dissection, radical parotidectomy), and the facial nerve was reconstructed with a cervical plexus graft. Within a year there was good recovery of facial nerve function, and the patient has been free of disease for seven years.

Fig. MS 53a–g. Carcinoma of the right auditory canal with involvement of the posterior bony ear canal. Radical resection was performed using a combined extra/intracranial extradural approach. The procedure involved a radical neck dissection, total parotidectomy, partial petrosectomy, and resection and reconstruction of the facial nerve.
a The anterior and posterior skin flaps have been developed, and the peripheral facial nerve branches are partially exposed. A Y-shaped incision was made around the auricle, which was left on a superior pedicle. The auditory canal is widely circumscribed, and the sternocleidomastoid muscle is divided. (*1*) Inlet of external auditory canal with carcinoma, (*2*) auricle with superior pedicle, (*3*) sternocleidomastoid muscle (divided), (*4*) peripheral facial nerve branches.
b The tumor block is mobilized from posteriorly to anteriorly. The dura of the middle and posterior fossae is exposed with the cutting burr. (*1*) Circumscribed auditory canal with tumor block, (*2*) middle fossa dura, (*3*) peripheral facial nerve branches (snared).
c Operative field following tumor removal and facial nerve grafting. (*1*) Jugular bulb, (*2*) internal carotid artery, (*3*) nerve graft at geniculate ganglion, (*4*) nerve grafts (branches), (*5*) hypoglossal nerve, (*6*) vagus nerve, (*7*) accessory nerve, (*8*) temporalis muscle, (*9*) common carotid artery.
d Anastomosis at the main trunk of the facial nerve.
e The temporal muscle is rotated inferiorly for cavity ablation. (*1*) Jugular bulb, (*2*) internal carotid artery, (*3*) facial nerve graft, (*4*) peripheral facial neuroanastomoses, (*5*) hypoglossal nerve, (*6*) vagus nerve, (*7*) accessory nerve, (*8*) temporal muscle.
f, g The patient six years postoperatively, with satisfactory facial nerve function

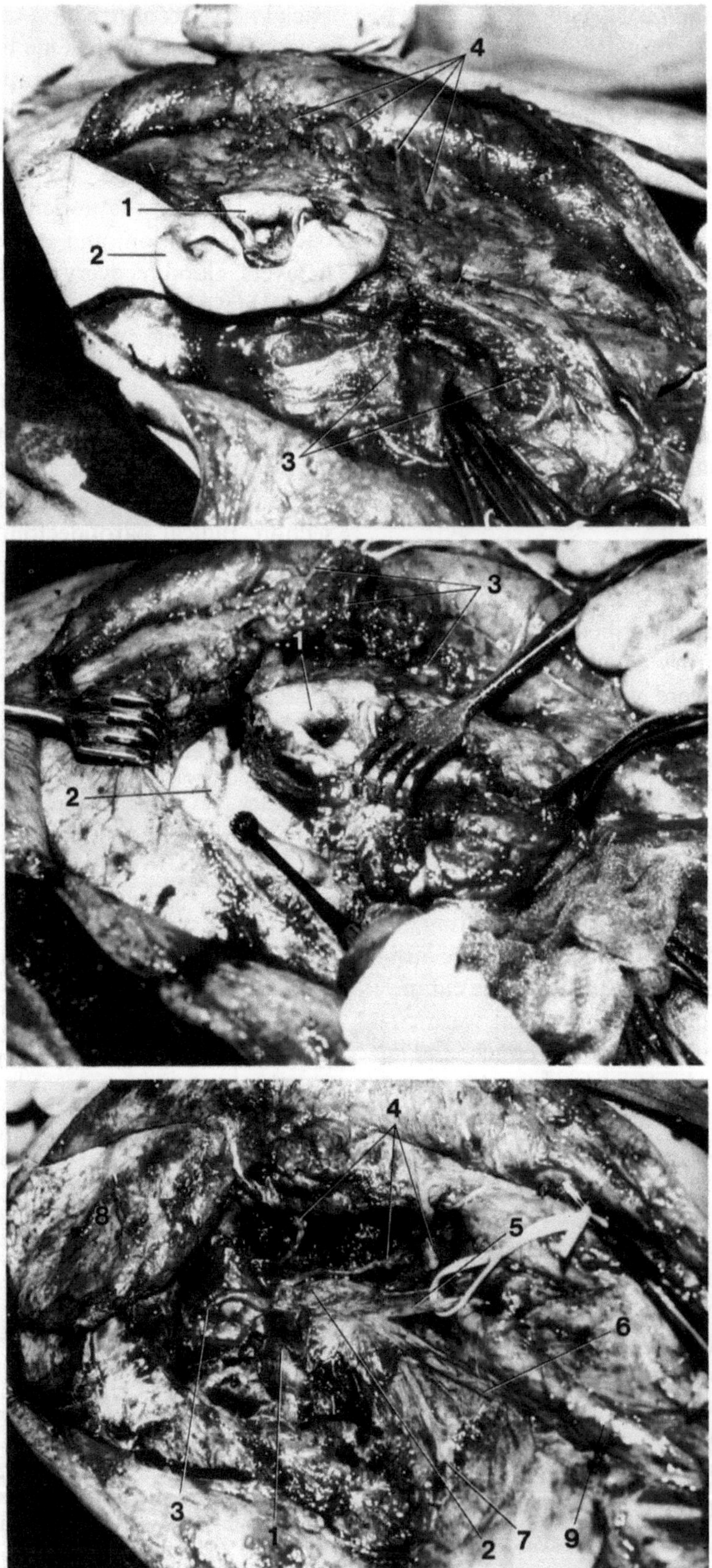

Fig. MS 53a–g
(Caption see p. 351)

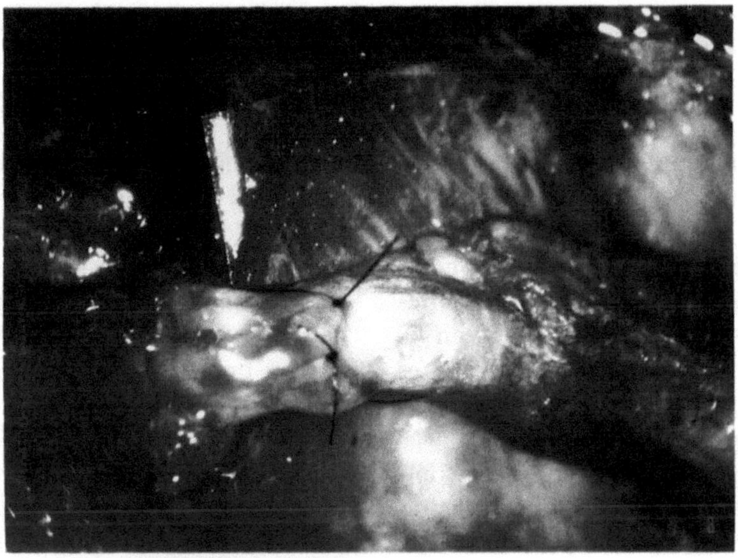
d

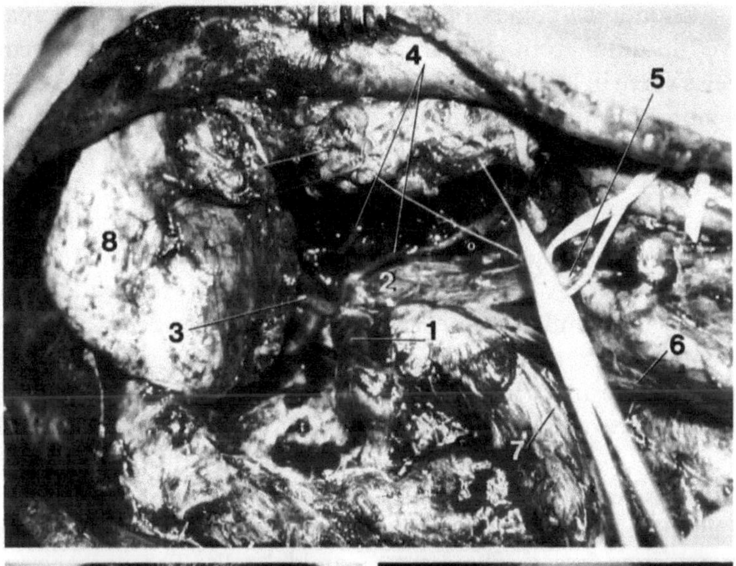

e

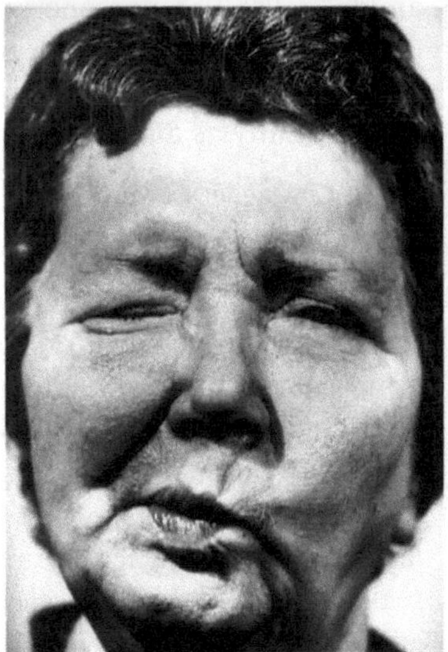
f

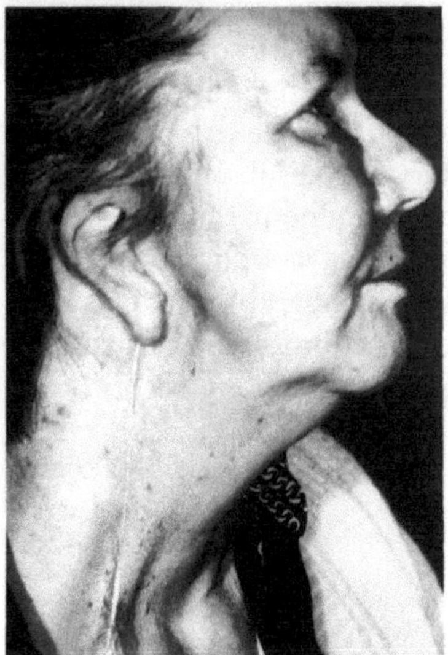
g

Chondrosarcoma of the Middle Skull Base

Chondrosarcoma is a malignant cartilaginous tumor that tends to arise de novo (primary chondrosarcoma) rather than from a preexisting benign cartilage tumor (secondary chondrosarcoma).

After osteosarcoma, it is the second most common malignant bone tumor in all large series (Dahlin 1978). It is most prevalent between 30 and 60 years of age, although sporadic cases in children and adolescents are reported.

Chondrosarcoma of the skull is rare in all large series. But the portion of the skull most commonly affected is the skull base, which is preformed in cartilage during embryonic development (Dahlin 1978). Chondrosarcomas of the skull base are believed to differ from chondrosarcomas occurring elsewhere in having a slower rate of growth and more sharply defined margins, implying a generally better prognosis (Minagi and Newton 1969).

Case Report. Chondrosarcoma of the right middle skull base (Fig. MS 54a–f). A 26-year-old male presented clinically with mild proptosis, widening of the palpebral fissure, abducens paresis, and subtle signs of hyposmia. The symptoms had developed a few weeks prior to hospitalization.

CT scans showed a mass lesion arising from the right middle skull base and extending far into the middle and posterior fossae. The mass was composed of a mixture of soft parts and areas of calcific density. Angiograms showed an upward and lateral, arcuate deflection of the internal carotid artery and displacement of the basilar artery to the left but no pathologic staining. While the CT scans gave a good appreciation of the tumor size, angiography gave useful information on the direction of tumor growth and on the destruction of the bony carotid canal.

Because the lesion was predominantly intracranial, a right temporal intracranial, intradural approach was used. The temporal lobe was elevated and the middle fossa was exposed to the tentorial margin, permitting identification of the structures of the tentorial incisure, the trigeminal, trochlear and oculomotor nerves, and the blood vessels. Having identified these structures, we incised the dura and the tumor capsule and began to debulk the tumor. While the soft part of the tumor was easily removed, the bony structures had to be removed with a diamond burr. The laterally displaced internal carotid artery traversed the center of the tumor, surrounded only by dura. It was freed of tumor tissue as far as the cavernous sinus. After coagulating and dividing the superior petrosal sinus, we continued the tumor removal caudally into the posterior fossa. There, too, the dura served to delimit the tumor capsule from brain structures. Apparently the tumor had displaced the dura as it grew and expanded, without penetrating it. The tumor capsule was found to be fused to the displaced basilar artery by calcium inclusions; since its removal might have ruptured the vessel, we decided to remove the soft tumor parts in this area and leave behind the calcified capsule wall.

To avoid cerebrospinal fluid leak, we used a pedicled temporal muscle flap to cover the large defect in the skull base, taking special care to seal off the eustachian tube and the opened pyramidal cells. The postoperative course was uneventful, and the patient experienced no further neurologic deficits. The lesion was identified histologically as a chondrosarcoma.

Comments: A rare chondrosarcoma of the middle skull base with predominantly intracranial, extradural growth was removed through an intracranial, intradural surgical approach. Angiograms gave important information on the displacement of major blood vessels. Because of the risk of vascular rupture, part of the calcified tumor capsule had to be left behind on the basilar artery. The opened pyramidal air cells were sealed with temporal muscle.

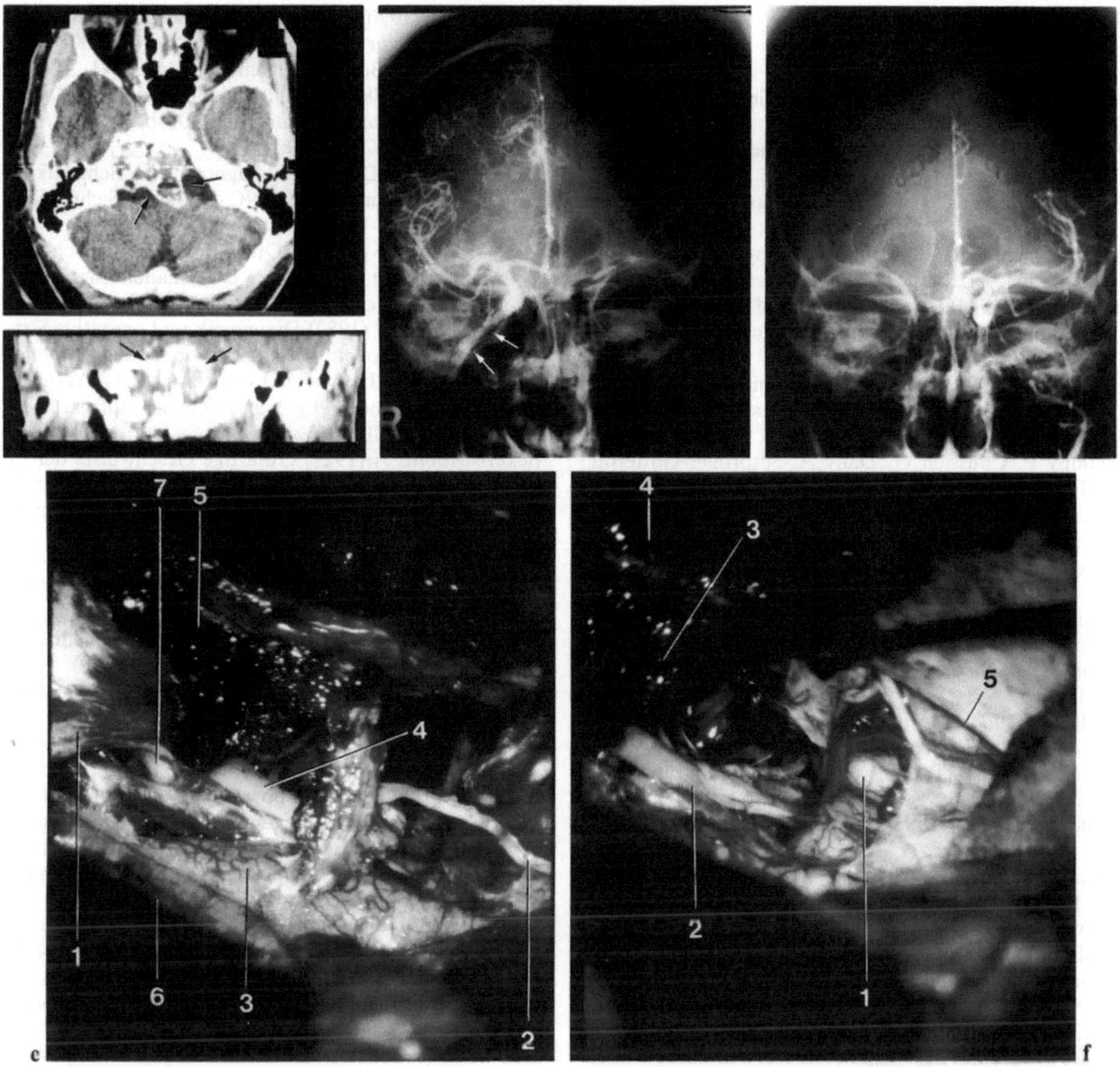

Fig. MS 54a–f. Chondrosarcoma of the middle skull base.
a, b Axial CT scans with coronal reconstruction show the large, predominantly intracranial mass lesion arising from the right middle skull base. The lesion is composed of soft parts and foci of calcified density (*arrows*).
c, d Bilateral carotid angiograms demonstrate superolateral displacement of the right internal carotid artery, signifying destruction of its bony canal by the tumor (*arrows*).
e Subtemporal intradural exposure of the middle fossa to the brain stem. The tentorial margin has been incised, and part of the tumor has been removed. (*1*) Tentorial margin, (*2*) Trochlear nerve, (*3*) brain stem, (*4*) oculomotor nerve, (*5*) residual tumor, (*6*) spatula, (*7*) posterior clinoid process.
f The posterior tentorial margin has been largely resected, and the lateral part of the tumor removed. Deep in the field, the medial part of the tumor is visible in the infratentorial space with the overlying dura. (*1*) Brain stem, (*2*) oculomotor nerve, (*3*) tumor in infratentorial space, (*4*) lateral cavity left by tumor resection, (*5*) tentorial margin

References

von Albertini A (1974) Histologische Geschwulstdiagnostik, 2nd edn. Thieme, Stuttgart

Arena S (1974) Tumour surgery of the temporal bone. Laryngoscope 84:645

Arena S, Hilal EY (1976) Neurilemomas of the infratemporal space. Arch Otolaryngol 102:180–184

Attenborough NR (1980) Maxillectomy via a temporal approach. J Laryngol Otol 94:149–162

Batsakis JG (1980) Tumors of the Head and Neck. Clinical and Pathological considerations. Williams and Wilkins. Baltimore, London

Bushe KA (1973) Unabweisbare neurochirurgische Akutsituationen im allgemeinen Krankenhaus. Langenbecks Arch Chir 334:336

Champy P, Coussien G, Dany A, Sesproges-Gotteron R (1964) Neurome du tron dechire posterior. Rev Laryngol 85:1034

Codman EA (1931) Epiphysical chondromatous giant cell tumors of the upper end of the humerus. Surg Gynec Obstet 52:543

Coleman CC Jr (1966) Removal of the temporal bone for cancer. Am J Surg 112:583–590

Columella B, Nicola G, Delzano G (1957) Champy et al. (1964)

Conley JJ (1963) The management of carotid body tumors. Surg Gynecol Obstet 117:722

Conley JJ (1964) Tumors of the infratemporal fossa. Arch Otolaryng 79:498

Conley JJ (1975) Salivary glands and the facial nerve. Thieme, Stuttgart

Conley JJ, Novack AJ (1960) The surgical treatment of malignant tumors of the ear and temporal bone. Arch Otolaryngol 71:635–652

Dahlin D (1978) Bone tumors: general aspects and data on 6221 cases. Thomas, Springfield, Ill

Dechaume M, Grellet M, Payen J, Gouggon C, Peri G, Dore P, Duhrville J (1968) Contribution a l'étude des syndromes des maxillaires. Rev Stomatol (Paris) 69:353

Denecke HJ (1959) Zur Chirurgie des N. facialis im Bereich der Parotis und der Schädelbasis. Wien Klin Wschr 71:180

Denecke HJ (1959/1960) Operationstechnische Probleme bei der Entfernung großer Neurinome im Bereich von Felsenbeinpyramide, N. facialis, Pharynx, Gefäßscheide, Ösophagusmund und Zunge. HNO 8:343

Denecke HJ (1966) Zur Chirurgie ausgedehnter Glomustumoren im Bereich des Foramen jugulare. Arch Otorhinolaryngol (NY) 187:656–662

Denecke HJ (1969a) Surgery of extensive glomus jugulare tumors of the ear. Rev Laryngol 90:265–270

Denecke HJ (1969b) Diskussionsbemerkung zu Gejrot und House. In: Hamberger C, Wersäll J (Ed) Disorders of the skull base region. Nobel Symposium 10, Stockholm 19 683.294

Denecke HJ (1970) Der infratemporale Zugangsweg zur Orbita und zur Fossa pterygoidea. Fortschr Kief und Gesichtschir Bd XIV. Thieme, Stuttgart 241–242

Denecke HJ (1978) Die Chirurgie ausgedehnter Tumoren des Felsenbeines und der Otobasis. Laryngol Rhinol Otol 57:287–290

Draf W (1974) Differentialdiagnose von Schädelknochenerkrankungen aus HNO-ärztlicher Sicht. HNO 22:14.23

Draf W, Samii M (1977) Otorhinolaryngologisch-neurochirurgische Probleme an der Schädelbasis. Laryngol Rhinol Otol 56:1007–1020

Draf W, Samii M (1982) Diagnostik und operative Strategie bei großen Glomustumoren der lateralen Schädelbasis. In: Majer H, Rieder Ch (eds) Aktuelles in der Otorhinolaryngologie. Thieme, Stuttgart New York, pp 61–70

Eckert-Möbius A (1929) Gutartige Geschwülste der inneren Nase und ihrer Nebenhöhlen. In: Denker A, Kahler O (eds) Handbuch der Hals-Nasen-Ohrenheilkunde. Vol 5. Springer, Berlin, p 107

Eneroth CM (1969) Histological aspects of parapharyngeal tumors. 10. Nobel Symposium Stockholm. Almquist and Wiksell

Eneroth CM (1976) Die Klinik der Kopfspeicheldrüsentumoren. Arch Otorhinolaryngol 213:61–110

Feinmann NL, Yakovac WC (1970) Neurofibromatosis in Childhood. J Pediatr 76:339

Fisch U (1977a) Die Mikrochirurgie des Felsenbeins. HNO 25:193–197

Fisch U (1977b) Infratemporal fossa approach for extensive tumors of the temporal bone and base of the skull. In: Silverstein H, Norell H (Eds.) Neurological surgery of the ear. Aesculapius, Birmingham AL pp 34–53

Fisch U (1983) The infratemporal fossa approach for nasopharyngeal tumors. Laryngoscope 93:36–44

Fisch U, Pillsbury HS (1979) Infratemporal fossa approach to lesions in the temporal bone and base of the skull. Arch Otolaryngol 105:99–107

Gacek RR (1976) Schwannoma of the jugulare foramen. Ann Otol 85:215

Gacek RR, Goodmann M (1977) Management of malignancy of the temporal bone. Laryngoscope 87:1622–1634

Gardner G, Cocke EW Jr, Robertson JT, Trumbull ML, Palmer RE (1977) Combined approach surgery for removal of glomus jugulare tumors. Laryngoscope 87:655–688

Gejrot T (1965) Surgical treatment of glomus jugulare tumors. With special reference to the diagnostic value of retrograde jugularography. Acta Otolaryngol 60:150–168

Gejrot T (1969) Jugular foramen syndromes. In: Hamberger CA, Wersäll J (eds) Disorders of the skull base region. Proceeding of the tenth Nobel Symposium Stockholm 1968. Almquist Wiksell Stockholm, pp 279–283

Glasscock ME, Harris PF, Newsons G (1974) Glomus tumors: Diagnosis and treatment. Laryngoscope 84:2006–2032

Grunert KA (1894) Die operative Ausräumung des Bulbus venae jugularis (Bulbusoperation) Arch Ohrenheilk 36:71
Guleke (1950) Allgemeine und spezielle chirurgische Operationslehre, 2nd edn, vol 2: Gehirn, Gehirnschädel, Wirbelsäule, Rückenmark. Springer, Berlin Göttingen Heidelberg, pp 428ff.
Heard G (1962) Nerve sheath tumors and von Recklinghausen's disease of the nervous system. Ann R Coll Surg 31:229
Hilding DA, Greenberg A (1971) Surgery for large glomus jugulare tumor. Arch Otolaryngol 93:227–231
Hilding DA, Selker R (1969) Total resection of the temporal bone for carcinoma. Arch Otolaryngol 89:636–645
Holt GR (1978) ENT Manifestations of von Recklinghausen's disease. Laryngoscope 88:1617–1638
Holt FJ, Wright EM (1948) Radiologic features of neurofibromatosis. Radiology 51:647
Hommerich KW (1977) Gutartige Geschwülste der Nase und der Nasennebenhöhlen. In: Berendes J, Link R, Zöllner F (Hrsg) Hals-Nasen-Ohren-Heilkunde in Praxis und Klinik Bd 2/Obere und untere Luftwege II Thieme, Stuttgart, S 120
Hunt JC, Pugh DG (1961) Skeletal lesions in neurofibromatosis. Radiology 76:1
Irons GB, Weiland LH, Bromm WL (1977) Paragangliomas of the neck: Clinical and Pathologic analysis of 116 cases. Surg Clin North Am 57:575
Jaffe HL, Lichtenstein L (1942) Benign chondroblastoma of bone. A reinterpretation of the so-called calcifying or chondromatous giant cell tumors. Amer J Pathol 18:969
Kempe L, Vanderark GD, Smith DR (1971) The neurosurgical treatment of glomus jugulare tumors. J Neurosurg 35:59–64
Kern E (1977) Chirurgische Behandlung maligner Weichteiltumoren. Dtsch Ärztebl 74:1757
Kleinsasser O (1975) Behavior and adequate treatment of epithelial tumors of the parotid gland. In: Conley JJ (ed) Salivary glands and the facial nerve. Thieme, Stuttgart
Kleinsasser O, Klein HJ (1968) Sekundäre Karzinome in primär gutartigen Mischtumoren der Speicheldrüsen. Arch Otorhinolaryngol 190:272
Klingler M (1951) Über Knorpelgeschwulst der Schädelbasis mit intrakranieller Ausdehnung. Acta Neurochir 1: 337–380
Lack EE, Cuhilla AL, Woodruff JM, Farr HW (1977) Paragangliomas of the head and neck region. A clinical study of 69 patients. Cancer 39:397
Landing BH, Tarber S (1956) Tumor of the cardiovascular system: Treatment. Atlas of Tumor Pathology Sect 3,6 asc 7,9
Lang I, Lanz T, Wachsmuth W (1979) Praktische Anatomie, part 1, vol 1: Kopf; part B: Gehirn und Augenschädel. Springer, Berlin Heidelberg New York
Lasjaunias P (1980) Embolisation in Tumors and vascular malformations of the head and neck. Ann Acad Med Singapore 9:332–341
Leroux R, Ennueyer A (1957) Les tumeurs malignes de l'oreille. Arnette, Paris
Lewin ML (1966) Non malignant maxillofacial tumors in children. Plast Reconstruct Surg 38:186
Lewis JS, Page R (1966) Radical surgery for malignant tumors of the ear. Arch Otolaryngol 83:114–119
Martin G, Kleinsasser O (1981) Neurogenic sarcomas of the neck in neurofibromatosis. Arch Otorhinolaryngol 232:273–283
Meacham WF, Capps JM (1960) Intracranial glomus jugulare tumor with successful surgical removal. J Neurosurg 17:157–160
Michelson RP, Connolly JE (1962) Removal of glomus jugulare tumor utilizing complete occlusion of the cerebral circulation. Laryngoscope 72:788–805
Miehlke A (1977) Diskussionsbemerkung zu Draf. 48. Jahresver d Dtsch Ges f HNO-Heilk Kopf- und Halschirurgie, Bad Reichenhall
Minagi H, Newton TH (1969) Cartilaginous tumors of the base of the skull. AJR 105:308–313
Mischke RE, Balbany TLJ (1980) Skull base approach to glomus jugulare. Laryngoscope 90:89–93
Mitterwallner FV (1955) Variationsstatistische Untersuchungen an den basalen Hirngefäßen. Acta Anat (Basel) 24:51–88
Neely JG (1979) Reversible compression neuropathy of the eighth cranial nerve from a large jugulare foramen schwannoma. Arch Otolaryngol 105:555–560
Obwegeser HL (1985) Temporal approach to the TMJ, the orbit and the retromaxillary-infracranial region. Head and Neck Surgery 7:185–199
Preston FW, Walsh WS, Clarke Th (1952) Cutaneous neurofibromatosis (von Recklinghausen's disease): clinical manifestations and incidence of sarcoma in 61 male patients. Arch Surg 64:813
Proctor B, Lindsay JR (1947) Tumors involving the petrous pyramid of the temporal bone. Arch Otolaryngol 46:180–194
Rand CW, Reeves DL (1943) Dermoid and epidermoid tumors (cholesteatomas) of the central nervous system. Report of twentythree cases. Arch Surg 46:350–376
Rehn E (1919) Die Freilegung der A. carotis interna in ihrem oberen Halsteil. Zentralbl Chir 46:25
Resler CR, Snow JB Jr, Williams GR (1966) Multiplicity and familial incidence of carotid body and glomus jugulare tumors. Ann Otol Rhinol Laryngol 75:114
Samii M (1974) Pneumoencephalo-Tomography. Ferdinand Enke Verlag, Stuttgart
Schwab W (1951) Über Myxome der Nasennebenhöhlen. HNO 2:285
Shapiro MJ, Neues DK (1964) Technique for removal of glomus jugulare tumors. Arch Otolaryngol 79:219–224
Tesarik J (1959) Myxome of the paranasal sinus. Cesk Otolaryngol 8:29
Tesarik J, Hubacek J (1968) Potentiell maligne Tumoren in Nase und Paranasalhöhlen. Acta Univ Palackianae Olomucen 48:125
Thoms OJ, Snow D, Trowbridge WV (1960) Glomus jugulare tumor. Report of a case with surgical removal. J Neurosurg 17:95–96

Ungerecht K (1963) Zur Chirurgie der Glomus jugulare Tumoren im Schläfenbein-Schädelbasisbereich. HNO 11:95–96
Ungerecht K (1966) Klinik und Therapie der Tumoren des Gesichtsschädels. Arch Klin Exp Ohr Nas Kehlk Heilk 187:1
Vollmar J (1975) Rekonstruktive Chirurgie der Arterien. 2nd edn. Thieme, Stuttgart
Voss EU, Vollmar J, Meister H (1977) Tumoren des Glomus caroticum. Thoraxchirurgie 25:1–12
Weille FL, Lane CS Jr (1951) Surgical problems involved in the removal of glomus-jugulare tumors. Laryngoscope 61:448–459
Wullstein HL, Wullstein SR (1976) Chirurgie der Tumoren des Mittelohres. In: Naumann HH (ed) Kopf- und Halschirurgie, vol 3: Ohrregion. Thieme, Stuttgart
Yasargil MG, Antic J, Laciga R, Jain KK, Hodosh RM, Smith RD (1976) Microsurgical pterional approach to aneurysm of the basilar bifurcation. Surg Neurol 6:83–91
Zehm S (1969) The surgical approach to the external part of the base of the skull related to the anterior and medial cranial fossa. Nobel Symposium 10. Almquist and Wiksell Stockholm
Zehm S (1970) Der retromaxilläre Raum. Thieme, Stuttgart
Zülch KJ (1956) Pathologische Anatomie der raumbeengenden intrakraniellen Prozesse. Handbuch der Neurochirurgie, vol 3. Springer, Berlin Göttingen Heidelberg

Surgery of the Posterior Skull Base (PS)

Surgery of the Internal Auditory Canal and Cerebellopontine Angle

General Operative Techniques

Introductory Remarks. The internal auditory canal and the structures of the cerebellopontine angle are accessible through three surgical approaches (Krmpotic et al. 1985):

1) The transtemporal extradural approach (Fisch 1976; House 1964).
2) The transmastoid translabyrinthine approach (Fisch 1976).
3) The lateral suboccipital (retrosigmoid) approach.

The selection of an approach is an interdisciplinary matter and should be based on individual pathoanatomic criteria and the anticipated surgical morbidity. The goal is the elimination of the pathological entity with minimal associated cosmetic and functional damage.

The Transtemporal Extradural Approach

This approach gives access to the bony walls of the internal auditory canal without opening the intradural space. The dura itself is not incised until the bony roof of the canal has been removed. This permits the surgeon to enter the internal auditory canal while preserving the cochleovestibular organ.

The Transmastoid Translabyrinthine Approach

In this approach the internal auditory canal is reached by removing the labyrinth and thus sacrificing cochleovestibular function. A craniotomy in the conventional sense is not required.

The Lateral Suboccipital (Retrosigmoid) Approach

This approach gives wide exposure of the structures of the cerebellopontine angle following incision of the dura and retraction of the cerebellum. The contents of the internal auditory canal also can be exposed by removing the posterior lip of the porus acusticus and the posterior wall of the canal. Anatomic factors are favorable for preserving the vestibulocochlear nerve and the facial nerve. The endolymphatic sac and the site of entry of the subarcute artery on the anterior surface of the pyramid may have to be sacrificed.

The transtemporal extradural approach and the transmastoid translabyrinthine approach were discussed previously (see p. 252), so here we shall describe only the technique of the lateral suboccipital approach.

Operative Technique
(Fig. PS 1 a, b)

The patient is placed in a semisitting position with the head tilted forward and turned 30° toward the affected side. The head is immobilized in a Mayfield frame. In the semisitting position, the venous pressure can be raised and the risk of air embolism decreased by elevating the leg to the level of the right atrium of the heart. Also, the microscopic field is easily surveyed without constant suction, thus avoiding trauma to small blood vessels and brain structures from the suction tip. A Doppler device is attached precordially so that blood flow turbulence can be constantly monitored throughout the operation. Any change in flow sounds caused by intravascular air is perceived as an audible signal,

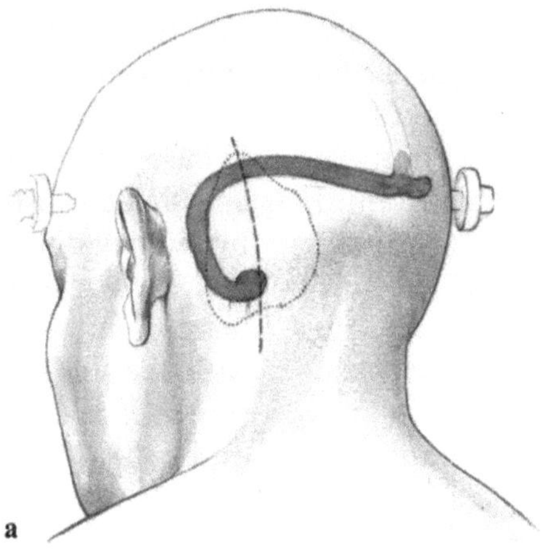

a

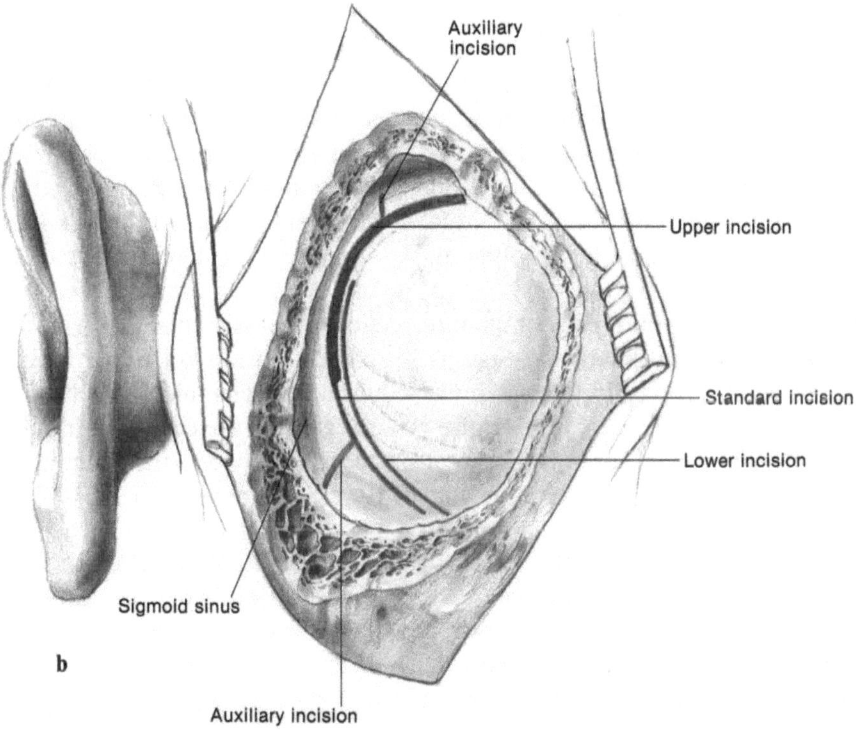

b

Fig. PS 1 a, b. The lateral suboccipital (retrosigmoid) approach to the internal auditory canal (IAC) and cerebellopontine angle.
a A vertical skin incision approximately 10 cm long is placed 1.5 – 2 cm medial to the mastoid. It extends superiorly to the level of the transverse sinus. Its inferior extent depends on whether the lesion is at the level of the superior or inferior cranial nerves.
b After retraction of the soft tissues and muscles, a burr hole is placed below the junction of the transverse and sigmoid sinuses and enlarged to 2–3 cm with a rongeur. The sigmoid sinus must be exposed, regardless of the extent of mastoid pneumatization. This improves vision of the cerebellopontine angle and minimizes retraction of the cerebellum. The possible dural incisions are indicated and depend on the surgical goal. The "standard incision" is for exposing the entire cerebellopontine angle from the tentorial incisure to the foramen magnum. The upper incision is for exposing the trigeminal nerve, the lower incision for exposing cranial nerves VII and VIII and the caudal nerve group. The "auxiliary" incisions create dural flaps that are retracted with holding sutures to improve access

and the embolus can be aspirated at once through a preoperatively placed right atrial catheter. For intraoperative measurement of auditory evoked potentials, we place an electrode over the mastoid on each side and attach a third electrode in the parietal area. An acoustic stimulus is delivered through headset plugs that are inserted into the external auditory canals in hearing-aid fashion. We routinely record evoked potentials to detect early auditory pathway irritation that might occur during the operation.

The skin is opened with a vertical incision placed 1.5–2 cm medial to the mastoid. The incision is about 10 cm long and extends superiorly to the level of the transverse sinus. The inferior limit of the incision depends on the necessary caudal extension of the dissection. The neck muscles are divided vertically, in line with the skin incision. If necessary a free muscle graft may be taken at this time for later use and stored in Ringer's solution. The muscles are retracted, and a burr hole is placed at the junction of the transverse and sigmoid sinuses. The hole is enlarged with a rongeur to make an opening 2–3 cm in diameter.

At least the border of the transverse sinus and sigmoid sinus should be visible at this stage as landmarks. The size of a cerebellopontine angle tumor has no influence on the size of the craniotomy. Indeed, with smaller tumors of the internal auditory canal it can be useful to extend the craniotomy medially somewhat to improve the angle of access to the fundus of the canal.

If a vascular decompression is planned, the craniotomy generally may be made somewhat smaller – about 2 cm in diameter – as there is no need for access to the internal acoustic meatus. It usually is not necessary to extend the craniotomy upward to reach the trigeminal nerve. The dura is opened as a C-shaped medially based flap, 2 mm distant from the transverse and sigmoid sinuses. Access is increased further by making oblique auxiliary incisions in the lateral dural margin to create a second, laterally based dural flap. This flap is retracted laterally with the dural sinus by means of traction sutures. Once the intradural structures have been exposed, the operating microscope is brought into place, and the procedure is continued using a 250-mm objective lens. The precision of surgical manipulations is improved and operator fatigue lessened by using an operating stool with supporting arm rests. Special microsurgical instruments are necessary and should include bayonet forceps, tumor grasping forceps, various microdissectors, microelevators, microscissors, and suction irrigators. Bipolar coagulating forceps with varying degrees of angulation should be available for hemostasis. Other necessary instruments are air-driven diamond burrs and the self-retaining Leyla retractor, which provides uniform, atraumatic pressure without intervention by assistants. Insertion of the retractor places tension on the bridging veins, so these should be coagulated and divided. The surgeon next opens the cerebrospinal fluid-filled cisterns located between the arachnoid and pia mater. Enough room is gained by withdrawing cerebrospinal fluid that the cerebellum and flocculus can be retracted medially without significant compression. The remaining steps in the procedure depend on the pathology and are described below.

Special Operative Techniques

Procedures on the Nerves of the Internal Auditory Canal and Cerebellopontine Angle

Transtemporal Extradural Resection of the Vestibular Nerve, Ganglion and the Cochlear Nerve

Introductory Remarks. The development and technique of this approach were discussed in some detail in the sections dealing with middle skull base trauma (see p. 252). Transtemporal resection of the meatal portion of the vestibular nerve, including the vestibular ganglion, is indicated in patients with Meniere's disease who do not respond to conservative therapy, to ablation of the vestibular system by intratympanic injection with gentamicin (Lange 1977), or to other procedures on the peripheral vestibular system such as a "saccotomy" to decompress the endolymphatic sac (Portmann 1927a, b; House 1962–1965). Transtemporal vestibular neurectomy is particularly recommended when residual hearing is present (Wigand 1979). In Wigand's series, hearing improved in a certain percentage of patients undergoing the transtemporal procedure. Choudard (1970) attributes this to an elimination of influences from the parasympathetic vestibulofacial anastomoses which tend to reduce the hearing. In patients who have severe tinnitus and a high degree of hearing loss, resection of the cochlear nerve may also be advised. The procedure generally recommended for deaf patients is vestibular and cochlear neurectomy performed by the translabyrinthine route.

Operative Technique
(Fig. MS 12a–n, Fig. PS 2a–e)

The internal auditory canal is exposed and entered, and the cranial nerves are identified. The facial nerve courses in the anterior superior compartment of the internal auditory canal. The superior part of the vestibular ganglion courses posterosuperiorly, the inferior part courses inferiorly, and the cochlear division of the vestibulocochlear nerve lies below and posterior to the facial nerve. The fundus of the internal auditory canal is divided into an upper and a lower compartment by a bony ridge called the transverse crest. The upper compartment contains the facial nerve anteriorly and the superior part of the vestibular ganglion posteriorly. The lower compartment houses the cochlear division of the vestibulocochlear nerve anteriorly and the inferior part of the vestibular ganglion posteriorly. In the upper compartment, the facial nerve is separated from the superior part of the vestibular ganglion by a bony ridge which House called the vertical crest (Bill's bar).

First the anastomotic connections between the vestibular nerve and facial nerve are divided with microscissors. Now the superior part of the vestibular nerve is raised on a 90° hook and divided with the neurectomy scissors as close to the fundus as possible. After the stump is aspirated, the branches of the inferior part of the vestibular nerve (posterior ampullary nerve and saccular nerve) become visible, deep in the field, and they also are divided. Next the tiny vessels leading to the vestibular ganglion are coagulated so that the vestibular nerve and ganglion can be removed far medially in the porus acusticus. The surgeon should watch for a possible loop of the anterior inferior cerebellar artery coursing between the vestibular nerve and cochlear nerve, to avoid injury to that vessel. If hearing is still present, the cochlear nerve is preserved by careful manipulations. In exceptional cases cochlear nerve section may be considered when tinnitus is severe. At the end of the procedure, the internal auditory canal and any opened air cells are sealed with a stored dural patch secured with fibrin glue. To avoid constricting scars, Wigand prefers to use a silicone sheet, onto which he glues a muscle-periosteal graft. Finally the temporal flap is replaced, the bone flap is reinserted, the temporal muscle is reapproximated, and the scalp is closed with all-layer sutures over a suction drain.

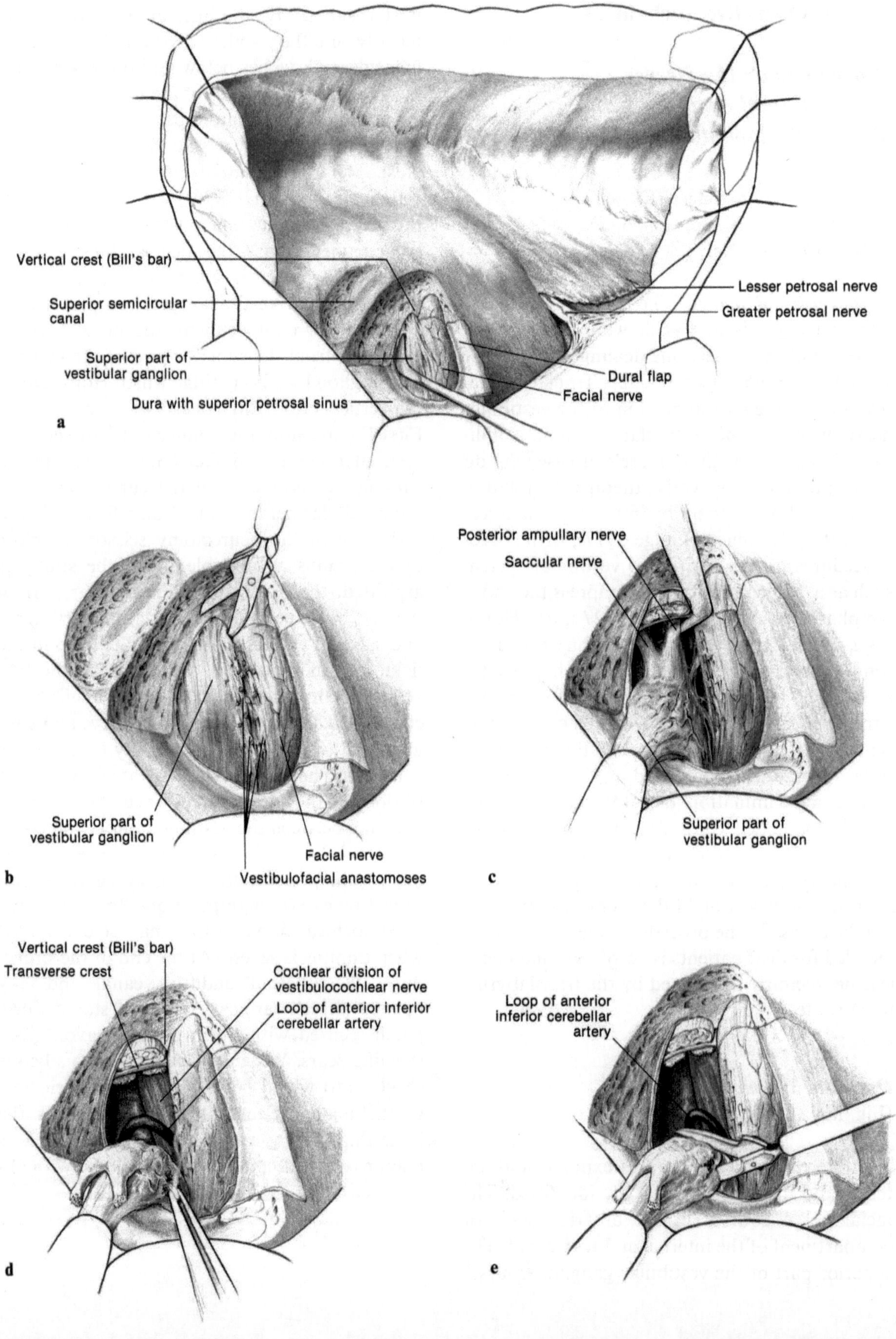
Vertical crest (Bill's bar)
Superior semicircular canal
Superior part of vestibular ganglion
Dura with superior petrosal sinus
Lesser petrosal nerve
Greater petrosal nerve
Dural flap
Facial nerve
a
Superior part of vestibular ganglion
Facial nerve
Vestibulofacial anastomoses
b
Posterior ampullary nerve
Saccular nerve
Superior part of vestibular ganglion
c
Vertical crest (Bill's bar)
Transverse crest
Cochlear division of vestibulocochlear nerve
Loop of anterior inferior cerebellar artery
d
Loop of anterior inferior cerebellar artery
e

Transmastoid Translabyrinthine Resection of the Vestibular Nerve, Ganglion and Cochlear Nerve

Introductory Remarks. The development of this approach and its technical fundamentals were discussed earlier in connection with middle skull base trauma (see p. 257). Neurectomy of the vestibular nerve and vestibular ganglion can be performed by this route with minimal surgical stress in the nearly deaf ear, because entry into the internal auditory canal requires ablation of most of the labyrinthine system with destruction of the inner ear structures. The transmastoid translabyrinthine approach to the internal auditory canal is generally preferred in the rare cases where cochlear neurectomy is proposed as a means of eliminating a severely disturbing, unilateral tinnitus.

Fig. PS 2a–e. Transtemporal vestibular neurectomy.
a The anterior surface of the pyramid is exposed after mobilizing the dura, and the self-retaining Fisch retractor is inserted. After the blue line of the semicircular canal and the greater petrosal nerve have been identified, the roof of the IAC is removed. The vertical crest (Bill's bar) appears laterally at the junction of the IAC fundus and fallopian canal as a bony ridge between the facial nerve and superior part of the vestibular ganglion. The roof of the IAC is burred away in the posteromedial direction along with the superior lip of the porus, giving a wide view of the IAC. The dura is opened with a trap-door flap based to protect the facial nerve.
b After the IAC has been opened, the vestibulofacial anastomoses are divided. The pars superior of the vestibular ganglion, which in this position lies above the transverse crest and posterior to Bill's bar, is severed by traction with a small hook.
c After retraction of the pars superior with the suction tip, the bipartite pars inferior of the vestibular ganglion can be seen below the transverse crest. This part of the ganglion likewise is bluntly severed with a hook, sparing the underlying cochlear division of the vestibulocochlear nerve.
d,e The entire vestibular ganglion is retracted to expose the cochlear division more clearly. Minute vessels passing to the vestibular ganglion are coagulated, and the vestibular division of the vestibulocochlear nerve is sectioned proximal to the ganglion. The surgeon should watch for the anterior inferior cerebellar artery, which may loop between the vestibular and cochlear divisions

Operative Technique
(Fig. MS 13a–e, Fig. PS 3a–e, Fig. PS 5a–c)

Following mastoidectomy, labyrinthectomy, and penetration into the internal auditory canal, the surgeon first locates the vertical crest (Bill's bar) marking the junction of the fallopian canal with the fundus of the internal auditory canal so that he can keep the facial nerve under control. The dura of the internal auditory canal is opened near the canal floor to avoid injury to the VII cranial nerve, and the vestibular nerve with its superior and inferior portions is visualized from behind. Vestibulofacial anastomoses are progressively divided with sharp instruments such as keratome knives and microscissors, taking care not to stretch the facial nerve. The risk of facial nerve injury during aspiration of cerebrospinal fluid is reduced by applying the suction over small cotton paddies. After the connections between the facial and vestibular nerves have been severed, the vestibular nerve is first divided close to the fundus. This must be done carefully and in a stepwise fashion. The vestibular nerve stump is then raised with the suction tip so that very small vessels passing to the vestibular ganglion can be coagulated and the vestibular nerve can be resected proximal to the porus of the internal auditory canal. When tinnitus is present, the more deeply situated cochlear nerve also is resected. When opening the dura and especially while dividing the vestibular nerves, the surgeon should watch for possible looping of the anterior inferior cerebellar artery, which must be kept intact (Fig. PS 5). Finally the dura is closed, the internal auditory canal is covered with stored dura, and the mastoid cavity, which has been cleared of mucosa, is obliterated with freshly obtained pieces of abdominal fat stuck together with fibrin glue. The wound is closed in layers in watertight fashion.

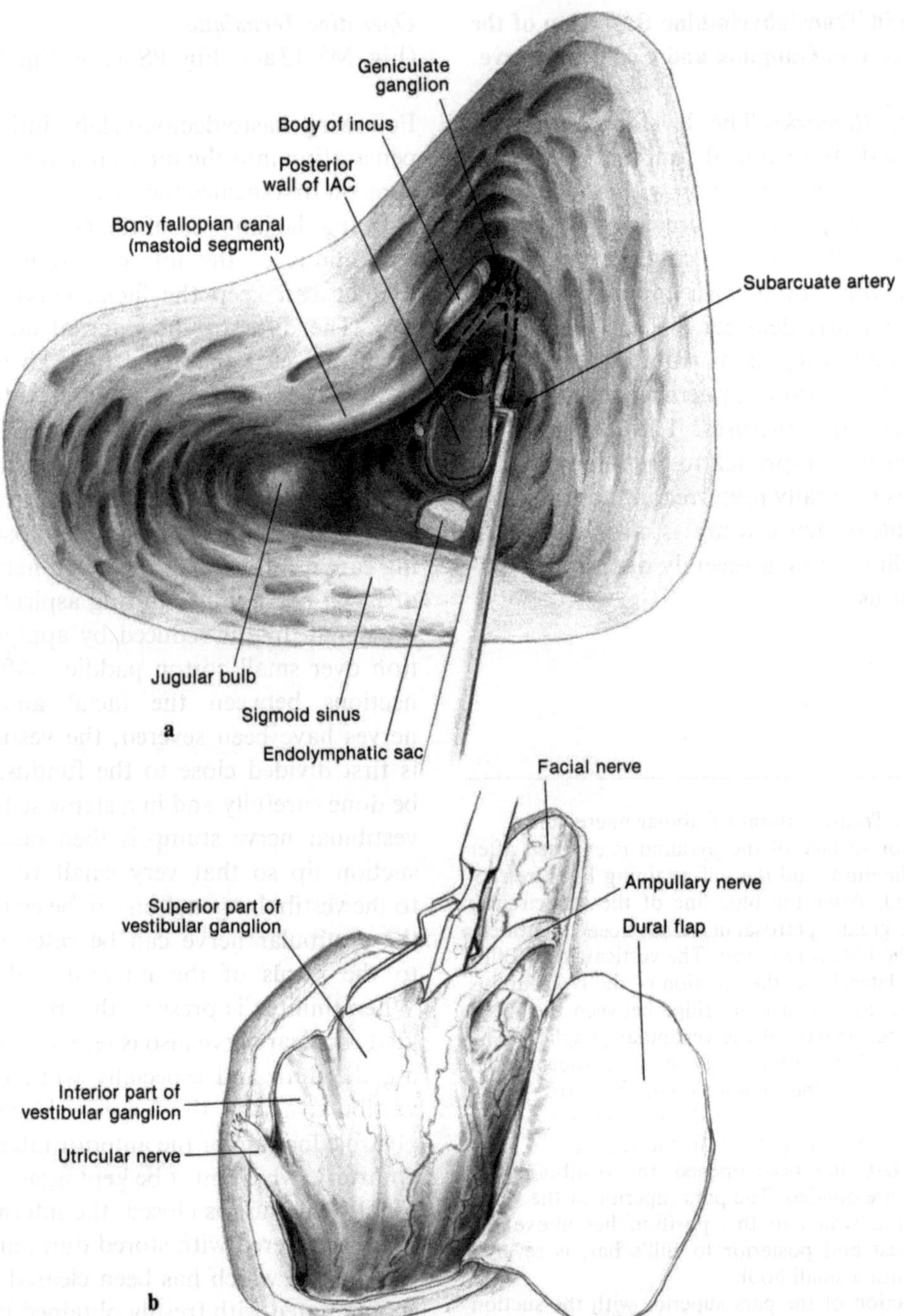

Fig. PS 3a–e. Translabyrinthine vestibulocochlear neurectomy.

a Mastoidectomy and labyrinthectomy have been carried out. The sigmoid sinus and mastoid segment of the facial nerve are covered by bone. The facial nerve is exposed from the geniculate ganglion to the IAC. The posterior wall of the IAC is thinned; a rectangular area has been outlined with the burr and if necessary can be elevated from the dura as a flap. The endolymphatic sac presents directly in front of the sinus; the endolymphatic duct was removed during the labyrinthectomy.

b A superiorly based dural flap is created, and the IAC is entered. The ampullary nerve, utricular nerve, and superior part of the vestibular ganglion are divided.

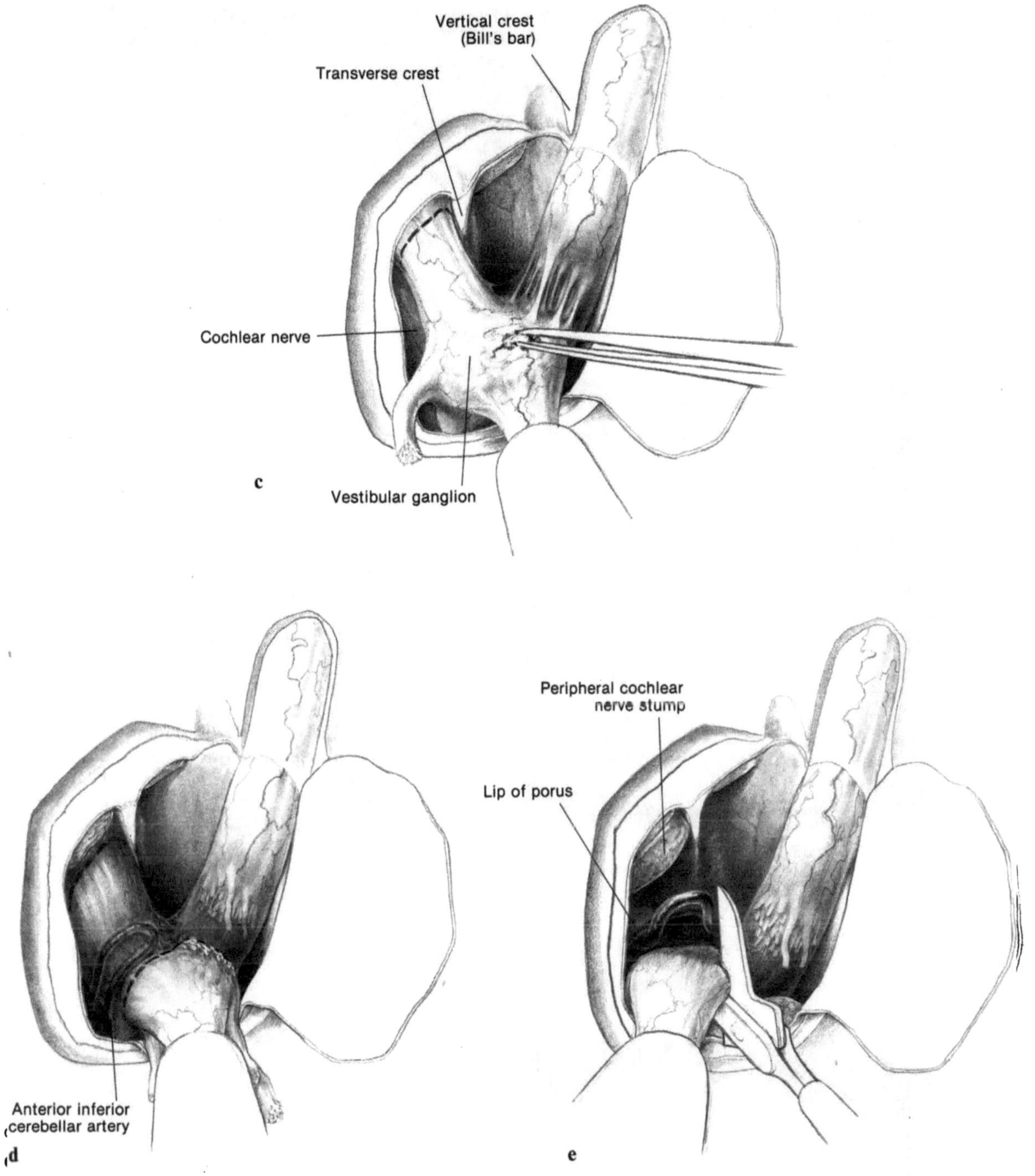

Fig. PS 3c–e.
c The inferior part of the vestibular ganglion is the next structure to be sectioned. The transverse crest and vertical crest (Bill's bar) appear as major surgical landmarks, and the cochlear nerve is visible deep in the field.
d The lateral part of the vestibular division is removed, allowing the anteroinferior lip of the porus acusticus to be identified. The vestibular division is now sectioned medial to the vestibular ganglion (– – –).
e Because hearing is sacrificed in the translabyrinthine approach, the cochlear division of the vestibulocochlear nerve usually is also resected to relieve tinnitus

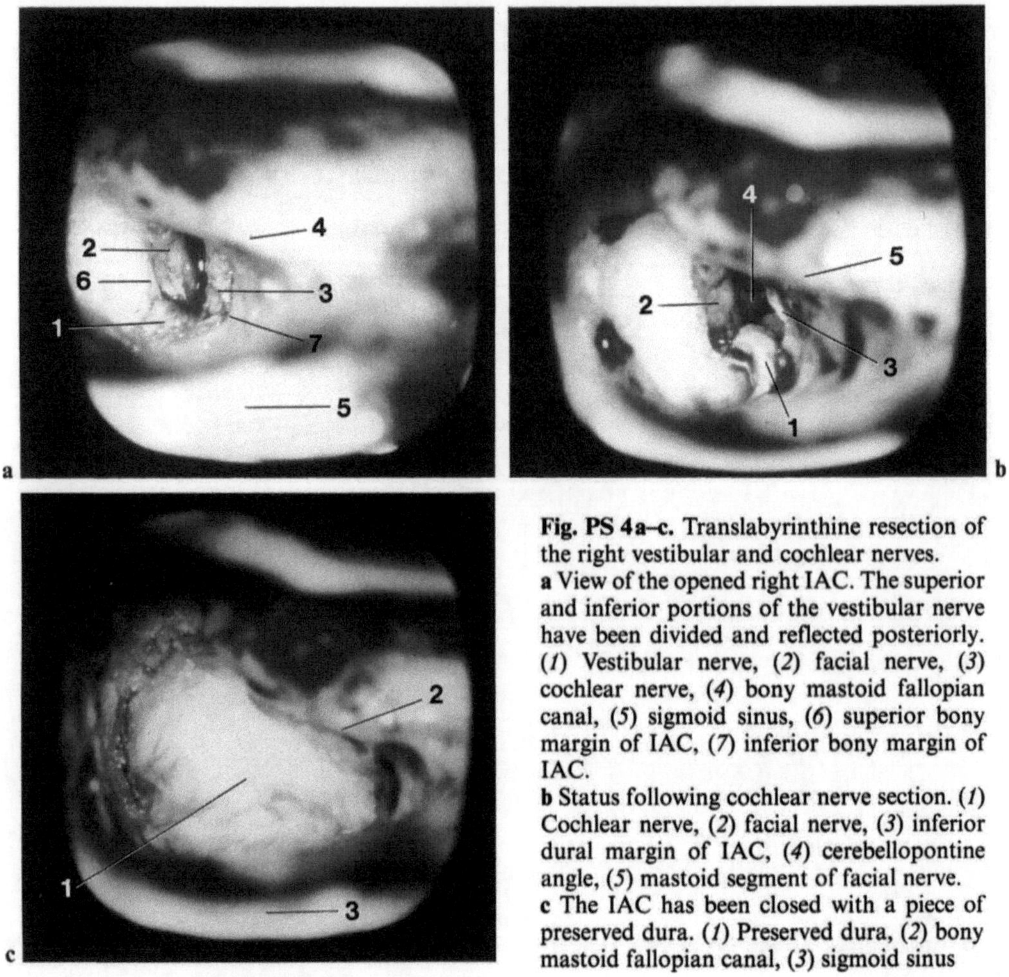

Fig. PS 4a–c. Translabyrinthine resection of the right vestibular and cochlear nerves.
a View of the opened right IAC. The superior and inferior portions of the vestibular nerve have been divided and reflected posteriorly. (*1*) Vestibular nerve, (*2*) facial nerve, (*3*) cochlear nerve, (*4*) bony mastoid fallopian canal, (*5*) sigmoid sinus, (*6*) superior bony margin of IAC, (*7*) inferior bony margin of IAC.
b Status following cochlear nerve section. (*1*) Cochlear nerve, (*2*) facial nerve, (*3*) inferior dural margin of IAC, (*4*) cerebellopontine angle, (*5*) mastoid segment of facial nerve.
c The IAC has been closed with a piece of preserved dura. (*1*) Preserved dura, (*2*) bony mastoid fallopian canal, (*3*) sigmoid sinus

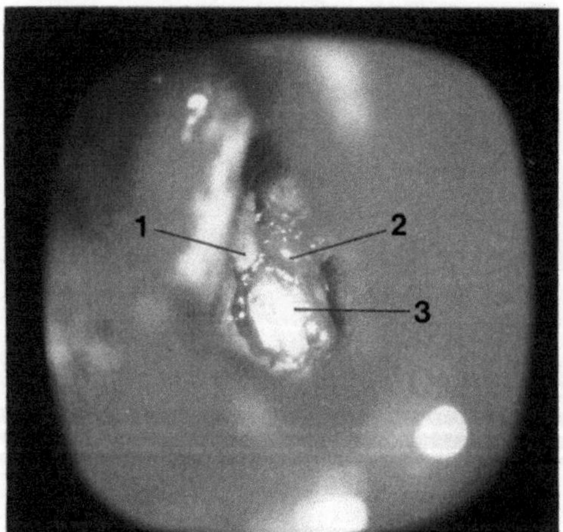

Fig. PS 5. Loop of the anterior inferior cerebellar artery in the IAC. (*1*) Facial nerve, (*2*) loop of anterior inferior cerebellar artery, (*3*) cochlear nerve

Vascular Decompression of the Cranial Nerves in the Cerebellopontine Angle

Introductory Remarks. The close anatomic relationship between the blood vessels and the peripheral nervous system holds true throughout the human body. In a 1934 issue of the *American Journal of Surgery*, Dandy was the first to suggest that compression of the trigeminal nerve in the cerebellopontine angle was a major cause of trigeminal neuralgia. In 215 patients undergoing occipital surgery, he unexpectedly found 12 tumors (6%), 11 angiomas (5%), 66 arterial loops and 30 venous loops (45%), and 9 other lesions causing compression of the trigeminal nerve root. Dandy himself removed the tumors that were found and divided the sensory nerve fibers without performing a vascular decompression.

The possible role of vascular compression of the facial nerve in the cerebellopontine angle in the pathogenesis of facial spasms was noted by Campbell and Keedy in 1947 and by Gardner in 1959 and 1962. Gardner, a pupil of Dandy, was the first, in 1959, to report on successful vascular decompression of the trigeminal root in the cerebellopontine angle without root resection.

The introduction of the operating microscope revolutionized the treatment of vascular nerve compression by enabling a systematic, microsurgical exploration of the cerebellopontine angle (Rand and Jannetta 1968). A pioneer in this area was Jannetta, who described the successful treatment of trigeminal neuralgia by vascular decompression and later reported on hundreds of successful outcomes in patients with facial spasm, vestibulocochlear dysfunction, and glossopharyngeal neuralgia (Jannetta 1967, 1970, 1976, 1977, 1981a, b). His outstanding results have since been confirmed by many other authors (Iwakuma et al. 1982; Rand 1981; Penzholz 1983; Samii 1983; Apfelbaum 1977).

The critics of vascular compression as an etiopathogenic mechanism of cranial neuropathy argue that a great many vessels in the human body are so closely related to peripheral and cranial nerves that nerve compression by blood vessels is an ever-present phenomenon and should not produce overt symptoms. The anterior inferior cerebellar artery, for example, is in close relation to cranial nerves VII and VIII

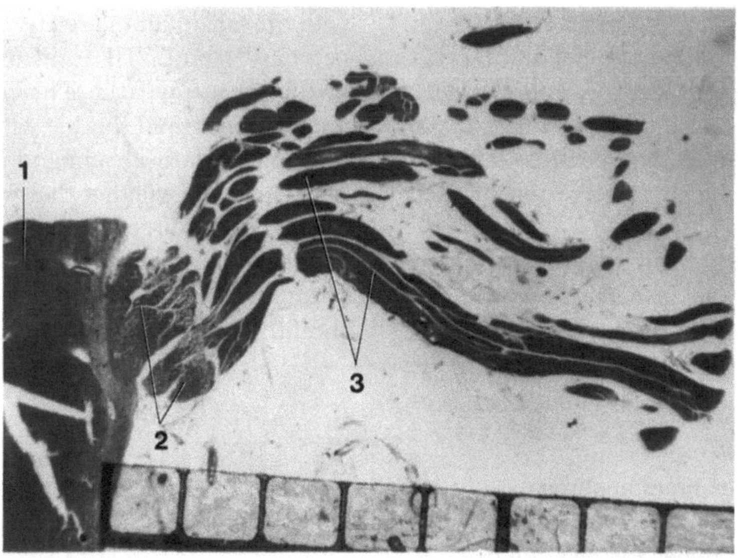

Fig. PS 6. Longitudinal section of the exit zone of the trigeminal nerve from the brain stem. The approximately 1.5-mm-long exit segment differs markedly in color (*lighter*) from the more peripheral parts of the nerve (*darker*). The central nerve fibers are surrounded by glial cells, and the more peripheral fibers by Schwann cells. (*1*) Brain stem, (*2*) central portion of trigeminal nerve, (*3*) peripheral portion of trigeminal nerve

(Mazzoni and Hansen 1970; Celis-Blaubach 1973). The branches of the artery may even pass between the nerve fascicles (Sunderland 1945). However, this line of reasoning neglects certain details of microneuroanatomy that are not widely known. On the microscopic level, some cranial nerves exhibit a central component and a peripheral component (Fig. PS 6). The central part of the facial and trigeminal nerve contains nerve fibers that are not accompanied by Schwann cells, as in the more peripheral part of the nerve, but by glial cells, which surround the nerve fibers over a distance of about 2 mm from the brain stem in the cerebellopontine angle. In 1962 Gardner proposed the term "junction zone" for the facial nerve segment that emerges from the brain stem and is covered by oligodendroglia. Jannetta (1977) pointed to this exit zone as the specific site of nerve irritation by vascular compression. It is assumed that this anatomically distinct zone has its own physiologic threshold of response to mechanical stimuli, and that changes in axonal metabolism are elicited in that segment with relative ease. The hypothetical explanation of the pathogenesis of facial spasm and trigeminal neuralgia is based on the phenomenon of "fiber interaction" at the compression site. It it likely that axonal short-circuits develop in the form of false synapses, which lead to an increased discharge of impulses causing spontaneous, involuntary facial movements or episodes of pain. Vascular decompression is a causal therapy which, unlike the many traditional destructive treatment methods, is aimed at the preservation of function.

The current definitive indications for microsurgical exploration of the cerebellopontine angle through the lateral suboccipital approach and concurrent vascular decompression of the affected cranial nerves, as required, are as follows:

1) "Idiopathic" trigeminal neuralgia.
2) Hemifacial spasm.
3) Disorders falling under the heading of "vestibulocochlear dysfunction".
4) Glossopharyngeal neuralgia.

It is extremely rare for vascular compression of the trigeminal nerve to coexist with an acoustic neuroma of the same or opposite side. Cases of this type are managed by vascular decompression and removal of the acoustic neuroma in one or two sittings (see p. 393).

It is possible that this pathogenetic mechanism underlies a number of other diseases involving the cranial nerves or brain stem, such as Bell's palsy (Jannetta and Bissonette 1978) and essential hypertension (Jannetta and Gendell 1979; Segal et al. 1979). Further experimental studies and critical evaluations of clinical outcomes are needed to resolve this question.

Operative Technique
(Fig. PS 7a–c, Fig. PS 8a, b)

Vascular Decompression of the Trigeminal Nerve. Vascular decompression of the trigeminal nerve is performed through the lateral suboccipital approach (see p. 360). The semisitting or supine position may be used. The craniotomy is placed relatively high at the junction of the transverse sinus and sigmoid sinus. The dura is opened along the transverse and sigmoid sinuses, bridging veins are coagulated, and the cerebellopontine angle is exposed just below the tentorium with the self-retaining retractor such that cranial nerves VII and VIII form the lower boundary of the operating field. The cisterns are opened, and cerebrospinal fluid is withdrawn. The location of the petrosal vein and its tributary vessels will determine whether the trigeminal nerve root exit zone is directly visible at this point, or whether the tributary veins will first have to be coagulated and divided. The petrosal vein itself should be spared if possible. In most cases of

Fig. PS 8a, b. Vascular decompression of the trigeminal nerve.
a The trigeminal nerve is exposed, and the vascular loop compressing it from below is identified. (*1*) Trigeminal nerve, (*2*) vascular loop, (*3*) vestibulocochlear nerve.
b A muscle graft is interposed between the vascular loop and trigeminal nerve. (*1*) Trigeminal nerve, (*2*) interposed muscle, (*3*) vestibulocochlear nerve

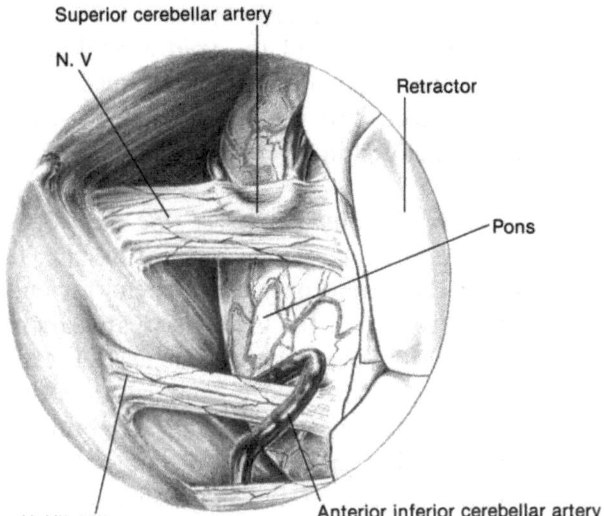

a

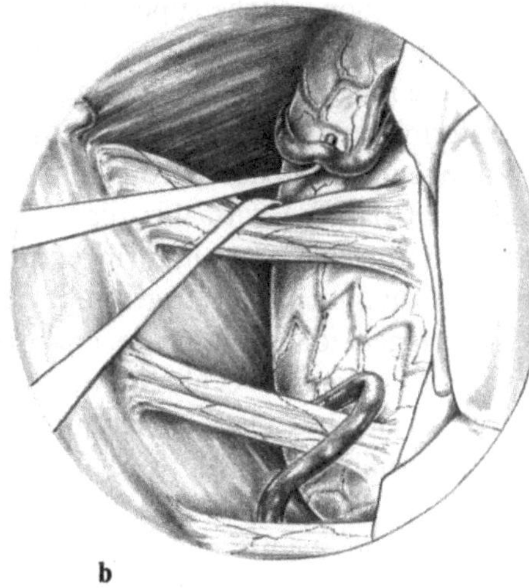

b

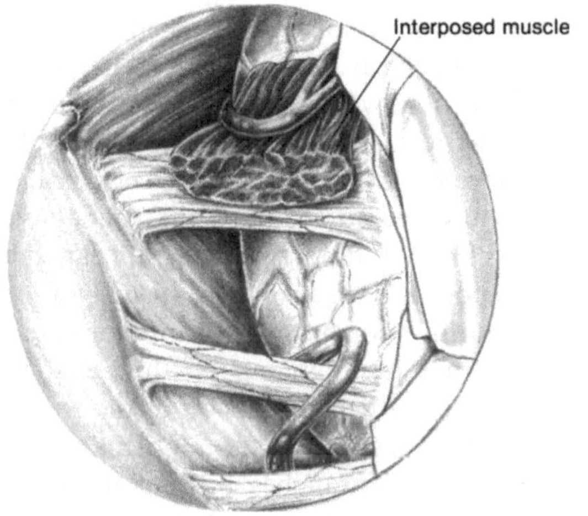

c

Fig. PS 7a–c. Vascular decompression of the trigeminal nerve.
a Compression of the trigeminal nerve at the brain stem by the superior cerebellar artery.
b The superior cerebellar artery is mobilized away from the trigeminal nerve. Cranial nerves VII and VIII and the anterior inferior cerebellar artery are visible in the lower part of the field.
c A sufficiently large piece of myofascia is interposed between the vessel and the trigeminal nerve at the brain stem

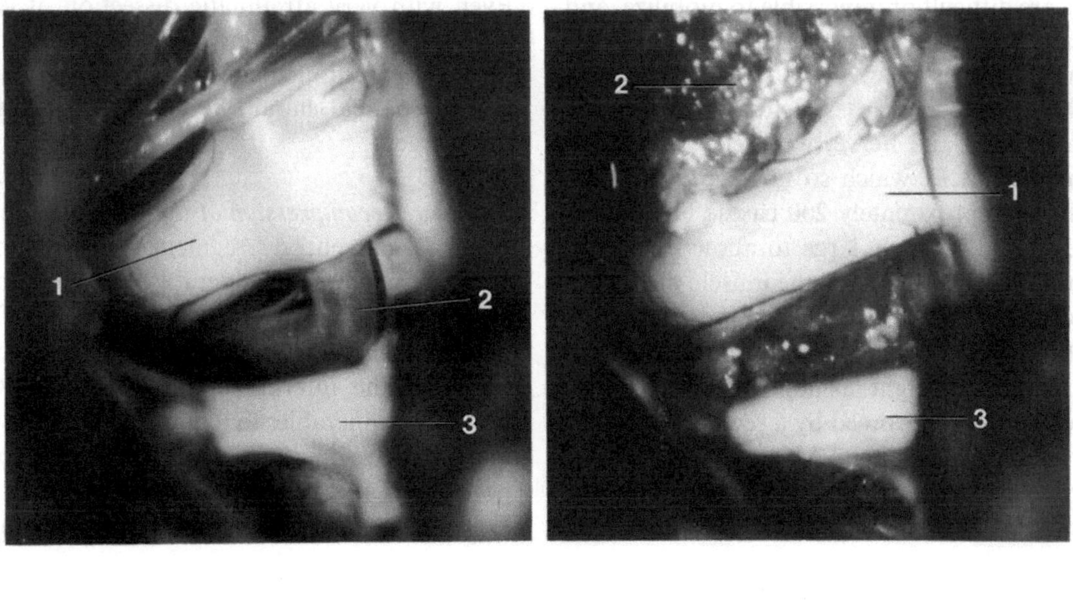

a b

trigeminal neuralgia, the surgeon will find several pulsating loops of the superior cerebellar artery in direct contact with the nerve. In rare cases there may be extreme looping of the anterior inferior cerebellar artery, causing the vessel to impinge upon the nerve from below. We have found that patients with this type of compression tend to have neuralgiform complaints in the third division of the trigeminal nerve. The classic trigger zones in the second trigeminal nerve division may be absent in these cases. Symptoms may be caused by venous loops alone or by a combination of arterial and venous loops.

The arachnoid membrane around the site of contact between the vascular loop and nerve may be thickened. The first step is to separate the arachnoid and push it aside far enough that material can be interposed between the vessel and nerve, while leaving enough arachnoid to help support the interposed material and keep it in place. Next the surgeon manipulates the offending vascular loop away from the nerve and attempts to transpose it onto a different plane. Tiny, hairlike vessels may occasionally be seen communicating between the vascular loop and brain stem. These branches can hinder mobilization of the vascular loop; they also pose a risk of hemorrhage and might even pull the loop back into its original position. Therefore they should be isolated, coagulated with bipolar forceps, and divided so that the vessel can be transposed without tension. Venous loops are difficult or impossible to mobilize, and in many cases there is no alternative to coagulating and dividing them.

While Jannetta interposes Gelfoam between the vascular loop and nerve, we prefer to use autogenous muscle, which so far has given good results in approximately 200 cases. The muscle piece should be fairly large to allow for subsequent shrinkage. Inserting the muscle piece concludes the actual vascular decompression. After careful removal of the brain retractor, the dura is closed in watertight fashion with simple interrupted sutures reinforced by a second over-and-over continuous stitch. Mastoid air cells, if opened, are occluded with bone wax or pieces of muscle to prevent cerebrospinal fluid leak through the pneumatic system of the ear and eustachian tube and to avoid ascending infection. The neck muscles are returned over the bone defect, and the subcutaneous tissue and skin are closed in layers.

Vascular Decompression of the Facial Nerve (Fig. PS 10a–c). For exposure of the facial nerve, the craniotomy must extend far enough inferiorly so that the facial nerve appears in the upper part of the field, i.e., the nerve is exposed from below. The field is bounded inferiorly by the caudal cranial nerves and vertebral artery. The fact that the cause of hemifacial spasm is located directly at the brain stem and not in the free course of the facial nerve in the cerebellopontine angle has an important bearing on the dissection technique. To avoid irritating the vestibulocochlear nerve and facial nerve during the dissection, we first expose the caudal cranial nerves by retracting the flocculus and displacing the choroid plexus upward. The vertebral artery is encountered in front of the caudal cranial nerves. From that point the surgeon can identify and expose the vascular loop (usually a looped posterior inferior or anterior inferior cerebellar artery) that is impinging on the facial nerve. As in vascular decompression of the trigeminal nerve, mobilization of the loop may be hampered by tiny branches passing to the brain stem. These should be isolated, coagulated, and if necessary divided. A muscle-fascia graft is interposed as described for the trigeminal nerve. Even with very atraumatic dissection, it is not always possible to avoid some degree of postoperative vestibulocochlear nerve dysfunction, and the patient should be informed of this before surgery.

Vascular Decompression of the Vestibulocochlear Nerve. The "central" segment of the vestibulocochlear nerve is considerably longer than the central portions of the trigeminal and facial nerves. It extends from the brain stem to the porus of the internal auditory canal. As the nerve is vulnerable to compression anywhere along this segment, a correspondingly longer portion of the nerve has to be exposed. The exposure technique is similar to that for the fa-

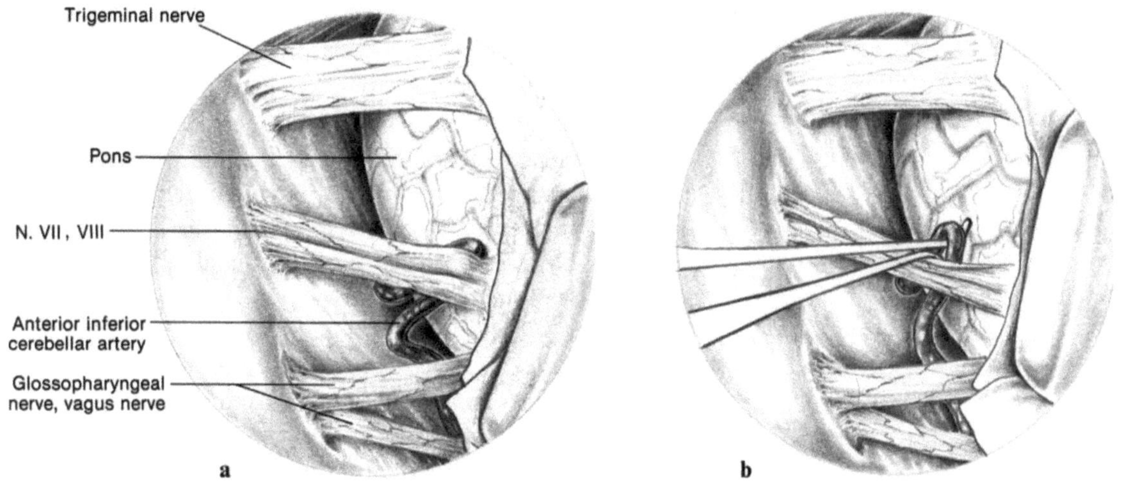

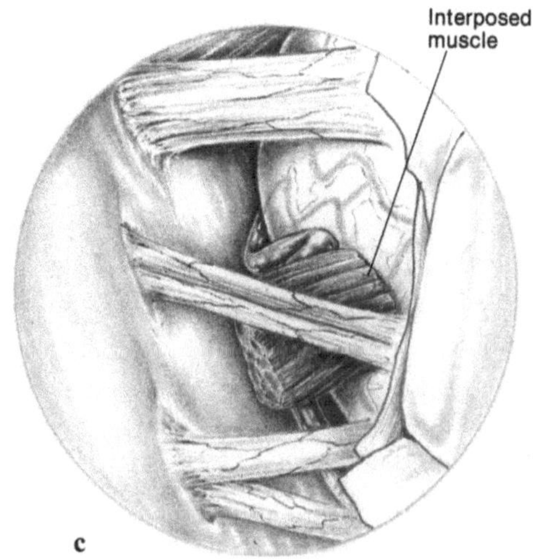

Fig. PS 9 a–c. Vascular decompression of the facial nerve.
a Exposure of the cerebellopontine angle. The field is bounded superiorly by the trigeminal nerve and inferiorly by the caudal cranial nerves. The facial nerve is being compressed at the brain stem by the anterior inferior cerebellar artery.
b Mobilization of the vascular loop.
c Interposition of myofascia

cial nerve, but the arachnoid is mobilized farther laterally to the opening of the internal acoustic meatus. A difficult situation arises when the offending vascular loop lies between the facial nerve and the vestibulocochlear nerve. We do not feel that it is appropriate to coagulate and divide an arterial loop of this kind, because we still know very little about the ability of the affected tissues to develop a collateral blood supply. In cases of this kind we prefer to leave the vascular loop alone, but we still try to "blanket" the nerves by wrapping a piece of muscle around the impinging loop (Samii et al. 1981).

Wigand et al. (1982 a, b) use an "extended transtemporal approach to the cerebellopontine angle for neurolysis of cranial nerves VII and VIII (Fig. PS 10 a, b). The first part of the exposure is similar to that described for middle skull base trauma (see p. 252), except that the skin incision is made in the shape of a gaussian bell curve based over the zygomatic arch. The center of the craniotomy flap lies 1.5 cm anterior to the external auditory canal and 2.5 cm over the root of the zygomatic arch. This ensures that the arcuate eminence will not obstruct the view of the internal auditory canal. The internal auditory canal is found by bisecting the angle between the greater petrosal nerve and the "blue line" of the superior semicircular canal, which usually equals 130°. Bone removal on this bisector leads to the roof of the internal auditory canal. While the classic approach of House (1961) provides only limited exposure of the cerebellopontine angle, a considerably broader view is obtained by additionally removing both lateral walls of

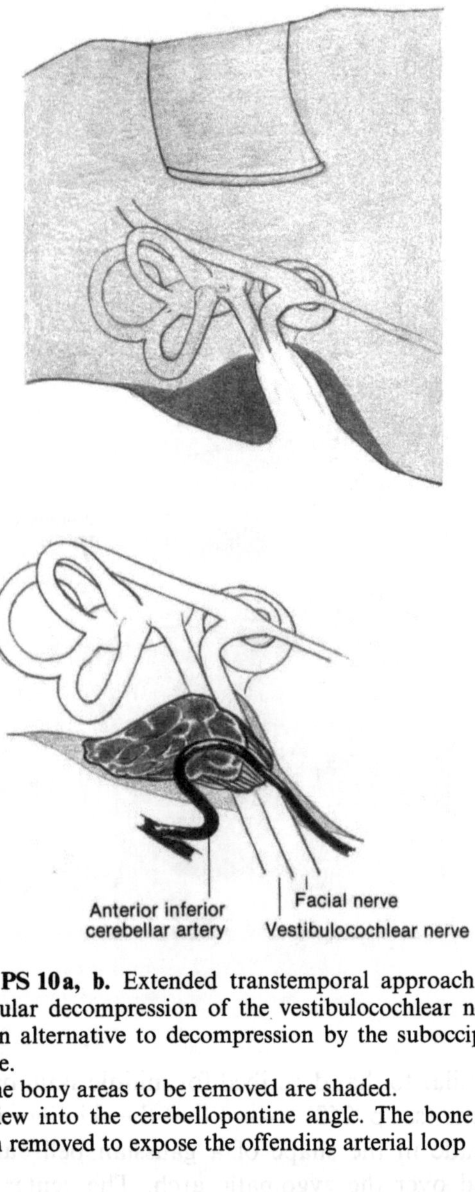

Fig. PS 10a, b. Extended transtemporal approach for vascular decompression of the vestibulocochlear nerve as an alternative to decompression by the suboccipital route.
a The bony areas to be removed are shaded.
b View into the cerebellopontine angle. The bone has been removed to expose the offending arterial loop

the internal auditory canal back to the superior semicircular canal and forward to the cochlea. Wigand ligates, clips, or coagulates the superior petrosal sinus to obtain a broader transdural approach after wide incision of the cerebellar and temporal dura. The meatal dura is slit in continuity with the cerebellar dural incision. At this stage it is possible to remove arachnoidal adhesions, decompress cranial nerves VII and VIII from arterial vessels, and interpose pieces of muscle and periosteum between the nerves and vessels. Good functional results with cessation of vertigo attacks demonstrate that Meniere-like symptoms can originate by arterial impingement on the cochlear and vestibular nerves. However, experience to date is insufficient to recommend vascular decompression as a routine treatment for vestibulocochlear dysfunction of undetermined etiology, as it may be recommended for hemifacial spasm and trigeminal neuralgia.

Vascular Decompression of the Caudal Cranial Nerves and Brain Stem. Vascular decompression of the caudal cranial nerves (IX-XI) has been proposed for the treatment of glossopharyngeal neuralgia (Jannetta 1977) and spastic torticollis (Freckmann et al. 1981). Only a few cases have been published to date, so we cannot yet judge the efficacy of this procedure. Since 1979, Jannetta and coworkers have discussed vascular decompression of the brain stem in the area of the medulla oblongata, from which cranial nerves IX and X arise, as a treatment for essential hypertension. There is both experimental and clinical evidence to show that patients with essential hypertension can benefit from this surgery (Jannetta and Gendell 1979; Segal et al. 1979).

In hypertensive patients who underwent vascular decompression for hemifacial spasm, we indeed found compression of the medulla oblongata by a displaced and markedly atherosclerotic vertebral artery or by the posterior inferior cerebellar artery arising from it. Our experience is illustrated by the following *case report* (Fig. PS 11a–d):

A 61-year-old man was hospitalized with a 6-year history of increasing right-sided hemifacial spasm, compounded later by the development of a slight facial paralysis in all three branches. The patient also manifested a bilateral conductive hearing loss, which was more pronounced in the right ear. He had been hypertensive for years, with systolic pressures of about 190 mmHg. CT scans demonstrated atypical looping of relatively large blood vessels, most notably of the vertebral artery and its branches in the cerebellopontine angle.

The cerebellopontine angle was explored through the lateral suboccipital approach in the

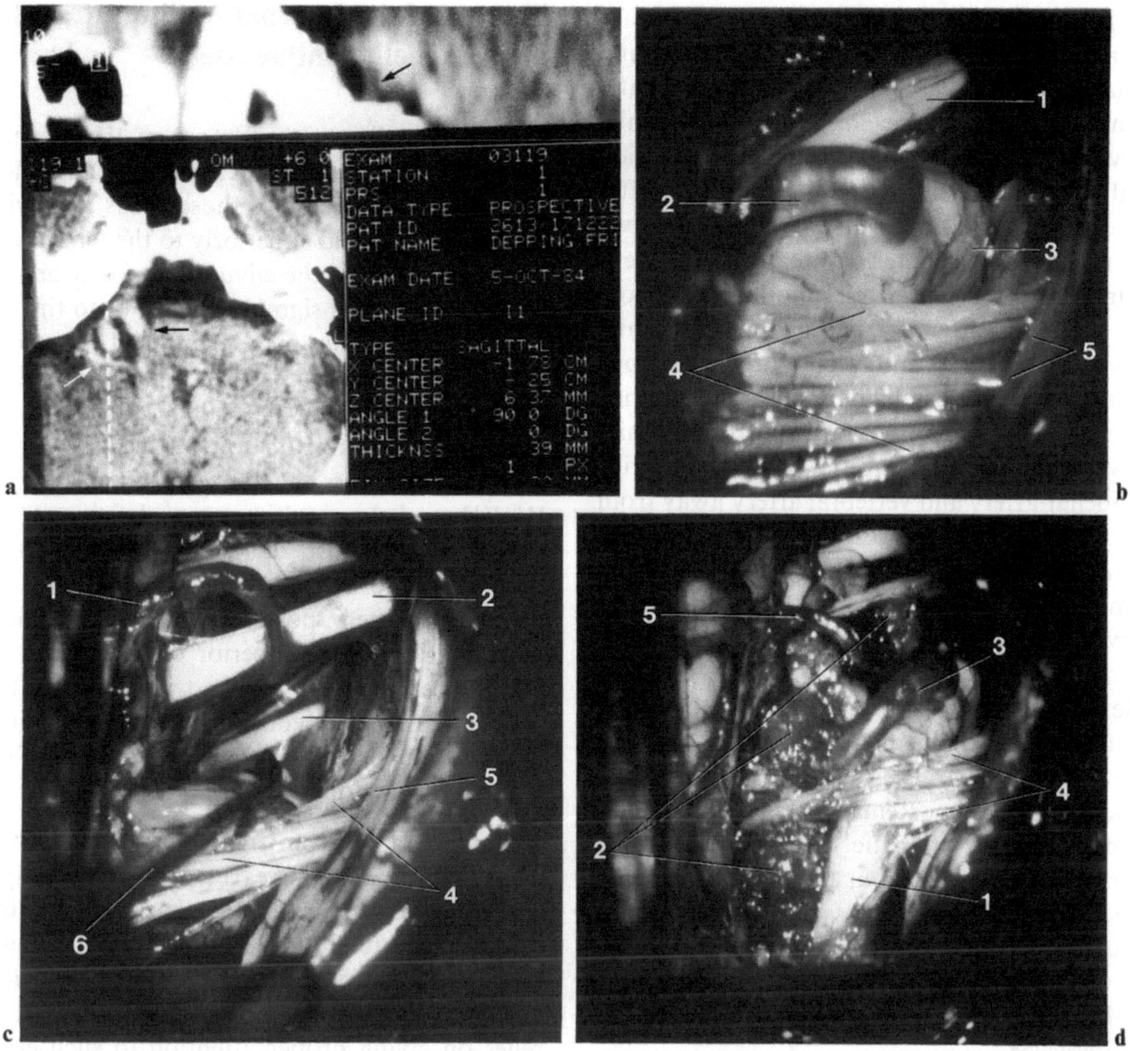

Fig. PS 11 a–d. Vascular decompression of the facial nerve and caudal cranial nerves in a 61-year-old man with right-sided hemifacial spasm and hypertension.

a Postcontrast axial CT scan with sagittal reconstruction shows the conspicuous vertebral artery and several large-caliber branching vessels in the right cerebellopontine angle.

b Lateral suboccipital exploration of the right cerebellopontine angle. The large-caliber vertebral artery with the origin of the posterior inferior cerebellar artery is visible in front of the caudal cranial nerves. (*1*) Vestibulocochlear nerve and facial nerve, (*2*) posterior inferior cerebellar artery, (*3*) vertebral artery, (*4*) caudal cranial nerves, (*5*) jugular foramen.

c A dissector displaces the posterior inferior cerebellar artery and vertebral artery downward to expose the part of the anterior inferior cerebellar artery impinging on the facial nerve. (*1*) Anterior inferior cerebellar artery, (*2*) vestibulocochlear nerve and facial nerve, (*3*) abducens nerve, (*4*) caudal cranial nerves, (*5*) jugular foramen, (*6*) dissector.

d At the end of the procedure cranial nerves VII and VIII, the caudal nerves, and the brain stem have been decompressed by the interposition of free muscle grafts. (*1*) Vertebral artery, (*2*) interposed muscle, (*3*) posterior inferior cerebellar artery, (*4*) caudal cranial nerves, (*5*) anterior inferior cerebellar artery semisitting position. The vertebral artery appeared enlarged with partial wall sclerosis and a mass-lesion effect. The brain stem was greatly compressed in the area of the caudal cranial nerves, and there was associated compression of the vestibulocochlear and facial nerves. After dissecting away the arachnoid, we found two arterial loops – the anterior inferior and posterior inferior cerebellar arteries, both arising from the vertebral artery – impinging on cranial nerves IX–XI, VII, and VIII. With meticulous dissection, we were able to mobilize the anterior inferior cerebellar artery away from cranial nerves VII and VIII, and the posterior inferior cerebellar artery and vertebral artery away from the caudal cranial nerves and brain stem. We then interposed several pieces of muscle to decompress the brain stem and affected cranial nerves. The wound was closed in standard fashion.

The hemifacial spasm that existed preoperatively disappeared immediately after the surgery, and the facial paralysis regressed slowly over a period of weeks. Remarkably, there was an immediate and dramatic fall of the systolic blood pressure from about 190 mm Hg to about 120 mm Hg. The blood pressure maintained this value several weeks after surgery, even though the patient had stopped taking antihypertensive medications. Hearing of the right ear could not be preserved.

Comments: The patient suffered extensive compression of the cranial nerves in the cerebellopontine angle and of the brain stem with hemifacial spasm, cochlear dysfunction, and essential hypertension. Surgical decompression of the cranial nerves from the anterior and posterior inferior cerebellar arteries and from the tortuous and calcified vertebral artery succeeded in curing the patient's hemifacial spasm, facial paralysis, and essential hypertension.

Tumors of the Internal Auditory Canal and Cerebellopontine Angle

Introductory Remarks. Tumors of the internal auditory canal and cerebellopontine angle are lesions that originate in those areas and with growth may extend superiorly to the tentorium, anteroinferiorly to the clivus, and posteriorly to the transverse and sigmoid sinuses or to the occipital bone and foramen magnum. The petrous bone with the structures of the inner and middle ear form a boundary laterally, while the pons and medulla oblongata form a medial boundary. These tumors may involve cranial nerves IV–XII, and the resulting nerve deficits are responsible for most of the symptoms which prompt diagnostic evaluation. The vertebral artery, basilar artery, posterior and anterior inferior cerebral arteries, superior cerebellar artery, and the petrosal vein and its tributaries are the vessels that must be considered during the diagnostic assessment and operative treatment of tumors in this region.

Symptoms range from signs of isolated cranial nerve irritation in an early phase to multiple cranial nerve deficits in later stages, culminating in the complete picture of an intracranial mass lesion with compression of the fourth ventricle and obstructive hydrocephalus. Early diagnosis relies on giving proper attention to such early symptoms as tinnitus; progressive, abrupt or fluctuant hearing loss; and disturbances of equilibrium such as postural, paroxysmal, and sustained vertigo. Such complaints may be early symptoms of a tumor primary to the internal auditory canal, but they can also represent late symptoms of a neoplastic process originating in the cerebellopontine angle. Other symptoms or syndromes like trigeminal neuralgia, facial paralysis, hemifacial spasm, glossopharyngeal neuralgia, vocal cord paralysis from vagal irritation, accessory nerve paralysis, or hypoglossal paralysis often signify a high degree of tumor expansion. That is because there is enough room in the cerebellopontine angle for the tumor to attain considerable size before producing symptoms. While trigeminal nerve irritation occurring some time after the appearance of vestibulocochlear nerve symptoms is considered evidence of an advanced acoustic neuroma, the primary occurrence of trigeminal nerve irritation can be an early symptom of a neuroma expanding into Meckel's cave or of a meningioma arising from that region. Sophisticated diagnostic techniques developed in recent years make it possible to detect acoustic tumors at an early stage with minimum patient risk and discomfort. These techniques include refined audiologic and vestibular tests, especially evoked potential audiometry, cochleomeatal scintigraphy (Bornemann et al. 1982–1983), high-resolution CT, air contrast studies of the cerebellopontine angle (computed pneumocisternography), and magnetic resonance imaging (MRI). Selective and superselective catheter angiography are of great value in determining the extent of vascular tumors. Also, superselective embolization of the tumor vessels can enhance the ease and safety of tumor removal and can even provide a definitive treatment in some cases (Debrun 1982; Lasjaunias 1983).

Approximately two-thirds of cerebellopontine angle tumors are neuromas arising from the vestibulocochlear nerve, known also as acoustic neuromas (or neurinomas). The prevalence is 79.2% in the series of Zülch, 65% in Yasargil, and 78% in our own material (Samii and Penkert 1984; Yasargil 1978; Zülch 1956). The incidence of meningiomas of this region is approximately 10%, and that of epidermoids is 3%–4%. Other tumors are quite rare and occur in fewer than 1% of the cases.

Acoustic Neuroma

Introductory Remarks. The historical development of acoustic neuroma surgery demonstrates clearly that the problem is an interdisciplinary one, and that the results depend critically on the technical aids and facilities that are available. A meaningful comparison of the advantages and disadvantages of the different approaches, familiar since the turn of the century, can be made only if the approaches are applied by expert surgeons using comparable technical aids.

As early as 1894, Ballance attempted to remove an acoustic neuroma by finger dissection through a *suboccipital* approach. Krause applied a similar approach in 1903, this time using brain spatulas. Significant advances are credited to Cushing (1917) and Dandy (1922, 1925, 1941) and to their respective groups. The high mortality accompanying the complete removal of acoustic neuromas prompted Cushing to enucleate the tumor only, leaving its capsule behind. This lowered the mortality to 10%–20%, but recurrence rates were high. By improving the operative technique, Dandy (1941) was able to effect complete tumor removal without increasing the mortality. However, he was able to preserve the facial nerve in only 1 of 45 patients. This contrasts with the series of Olivecrona (1940), who preserved the facial nerve in 18 of 23 patients. In a later review of 130 cases (Olivecrona 1967), the mortality rate was 18%. Late follow-ups of Olivecrona's patients (Horrax and Poppen 1949) showed, however, that half the patients either had developed a recurrence or had already died from one.

The *translabyrinthine approach* was first proposed by the otosurgeon Panse (1904), a contemporary of Krause, and Quix first used it in 1911 for removal of acoustic neuromas. Zange in 1915 described the translabyrinthine removal of acoustic and cerebellopontine angle tumors in greater detail. Already in 1905 Borchardt performed the first transsigmoidal resection of an acoustic neuroma.

The middle cranial fossa approach (transtemporal extradural approach) was used in the early part of the century by Jaboulay (1901; cited in Chavanne and Troullieur 1905) and Perry (1904) for vestibular nerve sectioning. It did not gain wide acceptance until after World War II, when various authors, aided by the operating microscope, used this approach to reach the superior semicircular canal (House 1961).

The microsurgical era of acoustic neuroma surgery was initiated by otologists in the early 1960s. In 1964 House reported on 54 cases. Working with the neurosurgeon Hitselberger (1964), he used the transtemporal approach and later changed predominantly to the translabyrinthine approach. He was followed by many other authors (Fisch 1970, 1978; Helms 1978; Pulec 1966 a,b; Sterkers 1971; Wigand 1976; etc.). The operating microscope, diamond burr, bipolar forceps, and suction irrigator were instruments that provided optimum vision with an absolute minimum of surgical trauma. They led to a drastic reduction in the 20%–30% mortality rate of the classic suboccipital neurosurgical procedure while also greatly reducing the surgical morbidity. Preservation of the facial nerve was possible in some 90% of the cases. In later years, facial nerve function became a key issue in the discussion between otosurgeons and neurosurgeons. It was reason enough for neurosurgeons to adopt the use of the operating microscope for acoustic tumor removal through the suboccipital approach, marking the start of the era of microneurosurgery (Rand and Kurze 1965; Rand 1969; Yasargil and Fox 1974; Rhoton 1974, 1976; MacCarty 1975; Malis 1975; Samii 1979; Di Tullio et al. 1978).

It was now possible to undertake the microsurgical removal of acoustic neuromas through the transtemporal and translabyrinthine routes and also through the suboccipital approach with comparable mortalities and with preservation of the facial nerve. Next came refinements of microsurgical technique which made it possible to preserve the anatomy and function of individual fascicles of the vestibulocochlear nerve through both the transtemporal approach (Cohen 1979; Cohen and Ransohoff 1981; Fisch 1978; Glasscock et al. 1978; Wigand 1979; Wigand et al. 1981) and the suboccipital approach (Koos 1977; Mackay and King 1977; Morrison and King 1984; Portmann 1975; Rand and Kurze 1968; Rhoton 1976; Samii and Ohlemutz 1981; Samii and Penkert 1984; Samii et al. 1985; Smith et al. 1973; Sterkers 1981; Sterkers et al. 1984; Di Tullio et al. 1978; Yasargil 1978).

Rand and Kurze (1965) listed the following advantages of the suboccipital, microsurgical removal of acoustic neuromas:

1) Wide exposure.
2) Direct visualization of the anterior inferior cerebellar artery and other brain stem vessels.
3) Dissection of the entire surface of the acoustic tumor, always under direct vision.
4) Identification of the facial nerve in the lateral angle of the internal auditory canal.
5) Ready access to the facial nerve when either anastomosis or graft reconstruction may be necessary.

Based on our own experience with the microsurgical removal of acoustic neuromas since 1968 and having tested the various approaches and their combinations in one or two stages, we can characterize the contemporary status of acoustic neuroma surgery as follows:

1) With small tumors confined to the internal auditory canal, it is possible to preserve the facial nerve and hearing by use of the transtemporal approach.
2) Small tumors extending beyond the internal auditory canal, larger tumors, and giant tumors can be completely removed through the microsurgical suboccipital approach with entry into the internal auditory canal. Facial nerve function can be preserved in most cases with this approach, and vestibulocochlear function can be preserved in a significant percentage of cases.
3) The translabyrinthine approach permits the complete removal of small tumors with moderate extension into the cerebellopontine angle while preserving the facial nerve. By the nature of the approach, salvage of hearing of the affected side is not possible.

In summary, then, we may say that the temporal extradural approach and lateral suboccipital approach are of equal value for small neuromas confined to the internal auditory canal, while suboccipital microsurgical removal is the method of choice for all larger tumors. The translabyrinthine approach may be considered in cases where the ear has been without useful auditory function for a prolonged period.

Transtemporal Extradural Approach for Removal of Acoustic Neuromas

Introductory Remarks. The technique for exposure of the internal auditory canal by this route was described in an earlier chapter (see pp. 252). W. F. House developed the "middle fossa approach" initially for the microsurgical extirpation of acoustic neuromas but later came to prefer the translabyrinthine route, as the latter is confined to the internal auditory canal. The extradural transtemporal approach enables preservation of the facial nerve and hearing and is fairly well tolerated. It is indicated for intrameatal neuromas. Selection of the approach is based on the results of high-resolution computed pneumocisternography, which also provides much information on fine anatomic details.

Operative Technique

(Fig. MS 12a–n, Fig. PS 12a, b, Fig. PS 13a–e)

The internal auditory canal is identified using one of the methods described earlier (see p. 254). For removal of a neuroma, it is essential that the bony roof of the fundus be removed to the lip of the porus and sufficiently far in the anterior and posterior directions before the dura of the internal auditory canal is opened. In the fundus area, care is taken to avoid injury to the cochlea anteriorly and injury to the superior semicircular canal and its ampulla posteriorly. The reddish luster of the tumor may become visible as the bone is thinned. The dura is incised in trap-door fashion over the tumor, creating a flap that serves to protect the facial nerve during further manipulations.
If the facial nerve is covered by tumor and cannot be readily identified, we recommend opening the tumor capsule after first coagulating any visible surface vessels. The tumor bulk is reduced by enucleation and careful coagulation to decompress the capsule and adjacent neural structures so that the facial nerve can be visualized and the tumor capsule can be separated from it with microscissors. At this stage we cover cranial nerve VII with a small cotton strip so that cerebrospinal fluid can be aspirated

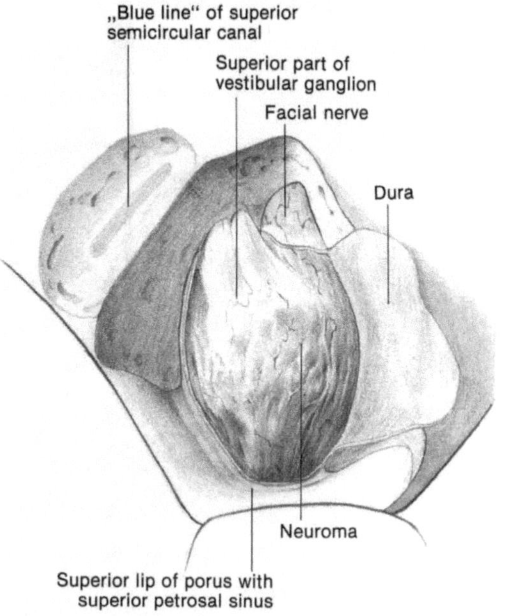

a

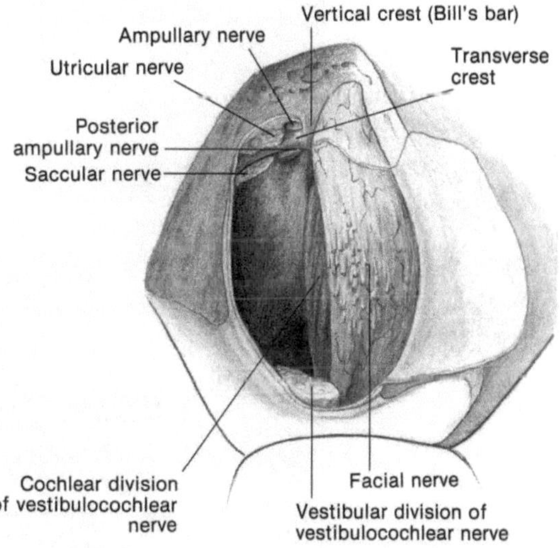

b

Fig. PS 12a, b. Removal of an intracanalicular acoustic neuroma by the transtemporal extradural approach (*left side*).
a The blue line of the superior semicircular canal is identified, and the IAC is entered by removing the bony roof and the superior lip of the porus and fashioning an anteriorly based dural flap. The neuroma, arising from the ganglion has displaced the facial nerve and bulges into the field.
b Situation following tumor removal. The stumps of the resected vestibular division of the vestibulocochlear nerve are visible. The facial nerve and cochlear nerve are intact. Major topographic landmarks are the vertical crest (Bill's bar) and the transverse crest

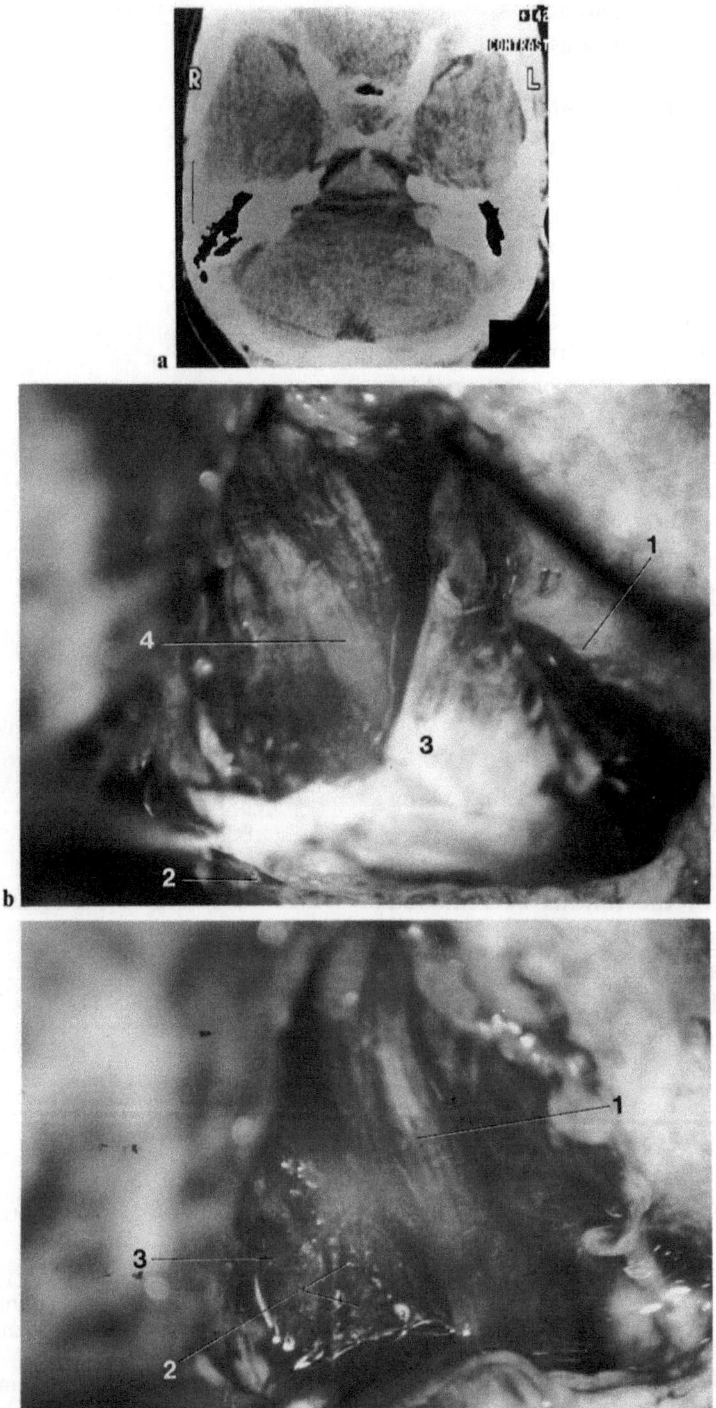
CONTRAST
R
L
a
4
1
3
2
b
1
3
2
c

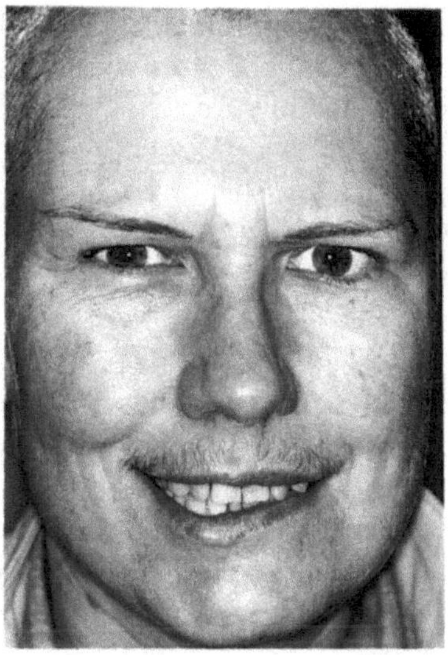

d

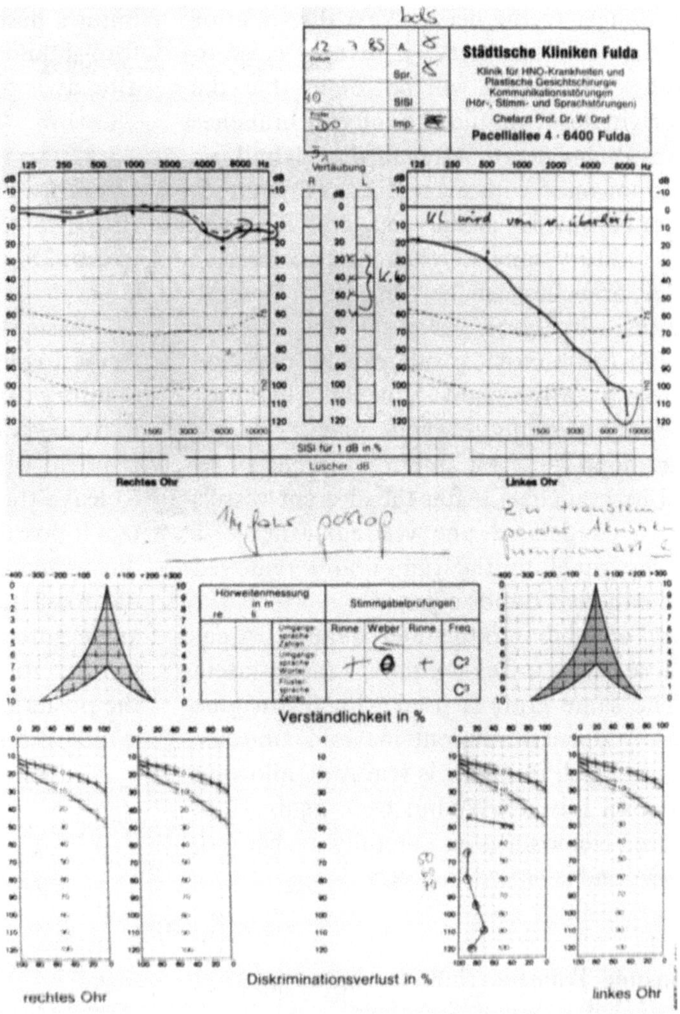

e

Fig. PS 13a–e. Transtemporal extradural removal of an acoustic neuroma with minimal extension beyond the IAC, preserving the facial nerve and cochlear nerve.
a Preoperative contrast-enhanced CT scan. The expansion of the left IAC and the tumor are clearly demonstrated.
b Status following transtemporal exposure of the tumor through the extended approach with mobilization of the superior petrosal sinus. The dural capsule over the tumor has been partially opened. (*1*) Anterior border of IAC, (*2*) superior petrosal sinus, (*3*) dural capsule, (*4*) tumor.
c Status following tumor removal. (*1*) Facial nerve, (*2*) arachnoid, (*3*) cochlear nerve.
d Eight days after surgery the patient had only minimal weakness in the oral branch of the facial nerve.
e Postoperative audiogram. Hearing in the left ear has not changed in comparison to the preoperative status

without danger to the nerve. Next the superior part of the vestibular nerve is divided close to the fundus. Usually it will be found that the tumor originates from the two inferior branches of the vestibular nerve. After further debulking of the tumor mass without torsion, as required, the tumor capsule is partially delivered from the internal auditory canal so that the two inferior vestibular branches can be transected close to the fundus with good vision of the cochlear nerve, and the tumor capsule can be removed completely from the auditory canal. This must be done very carefully to avoid injury to larger vascular loops (anterior inferior cerebellar artery and its branches). After the afferent vessels have been coagulated, the vestibular nerve is severed proximal to the tumor and removed with the adherent tumor capsule.

The dural opening into the internal auditory canal is closed with a free temporal muscle-fascia graft. The same graft is used with fibrin glue to seal any opened adjacent mastoid air cells. The House-Fisch retractor is removed, allowing the temporal lobe to expand back against the skull base. Hemostasis is carefully rechecked, and the wound is closed in layers.

Transmastoid-Translabyrinthine Approach for Removal of Acoustic Neuromas

Introductory Remarks. The technical fundamentals of this approach were described in an earlier chapter (see p. 257). The transmastoid-translabyrinthine approach permits the removal of acoustic neuromas that extend into the cerebellopontine angle, provided the degree of pneumatization and the anterior extent of the sigmoid sinus make adequate exposure of the posterior cranial fossa possible. The location and extent of the tumor are evaluated by high-resolution CT using air contrast enhancement and multi-plane reconstruction. Tumors that already impinge on the brain stem should not be approached by the translabyrinthine route, because it gives poorer exposure of the vessels between the tumor capsule and brain stem than the suboccipital approach. It should also be considered that the translabyrinthine approach implies destruction of the inner ear and therefore should be used only in cases where hearing already is profoundly impaired.

Operative Technique
(Fig. MS 13a–e, Fig. PS 14a–d, Fig. PS 15a–c) (see p. 257)

The basic steps in exposing the dura of the posterior fossa and posterior wall of the internal auditory canal following mastoidectomy and labyrinthectomy were previously described. For removal of acoustic neuroma, it is important to leave the bony shell of the sigmoid sinus intact if possible so that the sinus will be protected during manipulations deep in the field. The middle fossa dura is exposed from the sinodural angle anteriorly to the lip of the porus and inferiorly to the level of the jugular bulb. Then the posterior wall of the internal auditory canal is removed in the form of a bone flap, preferably

Fig. PS 14a–d. Transmastoid-translabyrinthine extirpation of acoustic neuroma.
a An extensive mastoidectomy has been performed. The mastoid segment of the facial nerve is covered by bone. The body of the incus is visible in the attic. The facial nerve is exposed from the geniculate ganglion to its entry into the fundus of the IAC. The jugular bulb marks the inferior limit of bone removal in the mastoid. The bony posterior wall of the IAC has been removed along with the bone covering the posterior fossa dura and the dural ridge at the posterior lip of the IAC. The proposed line of dural incision is coagulated to prevent bleeding from dural vessels.
b The dura has been opened, exposing the tumor. The tumor capsule is opened and the neuroma progressively enucleated by alternating between bipolar cautery and resection. The tumor has displaced the facial nerve superiorly. The cerebellum occupies the posterior part of the field.
c The tumor has been debulked. Tumor vessels arising from the anterior inferior cerebellar artery are coagulated. The bulbopontine sulcus formed by the pons and medulla is visible, and the resection site is indicated by a *dashed line*.
d Transection of the tumor stalk at the brain stem

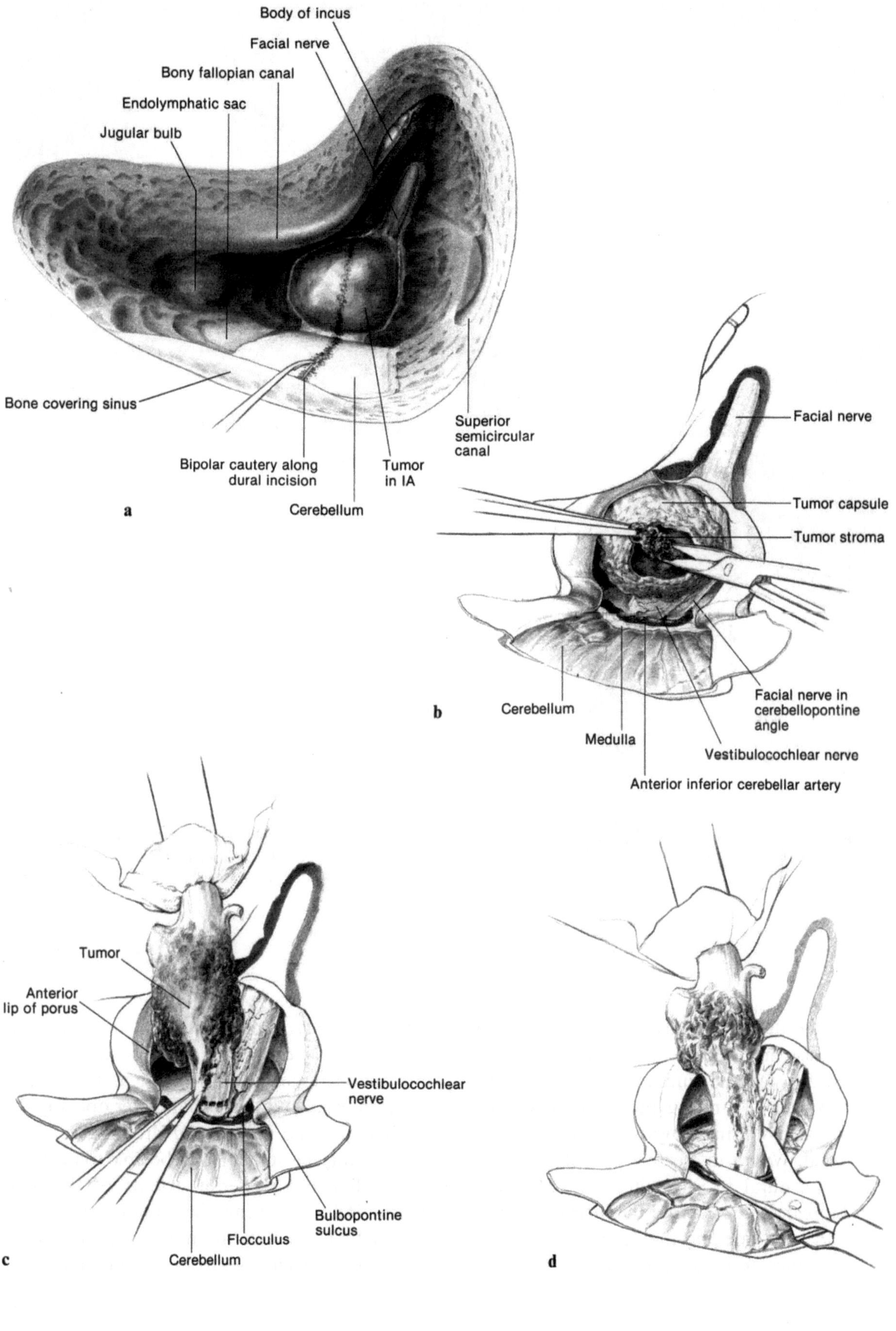

Body of incus
Facial nerve
Bony fallopian canal
Endolymphatic sac
Jugular bulb
Bone covering sinus
Bipolar cautery along dural incision
Cerebellum
Tumor in IA
Superior semicircular canal
a
Facial nerve
Tumor capsule
Tumor stroma
Cerebellum
Medulla
Facial nerve in cerebellopontine angle
Vestibulocochlear nerve
Anterior inferior cerebellar artery
b
Tumor
Anterior lip of porus
Vestibulocochlear nerve
Bulbopontine sulcus
Flocculus
Cerebellum
c
d

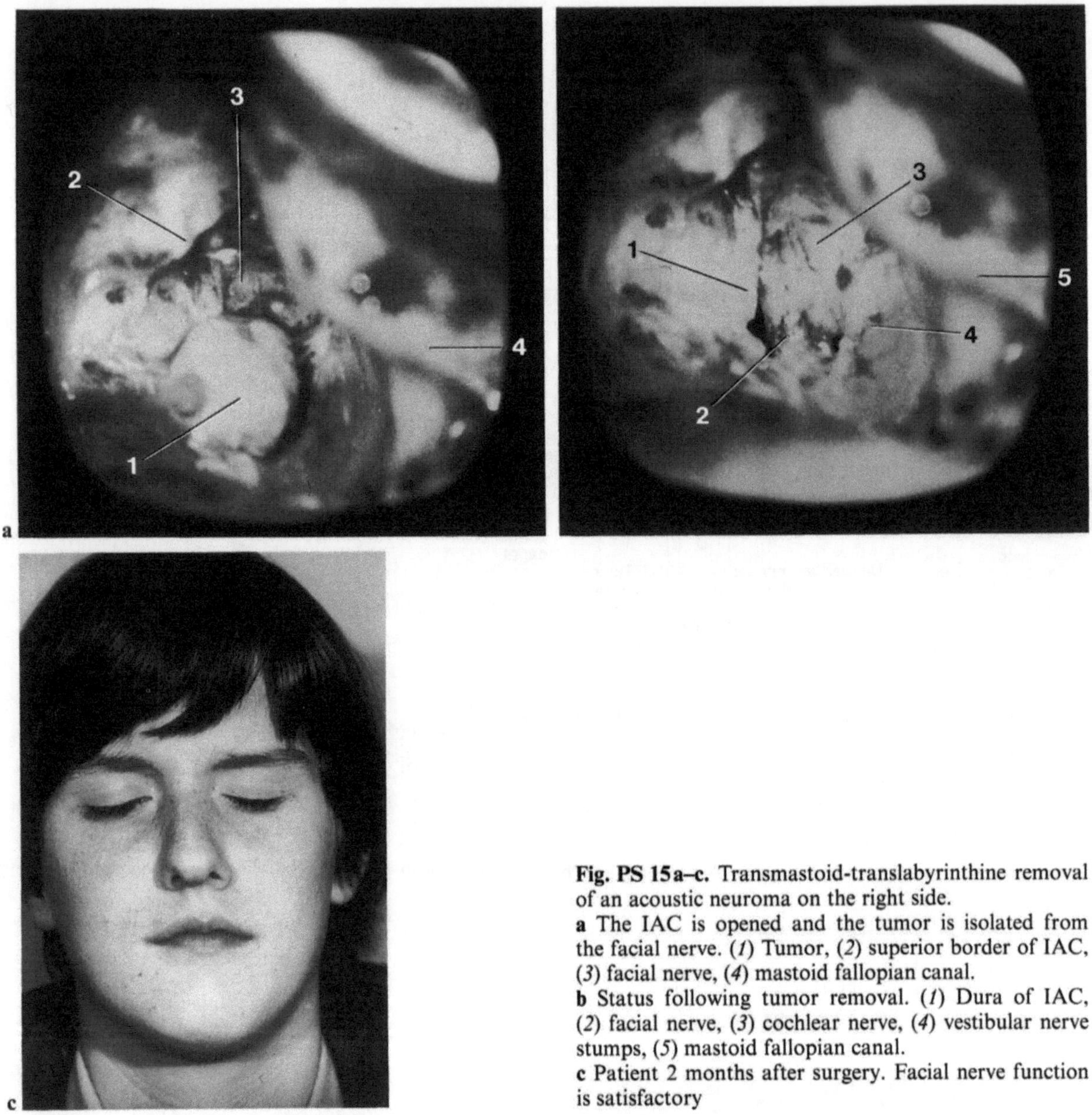

Fig. PS 15a–c. Transmastoid-translabyrinthine removal of an acoustic neuroma on the right side.
a The IAC is opened and the tumor is isolated from the facial nerve. (*1*) Tumor, (*2*) superior border of IAC, (*3*) facial nerve, (*4*) mastoid fallopian canal.
b Status following tumor removal. (*1*) Dura of IAC, (*2*) facial nerve, (*3*) cochlear nerve, (*4*) vestibular nerve stumps, (*5*) mastoid fallopian canal.
c Patient 2 months after surgery. Facial nerve function is satisfactory

leaving the dura primarily intact. The reddish tumor mass may become visible as the bone is thinned. We start the dural incision in the posterior fossa dura, carrying the incision forward from the sigmoid sinus toward the internal auditory canal. We try to create a pair of trap-door flaps. The dural incision sites are coagulated with bipolar forceps before the incision is actually made. On opening the dura, care is taken to avoid injury to large venous vessels that may course directly beneath it. The incision continues over the dural ring at the porus acusticus into the intrameatal dura as far as the fundus of the internal auditory canal. After opening the cerebellopontine cistern and draining cerebrospinal fluid, the surgeon will be able to evaluate the medial and posterior extents of the neoplasm. Before incising the tumor capsule, he should first visualize the junction point where the facial nerve emerges from the fallopian canal into the fundus of the internal auditory canal. The surgeon may then coagulate and incise the tumor capsule and proceed with piecemeal tumor removal, alternating constantly between enucleation and bipolar cautery. As this is done the tumor capsule will shrink appreciably, making it possible to coagulate feeding vessels close to the capsule surface. One should avoid undue traction on the capsule or torsion of the tumor during this time, as this might jeopardize the facial nerve or alter its position, making it difficult to control during the rest of the procedure. An effort is made to reduce the tumor bulk from all sides. This will enable the surgeon to follow the facial nerve from the lateral direction, i.e., from the fundus of the internal auditory canal, and also from the medial direction without actually touching the nerve. A larger tumor vessel, perhaps coming from the brain stem, can now be coagulated under reasonably good vision and divided. Finally the residual, thin tumor capsule is sharply separated from the facial nerve without traction.

The dural flaps are reunited with sutures as much as possible, and any residual defect is covered with one or two pieces of stored dura attached to the adjacent bone margins with fibrin glue. We have found freshly harvested pieces of abdominal fat to be excellent for ablating the surgical cavity. These are held together and in place with fibrin adhesive. Finally the wound is closed in layers.

Lateral Suboccipital Approach for Removal of Acoustic Neuromas

Operative Technique

(Fig. PS 16a–c, Fig. PS 19a–e)

The approach to the cerebellopontine angle and the craniotomy technique were described earlier (see p. 360). The cerebellopontine angle and the tumor are exposed after opening the cerebellopontine cisterns. Regardless of the tumor size, the internal auditory canal is opened first in order to define the lateral tumor boundary. After circular excision of the dura behind the posterior lip of the porus over an area of about 1 cm^2, the posterior wall of the internal auditory canal is progressively ablated with the diamond burr. We recommend starting with a larger burr 4–5 mm in diameter, which cuts more rapidly and is less apt to penetrate into the air cells or injure the soft tissues of the internal auditory canal. As the fundus is approached, progressively smaller burr sizes are employed. It is imperative that constant suction irrigation be maintained during the drilling. The roof of the internal auditory canal is the best landmark to use during removal of the posterior wall. The floor is kept intact if possible to avoid injury to a possibly high situated jugular bulb. Another critical factor is the very close proximity of the superior and posterior semicircular canals with the crus communis. If the tumor extends so far laterally that the fundus of the internal auditory canal has to be exposed, there is a potential for injury to the superior or posterior semicircular canal and the crus communis. This should be avoided because of a possible effect on residual hearing, although there is some question whether opening a semicircular canal will necessarily result in hearing impairment. Therefore we avoid drilling away the last bony strip before the fundus unless it is absolutely necessary after debulking of the tumor in the internal auditory canal. For this step we refer to the high-resolution preoperative CT scan to study the relation of the inner ear structures to the internal auditory canal (Fig. PS 17).

Magnetic resonance imaging provides extremely high-quality images of acoustic neuromas – especially the part of the tumor within the internal auditory canal – by eliminating the bony skull base (Fig. PS 18). This modality has nowadays replaced the more invasive computed pneumocisternography. Standard high-resolution CT continues to be important for preoperative assessment of the bony anatomy of the petrous pyramid.

In the area of the fundus, bone removal should proceed in a medial to lateral direction, rather than lateral to medial. In this way the bone between the internal auditory canal, the ampulla of the semicircular canal, and the jugular bulb can be thinned in 1/10 millimeter increments

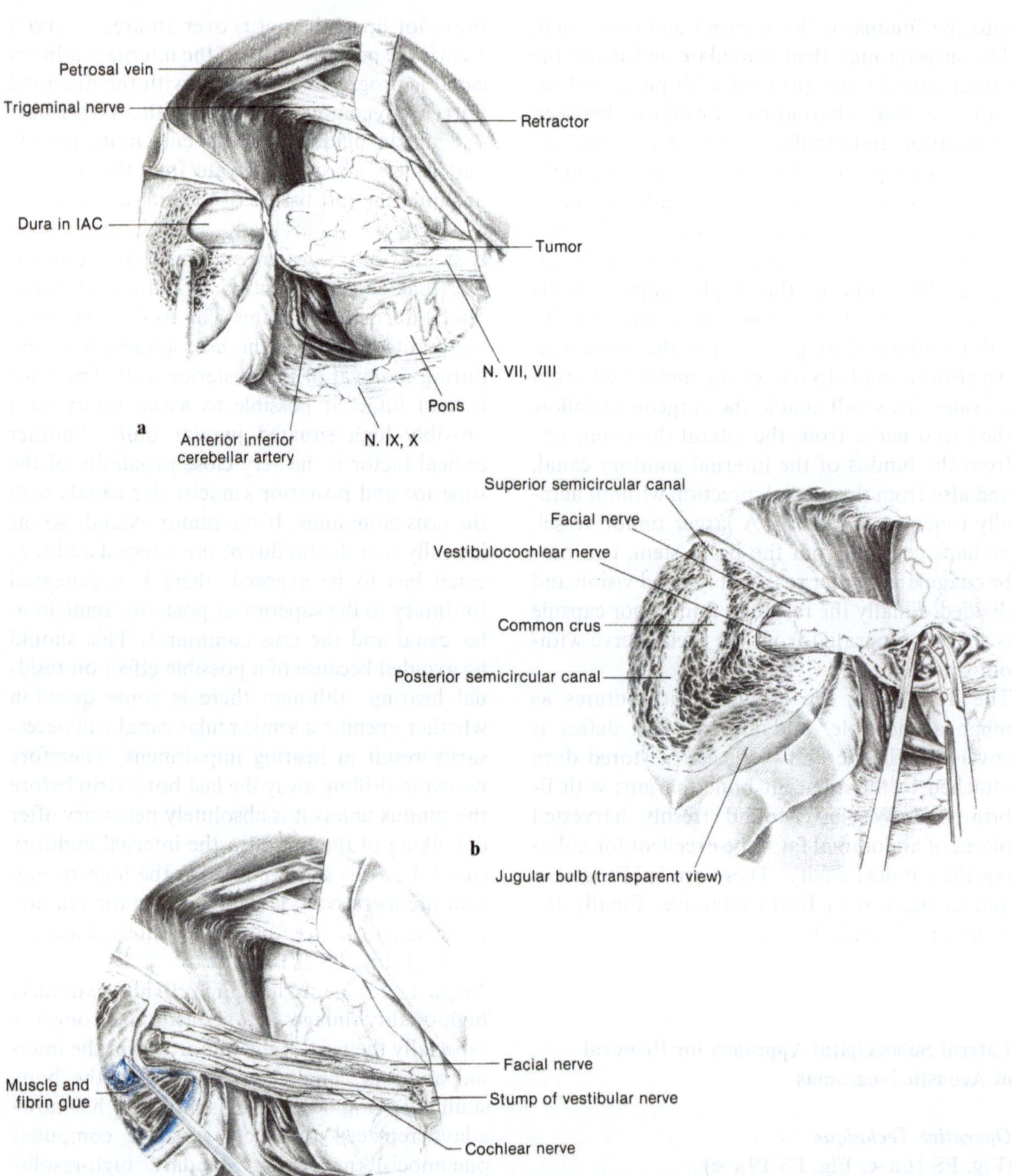

Fig. PS 16a–c. The lateral suboccipital approach for the removal of acoustic neuromas. Technique for "small tumors."
a The tumor is exposed in the cerebellopontine angle. The dura at the petrous bone is mobilized and resected, and the IAC is opened by burring away the posterior wall.
b When entering the IAC, care is taken not to open the ampulla of the semicircular canal or the jugular bulb. The dural sheath in the IAC is removed, then the tumor capsule is separated from the adjacent nerves.
c Status at the end of the procedure. The superior vestibular nerve (the site of tumor origin) is resected while the inferior vestibular nerve, facial nerve, and cochlear nerve are spared. Opened air cells are sealed with bone wax and a myofascial graft attached with fibrin glue to avoid cerebrospinal fluid leak through the eustachian tube

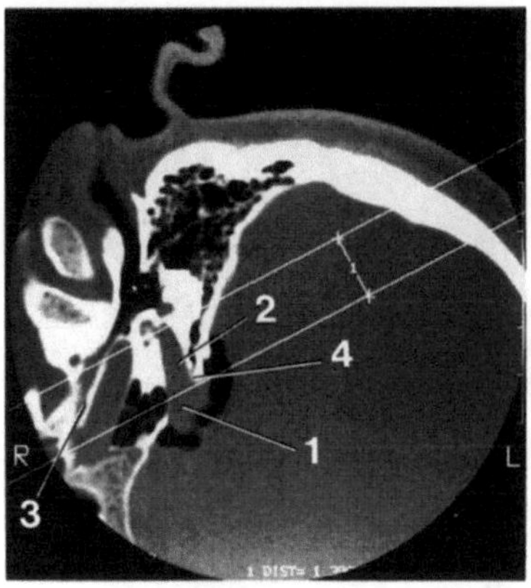

Fig. PS 17. Computed pneumocisternogram (right ear) gives a detailed image of the bony structures of the inner ear. (*1*) Acoustic neuroma, (*2*) IAC, (*3*) internal carotid artery (horizontal portion), (*4*) posterior lip of porus

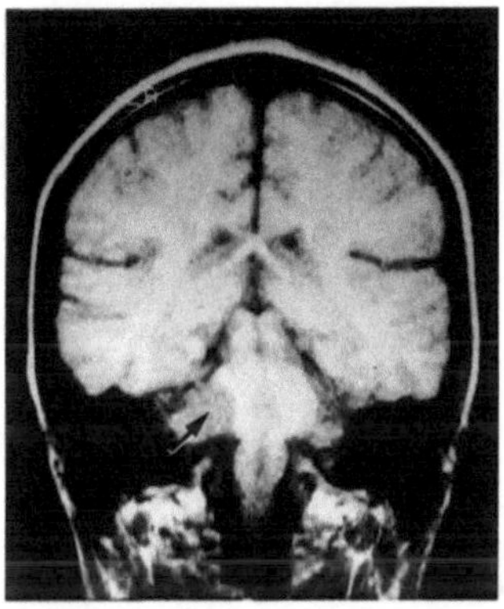

Fig. PS 18. Coronal MRI scan of an extensive acoustic neuroma that is compressing the pons (*arrow*)

with the diamond burr without causing injury to the peripheral vestibular apparatus itself or to the jugular bulb (Fig. PS 19a–e).

Opened air cells are occluded with wax and covered with a myofascial graft fixed with adhesive. This is necessary to prevent cerebrospinal fluid leak into the ear and through the eustachian tube and to eliminate the risk of ascending infection.

Further dissection will depend on whether the tumor is small and not yet in contact with the brain stem, or whether it is large and is already compressing the pons, displacing the trigeminal nerve, or impinging on the caudal cranial nerves.

Dissection of "Small" Tumors
(Fig. PS 19a–e)

These tumors may be entirely intracanalicular or may show varying amounts of extension into the cerebellopontine angle. Generally it is not difficult to identify the cranial nerves and vascular structures of the cerebellopontine angle at the brain stem before actual tumor removal is begun. First the facial nerve and vestibulocochlear nerve are identified medially close to the brain stem, and their relation to the medial tumor boundary is ascertained; the tumor-feeding vessels are also identified. The surgeon must be aware of two important facts before proceeding with the actual tumor dissection: first, even small tumors exert pressure on adjacent cranial nerves, usually nerves VII and VIII, which will show corresponding clinical signs of irritation. Second, there will be sites where firm adhesions exist between the tumor and the nerves VII and VIII. Hence it is inadvisable to try to dissect around the tumor mass and "roll" it, as the resulting pressure and tension will cause lesions and may produce total and immediate neurologic deficits, especially of the cochlear nerve. It is best to start by identifying a part of the tumor capsule that is free of neural contacts. The capsule is opened at that site, and piecemeal debulking of the tumor is begun, alternating constantly between enucleation and bipolar cautery. We use a round, angled microelevator to assist the tumor removal. As the tumor bulk is reduced, the capsule becomes lax, and pressure on surrounding cranial nerves is relieved. When dissecting the tumor capsule from the cranial nerves (not vice-versa!), we have found it helpful to dissect from all sides toward the point at which the capsule is most firmly adherent to the adjacent cranial nerves. The majority of tumors arise from the superior part of the vestibular nerve. The nerve components should be identified as soon as possible after they exit the brain stem, and the components from which the tumor arises should be divided. After the tumor has been debulked sufficiently, the corresponding nerve component is identified within the internal auditory canal and separated a sufficient distance from the tumor. At that point the last

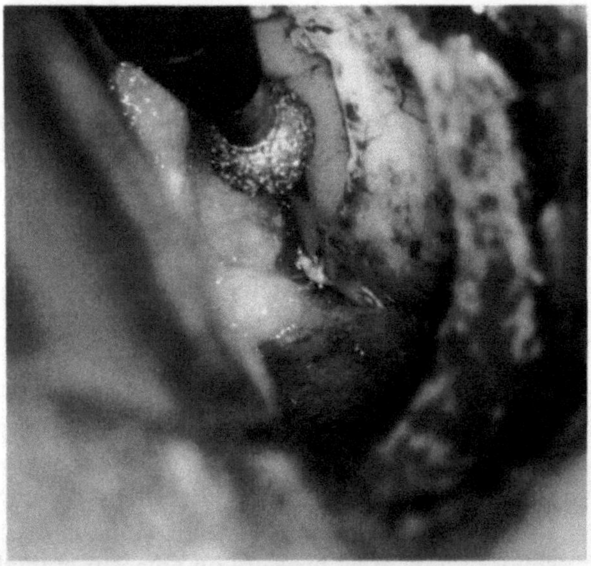

a

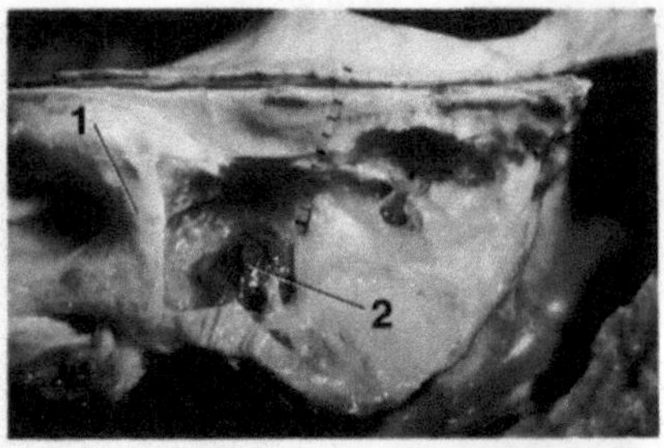

b

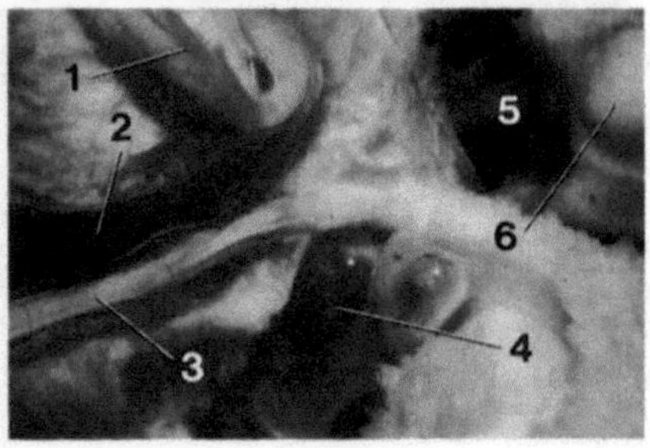

c

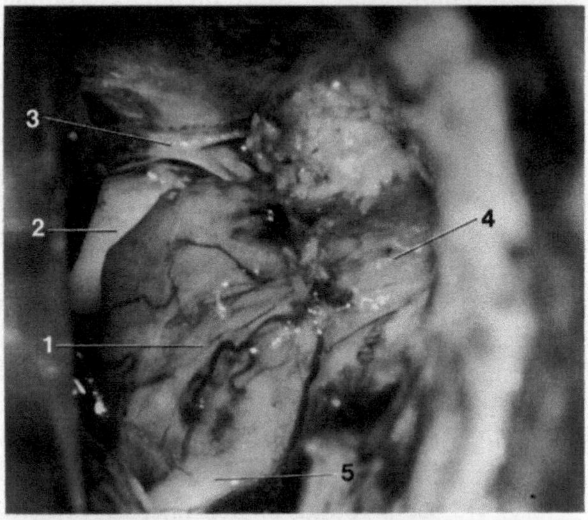

d

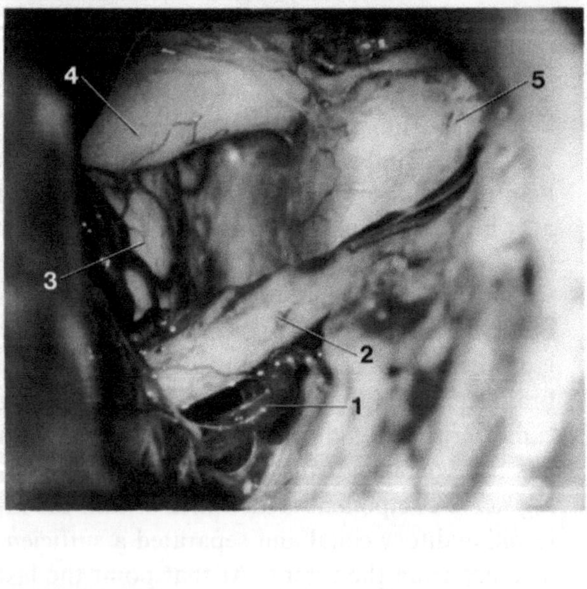

e

Fig. PS 19a–e. Suboccipital exposure of a "small" acoustic neuroma on the right side.
a The dura has been incised and reflected, and the IAC is opened from medially to laterally with the diamond burr.
b Anatomic specimen, viewed posteriorly, showing the relation of the IAC to the jugular bulb (suboccipital approach). (*1*) Posterior lip of porus, (*2*) jugular bulb.
c Anatomic specimen showing the relation of the IAC and its fundus to the vestibule of the inner ear. The facial nerve is reflected upward, the vestibular nerve is shown in correct relation to the semicircular canals, the bony ampulla of the posterior semicircular canal is opened, and the membranous ampulla is visible. (*1*) Facial nerve, (*2*) IAC, (*3*) vestibular nerve, (*4*) ampulla of posterior semicircular canal, (*5*) tympanic cavity, (*6*) ossicle.
d The IAC has been opened, exposing the tumor component in the internal meatus. (*1*) Tumor in cerebellopontine angle, (*2*) trigeminal nerve, (*3*) petrosal vein, (*4*) tumor in IAC, (*5*) vestibulocochlear nerve.
e View into the IAC following complete tumor removal. The facial nerve, cochlear nerve, and inferior vestibular nerve have been preserved. (*1*) Anterior inferior cerebellar artery, (*2*) seventh and eighth cranial nerve bundle, (*3*) brain stem, (*4*) trigeminal nerve, (*5*) fundus of IAC

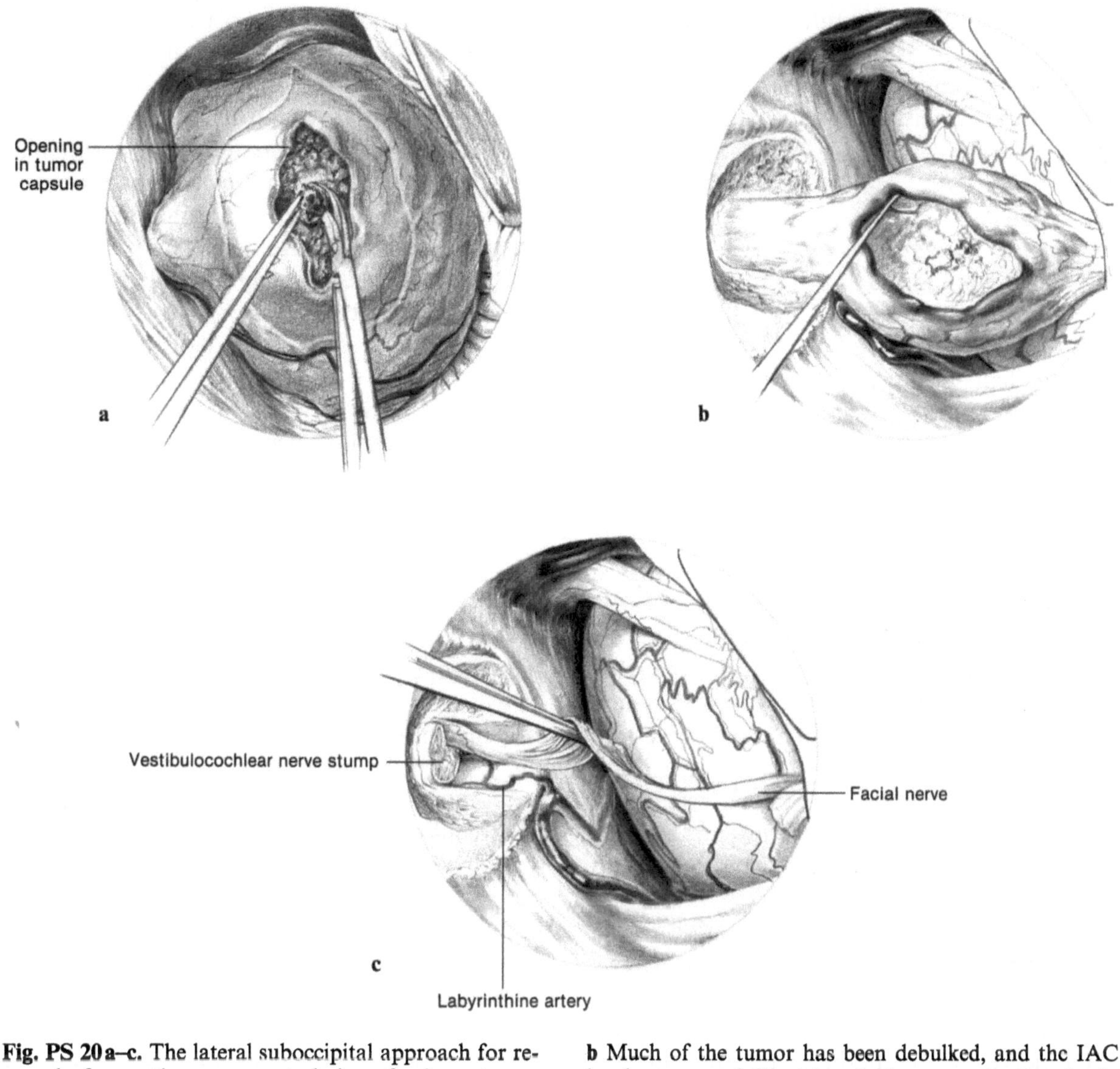

Fig. PS 20 a–c. The lateral suboccipital approach for removal of acoustic neuroma; technique for large tumor removal.
a The cerebellopontine angle is exposed and the tumor identified. The tumor capsule is opened, and the neuroma is enucleated piecemeal.
b Much of the tumor has been debulked, and the IAC has been opened. The trigeminal nerve and petrosal vein are dissected free in the upper part of the field, and the caudal cranial nerves and anterior inferior cerebellar artery in the lower part of the field. The brain stem has been partially decompressed.
c Status following complete tumor removal with facial nerve preservation

adhesion between the tumor and adjacent nerves is removed as atraumatically as possible by sharply sectioning the fibrous tissue connections with microscissors under high magnification.

Dissection of "Large" Tumors
(Fig. PS 20a–c, Fig. PS 21a–e)

With *large tumors,*which existed in three-fifths of the patients in our series, only the posterior part of the tumor is visible initially when the cerebellopontine angle is exposed. First the internal auditory canal is opened as described earlier. Next a large portion of the posterior tumor capsule is resected, and piecemeal enucleation is begun. We have never seen the facial nerve while working on the posterior part of the tumor; it is always displaced anteriorly. This means that enucleation can proceed fairly rapidly from the posterior aspect. After the tumor has been debulked, the caudal cranial nerves are identified, the tumor capsule is elevated away from them, and the nerves are protected with fibrin sponge. Then the anterior inferior cerebellar artery is identified, and the tumor-feeding vessels arising from it are coagulated, preserving the parent artery. Subsequent dissection of the tumor capsule from the cerebellum generally presents no serious difficulties. Before attempting to identify the vestibulocochlear nerve and facial nerve at the brain stem, the surgeon should enucleate and debulk the superior inferior portion of the tumor in order to expose the petrosal vein, the trigeminal nerve, and the angle between that nerve and the brain stem. The dissection should not be carried farther anteroinferiorly, because this would jeopardize the facial nerve. We apply two criteria in determining the salvageability of the vestibulocochlear nerve:

1) Preoperative auditory acuity.
2) Intraoperative morphologic findings.

If the ear has had no useful auditory acuity for some time (a period of months), and if the nerve is found to be markedly thinned out and discorored at operation, we do not consider it reasonable to attempt dissection of the vestibulocochlear nerve with the goal of achieving useful function. The operation can be greatly shortened in such cases by dividing the vestibulocochlear nerve close to the brain stem a sufficient distance from the tumor and then, having reduced the tension anterior to the tumor, identifying the facial nerve. On the other hand, if hearing has declined abruptly only a short time before the case comes to operation, and the surgeon finds no significant pathology of the vestibulocochlear nerve, every effort should be made to preserve it. With very meticulous dissection, we have seen a few instances of even improvement in preoperative auditory function. The rest of the dissection corresponds to the technique described for small tumors. Again, it is important for the surgeon to debulk the tumor from all sides as he works toward the site of maximum adhesion – usually between the facial nerve and tumor capsule just medial to the anterior lip of the porus.

It can occasionally be difficult to separate the tumor from the brain stem, especially when the brain stem is compressed, and this should not be attempted until the tumor bulk has been adequately reduced. At that point, final separation of the tumor from the brain stem involves nothing more than removing a thin layer of tumor capsule, which is carefully pulled laterally to expose the vessels communicating between the brain stem and capsule. (The high-power lens is used at this stage.) Vessels that pass into the tumor capsule are coagulated with bipolar forceps close to the capsule and divided with scissors. The vessels should not be torn, because very fine bleeders retracting into the brain stem can lead to severe neurologic deficits. With this technique, even tumors that are solidly fused to the brain stem can almost always be removed in toto with their capsule.

The suboccipital, total removal of a large acoustic neuroma is justified even in elderly patients, as the relatively mild stress of the operation relates very favorably to the radical extent of the removal (Fig. PS 22a–c).

With *cystic neuromas*, enucleation is easily and rapidly accomplished, but it can be difficult to develop a plane between the tumor capsule and

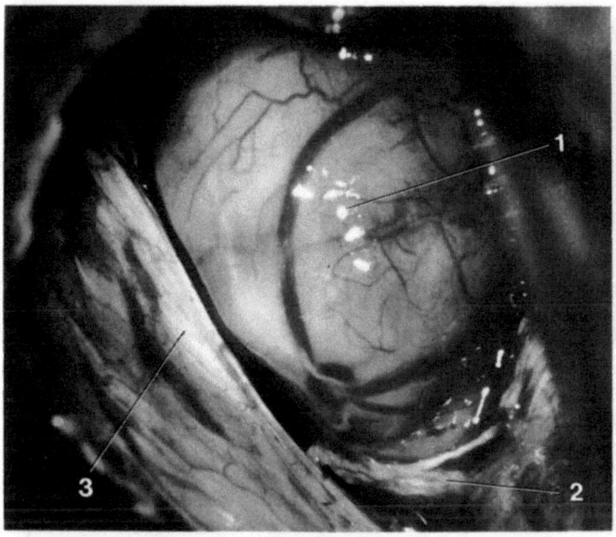

a

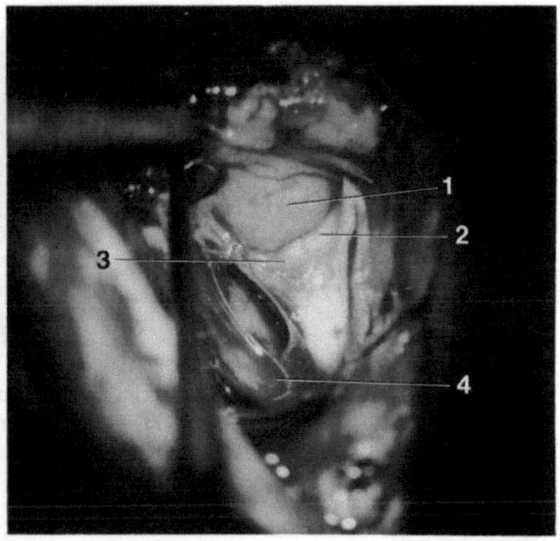

b

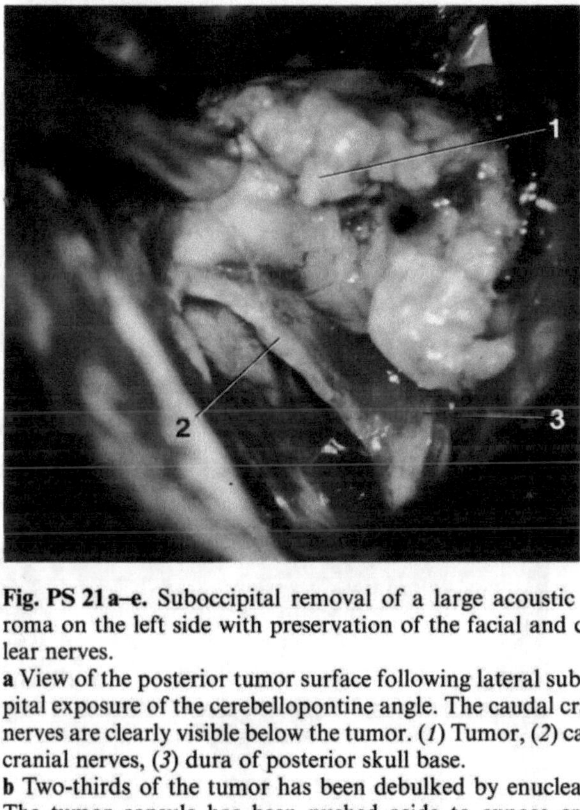

c

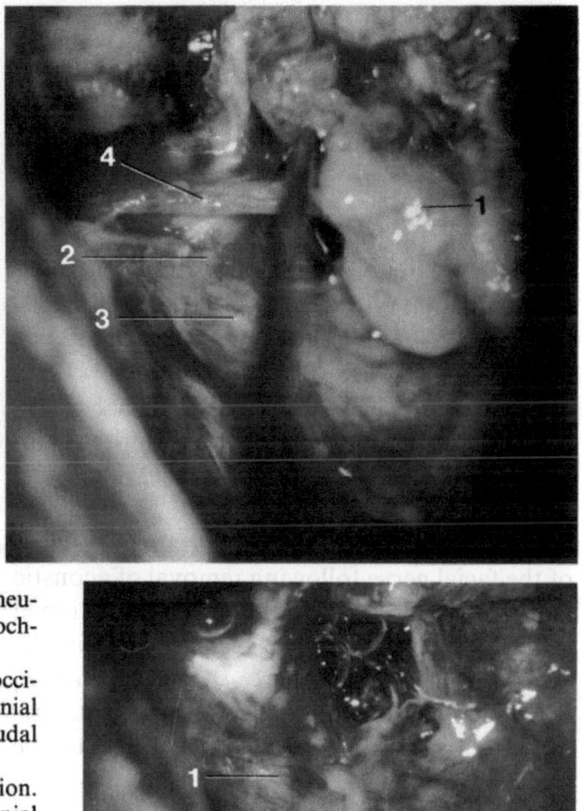

d

Fig. PS 21 a–e. Suboccipital removal of a large acoustic neuroma on the left side with preservation of the facial and cochlear nerves.

a View of the posterior tumor surface following lateral suboccipital exposure of the cerebellopontine angle. The caudal cranial nerves are clearly visible below the tumor. (*1*) Tumor, (*2*) caudal cranial nerves, (*3*) dura of posterior skull base.

b Two-thirds of the tumor has been debulked by enucleation. The tumor capsule has been pushed aside to expose cranial nerves VII and VIII as they exit the brain stem. (*1*) Tumor, (*2*) cranial nerve VII, (*3*) cranial nerve VIII, (*4*) arachnoid.

c The tumor is progressively separated from cranial nerve VIII (not vice-versa!). (*1*) Tumor, (*2*) cranial nerve VIII, (*3*) cranial nerve VII.

d View into the cerebellopontine angle and opened IAC. The site of tumor origin from the superior vestibular nerve is identified and resected with the capsule. (*1*) Tumor, (*2*) facial nerve, (*3*) cochlear nerve, (*4*) superior vestibular nerve.

e Status following complete tumor removal. The facial nerve, cochlear nerve and surrounding arachnoid have been preserved. (*1*) Facial nerve, (*2*) cochlear nerve

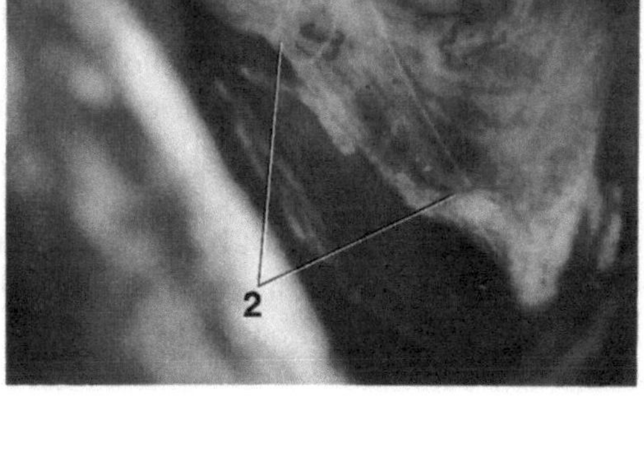

e

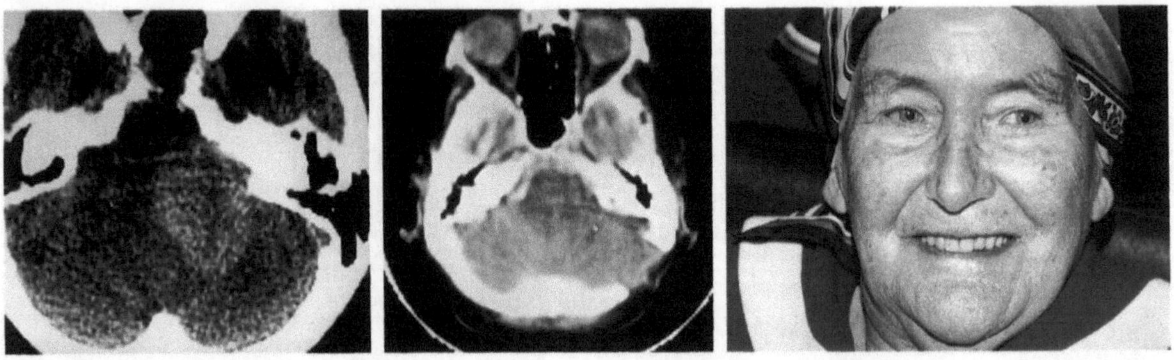

a, b c

Fig. PS 22a–c. Very large acoustic neuroma in a woman 84 years of age (!), preoperative and postoperative views.
a Preoperative CT scan shows a very large tumor displacing the brain stem.
b Postoperative CT scan.
c The patient 10 days after surgery

involved neural structures because of the intimate adhesions that usually form (Fig. PS 23a, b).

By applying the operative technique described, we have been able to preserve the anatomy and function of the *facial nerve* in approximately 90% of the cases. Careful, intraoperative electrical stimulation of the nerve can be done to confirm that it is intact functionally as well as anatomically.

If the neuroma has infiltrated the facial nerve, or in the rare cases where the tumor arises from that nerve, there is no way of preserving facial nerve continuity.

We feel it is important to ascertain the status of the facial nerve following removal of acoustic neuroma. If the facial nerve has been sectioned during surgery, it may be reconstructed in the same sitting or in an early second operation, depending on the extent of the nerve defect. Various techniques may be used according to the situation:

1) If the central and peripheral nerve stumps are identifiable in the cerebellopontine angle or internal auditory canal, can be sutured, and are of sufficient length, a primary end-to-end anastomosis may be performed (Malis 1977). If this cannot be done without tension, an interposition graft (usually from the sural nerve) should be used.

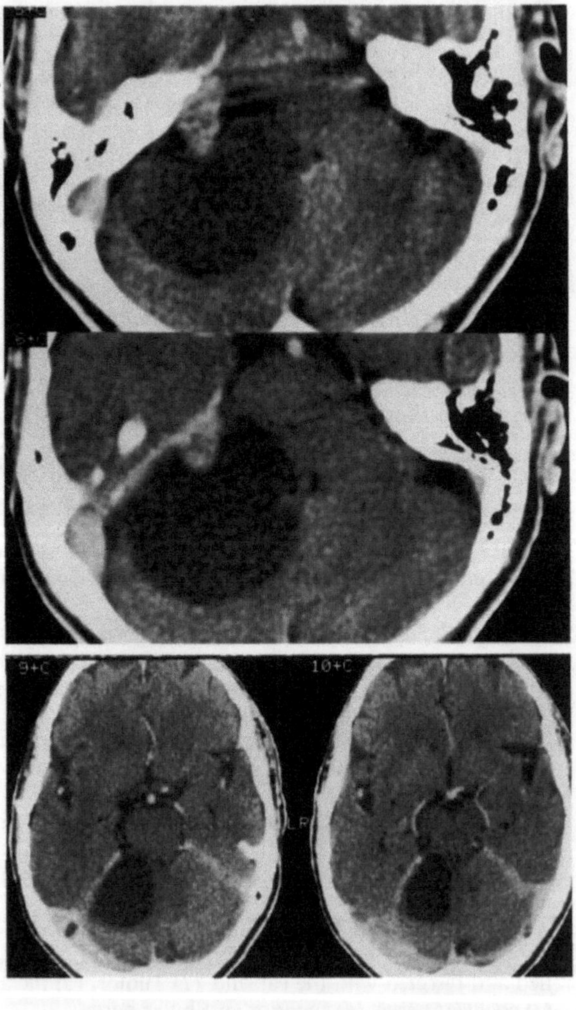

a

b

Fig. PS 23a, b. Neuroma of the cerebellopontine angle and IAC with an extremely large cyst before and after operative removal

2) If the central stump is present but the peripheral stump in the internal auditory canal is not usable, an intracranial-extratemporal anastomosis (Dott 1958) or an intracranial-intratemporal anastomosis (Samii 1979 may be performed in the same sitting (Fig. FN 7a, b, 8a, b).
3) If there is no usable central stump, a hypoglossal-facial anastomosis (Körte 1901), facio-facial anastomosis (Scaramella 1970/1971; Smith 1971), or a combination of both techniques (Stennert 1979) should be performed in a second operation at the earliest opportunity after removal of the acoustic neuroma.

Details on facial nerve reconstruction and rehabilitation are presented in Chapter 6 (see p. 473).

The possibility of *preserving cochlear nerve function* should be considered in the light of preoperative auditory function and the size of the neoplasm (Samii et al. 1985).

If we consider the total patient population, regardless of tumor size, we find that preoperative hearing could be preserved in about 28% of the cases using the operative technique outlined above. For tumors smaller than 3 cm, this percentage was approximately 40%. For tumors in the cerebellopontine angle larger than 3 cm, hearing could be salvaged in only 15% of the cases. Prognosis for preserving the hearing are most favorable in cases where the preoperative threshold of hearing at 2000 Hz is no less than 40–50 dB, and the discrimination is at least 50%. The total tumor size should not exceed 3 cm. When these criteria are met, hearing can be preserved in approximately 58% of the patients.

Bilateral acoustic neuromas account for 2%–3% of the cases. They differ from the typical unilateral tumor in several respects. Usually the diagnosis is greatly delayed. The preservation of cranial nerves VII and VIII is of major importance. Unfortunately, the technical problems posed by these neoplasms can be formidable. In contrast to unilateral neuromas, which develop from one aspect of the nerve sheath and displace surrounding neural structures, the neurofibromas in von Recklinghausen's disease result from an uncontrolled proliferation of Schwann's cells, connective tissue, and nerve tissue. They are lobulated and tend to envelop nerve fascicles or invade the interspaces between them. In addition, they manifest a multifocal occurrence in one or more nerves, which compounds the difficulty of complete removal. Even so, we have found it possible to preserve auditory function in 25%–30% of the cases and occasionally bilaterally (Fig. PS 24a–f). We prefer to remove the tumor first on the side that has the better hearing, as the chances for its preservation are more favorable.

In extremely rare cases *vascular compression of the trigeminal nerve may coexist with an acoustic neuroma* on the same or opposite side. This diagnosis should be considered when acoustic neuroma symptoms are accompanied by classic clinical features of trigeminal neuralgia. When the diseases are ipsilateral, operative treatment may consist of extirpation of the neuroma and vascular decompression of the trigeminal nerve in *one* sitting (Fig. PS 25a–d). If the vascular compression is contralateral to the neuroma, surgical treatment in separate stages is required.

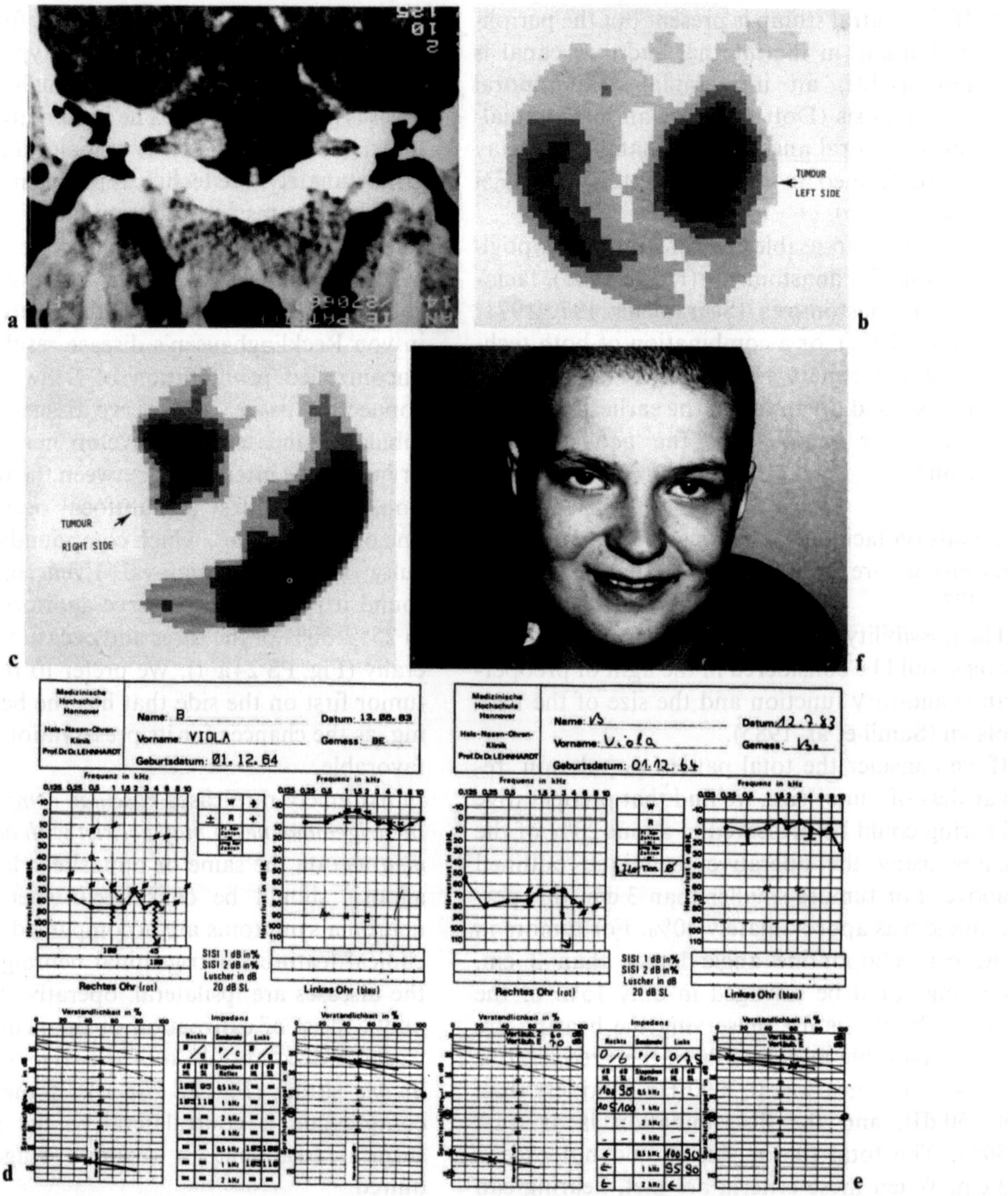

Fig. PS 24a–f. Bilateral acoustic neuromas in a 19-year-old female. Both tumors were completely removed with preservation of facial and auditory function.
a CT scan shows the larger tumor (2 cm in diameter) on the left, better hearing side and the smaller tumor on the right side, where hearing loss is severe.
b, c Appearance of the tumors on cochleomeatal scintigrams of the left and right sides.
d, e The pre- and postoperative audiograms are almost identical. The nearly normal hearing in the left ear was preserved.
f The patient several weeks after surgery, with normal facial nerve function

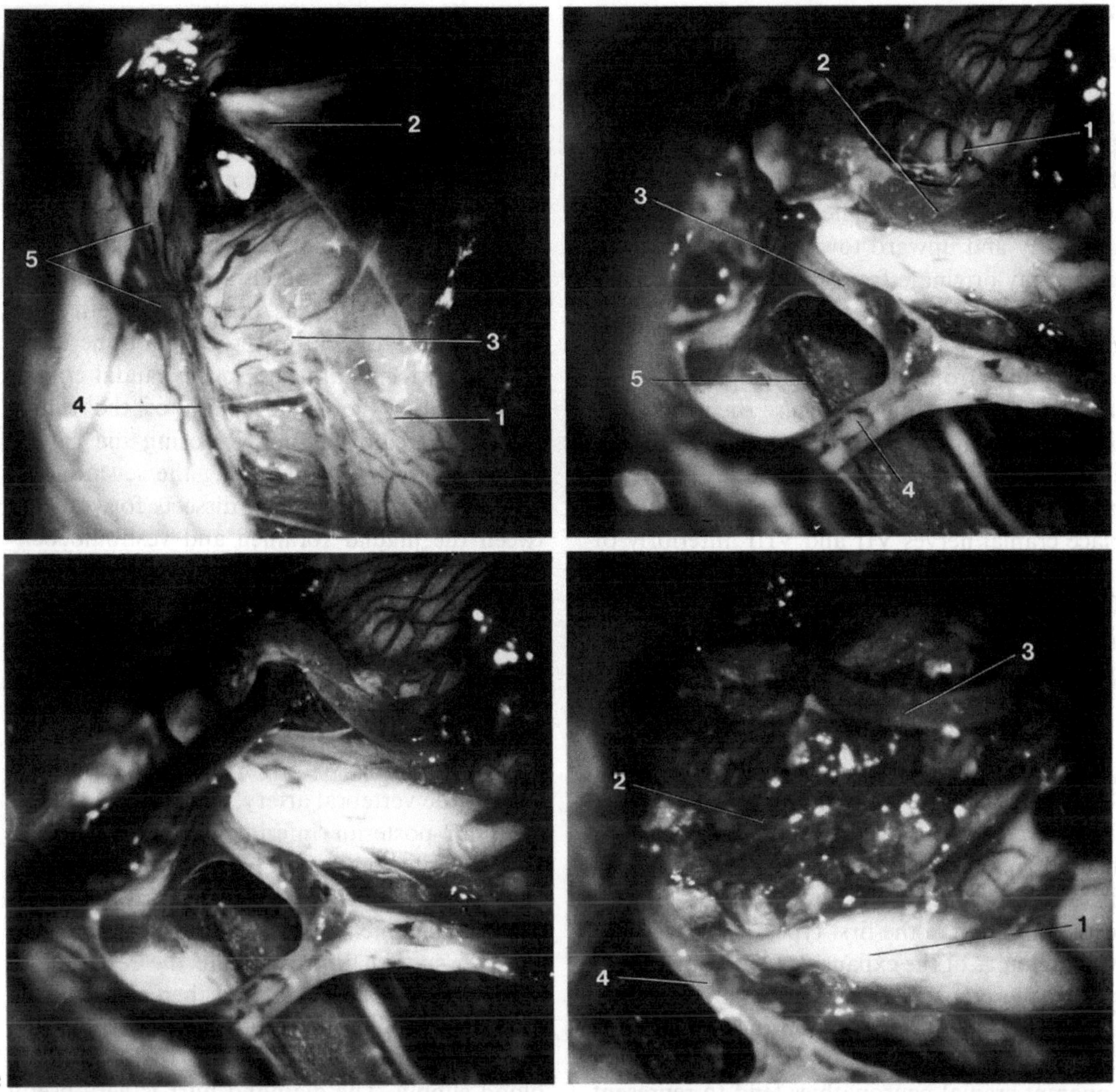

Fig. PS 25a–d. Acoustic neuroma on the right side combined with ipsilateral vascular compression of the trigeminal nerve. Four years before admission the patient experienced a rapid hearing loss followed later by recurring headaches and typical right-sided trigeminal neuralgia. CT demonstrated an acoustic neuroma on the right side. Operation disclosed a moderate-size acoustic neuroma having no direct contact with the trigeminal nerve, and compression of the trigeminal nerve by a branch of the superior cerebellar artery. The acoustic neuroma was removed and the trigeminal nerve decompressed in one operation. The patient experienced no further neuralgic symptoms following surgery. A moderate postoperative facial palsy regressed within a few weeks.
a The right cerebellopontine angle has been exposed through the lateral suboccipital approach, and the arachnoid-covered tumor is visualized. (*1*) Flocculus, (*2*) petrosal vein, (*3*) tumor, (*4*) porus of IAC, (*5*) pathologic dural vessels.
b The acoustic neuroma is completely removed along with its intrameatal extension. Compression of the trigeminal nerve by a branch of the superior cerebellar artery is apparent. The still-intact arachnoid over the trigeminal nerve indicates that the tumor has no direct contact with this nerve. (*1*) Brain stem, (*2*) superior cerebellar artery, (*3*) facial nerve, (*4*) cochlear nerve, (*5*) porus of IAC.
c The vascular loop impinging on the trigeminal nerve is elevated.
d Status at the end of the operation with a free muscle graft interposed between the trigeminal nerve and superior cerebellar artery. (*1*) Trigeminal nerve, (*2*) muscle graft, (*3*) superior cerebellar artery, (*4*) facial nerve

Meningiomas of the Cerebellopontine Angle

Introductory Remarks. These meningiomas may develop anterior or posterior to the internal auditory canal and may extend in the cranial or caudal direction. Meningiomas that extend far anteriorly and upward toward the tentorial incisure may originate from the dura of Meckel's cave, from the clivus, or from the tentorial margin. Tumors occurring behind the porus acusticus originate from the dura of the petrous bone to the jugular foramen. Because their direction of growth is highly variable, the relations of the cranial nerves and vascular structures to the tumor are extremely diverse. The tumor may displace cranial nerves VII and VIII anteriorly or posteriorly, depending on its site of origin. These structures also may traverse the center of the tumor in some instances. One of two types of tumor morphology can occur:

1) An expansive type that displaces surrounding structures as it grows.
2) An enplaque type that grows along neighboring structures and envelops them.

The second type requires a far more exacting dissection technique, but fortunately it is much less common than the first type.
Meningiomas of the expansive type displace and stretch the cranial nerves much the same way that acoustic neuromas do, but they are less apt to form adhesions with them. Thus, clinically apparent cranial neuropathies tend to represent functional, neurapraxic disorders rather than permanent pathoanatomic changes, and good functional recovery – even of the vestibulocochlear nerve – is the rule following tumor removal. So the question of facial and vestibulocochlear nerve preservation is not a problem issue with these neoplasms. We have seen patients with profound preoperative hearing loss experience an almost complete recovery of hearing following the removal of the meningioma.

Operative Technique

The lateral suboccipital approach using microsurgical technique has dramatically improved outcomes in terms of mortality as well as morbidity. The foremost dissection technique consists of piecemeal tumor removal, relying heavily on the use of bipolar cautery. Tumor emulsification with the Caviton ultrasonic surgical aspirator (CUSA) also has proven very effective. If tumor fills the entire cerebellopontine angle from the trigeminal nerve to the caudal cranial nerve group, the lateral parts of the tumor should be removed first, exposing the caudal cranial nerves. After exposing the seventh and eighth nerves, the surgeon dissects forward between the jugular foramen and vestibulocochlear nerve and between the facial nerve and trigeminal nerve to remove the anterior portions of the tumor. Care is taken that the cranial nerves, which form the access sites for the dissection, are not traumatized by the instruments, especially the bipolar forceps. Of course special attention is also given to the vascular structures, such as the vertebral artery, basilar artery, anterior and posterior inferior cerebellar arteries, and superior cerebellar artery, which may be encased in tumor. When removing the area of tumor attachment on the bony skull base, the surgeon should first coagulate the residual tumor with bipolar current and then circumscribe it with a knife to separate it from the bone. It is not unusual for this area to have a rich blood supply. The diamond burr is very useful in this, for it not only ensures the complete removal of meningioma that has infiltrated the bone but also provides effective hemostasis. Separation of the tumor capsule from the brain stem employs the same technique as for acoustic neuroma but generally is more easily accomplished.

Case Presentations

Case Report. Meningioma of the left cerebellopontine angle arising from the tentorium (Fig. PS 26a, b). A 44-year-old woman complained for months of increasing, menses-relat-

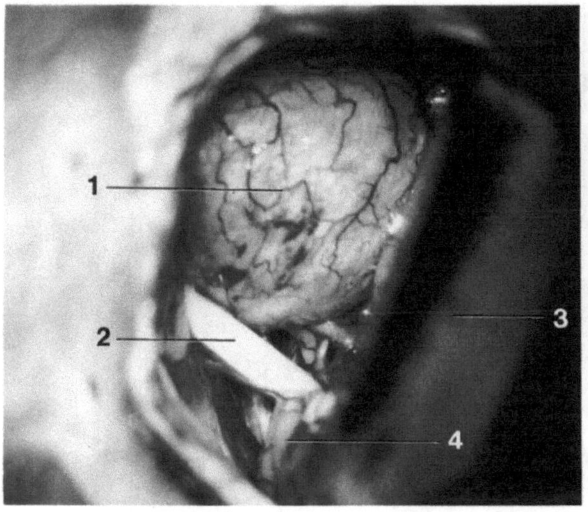

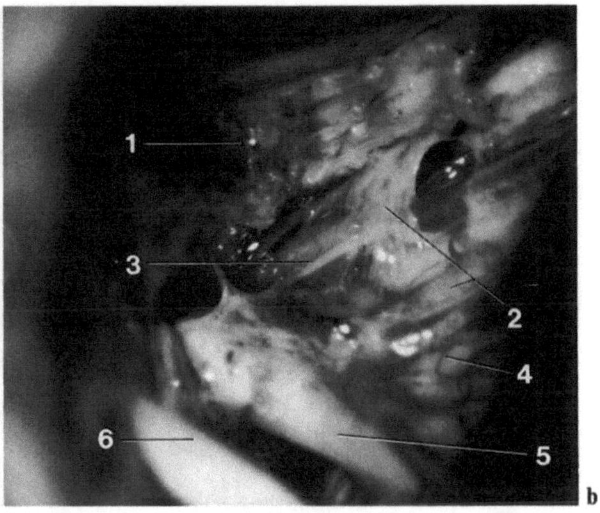

Fig. PS 26 a, b. Meningioma of the left cerebellopontine angle originating from the tentorium.
a Status following lateral suboccipital exposure of the cerebellopontine angle. The smooth, globular tumor occupies the space between the tentorium above, the brain stem medially, nerves VII and VIII below, and the posterior surface of the pyramid. The trigeminal nerve and trochlear nerve are covered by the tumor. (*1*) Tumor, (*2*) cranial nerves VII and VIII, (*3*) brain spatula, (*4*) flocculus.
b Status following tumor removal. The tentorial attachment of the tumor is coagulated before the tumor is removed. The major neurovascular structures of the cerebellopontine angle are exposed. (*1*) Tumor attachment on tentorium, (*2*) branches of superior cerebellar artery, (*3*) trochlear nerve, (*4*) brain stem, (*5*) trigeminal nerve, (*6*) cranial nerves VII and VIII

ed pain in the left mastoid area and migraine-like headaches and facial pain also on the left side. A neurologic examination showed no definite signs of cranial neuropathy. CT scan demonstrated a large mass lesion in the posterior cranial fossa riding on a large area of the petrous pyramid. Examination by an otorhinolaryngologist revealed normal hearing and vestibular findings. Under a presumptive diagnosis of posterior fossa meningioma, the cerebellopontine angle was exposed through the lateral suboccipital approach. A meningioma approximately 1.5 × 2.5 cm in size was found anterior to cranial nerves VII and VIII. It extended to the tentorium and had caused marked compression of the trigeminal nerve. Using microsurgical technique, we were able to reduce the tumor bulk piecemeal and dissect it free from the surrounding nerves. The tumor origin was on the tentorium, so a half-dollar-size area (about 2.5 cm diameter) of the tentorium was included in the resection to ensure a radical excision. The postoperative course was uncomplicated. Hearing and other cranial nerve functions were normal, as before surgery.

Comments: A meningioma arising from the tentorium and extending into the cerebellopontine angle between cranial nerves V and VII/VIII and the brain stem was microsurgically removed with preservation of cranial nerve functions.

Case Report. Meningioma of the right cerebellopontine angle and fourth ventricle (Fig. PS 27 a–d). The 35-year-old patient had a 7-month history of imbalance that began after he sustained a muscle tear in the right thigh. The imbalance was not accompanied by hearing loss or tinnitus. Vestibular testing showed a spontaneous positional nystagmus to the right, and electronystagmography showed a brisk response with a slight left-sided predominance. Tone and speech perception were normal. Evoked potential audiometry showed a prolonged P_6 latency

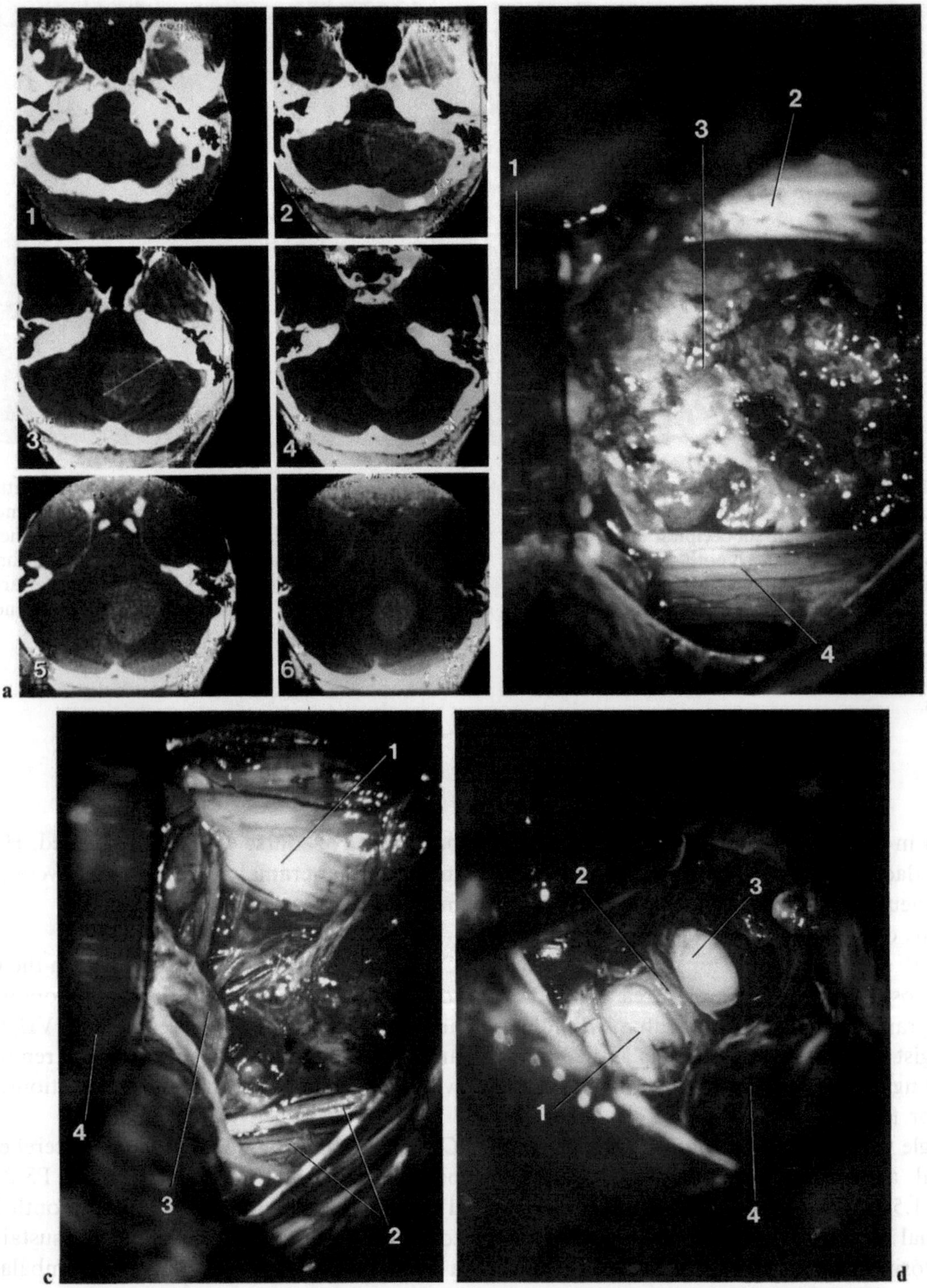
1
2
3
4
5
6
a
1
2
3
4
b
1
2
3
4
c
1
2
3
4
d

on the right side. The tentative diagnosis of a posterior cranial fossa tumor was confirmed by CT scans, which delineated a 4-cm mass in the right posterior fossa that extended across the midline from the posterior surface of the petrous bone and completely filled the fourth ventricle. The tumor was exposed through a lateral suboccipital craniectomy. It completely occupied the cerebellopontine angle, displacing the facial and vestibulocochlear nerves forward and upward and the caudal cranial nerves downward. The tumor had led to atrophy of the right cerebellum and was covered only by a thin sheet of cerebellar tissue. This was incised, the tumor was debulked piecemeal, and the capsule was progressively dissected from surrounding structures, to which it had become adherent. The lesion was heavily vascularized and appeared to derive its major supply from the anterior inferior cerebellar artery. The feeding arteries were coagulated and divided. The caudal cranial nerves were very firmly adherent to the tumor capsule between the blood vessels, but we were able to preserve them while removing the capsule. The tumor had invaded the fourth ventricle through its lateral wall and extended to the aqueduct, mimicking a plexus papilloma. We finally succeeded in removing the tumor completely while preserving all the nerves of the cerebellopontine angle and the blood vessels transversing it. The fourth ventricle remained widely open laterally. The wound was closed in standard fashion. Histology identified the lesion as a fibroblastic meningioma.

The postoperative course was uneventful, and after 10 days the patient was discharged in excellent condition. By that time his vertiginous complaints had improved considerably.

Comments: This case involved a rare meningioma arising from the fourth ventricle. It had filled the entire fourth ventricle to the aqueduct and had then grown laterally through the ventricle wall and foramen of Luschka into the cerebellopontine angle, extending to the posterior surface of the petrous pyramid. Neuroradiologic studies did not provide a definitive diagnosis because of the localization and extent of the lesion. Plexus papilloma was considered in addition to meningioma because of the ventricular involvement. Lack of involvement of the posterior fossa dura was consistent with a diagnosis of primary intraventricular meningioma.

Fig. PS 27a–d. Meningioma of the right cerebellopontine angle and fourth ventricle.
a *(1–6)* Mass lesion of the right posterior cranial fossa 4 cm in diameter extending across the midline from the posterior surface of the petrous pyramid and completely filling the fourth ventricle.
b The tumor is exposed in the cerebellopontine angle between the trigeminal nerve above and the vestibulocochlear and facial nerves below. (*1*) Spatula, (*2*) trigeminal nerve, (*3*) tumor, (*4*) cranial nerves VII and VIII.
c The cerebellopontine angle has been cleared of tumor, permitting identification of cranial nerves VII and VIII, the anterior inferior cerebellar artery, and the caudal cranial nerve group. (*1*) Cranial nerves VII and VIII, (*2*) caudal cranial nerves, (*3*) anterior inferior cerebellar artery, (*4*) brain spatula.
d The intraventricular tumor component has been removed from the fourth ventricle. This picture shows a view from the right lateral aspect through the enlarged foramen of Luschka onto the floor and opposite lateral wall of the fourth ventricle. (*1*) Floor of fourth ventricle, (*2*) loop of posterior inferior cerebellar artery, (*3*) cerebral aqueduct, (*4*) cerebellum

Epidermoid Tumor of the Cerebellopontine Angle

Introductory Remarks. Epidermoids are true neoplasms, generally of embryologic origin, that arise from heterotopic germ cells. In otorhinolaryngology these lesions are known as true cholesteatomas.

Epidermoids are the third most common tumor type in this region. Initial symptoms are nonspecific. Some patients experience classic trigeminal neuralgic attacks or a constant trigeminal pain. Others seek medical help because of vestibulocochlear symptoms. Early CT scans show a low-density cystic mass with irregular margins in the cerebellopontine angle. In many cases densitometry at this stage is sufficient to provide a preoperative diagnosis. Symptoms usually remain subtle for quite some time, even when the tumor is large. Occasionally the disease becomes bilateral by spreading from the pons to the contralat-

eral side or by invading the third ventricle through the foramen of Luschka.
Epidermoids (true cholesteatomas) are different from the "false" cholesteatomas of the otorhinolaryngologist. Epidermoids can originate in the cerebellopontine angle, whereas false cholesteatomas may gradually invade the middle or posterior cranial fossa over a period of years or decades by way of the middle ear and petrous bone. The latter should be removed in a combined otosurgical-neurosurgical operation. Even when the middle and inner ear have been cleared of disease, trauma or inflammation can occasionally lead to a recurrence of cholesteatoma in the middle or posterior cranial fossa.

Operative Technique
(Fig. PS 28 a–d)

As for neuromas and meningiomas, the cerebellopontine angle is exposed through the lateral suboccipital approach. The lesion presents as a soft, pearly, globular mass with irregular borders. The tumor capsule is usually very thin and adherent to the arachnoid at multiple sites; it is removed in large pieces. The strategy is to clear one region of tumor completely before moving to the next region so that small remnants of capsule will not be left behind. An effective technique is to open the capsule and debulk the tumor first, so that the matrix can be atraumatically separated from the surrounding neurovascular structures under optimum vision. As a final step, all the corners of the cerebellopontine angle should be carefully inspected, and the surgical cavity should be irrigated to ensure removal of residual tumor cells, for even tiny remnants of epithelium or matrix can incite a recurrence. It is possible through microsurgical technique to normalize functional hearing losses that were caused by tumor compression.

Case Presentations

Case Report. (F. K.) Epidermoid of the left cerebellopontine angle (Fig. PS 28 a–d). Ten years before he was hospitalized, the patient noticed a gradually progressive hearing loss. For the past 3 years he had also experienced unsteadiness of gait. A thorough diagnostic workup performed 10 years after symptom onset showed a significant hearing loss in the left ear, decreased excitability of the left peripheral vestibular apparatus, and mild facial weakness. There was marked expansion of the left internal auditory canal in the plain skull X-ray films. CT scans showed a 5-cm mass in the left cerebellopontine angle causing compression of the fourth ventricle. Examination just prior to surgery disclosed facial weakness, severe hearing loss in the left ear, slight sway in the Romberg test with no directional predominance, deviation of the gait to the left during blind walking, a large-amplitude nystagmus on left gaze, a small-amplitude component on right gaze, and vertical nystagmus on upward gaze. There was no evidence of caudal cranial neuropathy, the soft palate was in place, and pharyngeal sensitivity was equivalent on both sides.
The cerebellopontine angle was exposed through the lateral suboccipital approach. The cerebellum was elevated and the cisterna magna was opened, exposing a large epidermoid. The tumor extended superiorly to the tentorium and inferiorly to the foramen magnum. The caudal cranial nerves were adherent to the tumor cap-

→

Fig. PS 28 a–d. Large epidermoid of the left cerebellopontine angle. Hearing improved following total removal of the lesion.
a The cerebellopontine angle was exposed through the lateral suboccipital approach, uncovering a pearly, globular tumor causing elevation of the caudal cranial nerves and of nerves VII and VIII passing into the porus acusticus. (*1*) Vestibulocochlear nerve and facial nerve, (*2*) caudal cranial nerves, (*3*) tumor.
b The tumor has been partially removed. Essential microanatomic details of the cerebellopontine angle can be appreciated. (*1*) Cranial nerves VII and VIII, (*2*) abducens nerve, (*3*) brain stem vessels, (*4*) residual tumor at brain stem.
c View into the cerebellopontine angle following complete tumor removal. (*1*) Porus acusticus, (*2*) cranial nerves VII and VIII, (*3*) pons.
d Pre- and postoperative audiograms. The drop at higher frequencies caused by tumor compression is no longer apparent after surgery

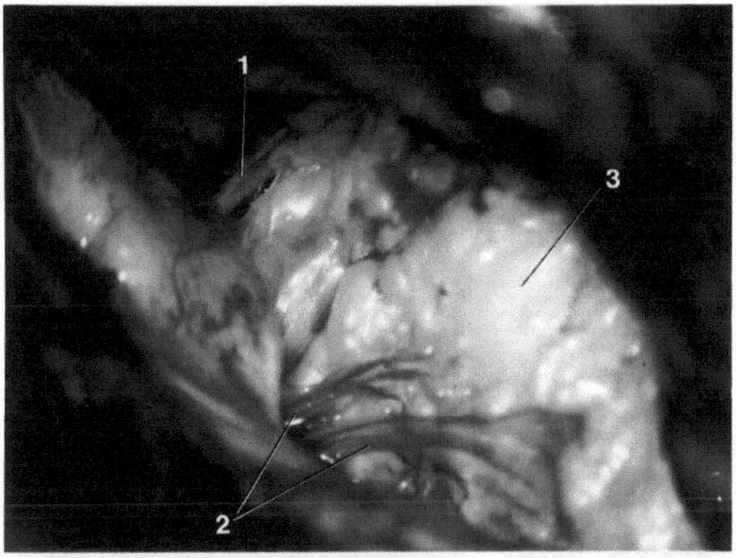

a

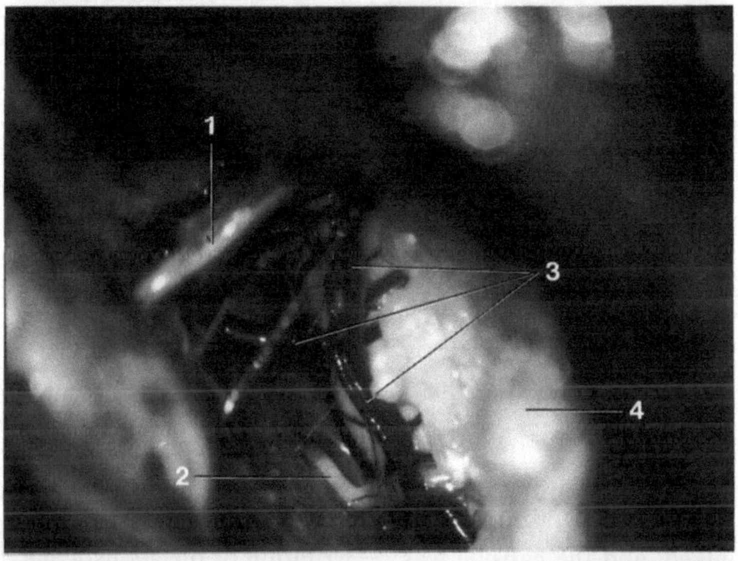

b

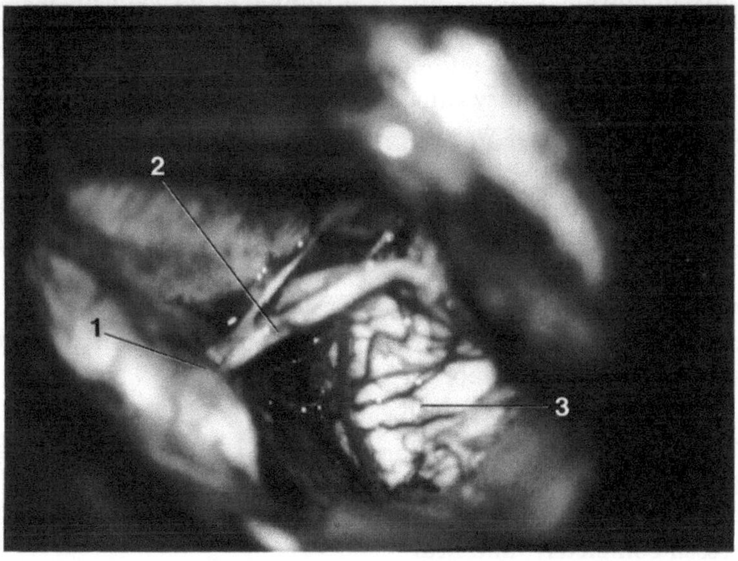

c

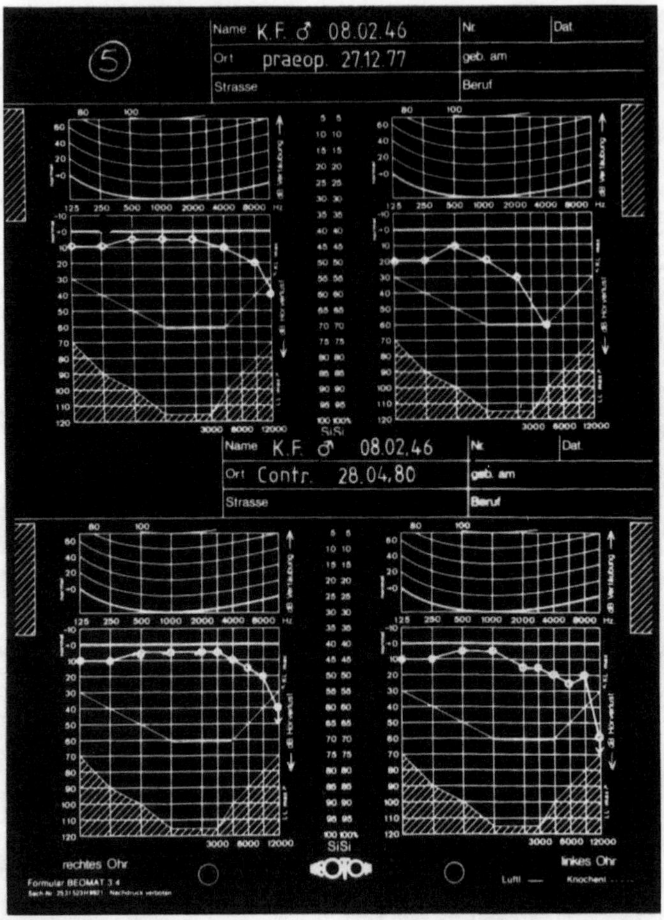

Fig. PS 28d

sule. The tumor extended laterally into the internal auditory canal. First the lateral portions of the tumor were debulked, and the capsule was separated from the caudal cranial nerves. We were then able to identify the facial and vestibulocochlear nerves in the internal auditory canal and dissect the tumor from them. This was followed by progressive debulking of the main tumor mass. The pons was greatly compressed. The matrix was separated at that site and progressively followed to the medulla oblongata, dissecting it away from the anterior inferior cerebellar artery. To remove the medial part of the tumor, it was necessary to resect the cerebellar tonsil and open the lateral wall of the fourth ventricle. Finally we were able to effect a complete removal. The postoperative course was uncomplicated. Within a few months after surgery the facial palsy regressed completely, and hearing returned almost to normal (!). Apparently the hearing loss resulted from simple functional irritation of the acoustic nerves by the tumor.

Comments: This case illustrates the insidious nature of epidermoid symptoms, the difficulty of mobilizing the tumor capsule, and the potential for hearing improvement following the removal of cerebellopontine angle tumors causing simple compressive nerve irritation when atraumatic microsurgical dissection is used. The duration of hearing impairment appears to have little bearing on the potential for recovery.

Other Cerebellopontine Angle Tumors

Introductory Remarks. In principle, any type of space-occupying lesion can occur in the cerebellopontine angle. The diagnosis of cerebellopontine angle lesions has benefitted greatly in recent years from radiologic procedures such as high-resolution CT, MRI, and superselective angiography. Even so, it is not possible to make a definitive preoperative diagnosis in all cases. The spectrum of space-occupying lesions in this area includes neuromas arising from other cranial nerves (trigeminal, facial, glossopharyngeal, etc.), angiomas, aneurysms, ependymomas, plexus papillomas, spongioblastomas, medulloblastomas, chordomas, chondromas, arachnoidal cysts, and recurrences of tumors that were removed from the outer skull base but have penetrated into the cerebellopontine angle (e.g., glomus tumors). Metastases from various primary malignancies also can occur in the cerebellopontine angle. Diagnosis in these cases relies heavily on accurate history taking and a thorough clinical evaluation.

The principles of operative treatment are the same as for the tumor types previously discussed.

Functionally important structures may be sacrificed to accomplish a total removal, but this should be considered only if the prognosis is favorable.

Case Presentations

Case Report. Arteriovenous angioma in the internal auditory canal (Fig. PS 29a–f). An otherwise healthy woman 50 years of age experienced a sudden gait disturbance in the summer of 1981 with imbalance and intermittent vertigo, prompting consultation with an ENT physician. She also had neck pain radiating to the right postauricular region and right facial muscle weakness with disturbed taste sensation on the right half of the tongue. The symptoms remitted in about 10 weeks. In February of 1982 the patient again experienced imbalance, vertigo without nausea, and a ringing tinnitus in the right ear of varying intensity. This was accompanied by a slight hearing loss in the right ear, a furry sensation on the right side of the face, and pain in the right eye.

Initial examination on March 1, 1982, disclosed a slight hypesthesia of the right facial half with an obtunded corneal reflex and very slight facial nerve palsy on the right side with reduced voluntary activity in the electromyogram and abnormal regeneration potentials. Otoscopic and laryngoscopic findings were normal. The stimulated reflex response of the facial muscles was markedly prolonged on the right side. Taste sensation on the right half of the tongue was diminished. Cranial nerves VI, IX, X, and XII functioned normally. In the ensuing weeks an increasing sensorineural hearing loss developed in the right ear. Brain stem audiometry showed a slightly prolonged P_5 latency. Vestibular testing showed a small-amplitude spontaneous nystagmus beating to the left, a nonlocalizing gaze nystagmus, a localizing positional nystagmus, and no caloric response of the right labyrinth with a concurrent disturbance of the vestibulospinal responses and of slow eye tracking. Overall, the combination of a peripheral and central vestibular disorder together with the hearing deficit and prolonged auditory brain stem response was consistent with a diagnosis of acoustic neuroma. However, CT examination before and after i.v. contrast enhancement showed no evidence of disease in the posterior fossa. Therefore, computed pneumocisternography was performed in March of 1982 to establish a diagnosis. The right internal auditory canal was slightly expanded and contained a smooth-bordered mass that projected several millimeters from the porus into the cerebellopontine cistern. A right intrameatal tumor was diagnosed. The internal auditory canal was approached transtemporally and the meatal dura was incised, exposing a pulsating mass that had displaced the facial nerve and the eighth cranial nerve group anteriorly downward. As the vascular supply of the mass could not be visualized, the operation was discontinued, and the patient was referred to us for a lateral suboccipital exposure – the only approach that would enable the vascular connections of the lesion to be eval-

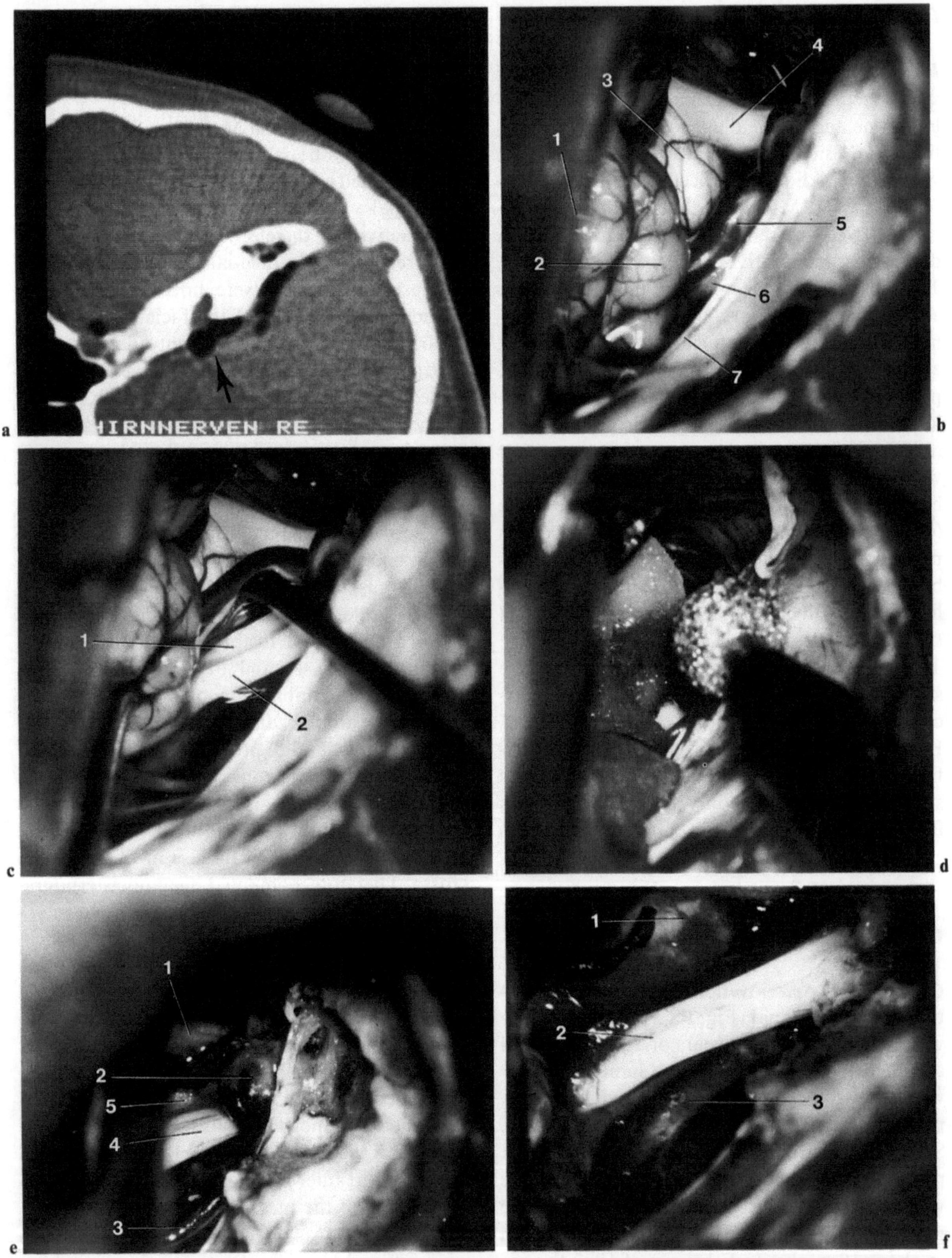
HIRNNERVEN RE.
a
3
4
1
5
2
6
7
b
1
2
c
d
1
2
5
4
3
e
1
2
3
f

uated. Following lateral suboccipital exposure of the cerebellopontine angle, we identified cranial nerves VII and VIII, and we could see the dome of the vascular malformation protruding from the auditory canal. We also saw a relatively large-caliber pathologic vessel entering the lesion and compressing cranial nerves VII and VIII from above. A branch of the inferior cerebellar artery also entered the lesion from the caudal side. To improve exposure, it was necessary to drill open the posterior wall of the internal auditory canal with the diamond burr. Multiple adhesions were present between the vascular malformation and the meatal dura. We coagulated the branch of the anterior inferior cerebellar artery supplying the tumor from below and also the pathologic vessel (carrying mixed blood) entering the lesion above the facial and vestibular nerves. Then we carefully separated the intrameatal vascular dysplasia from the fascicles of cranial nerves VII and VIII and removed it.

The patient complained of severe, unremitting vertigo shortly after surgery. Subtotal facial paralysis with incomplete lid closure persisted initially despite the microsurgical dissection and preservation of the nerve fascicles but improved within three weeks until only a slight residual palsy of the oral branch remained. Deafness in the right ear could not be avoided; this may be related to an atypical blood supply of the cochlear nerve. The vertiginous symptoms gradually regressed. Several months postoperatively facial function was normal except for a slight synkinesis.

Comments: An arteriovenous malformation of the internal auditory canal mimicking an intrameatal acoustic neuroma was removed through the suboccipital approach, which gives the best and safest exposure of the vessels supplying the lesion. Preservation of function of the cranial nerves VII and VIII is difficult, because they may have an atypical blood supply (Penkert 1985).

Case Report. Metastatic clear-cell adenocarcinoma in the right cerebellopontine angle (Fig. PS 30a, b). Slightly more than one year before his operation, the patient complained of tinnitus and increasing hearing impairment in the right ear. The hearing loss did not respond to infusion therapy. Seven months later an increasing right facial weakness supervened that was more pronounced around the mouth. Next the patient developed vertigo with hypoexcitability of the right labyrinth and nystagmus elicited by head shaking. Audiometric tests two months later showed complete deafness in the right ear. CT scans were ordered at this point and showed multiple low-density foci in the right cerebral hemisphere and a mass lesion in the right cerebellopontine angle with impending brain stem compression. Metastatic growths and von Recklinghausen's neurofibromatosis were considered in differential diagnosis. The patient was referred to us for further evaluation and for removal of the mass in the cerebellopontine angle. A comprehensive, preoperative internal examination showed no evidence of a primary tumor. The right cerebellopontine angle was exposed in standard fashion through a lateral suboccipital craniotomy. A reddish, cauliflower-like growth was found in the cerebellopontine angle and was dissected free from the anterior inferior cerebellar artery and cranial nerves VII and VIII. On opening the internal auditory canal, it was found that the tumor had reached the

Fig. PS 29a–f. Angiomatous malformation of the IAC in a woman 50 years of age (Penkert et al. 1985).
a Computed pneumocisternogram of the right cerebellopontine angle (after lumbar injection of 2 ml air) shows a mass lesion in the IAC presenting a smooth interface with the air bubble in the cistern.
b Intraoperative view of the right cerebellopontine angle. (*1*) Spatula, (*2*) flocculus, (*3*) pons, (*4*) trigeminal nerve, (*5*) angioma, (*6*) vestibulocochlear nerve, (*7*) dural margin.
c Venous drainage has been interrupted. (*1*) Facial nerve, (*2*) vestibulocochlear nerve.
d Status following excision of the petrosal dura and initial opening of the IAC with the diamond burr.
e Opening of the IAC has been completed. (*1*) Trigeminal nerve, (*2*) angioma, (*3*) feeding artery, (*4*) vestibulocochlear nerve, (*5*) draining vein.
f Status after coagulation of the feeding and draining vessels and removal of the arteriovenous angioma. (*1*) Trigeminal nerve, (*2*) vestibulocochlear nerve, (*3*) anterior inferior cerebellar artery

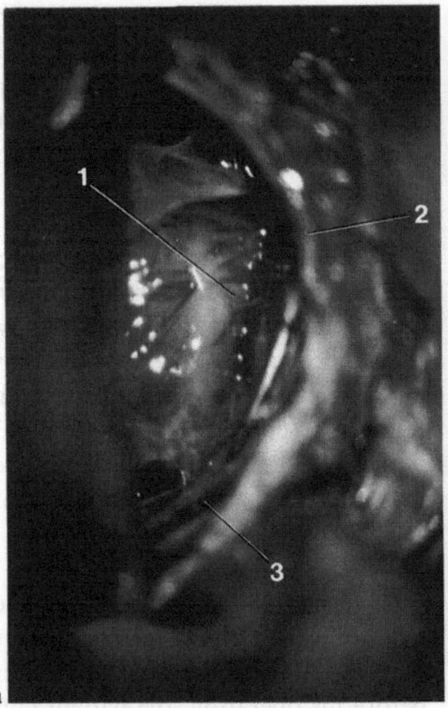

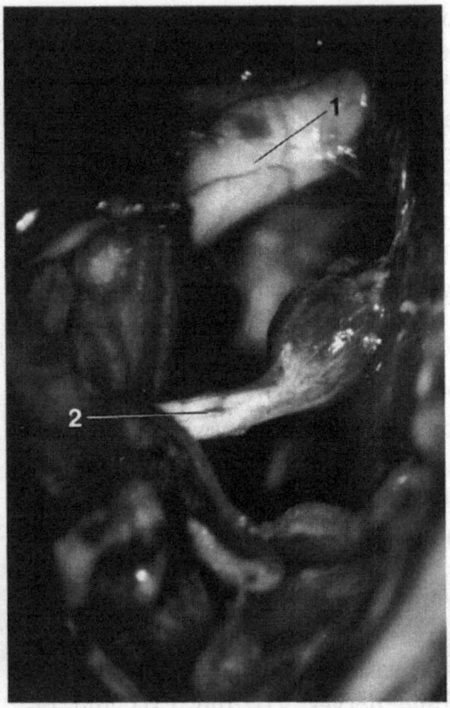

Fig. PS 30 a, b. Multifocal mass lesions in the right cerebral hemisphere and right cerebellopontine angle in a man 55 years of age. Differential diagnosis: malignant metastases or Von Recklinghausen's disease (neurofibromatosis). Though a primary tumor could not be found initially, histology confirmed metastatic adenocarcinoma.

a Exposure of the right cerebellopontine angle through the lateral suboccipital route. (*1*) Tumor, (*2*) porus acusticus, (*3*) caudal cranial nerves.
b Most of the tumor has been removed, and there is obvious infiltration of the facial nerve in the porus. Frozen section revealed adenocarcinoma, so the nerve was not reconstructed. (*1*) Trigeminal nerve, (*2*) facial nerve

fundus. As the tumor was debulked, it became apparent that the facial and vestibulocochlear nerves were completely infiltrated and no longer contained normal fascicles. These nerves were transected at the brain stem, and thc tumor was completely removed down to the fundus. Frozen-section examination disclosed metastatic adenocarcinoma, so nerve grafting was not performed in view of the multiple metastatic processes.

Comments: This case involved a metastatic adenocarcinoma in the cerebellopontine angle from an unknown primary tumor. The multiple intracranial masses were consistent with von Recklinghausen's disease. The nature of the disease was established by lateral suboccipital exploration.

References

Apfelbaum RI (1977) A comparison of gerrutaneous radiofrequency trigeminal neurolysis and microvascular decompression of the trigeminal nerve for the treatment of tic douloureux. Neurosurgery 1:16–21
Ballance CA (1894) Cited in Glasscock (1968)
Ballance CA (1907) Some points in the surgery of the brain and its membranes. Macmillan, London
Borchardt M (1905) Zur Operation der Tumoren des Kleinhirnbrückenwinkels. Berl Klin Wschr 42: 1033–1035
Bornemann H, Hundeshagen H, Franke KD (1982) Digitale Szintigraphie des Mittel- und Innenohres. Radioaktive Isotope. Klin Forsch 15:403
Bornemann H, Franke KD, Bornemann C, Hundeshagen H (1983) Die Bedeutung der cochleomeatalen Szintigraphie zur Diagnostik des Akustikusneurinomes. Arch Otorhinolaryngol Suppl 1983/II, p 314–316
Campbell E, Keedy C (1947) Hemifacial spasm: a note on the etiology in two cases. J Neurosurg 4:342–347

Celis-Blaubach A (1973) La boucle vasculaire du conduit auditif interne. Ann Otolaryngol 90:717–722
Chavanne F, Troullieur (1905) De la section intra-cranienne du nerf auditif. Bulletins et Memoires de la Société Française d'Otologie et de Laryngeologie. Tome XXI, Maloine Edit, Paris
Choudard CH (1972) Recherche sur l'organisation intraaxiale des formations motrices et parasympathiques du nerf facial. These Med Paris 264:93 (III)
Cohen N (1979) Acoustic neuroma surgery with emphasis on preservation of hearing. Laryngoscope 89:886–896
Cohen NL, Ransohoff J (1981) Preservation of hearing in acoustic neurinoma surgery. In: Samii M, Jannetta PJ (eds) The cranial nerves. Springer, Berlin Heidelberg New York, p 561–568
Cushing H (1917) Tumors of the nervus acusticus and the syndrome of the cerebellopontine angle. WB Saunders Philadelphia London
Dandy WE (1922) An operation for the total exstirpation of tumors of the cerebellopontine angle: a preliminary report. Bull Hopkins Hosp 33:344–345
Dandy WE (1925) An operation for the total removal of cerebellopontine (acoustic) tumors. Surg Gynecol Obstet 41:129–148
Dandy WE (1934) Concerning the cause of trigeminal neuralgia. Am J Surg 24:447–455
Dandy WE (1941) Results of removal of acoustic tumors by the unilateral approach. Arch Surg 42:1026–1033
Debrun G (1982) Treatment of certain intracerebral vascular lesions with balloon catheters. In: Schmideck HH, Sweet WH (eds) Operative neurosurgical techniques, vol 2. Grune & Stratton, New York, p 789
Di Tullio MV Jr, Malkasian D, Rand RW (1978) A critical comparison of neurosurgical and otolaryngological approaches to acoustic neuromas. J Neurosurg 48:1–12
Dott NM (1958) Facialis paralysis-restitution by extrapetrous nerve graft. Proc Roy Soc Med 51:900–902
Fisch U (1970) Transtemporal surgery of the internal auditory canal. Adv Otorhinolaryngol 17:203–240
Fisch U (1976) Chirurgie im inneren Gehörgang und an benachbarten Strukturen. In: Naumann HH (ed) Kopf- und Hals-Chirurgie Bd 3, S 457–543
Fisch U (1978) Otochirurgische Behandlung des Akustikusneurinoms. In: Plester D, Wende S, Nakayama N (eds) Kleinhirnbrückenwinkeltumoren. Springer, Berlin Heidelberg New York
Freckmann N, Nagenah R, Hermann HD, Müller D (1981) Treatment of neurogenic torticollis by microvascular lysis of the accessory nerve roots – indication, technique and first results. Acta Neurochirurgica 59:167–175
Gardner WJ (1962) Concerning the mechanism of trigeminal neuralgia and hemifacial spasm. J Neurosurg 19:947–957
Gardner WJ, Miklos MV (1959) Response of trigeminal neuralgia to "decompression" of the sensory root. J Am Med Ass (JAMA) 170:1773–1776
Glasscock ME (1968) History of the diagnosis and treatment of acoustic neuroma. Arch Otolaryng 88:578
Glasscock ME, Hays JW, Miller GW, Drake FD, Kanok MM (1978) Preservation of hearing in tumors of the internal auditory canal and cerebellopontine angle. Laryngoscope 88:43–55
Helms J (1978) Zur chirurgischen Anatomie des Felsenbeines. In: Plester D, Wende S, Nakayama N (eds) Kleinhirnbrückenwinkeltumoren. Springer, Berlin Heidelberg New York
Horrax G, Poppen JL (1949) The End Results of Complete Versus Intracapsular Removal of Acoustic Tumors. Ann Surg 130:567–575
House WF (1961) Surgical exposure of the internal auditory canal and its contents through the middle cranial fossa. Laryngoscope 71:13-63-1385
House WF (1962) Subarachnoid shunt for drainage of endolymphatic hydrops: A preliminary report. Laryngoscope 72:713
House WF (1964) Evalution of transtemporal removal of acoustic neuromas. Arch Otolaryngol 80:731–750
House WF (1964) Monograph transtemporal bone microsurgical removal of acoustic neuromas. Arch Otolaryngol 80:597–730
House WF (1965) Subarachnoid shunt for drainage of hydrops. A report of 146 cases. Laryngoscope 75:1547–1551
House WF (1976) Cited in Jongkees LBW Chirurgie des Mastoids und der Pyramidenspitze sowie des intratemporalen Nervus facialis. In: Naumann HH (ed) Kopf- und Halschirurgie Bd 3, S 162ff.
House WF, Hitselberger WE (1964) Morbidity and mortality of acoustic neuromas. Arch Otolaryngol 80:752–757
House WF, Hitselberger WE (1964) Transtemporal bone microsurgical removal of acoustic neuromas. Total versus subtotal removal of acoustic tumors. Arch Otolaryngol 80:751–752
Iwakuma T, Matsumoto A, Nakamura N (1982) Hemifacial spasm. Comparison of three different operative procedures in 110 patients. J Neurosurg 57:753–756
Jannetta PJ (1967) Structural mechanism of trigeminal neuralgia: Arterial compression of the trigeminal nerve at the pons in patients with trigeminal neuralgia. J Neurosurg 26(II):159–162
Jannetta PJ (1970) Microsurgical exploration and decompression of the facial nerve in hemifacial spasm. Curr Top Surg Res 2:217–220
Jannetta PJ (1976) Microsurgical approach to the trigeminal nerve for Tic douloureux. Progr Neurol Surg 7:180–200
Jannetta PJ (1977) Observations on the etiology of trigeminal neuralgia, hemifacial spasm, acoustic nerve dysfunction and glossopharyngeal neuralgia. Definitive microsurgical treatment and results in 117 patients. Neurochirurgia 20:145–154
Jannetta PJ (1981a) Vascular decompression in trigeminal neuralgia. In: Samii M, Jannetta PJ (eds) The cranial nerves. Springer, Berlin Heidelberg New York, pp 331–340
Jannetta PJ (1981b) Hemifacial spasm. In: Samii M, Jannetta PJ (eds) The cranial nerves. Springer, Berlin Heidelberg New York, pp 484–493

Jannetta PJ, Bissonette DJ (1978) Bell's Palsy: a theory as to etiology. Observations in six patients. Laryngoscope 88:849–8545

Jannetta PJ, Gendell HM (1979) Clinical observations on etiology of essential hypertension. Surg Forum 30:431–432

Körte W (1903) Ein Fall von Nervenpfropfung des N. facialis auf den N. hypoglossus. Dtsch Med Wschr 29:293–295

Koos W (1977) Die Mikrochirurgie als Voraussetzung für Fortschritte in der Behandlung des Akustikusneurinoms. Wien Med Wochenschr 8:246–249

Krause F (1903) Zur Freilegung der hinteren Felsenbeinfläche und des Kleinhirns. Beitr Klin Chir 37:728–764

Krmpotic J, Draf W, Helms J (1985) Chirurgische Anatomie des Kopf-Hals-Bereiches. Springer, Berlin Heidelberg New York

Lange G (1977) Die intratympanale Behandlung des Morbus Meniere mit ototoxischen Antibiotika. Laryngol Rhinol Otol 56:409–414

Lasjaunias PL (1983) Craniofacial and upper cervical arteries. Williams & Wilkins, Baltimore/London

MacCarty CS (1975) Acoustic neuroma and the suboccipital approach (1967–1972). Mayo Clin Proc 50:15–16

Mackay IS, King IJ (1977) Pre- and postoperative brainstem responses in a case of acoustic neuroma, sparing the VIII nerve. Clinical Otolaryngology 2:233–238

Malis LI (1975) Microsurgical treatment of acoustic neurinomas. In: Handa H (ed) Microsurgery. Igaku Sho, Tokyo

Malis LI (1977) Nerve grafting by microscope in the cranium. In: Rubin LR (ed) Reanimation of the paralyzed face. Mosby, St. Louis, p 211–216

Mazzoni A, Hansen CC (1970) Surgical anatomy of the arteries of the internal auditory canal. Arch Otolaryng 91, 128

Morrison AW, King TT (1984) Space-occupying lesions of the internal auditory meatus and cerebellopontine angle. Adv Otorhinolaryngol 121–142

Olivecrona H (1940) Acoustic tumors. J Neurosurg Psychiat 3:141–146

Olivecrona H (1967) Acoustic tumors. J Neurosurg 26:6–13

Panse R (1904) Ein Gliom des Akustikus. Arch Ohrenheilk 61:251

Penkert G, Samii M, Haid T, Rettinger G (1985) Angiomatöse Fehlbildung des inneren Gehörgangs mit den Leitsymptomen Schwindel und Ohrensausen. HNO 33:17–22

Penzholz H (1983) Die operative Behandlung der Trigeminusneuralgie. Neurol 10:29–34

Perry RH (1904) A case of tinnitus and vertigo treated by division of the auditory nerve. J Laryngol Otol 19:402–403

Portmann G (1927a) The saccus endolymphaticus and an operation for draining the same for the relief of vertigo. J Laryngol Otol 42:809

Portmann G (1927b) Vertigo: Surgical treatment by opening the saccus endolymphaticus. Arch Otolaryngol 6:309

Portmann G (1932) Traite de techniques operatoire otorhinolaryngologique. Masson Paris

Portmann M (1975) Tumors of the Internal Auditory Meatus and Surrounding Structures. In: Portmann M et al. (eds) The Internal Auditory Meatus. Churchill Livingstone, Edinburgh, p 219

Pulec JL (1966a) Symposium on acoustic neuroma – Diagnosis and management of acoustic neuroma. Laryngoscope 76:1097–1103

Pulec JL (1966b) Comments on translabyrinthine approach to acoustic neuromas. Arch Otolaryngol 83:592–594

Quix F (1911) Ein Akustiktumor. Arch Ohrenheilk 84:252

Rand RW (1969) Microneurosurgery for acoustic tumors. In: Rand RW (ed) Microneurosurgery. St. Louis, Mosby, p 126–155

Rand RW (1981) The Gardner neurovascular decompression operation for trigeminal neuralgia. Acta Neurochir 58:161–168

Rand RW, Jannetta PJ (1968) Microneurosurgery: application of the binocular surgical microscope in brain tumors, intracranial aneurysm, spinal cord disease and nerve reconstruction. Proc Congr Neurol Surg. In: Clinical Neurosurgery Chapter XIV. Williams and Wilkins, Baltimore, pp 319–342

Rand RW, Kurze T (1965) Microneurosurgical resection of acoustic tumors by a transmeatal posterior fossa approach. Bull Los Angeles Neurol Soc 30:17–20

Rand RW, Kurze T (1968) Preservation of vestibular, cochlear and facial nerves during microsurgical removal of acoustic tumors. Report of two cases. J Neurosurg 28:158–161

Rhoton AL (1974) Microsurgery of the internal acoustic meatus. Surg Neurol 2:311–318

Rhoton AL (1976) Microsurgical removal of acoustic neuromas. Surg Neurol 6:211–219

Samii M (1979) Neurochirurgische Gesichtspunkte der Behandlung der Akustikusneurinome mit besonderer Berücksichtigung des N. facialis. 2 Laryngol Rhinol Otol 58:97–106

Samii M (1983) Pathogenese und operative Behandlung des Spasmus facialis. Akt Neurol 10:11–17

Samii M, Ohlemutz A (1981) Early experience in vascular decompression for vestibulo-cochlear malfunction. In: Samii M, Jannetta PJ (eds) The cranial nerves. Springer, Berlin Heidelberg New York, pp 556–558

Samii M, Ohlemutz A (1981) Preservation of eighth cranial nerve in cerebello-pontine angle tumors. In: Samii M, Jannetta PJ (eds) The cranial nerves. Springer, Berlin Heidelberg New York, p 586–587

Samii M, Penkert G (1984) 100 mikrochirurgische Tumorentfernungen im Kleinhirnbrückenwinkel unter besonderer Berücksichtigung der Hörfunktionserhaltung. Zbl Neurochir 45:7

Samii M, Turel KE, Penkert G (1985) Management of Seventh and Eighth Nerve. Involvement by Cerebellopontine Angle Tumors. Clin Neurosurg 32:242–272

Scaramella L (1970) Preliminary reports on facial nerve anastomosis. Thirn Int. Symposium on Facial Nerve Surgery. Osaka, Sept. 27–30

Scaramella L (1971) L'anastomosi tra i due nervi faciali. Arch Ital Otol 28:207–215

Segal R, Gendell HM, Canfield D, Dujovny M, Jannetta PJ (1979) Cardiovascular response to pulsatile pressure applied to ventrolateral medulla. Surg Forum 30:433–435

Smith JW (1971) A new technique of facial animation. Transactions Fifth International Congress Plastic and Reconstructive Surgery. Butterworth, Melbourne, p 83–84

Smith MFW, Miller RN, Cox DJ (1973) Suboccipital microsurgical Removal of Acoustic Neurinomas of All Sizes. Trans Am Otol Soc p 119

Stennert E (1979) Combined approach in extratemporal facial nerve reconstruction. Clin Plast Surg 6:481–486

Sterkers JM (1971) Chirurgie du conduit auditif interne, neurotomies et tumeurs (55 cas). Société Française d'Otorhinolaryngologie, 68ᵉ Congres Paris. Arnette, Paris

Sterkers JM (1981) Retro-sigmoid approach for preservation of hearing in early acoustic neuroma surgery. In: Samii M, Jannetta PJ (eds) The cranial nerves. Springer, Berlin, pp 579–585

Sterkers JM, Sterkes O, Mandelonde C, Corlien P (1984) Preservation of Hearing by the Retrosigmoid Approach in Acoustic Neuroma Surgery. Adv Otorhindaryngologie 34:187–192

Sunderland S (1945) The arterial relations of the internal auditory meatus. Brain 68:23–27

Wigand ME (1976) Schwindel, ein Leitsymptom der Felsenbeinneurinome. Neutrol Psychiat 2:307–313

Wigand ME (1979) Der transtemporale Zugang zur Operation des kleinen Octavusneurinomes. Course on surgery of the skull base, Hannover

Wigand ME (1979) Die transtemporale, extradurale Chirurgie des inneren Gehörganges. Course lecture, Surgery of the skull base, Hannover

Wigand ME, Haid T, Berg M, Rettinger G (1981) Early diagnosis and transtemporal removal of small nerve VII and VIII tumors. In: Samii M, Jannetta PJ (eds) The cranial nerves. Springer, Berlin Heidelberg New York, p 549–574

Wigand ME, Hait T, Berg M, Rettinger G (1982a) Otochirurgische Neurolyse des VIII. Hirnnerven bei progressiven, cochleovestibulären Störungen. Arch Otorhinolaryngol 235:531–534

Wigand ME, Haid T, Berg M, Rettinger G (1982b) The enlarged transtemporal approach to the cerebellopontine angle. Technique and indications. Acta otorhinolaryngol Ital 2:571–582

Yasargil MG, Fox JL (1974) The microsurgical approach to acoustic neurinomas. Surg Neurol 2:393–398

Zange G (1915) Translabyrinthäre Operationen von Akustikus- und Kleinhirnbrückenwinkeltumoren. Berl Klin Wochenschr 52:1334

Yasargil MG (1978) Mikrochirurgie der Kleinhirnbrükkenwinkel-Tumoren. In: Plester D, Wende S, Nakayama N (eds) Kleinhirnbrückenwinkeltumoren. Springer, Berlin Heidelberg New York, p 215–257

Zülch KJ (1956) Pathologische Anatomie der raumbeengenden intrakraniellen Prozesse. Handbuch der Neurochirurgie, vol 3, Springer, Berlin Göttingen Heidelberg

Surgery of Tumors of the Lateral Posterior Skull Base and Petrous Bone

General Operative Techniques

Tumors of the lateral posterior skull base most commonly extend into the middle skull base. The symptoms, diagnosis, and operative strategy were discussed previously (see p. 296).
The posteroinferior approach is the preferred extracranial route to the posterior lateral skull base. It can provide exposure of the lateral middle skull base, outer posterior skull base, and adjacent dura (see p. 300).
If dural infiltration is discovered, the primary extracranial procedure is converted to an intracranial operation in the same sitting (see p. 416).

Special Operative Techniques

Introductory Remarks. The petrous bone, or petrous portion of the temporal bone, is an important connecting and boundary structure between the middle and posterior cranial fossae. Viewed externally, it represents a major component of the middle and posterior skull base. Because it contains the sensory organs of the inner ear as well as the facial nerve, the petrous bone is a key element in the determination of operative strategy. The *jugular foramen* of the posterior skull base, which is transversed by important neurovascular structures like the jugular bulb, cranial nerves IX-XI and the hypoglossal nerve, can constitute the origin for primary extradural processes of the posterior skull base. The principal lesions of this area are, in order of frequency, neuromas, chemodectomas (glomus tumors), and carcinomas of various origins that involve the skull base.

Neuromas of the Jugular Foramen and Hypoglossal Nerve

Introductory Remarks. The tumors can grow far into the cerebellopontine angle by destroying the bony skull base, pushing the dura ahead as they expand. Often it cannot be determined preoperatively whether the dura is intact and demarcates the tumor from the cranial interior, or whether dural infiltration has occurred. Thus, one should always be prepared for the necessity of converting a primary extracranial, extradural operation into an intracranial, intradural one. With preoperative interdisciplinary planning, this should present no difficulties. Extracranial neuromas, too, can be dissected atraumatically by combining macro- and microsurgical techniques and by enucleating the tumor to diminish its bulk.

Case Presentations

Case Report. Extradural neuroma of the left jugular foramen (Fig. PS 31 a–g). Laryngoscopic examination in a 15-year-old boy with hoarseness showed left vocal cord paralysis, which was initially interpreted as idiopathic recurrent laryngeal nerve palsy in the presence of normal thyroid and mediastinal findings. Three years later the patient additionally developed a sensorineural hearing loss and slight palsy in the oral branch of the left facial nerve. X-rays showed an extensive tumor that apparently had developed from the jugular foramen far into the petrous bone. CT scans showed tumor extension into the cerebellopontine angle. The tumor was exposed through a combined cervical-transmastoid approach after identifying cranial nerves

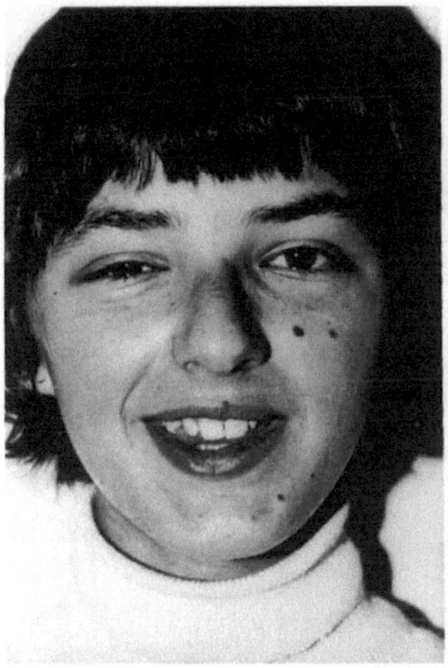

a

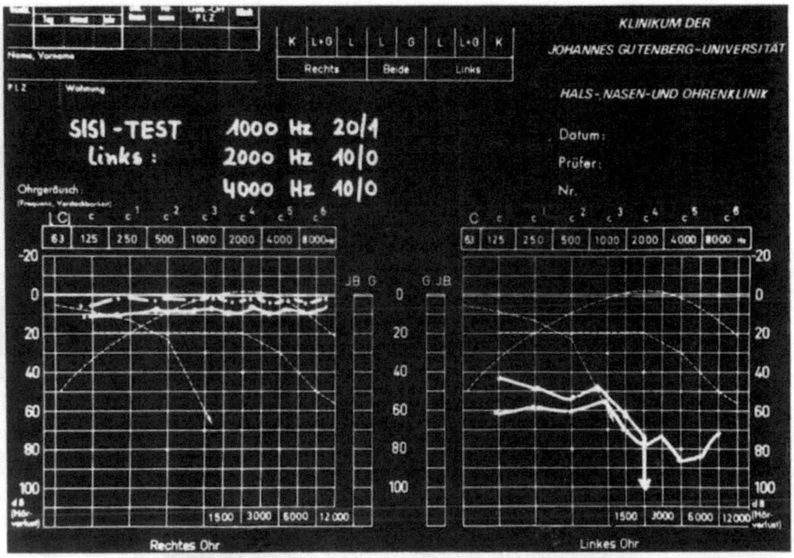

b

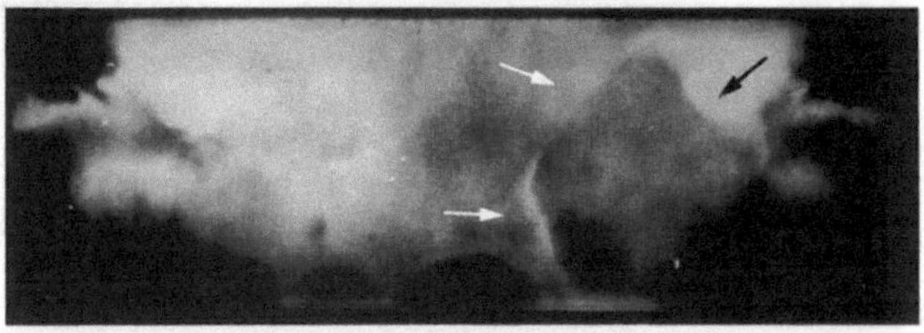

c

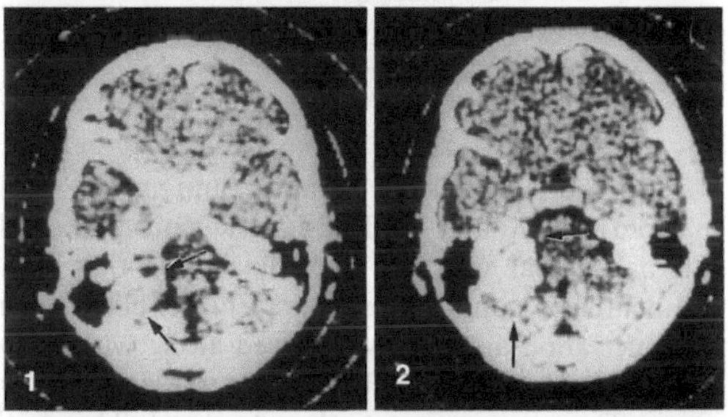

d

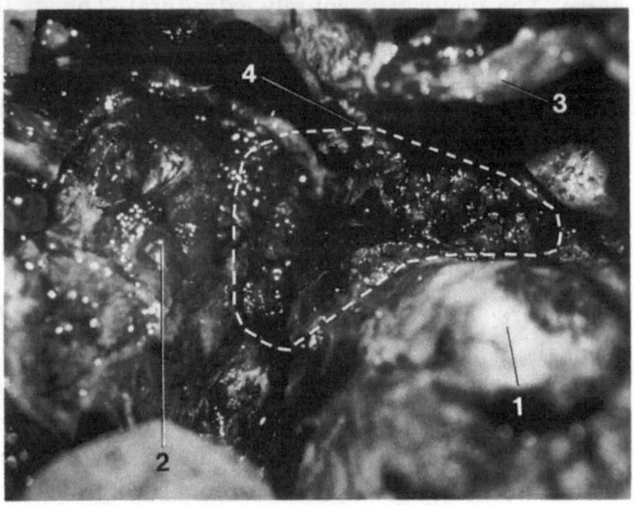

e

Fig. PS 31 a–g. Extradural neuroma of the left jugular foramen.
a Boy 15 years of age with mild facial palsy on the left side.
b Tone threshold audiogram indicates sensorineural hearing loss on the left side.
c PA tomogram of the petrous bone shows sharply circumscribed destruction of the left skull base extending to the IAC. The reactive margin is evidence of slow tumor growth.
d CT scans with (*1*) and without (*2*) contrast enhancement show tumor extension into the left cerebellopontine angle (*arrow*) with compression of the pons and cerebellum.
e The tumor was exposed through the posteroinferior approach. The facial nerve is partially exposed and is compressed by tumor. (*1*) Sigmoid sinus, (*2*) jugular vein, (*3*) facial nerve, (*4*) tumor

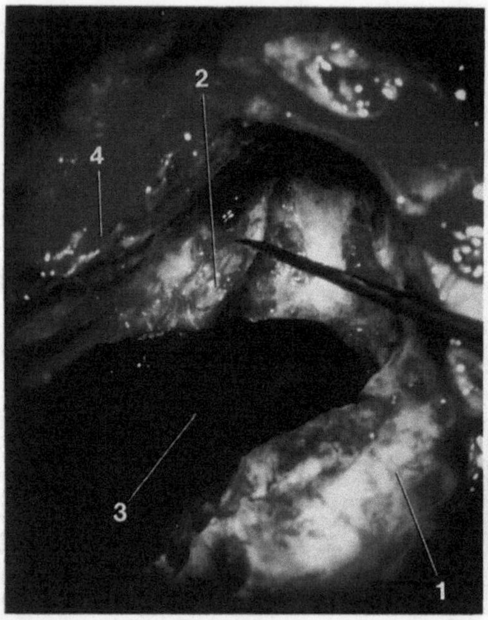

f

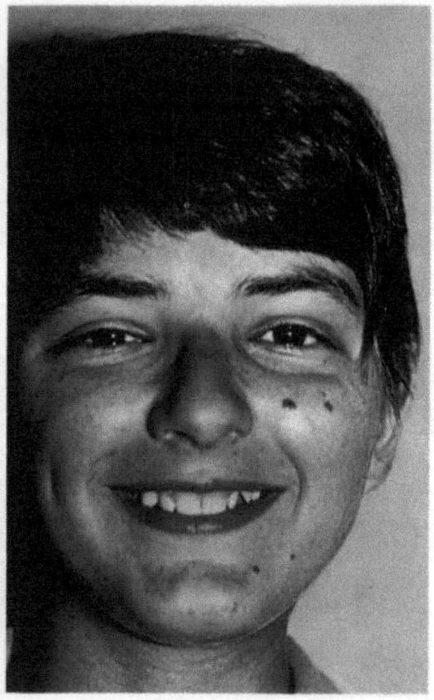
g

Fig. PS 31 f, g.
f Status following complete removal of the tumor, which was entirely extradural. (*1*) Sigmoid sinus, (*2*) facial nerve, (*3*) view of the posterior fossa dura, displaced posteromedially by tumor, (*4*) posterior meatal wall.

g The patient six days after surgery, showing complete regression of the facial palsy

VII (at the stylomastoid foramen and in the mastoid), IX, X, and XI. The sigmoid sinus and internal jugular vein had to be ligated so that the neoplasm could be progressively debulked by enucleation and finally removed along with the attached jugular bulb, sparing the facial nerve. The tumor was entirely extradural. The resection resulted in a large cavity extending into the cerebellopontine angle and lined by healthy dura. By the sixth postoperative day the facial palsy had regressed completely, indicating that the deficit had been caused by a simple neurapraxic disturbance. The recurrent nerve palsy persisted.

Comments: A large neuroma, probably arising from the neural structures of the jugular foramen, was totally removed with preservation of the surrounding cranial nerves. Facial nerve palsy had existed only a short time and resolved soon after surgery. The recurrent laryngeal nerve palsy had existed for several years and was irreversible. The cranial nerves formed a dense plexus in the area of the jugular foramen, and we were unable to identify the particular nerve from which the tumor arose. The completely extradural growth was removed by enucleation and total resection of the capsule through a posteroinferior approach.

Case Report. Neuroma of the right hypoglossal nerve close to the skull base (Fig. PS 32a–d). Dysphagia and speech slurring developed over a period of months in a 49-year-old man due to right hypoglossal nerve palsy. This was accompanied by medial displacement of tonsillar structures on the right side. Radiologic studies demonstrated a large tumor of the lateral posterior and middle skull base extending into the infratemporal fossa. The neoplasm was approached posteroinferiorly from the neck, also exposing the afferent cranial nerves. By enucleating the tumor and then resecting its capsule, we were able to accomplish total removal

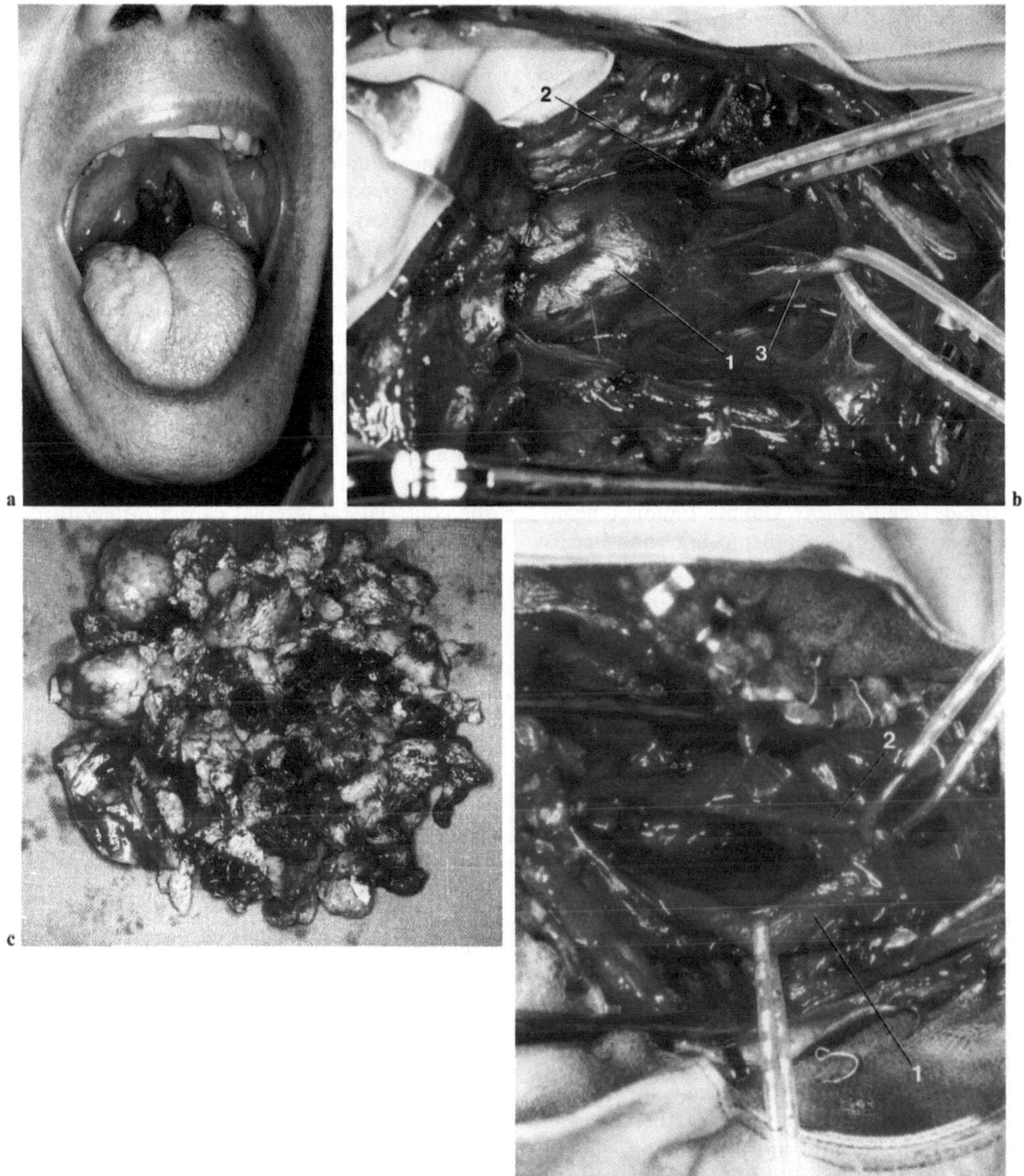

Fig. PS 32a–d. Neuroma of the right hypoglossal nerve at the skull base.
a Tumor has caused medial displacement of right tonsillar structures, and the right half of the tongue is atrophied due to hypoglossal paralysis.
b Exposure of the neoplasm through the posteroinferior approach. (*1*) Tumor, (*2*) hypoglossal nerve, (*3*) vagus nerve.
c Tumor particles.
d Status following tumor removal. (*1*) Internal carotid artery, (*2*) hypoglossal nerve

of the neuroma (as it was identified by histology) without extensive resection of the bony skull base and without sacrifice of cranial nerve structures.

The patient recovered normal hypoglossal nerve function within a few weeks after surgery.

Comments: A large neuroma arising from the hypoglossal nerve at the skull base was completely removed microsurgically using the enucleation technique with preservation of the surrounding cranial nerve structures and without additional resection of the bony skull base.

Glomus Tumors

Introductory Remarks. Glomus tumors (chemodectomas) have been a therapeutic challenge for otorhinolaryngologists, neurosurgeons, and radiologists since they were first recognized as a separate entity in the 1940s (Guild 1941; Robertson et al. 1982; Rosenwasser 1969, 1968). This is because the tumor, which is benign in more than 90% of cases, is unique in its pathoanatomic features and growth. It is extremely well vascularized and bleeds considerably during surgery. It tends to form fingerlike projections that invade the various fissures and canals of the skull base, and the tumor can infiltrate and destroy bone as well as dura. Concomitant extra- and intracranial involvement is possible when growth is extensive. The development of glomus tumor surgery reflects the problems associated with the diagnosis and treatment of these lesions (Gardner et al. 1977; Graf et al. 1979; Kleinsasser 1963; Mündnich 1966; Ungerecht 1963; Zak 1954). *Clinically*, the presence of a reddish, pulsating mass in the ear canal is diagnostic for this type of tumor. Bulging of the lateral pharyngeal wall signifies that the tumor involves not only the otobase (Wullstein 1972) but also the cervical region. The presence of recurrent laryngeal nerve palsy, paralysis of the soft palate, "backdrop phenomenon" of the posterior pharyngeal wall, and hypoglossal nerve palsy signify that the tumor envelops the jugular foramen and very likely has spread to the cranial cavity.

Defining the extent of these tumors requires all the resources of modern radiology. Besides plain skull X-rays in multiple projections (including the oblique Stenver view of the petrous bone), high-resolution CT scans, MRI, and cranial angiography are indispensable aids. Selective and superselective catheterization of the external carotid, internal carotid, and vertebral arteries and their major branches on both sides can demonstrate pathologic vessels and arteriovenous anastomoses and provide information on the extent of the tumor and its blood supply. By compression of the common carotid artery on the involved side and angiography of the internal carotid artery on the opposite side, one can assess the functional capacity of the circle of Willis and the potential blood supply from the contralateral internal carotid artery to the tumor-involved hemisphere. The hemodynamic importance of the vertebrobasilar system can be similarly assessed.

Veldman et al. (1980) remind us of the familial and multicentric occurrence of glomus tumors on one or both sides and the possible coexistence of carotid body and glomus jugulare tumors. They also note the potential value of radionuclide angioscintigraphy for noninvasive early diagnosis.

The studies of Van Baars et al. (1981) indicate that two or more glomus tumors can be found in 38% of patients with familial, nonchromaffin paragangliomas (Fig. PS 33). Parkin (1981) recommends that angiography be used in patients with familiar glomus tumors to screen for occult pheochromocytomas so that intraoperative blood pressure fluctuations will not take the surgeon by surprise.

Glomus tumors in the area of the petrous bone may arise from the glomus jugulare as well as from the glomus tympanicum and several other nonchromaffin paraganglia (Fig. PS 34).

Since Seiffert (1934; cited in Lundgren 1949), many authors have addressed the problems associated with glomus tumor surgery (Capps 1952; Lundgren 1949; Meacham and Capps 1960; Semmes 1953; Thoms et al. 1960; Weille and Lane 1951). A common feature of these early studies is that either otorhinolaryngologic or neurosurgical techniques were employed to

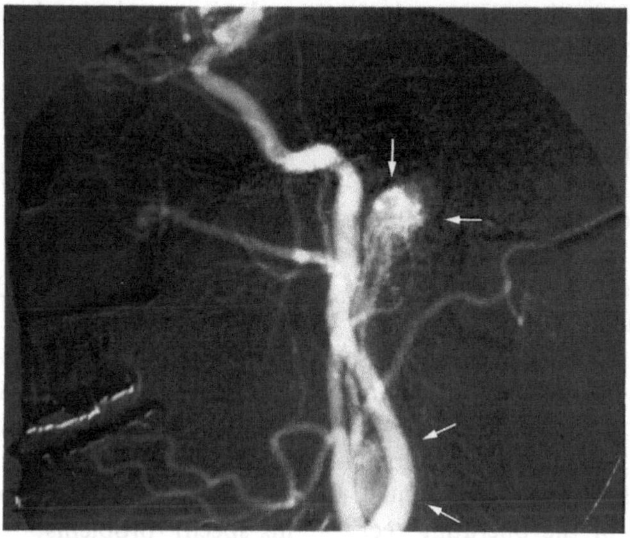

Fig. PS 33. Multifocal glomus tumors in a 19-year-old female. Angiograms demonstrated tumors in the left carotid bifurcation and jugular foramen and a carotid body tumor on the right side. The three tumors were completely removed in two operations

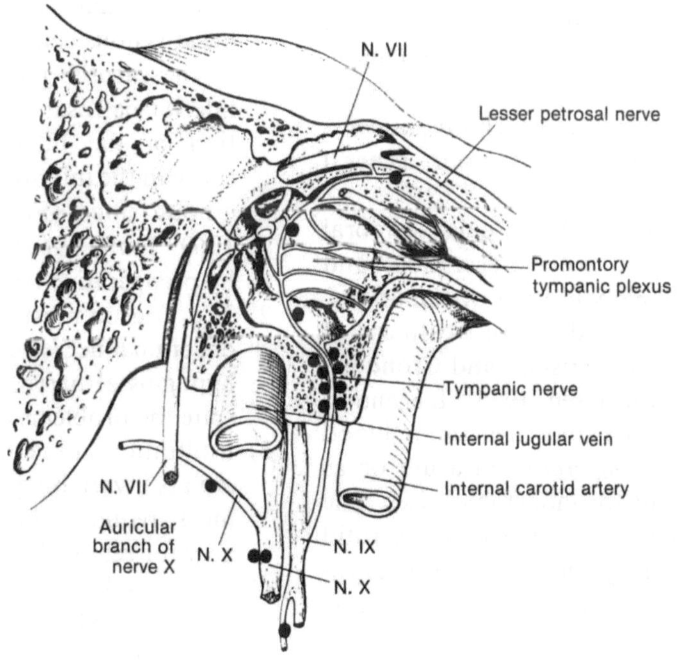

Fig. PS 34. Nonchromaffin paraganglia of the skull base region, from which glomus tumors can arise (after Draf, from Krmpotić/Draf/Helms 1988)

remove the tumor as far as the adjacent dura, leaving part of the tumor behind in some cases. Improvements in anesthetic techniques and the development of a common otosurgical-neurosurgical strategy initiated the modern surgical management of glomus tumors. Increasingly acceptable results were achieved in terms of the completeness of tumor removal and the resulting morbidity (Denecke 1966, 1969, 1978; Draf and Samii 1982; Gardner et al. 1977; Gejrot 1965; Hilding and Greenburg 1971; House 1968; House and Hitselberger 1976; Shapiro and Neues 1964). Authors such as Fisch (1977), Glasscock et al. (1974), Mischke and Balbany (1980), and Spector et al. (1973) have contributed to the refinement of the operating technique.

The *radiotherapy* of glomus tumors was recommended by Walsh in 1955 and has been a frequent topic of discussion (Maruyama 1972; Silverstone 1973). Opinions differ as to whether radiotherapy is capable of arresting tumor growth or providing regression. In our view, the only reliable treatment option is surgical removal. Radiotherapy may be appropriate as a palliative measure for those cases which are inoperable because of the patient's poor general health.

The *embolization* of highly vascular cerebral malformations began with Lüssenhop and Spence (1960). The embolization of tumor vessels has also been applied to the treatment of glomus jugular tumors (Brismar and Cronquist 1978; Hilal and Michelsen 1975; Lasjaunias 1983). The goal is to reduce the tumor blood supply either as a *preoperative* measure or as a *palliative* treatment for inoperable cases. The preoperative embolization of external carotid branches, most notably the ascending pharyngeal artery, maxillary artery and facial artery, can facilitate surgical removal by greatly decreasing the bleeding tendency of the tumor. Occluding the branches of the internal carotid or vertebral artery is not recommended, as it carries the risk of cerebral arterial embolization. In all cases the embolization should be performed by a highly experienced neuroradiologist. The use of preoperative embolization, combined with surgical extirpation using macro- and microsurgical techniques, has demonstrated its ability to improve the overall surgical results.

Operative Technique
(Fig. PS 35a–e)

The technique described below has served us well for the removal of very large glomus tumors with anterior extension into the horizontal carotid canal and wide infiltration of the dura with invasion of the middle and posterior fossae (Krmpotic et al. 1988).

The surgeon must give attention to the following specific problems:

1) *Bleeding* from the tumor itself, from the often heavily vascularized adjacent bone, and from large venous channels like the sigmoid sinus and transverse sinus, which usually have been invaded by the larger tumors. Also, the tumor may grow through the transbasal venous channels from the jugular bulb to the carotid genu, through the accessory inferior petrosal sinus to the horizontal portion of the internal carotid artery, and through the inferior petrosal sinus to the cavernous sinus (Fig. PS 36) (Denecke 1966, 1969; Teufel 1964). Bleeding can be reduced by preoperative embolization.
2) The surgeon must strive to preserve the caudal cranial nerves in the jugular foramen, the hypoglossal nerve, and the facial nerve despite the problems caused by bleeding.
3) Infiltration of the middle and posterior fossa *dura* is invariably present in large glomus tumors, requiring intracranial, intradural surgery for removal of the involved dura.
4) At the end of the operation, *infection* must be prevented by occluding the eustachian tube and ear canal. The principle of the operation corresponds to the *posteroinferior approach* (see p. 300).

The tumor is exposed through a Y-shaped or C-shaped skin incision (Fisch 1978) that provides a wide pedicle for the auricle. The incision extends inferiorly along the anterior border of the sternocleidomastoid muscle as far as the cla-

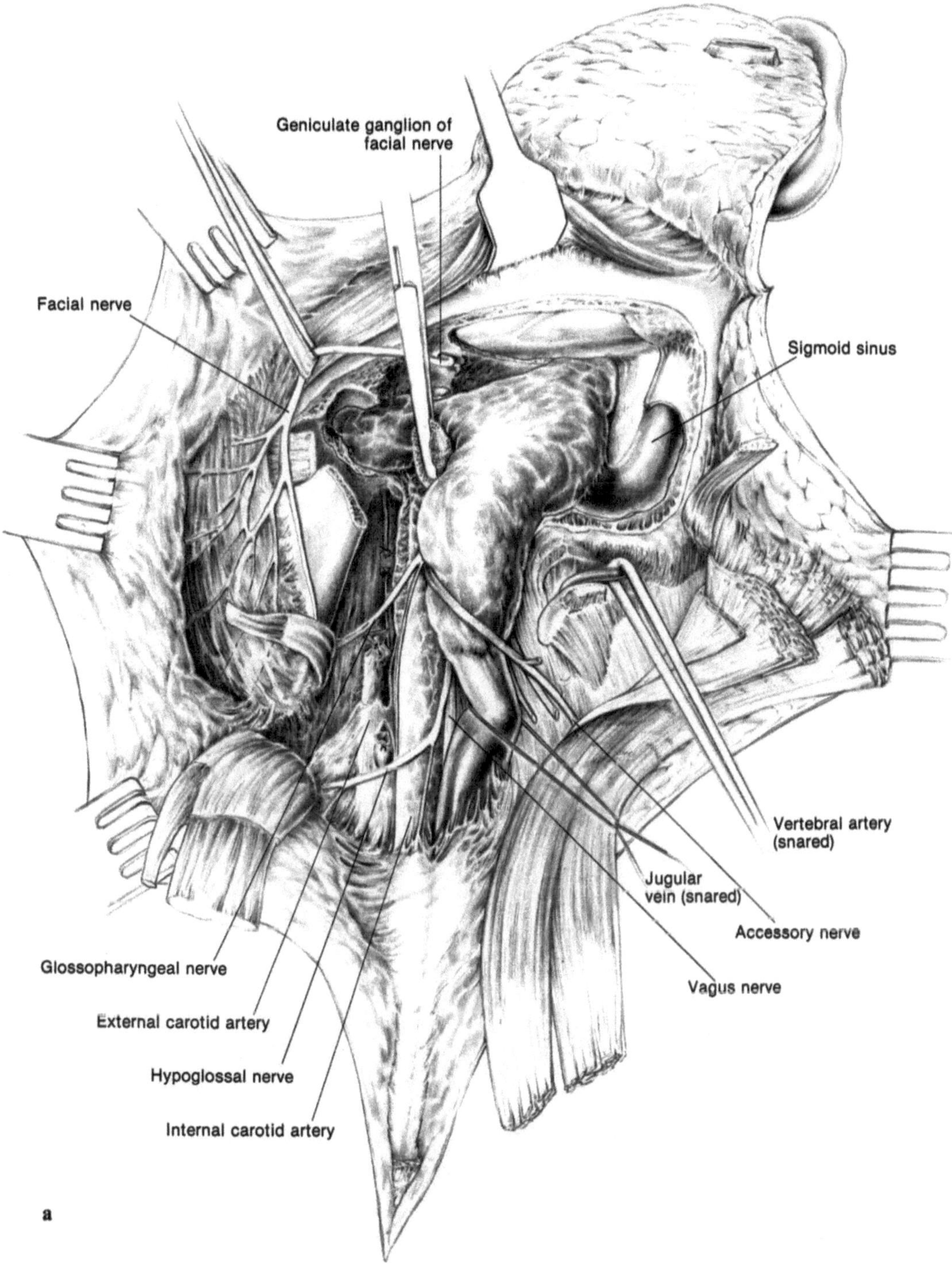

Fig. PS 35a–e. Extirpation of a large glomus tumor arising from the jugular bulb (*left side*).

a The auricle is reflected superiorly, the skin flaps are developed, mandibular condylectomy is performed, and the major neurovascular structures of the skull base and the sigmoid sinus are exposed in the neck (see also Fig. 33a-h, posteroinferior approach to the lateral middle skull base, see p. 300) to obtain wide exposure of the neoplasm. A difficult step in the operation is to follow the tumor extension along the internal carotid artery to its horizontal portion. If the tumor is found to encase the carotid genu and the horizontal limb as far as the cavernous sinus, optimum exposure of this vessel and of the facial nerve is achieved in minimum time by performing parotidectomy and mandibular condylectomy at the start of the operation. The sternocleidomastoid muscle is isolated during dissection of the skin flaps, released from the clavicle, and mobilized in its inferior two-thirds. It is left on a cutaneous pedicle superiorly after detaching it from the mastoid so that it can be utilized for cavity ablation and hemostasis

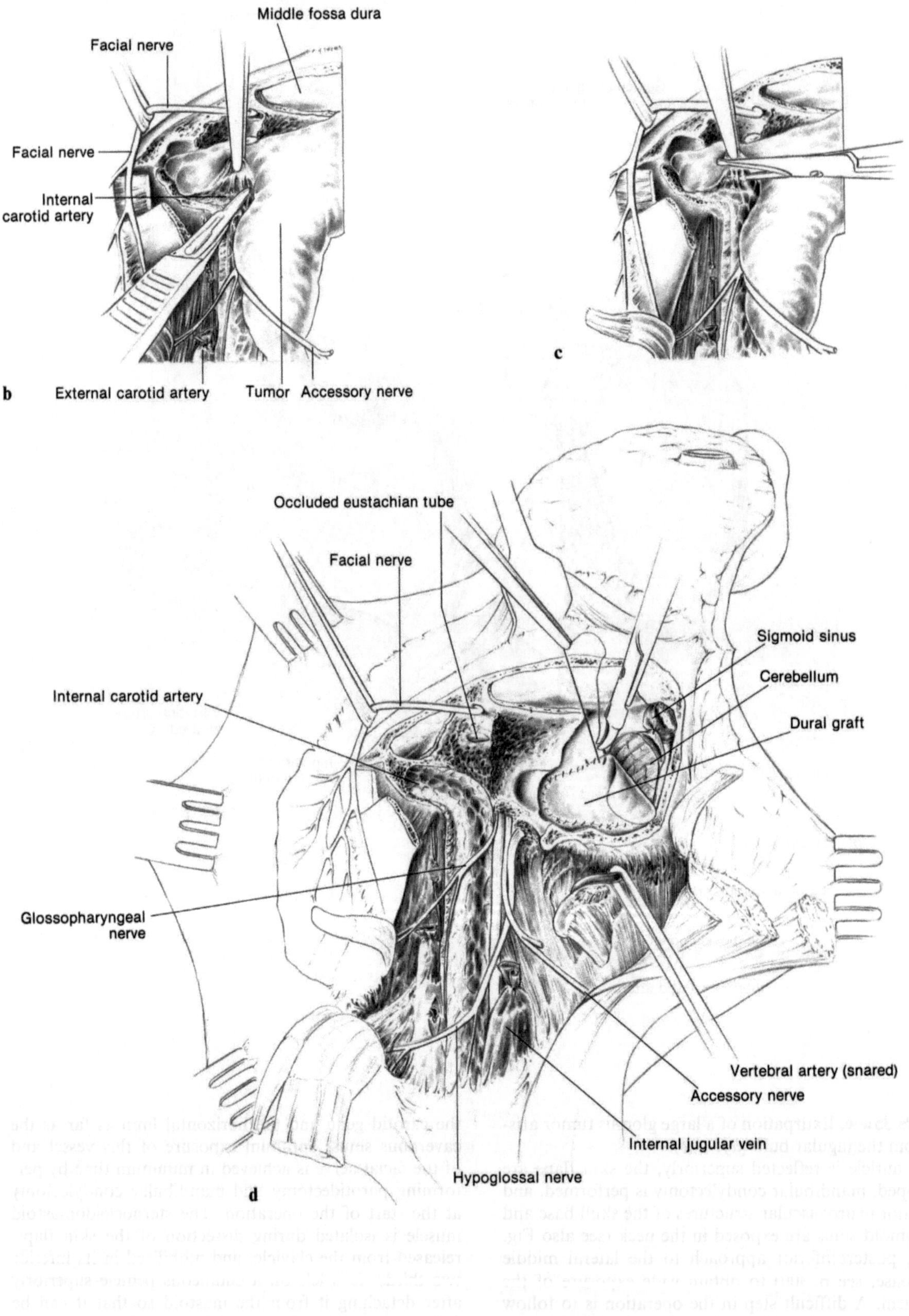
Middle fossa dura
Facial nerve
Facial nerve
Internal carotid artery
b
External carotid artery
Tumor
Accessory nerve
c
Occluded eustachian tube
Facial nerve
Sigmoid sinus
Cerebellum
Dural graft
Internal carotid artery
Glossopharyngeal nerve
Vertebral artery (snared)
Accessory nerve
Internal jugular vein
Hypoglossal nerve
d

Fig. PS 35b–e.
b, c The difficult dissection of the horizontal portion of the internal carotid artery is done microsurgically using sharp scalpel dissection combined with traction on the tumor. In most cases the tumor can be separated from the vessel atraumatically on the subadventitial plane using this technique (**b**). Another technique employs blunt-tipped scissors, which likewise are used to open the tumor and separate it from the blood vessel.
d Status following tumor removal. The internal jugular vein is ligated at the neck, the sigmoid sinus is ligated at its junction with the transverse sinus, and the intervening sinus is removed along with the jugular bulb. Cranial nerves VII, IX, X, XI, and XII are preserved. The posterior fossa dura resected with the tumor is replaced by a dural graft. To avoid ascending infection via the eustachian tube, the tube orifice is sealed with an ossicle and a small dural graft.
e At the end of the operation the large surgical cavity is obliterated with the sternocleidomastoid muscle and fibrin glue

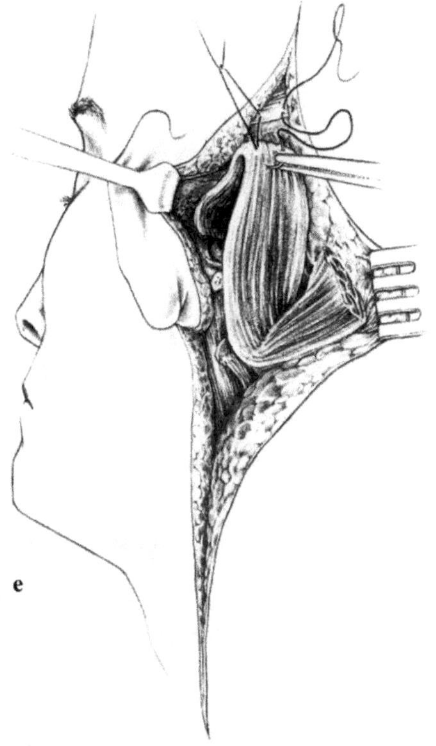

e

vicle, depending on the tumor size. The tumor is initially exposed from all sides before the lesion is attacked. This involves placing a craniectomy opening in the region of the middle and posterior fossae, remaining outside the dura, and exposing the carotid sheath above the clavicle. If the tumor is found to envelop the carotid genu and the horizontal portion of the internal carotid artery as far as the cavernous sinus, a time-saving dissection and optimum exposure of this vessel and facial nerve is achieved by starting the operation with a parotidectomy and mandibular condylectomy. The sternocleidomastoid muscle is isolated during dissection of the skin flaps, detached from the clavicle, and mobilized in its inferior two-thirds. Superiorly it is stripped from the mastoid tip but remains attached to the skin covering the mastoid so that it can be used later to ablate the surgical cavity (Denecke 1966, 1969, 1978). Next the tumor is prepared from the neck. For this step we have found the scalpel to be least traumatizing for dissection of the major vessels, especially the carotid artery, and the cranial nerves. Another key instrument is once again the bipolar cautery, which provides for rapid, tissue-sparing hemostasis. The surgeon mobilizes the tumor farther superiorly while progressively ligating the feeding vessels from the external carotid artery, especially the ascending pharyngeal artery, which usually is greatly enlarged and may arise from the *medial* aspect of the carotid bifurcation. The internal carotid artery is freed of tumor on the adventitial plane, using the diamond burr for the petrosal segment. Next the part of the tumor in the mastoid and petrous bone is encompassed. The neck muscles inserting on the mastoid are released medial to the attachment of the sternocleidomastoid, and the transverse process of the atlas is identified to avoid injury to the vertebral artery during the rest of the procedure. Access to the petrous bone is expanded by releasing the posterior portion of the digastric muscle from the digastric groove, reflecting the stylohyoid muscles forward and downward, and removing the styloid process, a key landmark lateral to the internal carotid artery. The mastoid process and petrous bone are removed as the tumor extent requires, exposing and mobilizing the facial nerve and surrounding fibrous tissue sheath. To avoid venous reflux from the internal jugular vein ligature, the transverse sinus is ligated or clipped before its junction with the sigmoid sinus. The tumor-

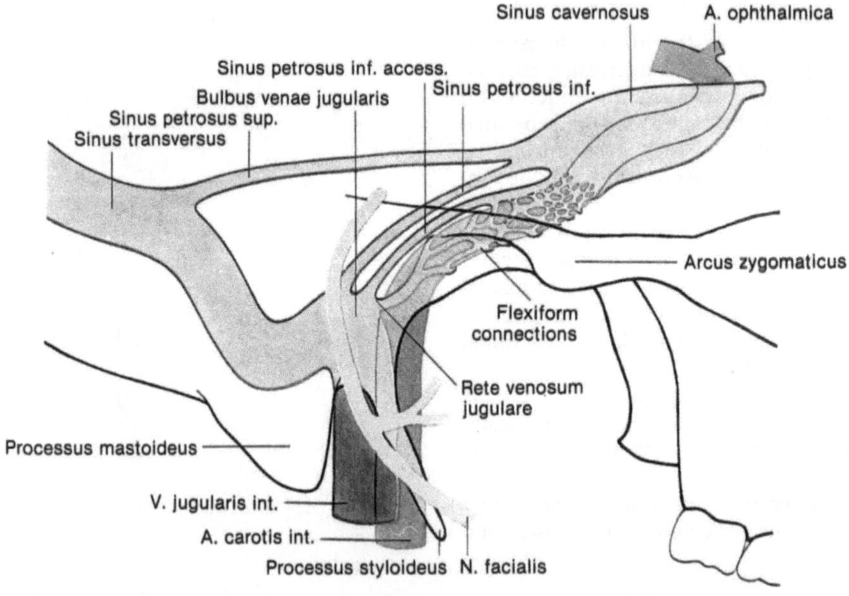

Fig. PS 36. The transbasal venous pathways (after Zak, from Krmpotić/Draf/Helms 1988)

involved dura is prepared from behind, forward, and the vessels supplying the tumor from the medial aspect are dealt with under direct visual control. At this point the glomus tumor can be mobilized anteriorly together with the sigmoid sinus, jugular bulb, and the superior portion of the ligated internal jugular vein. Strong bleeding from the inferior petrosal sinus is controlled with Surgicel.

Care is taken to preserve cranial nerves IX–XI in the anterior part of the jugular foramen. The mobilized portion of the tumor is removed, and residual tumor along the horizontal portion of the internal carotid artery is traced while removing the bony canal wall. The surgeon is cautioned against removing the mobilized petrous apex in one piece, because tilting of the petrous tip can easily cause injury to the internal carotid artery. If necessary, the internal carotid artery is exposed to its site of entry into the cavernous sinus. Removal of the tumor results in a wide communication with the middle and posterior cranial fossae, which must be sealed off in the final reconstructive phase. The dural defect is patched with a piece of stored dura attached with a simple continuous or interrupted suture line to obtain a watertight closure. The suture line may be reinforced with fibrin glue.

Fig. PS 37 a–m. Glomus tumor of the right temporal bone and right cervical region with intracranial extension.
a View into the oral cavity. The tonsillar displacement signifies extensive parapharyngeal tumor growth.
b, c Vertebral angiograms show the pronounced vascularization and extent of the glomus tumor.
d Axial CT scan demonstrates tumor invasion of the middle and posterior fossae with destruction of the bony petrosal skull base.
e Y-shaped skin incision
f The cervical part of the tumor is mobilized and reflected upward. (*1*) Tumor, (*2*) hypoglossal nerve (snared), (*3*) external carotid artery (ligated), (*4*) common carotid artery, (*5*) vagus nerve, (*6*) internal carotid artery, (*7*) accessory nerve.
g Status following complete tumor removal with resection of a 6×4-cm area of the posterior fossa dura. (*1*) Facial nerve, (*2*) hypoglossal nerve, (*3*) stump of external carotid artery, (*4*) common carotid artery, (*5*) vagus nerve, (*6*) internal carotid artery, (*7*) accessory nerve, (*8*) dural defect (– – –).
h The dural defect has been closed with a stored dural graft (*arrows, dotted line*)
i The eustachian tube is occluded with the incus and stored dura, and the surgical cavity is ablated with the sternocleidomastoid muscle flap based superiorly on the retromastoid skin and with the remaining parts of the temporal muscle.
k At the end of the operation the ear canal is closed with a double suture row after resecting part of the cavum cartilage.
l, m The patient one year after surgery. The wound healed well, and facial nerve function is satisfactory

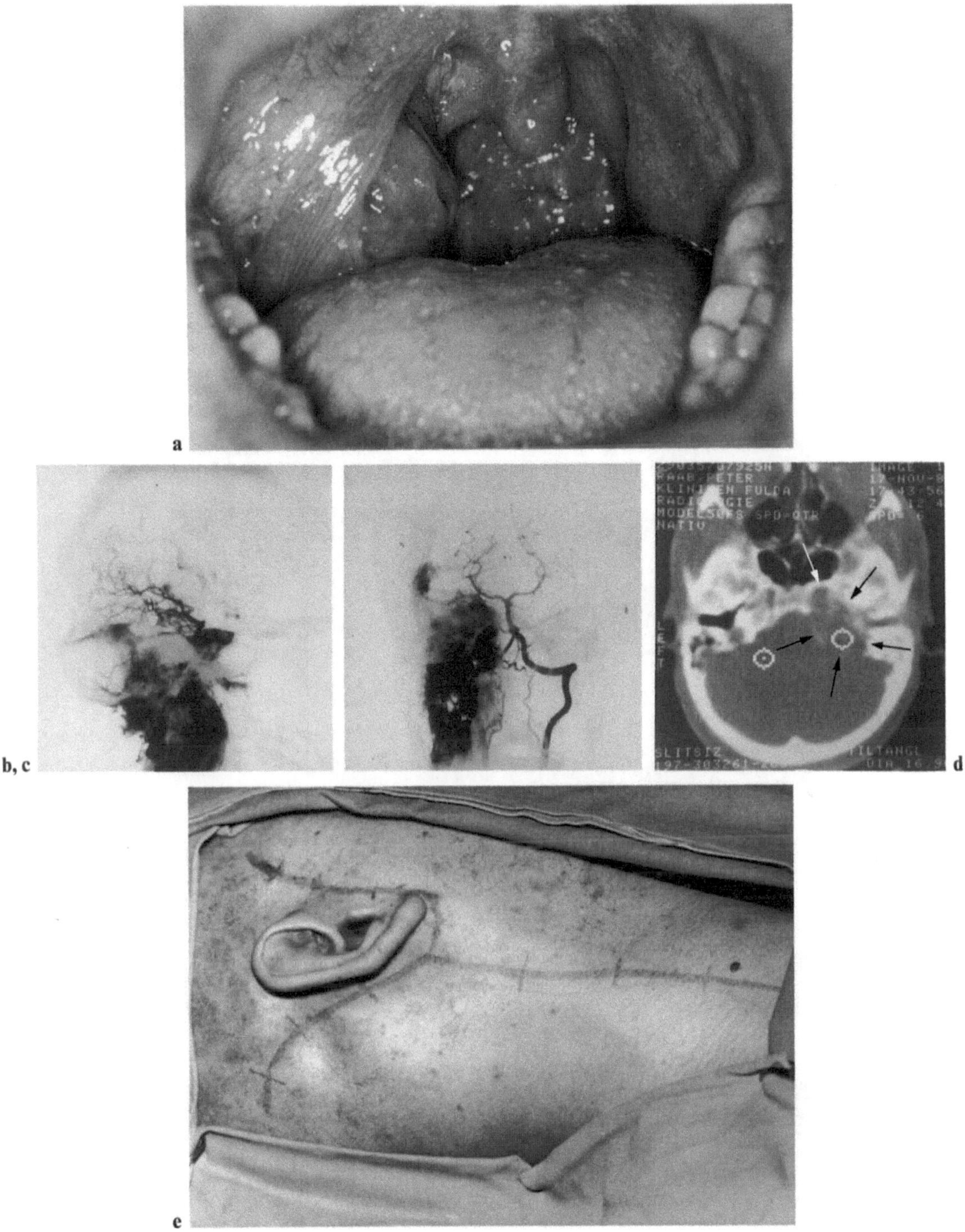
a
b, c
d
e

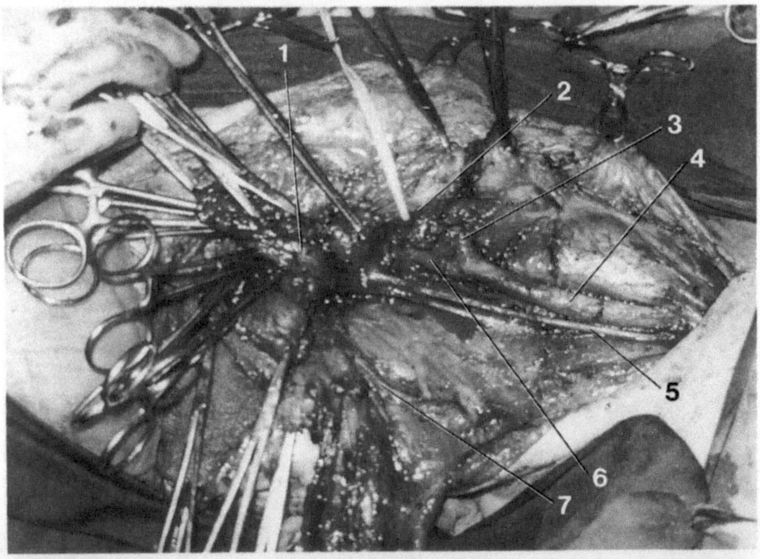

f

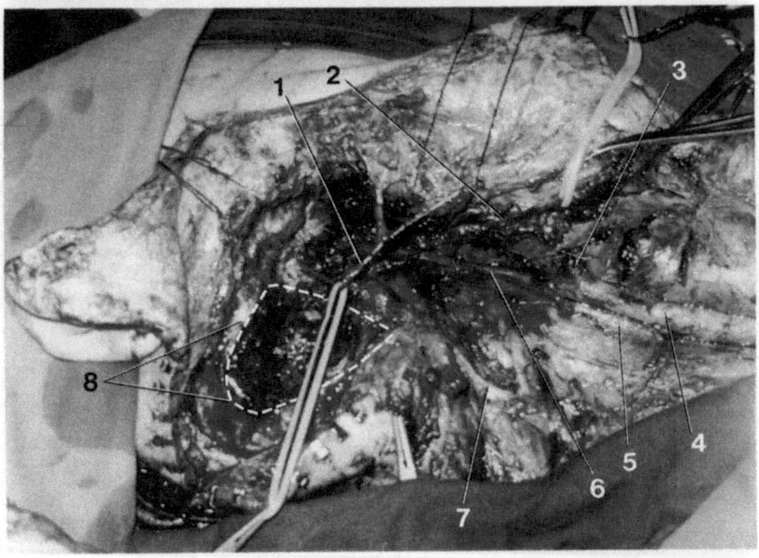

g

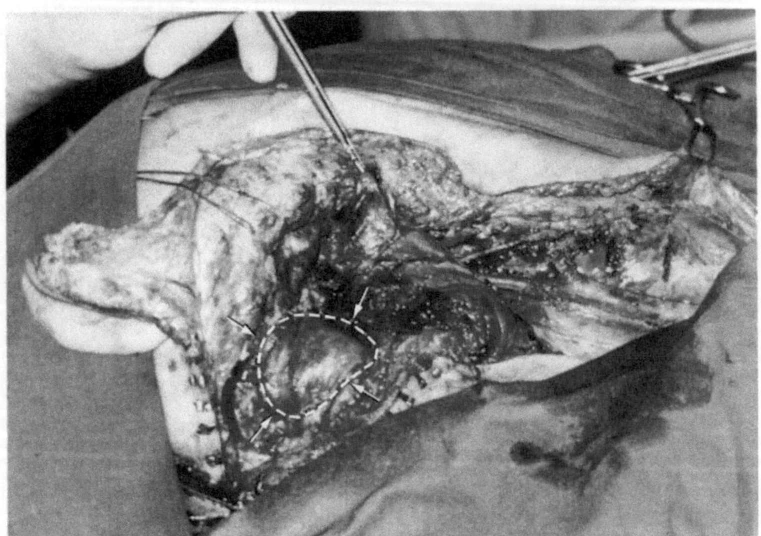

h

Fig. PS 37f–m

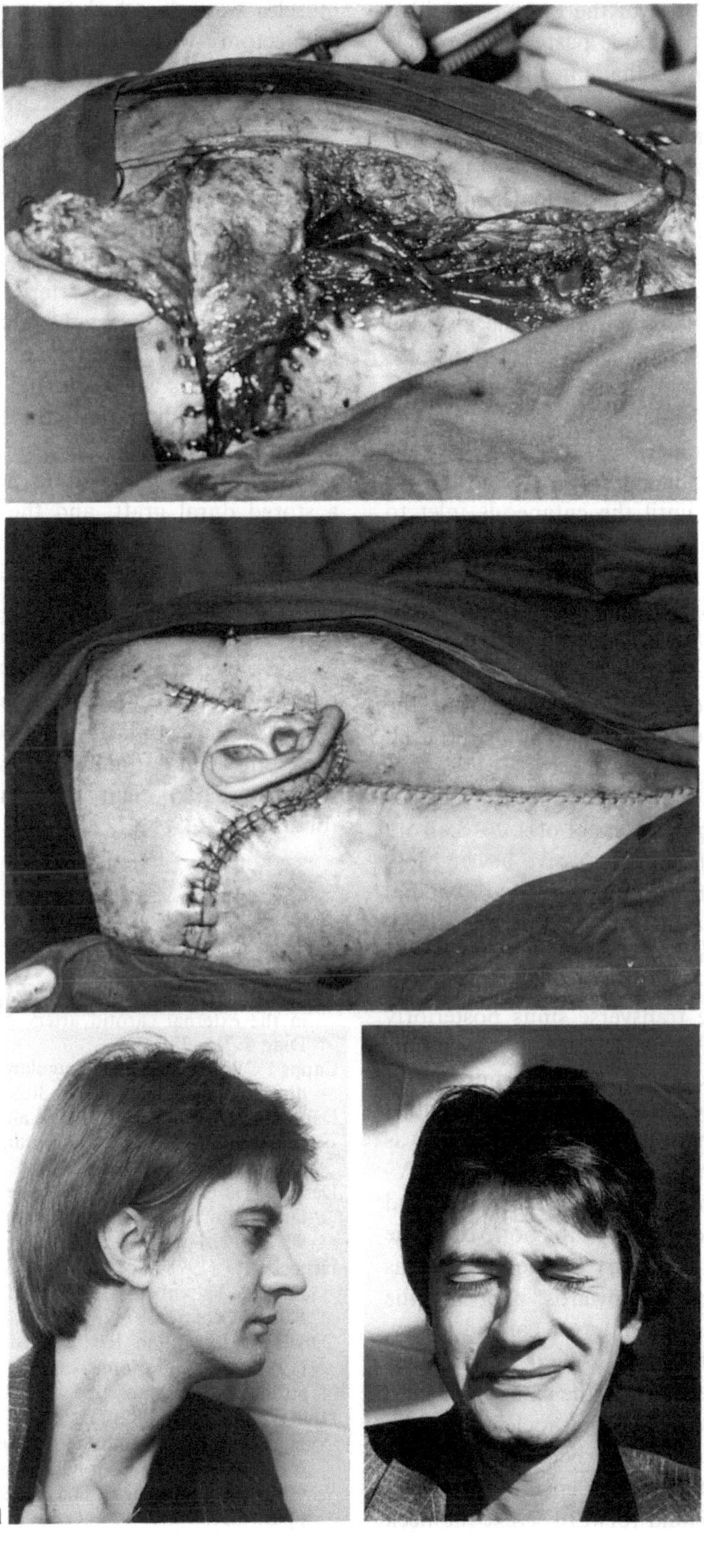

i

k

l

m

The remaining portion of the bony eustachian tube is occluded with bone paste or an ossicle (incus) to avoid ascending infection from the nasopharynx. It is additionally sealed with a graft of stored dura. The posterior meatal wall and tympanic membrane generally are sacrificed during the petrosectomy. For final hemostasis and cavity obliteration, the superiorly based sternocleidomastoid muscle flap is placed into the surgical cavity and attached with sutures and fibrin glue. The temporal muscle also can be swung into the surgical cavity if required.
Before the auricle is sutured back into place, the inlet to the ear canal, transected at the start of the operation, must be sealed. This is done by resecting the cartilaginous portion of the ear canal and cavum until the cutaneous inlet to the ear canal can be closed with tension-free everting sutures. Then the auricle is replaced and the wound closed in layers after inserting two large-bore suction drains.

Case Report. Extensive glomus tumor of the right temporal bone and right side of the neck with intracranial extension (Fig. PS 37a–m). Clinical examination revealed a reddish, pulsating mass in the right ear canal of a 24-year-old man who had suffered progressive hearing loss and a pulsatile tinnitus for several years. Medial displacement of the right tonsil was also noted. Subtraction angiography showed a tumor extending from the jugular bulb through the sigmoid sinus to the transverse sinus posteriorly and to the cavernous sinus anteriorly with wide involvement of the skull base. It extended inferiorly to the clavicle. Axial CT defined the intracranial extent of tumor growth. The tumor was approached in standard fashion through a Y-shaped skin incision around the auricle and transection of the ear canal at the bone-cartilage junction. The cervical part of the tumor was developed from below upwards, exposing the common carotid artery, internal carotid artery, jugular vein, and caudal cranial nerves. The feeding vessels arising from the external carotid artery were ligated. The sternocleidomastoid muscle was reflected superiorly on its cutaneous pedicle, and the tumor was encompassed and mobilized from behind forward. Next the neck muscles were detached from the skull base, a craniectomy was performed, the transverse sinus was ligated at its junction with the sigmoid sinus, the internal jugular vein was ligated, and the glomus tumor was prepared anteriorly with concomitant removal of the infiltrated dura. Further mobilization of the tumor was obtained by subtotal petrosectomy with exposure of the facial nerve. On reaching the horizontal portion of the internal carotid artery, we removed the tumor specimen dissected to that point and also removed the last, large tumor extension to the cavernous sinus while ablating the bony carotid canal with the diamond burr. The resection left a dural defect 10 × 12 cm in size. The facial nerve was intact. The dura was patched with a stored dural graft, and the eustachian tube was sealed with the incus and a small dural graft before obliterating the surgical cavity with the sternocleidomastoid and temporal muscles. Finally the cutaneous ear canal was closed, and wound closure was effected in layers. Postoperative angiography and CT confirmed total removal of the neoplasm. One year after surgery the cosmetic and functional result appeared satisfactory. The patient has been free of disease for six years.

References

Brismar J, Cronquist S (1978) Therapeutic embolization in the external carotid artery region. Acta Radiol Diag 5:715–731
Capps FCW (1952) Glomus jugulare tumors of the middle ear. J Laryngol Otol 66:302–314
Denecke HJ (1966) Zur Chirurgie ausgedehnter Glomustumoren im Bereich des Foramen jugulare. Arch Otorhinolaryngol 187:656–662
Denecke HJ (1969) Surgery of extensive Glomus jugulare tumors of the ear. Revue de Laryngologie 90:265–270
Denecke HJ (1978) Die Chirurgie ausgedehnter Tumoren des Felsenbeines und der Otobasis. Z Laryng Rhinol Otol 57:287–290
Dickens WJ, Million RR, Cassisi RJ, Singleton GT (1962) Chemodectomas arising in temporal bone structures. Laryngoscope 92:189–191
Draf W, Samii M (1982) Diagnostik und operative Strategie bei großen Tumoren der lateralen Schädelbasis. In: Majer EH, Rieder CH (eds) Aktuelles in der Otorhinolaryngologie. Thieme, Stuttgart New York, pp 61–70

Fisch U (1977) Infratemporal fossa approach for extensive tumors of the temporal bone and base of the skull. In: Silverstein H, Norrell H (eds) Neurological Surgery of the Ear. Aesculapius, Birmingham, pp 34–53

Fisch U (1978) Infratemporal fossa approach to tumors of the temporal bone and base of the skull. J Laryngol Otol 92:949–967

Gardner G, Cocke E, Robertson JT et al (1977) Combined approach surgery for removal of glomus jugulare tumors. Laryngoscope 87:655–688

Gejrot T (1965) Surgical treatment of glomus jugulare tumors. With special reference to the diagnostic value of retrograde jugularography. Acta Otolaryngol 68:150–168

Glasscock, Harris FF (1974) Glomus tumors. Diagnosis and treatment. Laryngoscope 84:2006–2032

Graf K, Fisch U (1979) Geschwülste des Ohres und des Felsenbeines. In: Berendes J, Link R, Zöllner F (eds) Hals-Nasen-Ohrenheilkunde in Praxis und Klinik Bd 5/III Thieme, Stuttgart

Guild S (1941) Hitherto unrecognized structure, the glomus jugulare in man. Anat Rec Suppl 2, 79:28

Hilal K, Michelsen L (1975) Therapeutic percutaneous embolization for extra-axial vascular lesions of the head, neck and spine. J Neurosurg 5:275–287

Hilding DA, Greenburg A (1971) Surgery for large glomus jugulare tumors. Arch Otolaryngol 93:227–231

House W (1968) Panel discussion McCabe BF, moderator, Rosenwasser H, House W, Witten RH, Hamberger CA: Management of glomus tumors. Arch Otolaryngol 89:170–178

House W, Hitselberger WE (1976) The transcochlear approach to the skull base. Arch Otolaryngol 102:334–342

Kleinsasser O (1963) Diskussionsbemerkungen zu Ungerecht. HNO 11:95–96

Krmpotic-Nemanic J, Draf W, Helms J (1988) Surgical Anatomy of Head and Neck. Springer, Berlin Heidelberg New York Tokyo

Lasjaunias RG (1983) Craniofacial and upper cervical arteries. Williams and Wilkins, Baltimore London

Lundgren N (1949) Tympanic body tumors in the middle ear-tumors of carotid body type. Acta Otolaryngol 37:366–379

Lussenhop AJ, Spence WT (1960) Artificial embolization of cerebral arteries: Report of use in case of arteriovenous malformation. JAMA 172; 1153–1155

Maruyama Y (1972) Radiotherapy of tympanojugular chemodectomas. Radiology 165:659–663

Meacham WF, Capps JH (1960) Intracranial glomus jugulare tumor with successful surgical removal. J Neurosurg 17:157–160

Mischke RE, Balbany ThJ (1980) Skull base approach to glomus jugulare. Laryngoscope 90:89–93

Mündnich (1966) Diskussionsbemerkungen zu Denecke. Arch Otorhinolaryngol (NY) 197:661

Parkin JL (1981) Familiar multiple tumors and pheochromocytomas. Ann Otol 90:6–63

Robertson J, Gardner G, Cocke BW, Gerald SB, Trumbull ML, Palmer RE (1982) Glomus jugulare tumors. In: Schmidek HH, Sweet WH (eds) Operative Neurosurgical techniques. Grune & Stratton, New York London, Vol 1, pp 649–670

Rosenwasser H (1968) Carotid body tumor of the middle ear and mastoid. Arch Otolaryngol 41:64–67

Rosenwasser H (1969) Glomus jugulare tumors. Long term results. Arch Otolaryngol 89:160–166

Semmes RE (1953) Discussion of paper by Alexander E Jr, Adams S Tumors of the glomus jugulare. Follow-up study two years after roentgentherapy. J Neurosurg 16:672–674

Shapiro MJ, Neues DK (1964) Technique for removal of glomus jugulare tumor. Arch Otolaryngol 79:219–224

Silverstone S (1973) Radiation therapy of glomus jugulare tumors. Arch Otolaryngol 25:43–48

Spector CJ, Paisel R, Ogura J (1973) Glomus tumors in the middle ear. I. An analysis of 46 patients. Laryngoscope 83:1652–1672

Teufel J (1964) Einbau der A. carotis in den Canalis caroticus unter Berücksichtigung des Venenabflusses. Gegenbauers Morphol Jahrb 106:188–274

Thoms OJ, Shaw DT, Trowbridge WV (1960) Glomus jugulare tumor. Report of a case with survival removal. J Neurosurg 17:500–504

Ungerecht K (1963) Zur Chirurgie der Glomus jugulare Tumoren im Schläfenbein-Schädelbasisbereich. HNO 11:95–96

Van Baars F, Van den Broek P, Cremers C, Veldman J (1981) Familial nonchromaffinic paragangliomas (glomus tumors): Clinical aspects. Laryngoscope 91:988–996

Veldman TE, Mulder PHM, Ruijs SHG, de Haas G, van Waes PFGM, Hoekstra (1980) Early detection of asymptomatic hereditary chemodectomas with radionuclide scintiangiography. Arch Otolaryngol 106:547–552

Walsh TE (1955) Discussion of paper by Williams HL et al. Chemodectomas of the glomus jugulare (nonchromaffin paragangliomas) with especial reference to their response to roentgen therapy. Trans Am Otol Soc 43:264–290

Weille FL, Lane C Jr (1951) Surgical problems involved in the removal of glomus jugulare tumors. Laryngoscope 61:483–459

Wullstein HL (1972) Hat Terminologie zur Definition unseres Faches eine Bedeutung? HNO 20:259–261

Zak FG (1954) An expanded concept of tumors of glomic tissue. NY State J Med 54:1153

On the Problem of Paralytic Dysphagia Caused by Posterior Skull Base Tumors

Introductory Remarks. Intracranial mass lesions of the cerebellopontine angle and jugular foramen, extracranial masses at the skull base, trauma to the skull base and neck, and the surgical removal of tumors in this region can result in a unilateral vagus nerve deficit with paralysis of the soft palate and pharynx and, through loss of the superior and inferior laryngeal nerves, paralysis of the ipsilateral vocal cord.

Patients who develop paralysis of the X-cranial nerve slowly because of a tumor generally adapt well to the palatal and pharyngeal paralysis. In these cases dysphagia and aspiration, the major clinical signs of vagus dysfunction, remain subtle, and the chief complaint is hoarseness.

When vagus nerve paralysis occurs suddenly, as after a surgical procedure, the full picture of paralytic dysphagia becomes evident. During deglutition, muscular contractions on the healthy side of the pharynx raise the intrapharyngeal pressure and cause an *indentation of the paralyzed pharyngeal wall*, which fills with ingested food. Ingesta also is pushed through the incompetent glottis into the trachea and, because of the palatal incompetence, into the nasopharynx. *At the end of deglutition* the paralyzed side of the pharynx is still filled with ingesta, and as the pressure subsides, this material drops into the laryngeal inlet and passes through the *incompetent glottis into the lower airways*. This problem is compounded by the fact that the patient is unable to cough effectively due to incomplete glottic closure. The danger of *deglutition pneumonia* is always present (Denecke 1961, 1980).

Besides *hoarseness*, patients experience a significant *loss of air during speech*. Sleep is repeatedly interrupted by paroxysms of coughing caused by salivary drainage into the larynx, which is open for respiration.

Building on the early experiments of Kaplan (1951) and Naffziger et al. (1948), Denecke (1961) has developed a complex surgical procedure for the rehabilitation of swallowing and speech that can restore patients to full occupational and social fitness.

The decision to undertake the operation and its timing depend on the degree of damage to the vagus nerve. If the nerve or its center has been merely compressed by retractor pressure or during dissection of the nerve, spontaneous recovery should occur within a few weeks. With complete transection or more severe damage to the vagus nerve or its center, the swallowing and speech difficulties usually will not regress. In these cases we advise early surgical intervention to spare the patient prolonged infirmity with the risk of recurring bronchopneumonia, particularly since the operation does not cause extra morbidity.

The Denecke Operation to Restore Swallowing and Speech in Unilateral Vagus Nerve Paralysis

The operation consists basically of *four parts*, which are performed in one or two stages:

1) Myotomy of the cricopharyngeal muscle with division of the adjacent esophageal musculature.
2) Correction of glottic closure with rotation of the arytenoid cartilage and cartilage implantation into the paralyzed vocal cord.
3) Resection of the paralyzed pharyngeal wall from the mouth of the esophagus to the level of the inferior tonsillar pole and closure of the resulting pharyngeal defect.

4) Fixation of the soft palate to the posterior pharyngeal wall.

In all cases the surgeon should observe the swallowing act fluoroscopically prior to surgery so that he can appreciate its pathophysiology and gain an accurate impression of the extent of the pathoanatomic and pathophysiologic disturbances and their surgical implications. He should observe deglutition again after surgery to determine the efficacy of the procedure.

With acute, bilateral paralysis of the vagus nerve, cricopharyngeal myotomy facilitates salivary drainage above the mouth of the esophagus but does not permit satisfactory deglutition. As a last recourse in these patients, Denecke recommends subtotal occlusion of the rima glottidis, leaving a small speech fistula in the anterior commissure. Experience has shown that the patients can manage some speech by digital closure of the tracheostomy, which is always necessary. Also, acceptable deglutition can be achieved without significant aspiration problems.

Details on operative technique may be found in Denecke (1980).

References

Denecke HJ (1961) Korrektur der Schluck- und Stimmstörung bei partieller Lähmung der Pharynx- und Larynxmuskulatur. Arch Ohr-, Nas-Kehlk Heilk 178:538–539

Denecke HJ (1980) Die otorhino-laryngologischen Operationen im Mund- und Halsbereich. Springer, Berlin Heidelberg New York, pp 678ff

Kaplan S (1951) Paralysis of deglutition. Ann Surg 133:572–573

Naffziger HC, Davis C, Bell HG (1948) Paralysis of deglutition. Ann Surg 128:732–742

Surgery of the Clivus (CL)

Introductory Remarks. Because the clivus occupies a central location in the skull base, it is subject to involvement by numerous diseases. Advanced neuroradiologic imaging procedures such as high-resolution CT, superselective angiography, and MRI enable lesions of this area to be accurately delineated.

The relative inaccessibility of the clivus and its close proximity to the brain stem and surrounding structures meant that, until recently, even benign lesions of this region were often considered to be inoperable.

Advances in the surgery of this region were made possible by an integrated application of the experience of interested disciplines relating to skull base surgery. This made it possible to devise an optimum approach to a particular problem without regard to specialty-imposed surgical boundary lines. Another important factor in the development of clivus surgery is the microsurgical operating technique, which enables the excision of pathological entities with maximum preservation of function and low morbidity even in anatomically complex areas.

A detailed knowledge of microsurgical anatomy is an absolute prerequisite for success. Topographic anatomic relationships will vary with the disease and with the route of surgical access:

In the midline the clivus is closely related superiorly to the sphenoid sinus, the floor of the sella turcica, and the dorsum sellae. Inferiorly it relates closely to the foramen magnum, the atlas, and the dens of the axis. Extracranially the clivus borders anteriorly on the mucosal lining of the pharyngeal roof and the posterior wall of the nasopharynx and oropharynx. The vertebrobasilar vascular system courses intracranially, just behind the dura, and posterior to it are the pons and medulla oblongata.

Intradurally the clivus is bordered superolaterally by the petrous apex, the floor of the middle fossa, and the structures in the tentorial incisure. It is bordered inferolaterally by the cerebellopontine angle and jugular foramen. Extradurally, the clivus is bounded superiorly by the sphenoid sinus, ethmoid cells, frontal sinus, the choanal openings and the nasal cavities, and laterally by the pterygoid process and the infratemporal fossa with its neurovascular and muscular structures.

The topographic anatomy of the clivus makes a number of surgical approaches feasible (Fig. CL 1):

The *primary extracranial approaches* are, from anteriorly to posteriorly, the transsphenoidal, the transoral, the transcervical, the lateral infratemporal, and the posteroinferior.

Primary intracranial approaches consist of the transfrontal, frontotemporal (or subtemporal), lateral suboccipital, and medial suboccipital.

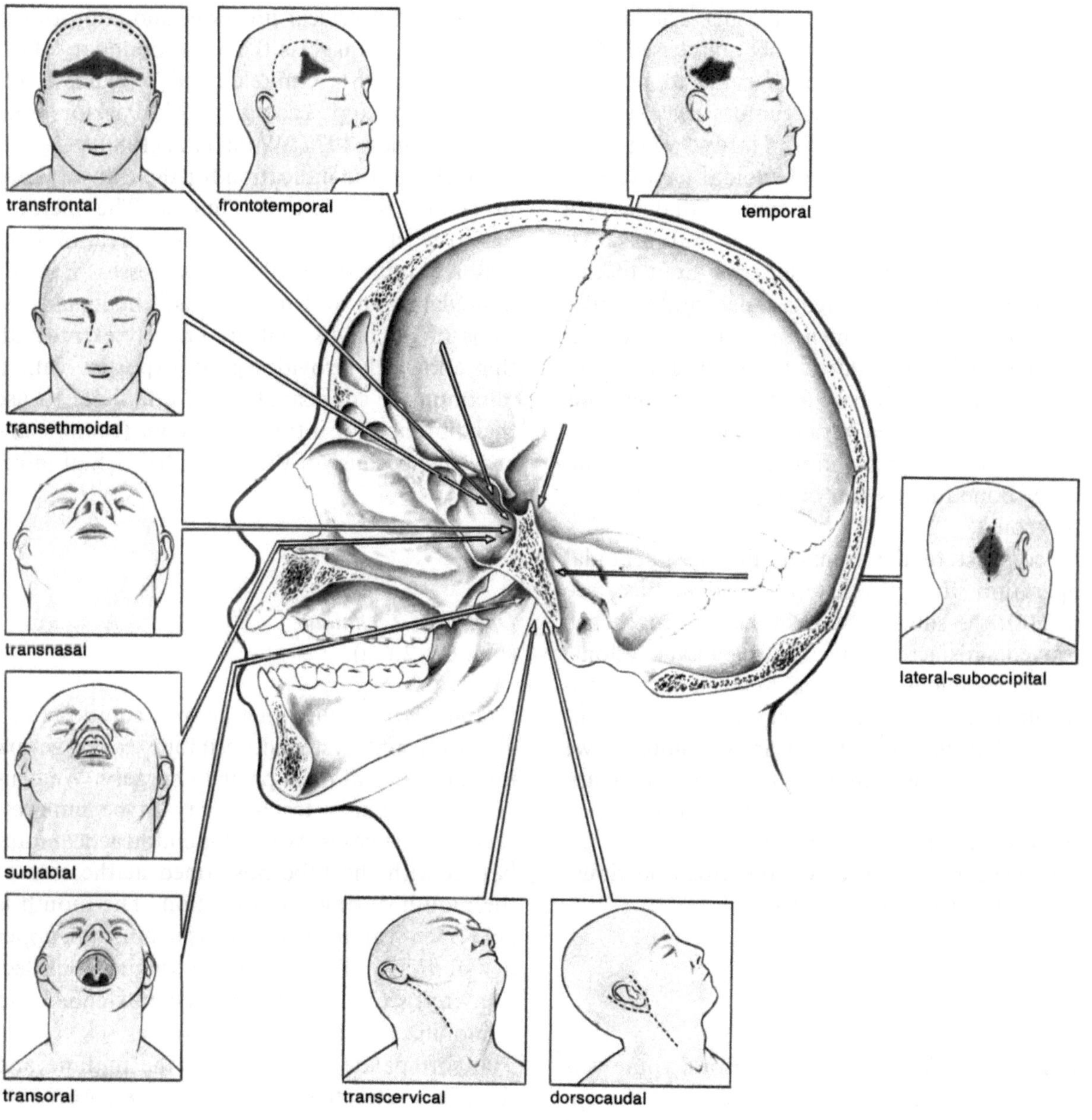

Fig. CL 1. Overview of surgical approaches to the clivus

General Operative Techniques

Extracranial Approaches

Transsphenoidal Approach
(Fig. MS 17a, b)

The transsphenoidal approach was originally developed as a primary extradural approach for the removal of pituitary neoplasms. The historical aspects were previously discussed (see p. 274). Later this approach came to be used for the removal of clivus tumors (Decker and Malis 1970; Derome 1979; Hardy 1977; Rougerie et al. 1967). Transsphenoidal exposure of the clivus is indicated for tumors that involve the clivus as well as the adjacent paranasal sinuses and pharynx. The superior limit of this approach is the diaphragma sellae, and the inferior limit is the foramen magnum. Dissection can be carried laterally as far as the bony limit of the middle skull base (carotid canal, petrous apex, etc.). Besides pituitary tumors, interosseous meningiomas, fibrous dysplasia, and other bone tumors can be approached through this route.

In contrast to the transseptal-transsphenoidal operation for pituitary microadenomas (see p. 274), the sublabial-transseptal approach has proved satisfactory for extensive clivus lesions. It is amenable to extension, and the narrow nasal inlet is not a limiting factor. For clivus tumors that involve the paranasal sinuses, we prefer the transethmoidal-transsphenoidal approach using a standard or extended paranasal rhinotomy incision (see p. 160).

The *operative technique* was described previously in some detail (see p. 160).

Transoral Approach

Introductory Remarks. The transoral route was long used as an orthopedic approach to the upper cervical spine for the treatment of extradural processes such as tuberculosis and osteomas (Fang and Ong 1962). Mullan et al. (1966) showed that surgical removal of an epidural sarcoma also was feasible through the transoral route. Reports followed on the successful clipping of basilar artery aneurysms located in the midline (Drake 1969; Laine et al. 1977; Pia and Lorenz 1980). A lethal infection later caused Drake to abandon this approach, however (Drake 1973, 1978). Most reports on successful operations have concerned extradural processes such as basilar invagination, dens resections, fusions at the C1/C2 or C2/C3 level, anomalies of the craniocervical junction, and chordomas, which may transgress the dural boundary (Delgado et al. 1981; Gutkelch and Williams 1972; Krayenbühl and Yasargil 1975; Pasztor et al. 1984; Verbiest 1977; Wood et al. 1980).

We feel that the indication for the transoral approach for these lesions is limited. The operator has to work through an unsterile area, and access is confined to midline processes. But for limited benign and in rare cases malignant lesions of the clivus that are entirely extradural, this approach provides good exposure with a minimum of surgical stress. We hesitate to use the approach for intradural lesions (tumors, aneurysms) because of the associated risk of infection.

Operative Technique
(Fig. CL 2a–g)

Oral irrigations with an antiseptic solution (e.g., Hexoral) and systemic antibiotic coverage are initiated several days prior to surgery. We consider preliminary tracheotomy to be unnecessary in most cases. We prefer endotracheal intubation with the tube positioned at the side of the mouth during the operation. The mouth is held open with a gag that rests against the upper dental arch and depresses the tongue (tonsillectomy retractor). The head is hyperextended and immobilized in the Mayfield frame.

The soft palate is incised on the midline and the edges retracted with stay sutures. Access to C1 and C2 can be gained by retracting the soft palate with two soft suction catheters that are passed through the nasal cavities, brought out through the mouth, and secured with clamps. The posterior wall of the pharynx is opened with

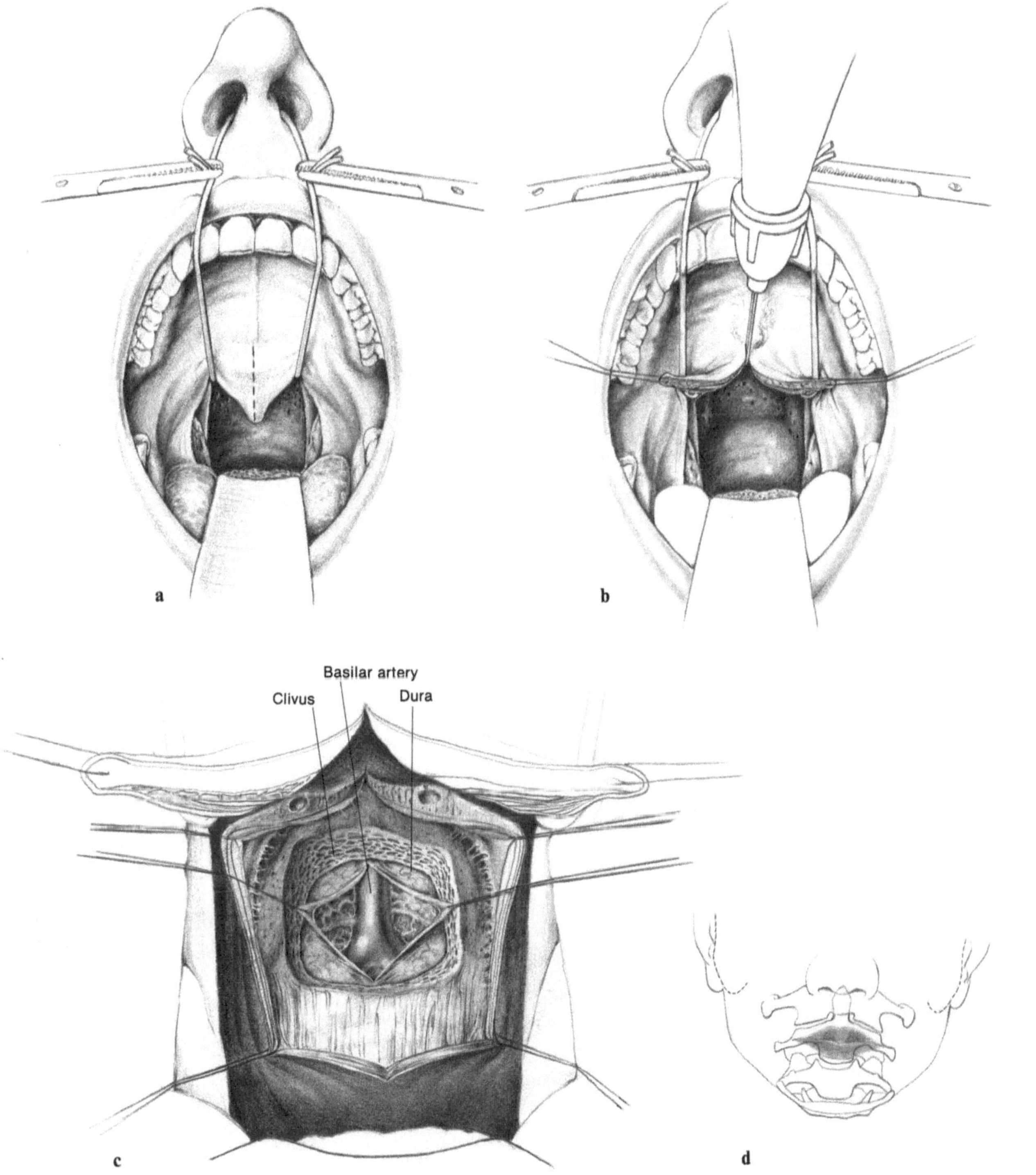

Fig. CL 2a–g. The transoral approach to the clivus.
a Incision of the uvula and soft palate. The blade of the mouth gag depresses the tongue.
b Midline incision of the soft palate
c The soft tissues of the posterior pharyngeal wall are incised on the midline from the roof of the nasopharynx to the arch of the atlas, and the clivus is fenestrated with the diamond burr. Subjacent dura is vertically incised to expose the basilar artery.
d Schematic view: dissection can be carried inferiorly to the level of C3 through the transoral approach

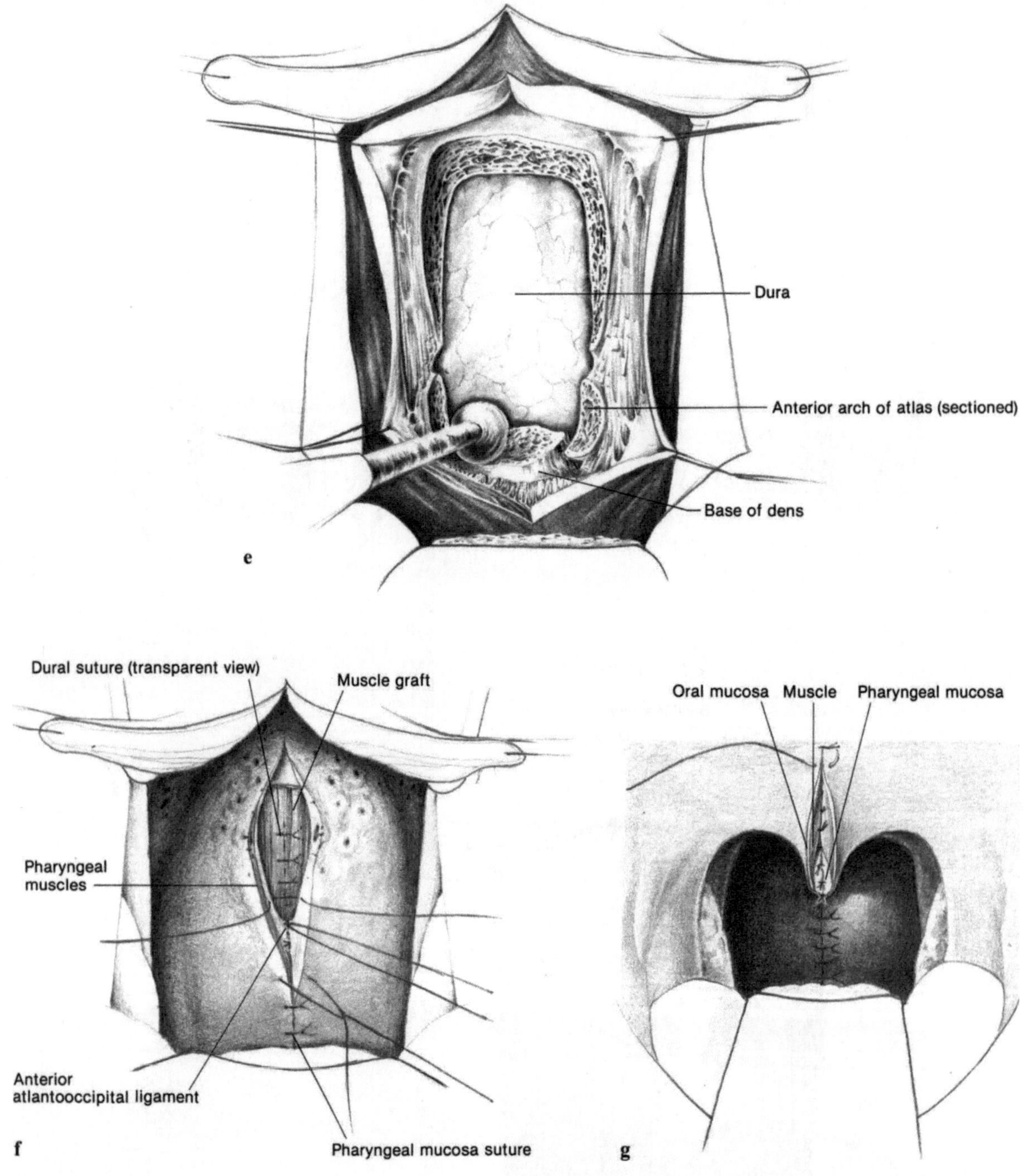

Fig. CL 2e–g.
e Extension of the approach at the craniocervical junction by removing the anterior arch of the atlas and the dens.
f Closure in layers: 1) Dural closure with interrupted sutures. The stiffness and poor mobility of the dura in this area often exclude a primary watertight closure, so the duraplasty (stored dural graft) is reinforced by covering it with free myofascial or fat graft attached with glue. 2) Reapproximation of the pharyngeal muscles including the anterior longitudinal ligament. 3) Closure of the mucosa with simple interrupted sutures.
g The soft palate is closed in three layers (pharyngeal mucosa, muscles, oral mucosa) to avoid dehiscence

a vertical midline incision, which may extend from the pharyngeal roof to C3 depending on the extent of the lesion.

The prevertebral muscles are carefully dissected from the lower clivus, the arch of the atlas, and the anterior surface of C2 on the subperiosteal plane for later use during wound closure. The operating microscope is brought into position, and the arch of the atlas and dens of the axis are drilled away. This will expose the anterior rim of the foramen magnum and the lowermost portion of the clivus. A tumor at this site is removed by enucleation and subsequent resection of its capsule. If the lesion has penetrated the dural boundary, the primary extradural procedure is expanded to an intradural operation, and the dura will be lacking as a protective layer for the vertebral and basilar arteries with their perforating brain stem vessels. It is difficult to achieve a direct dural closure in the small confines of the transoral cavity. Even when there is not a true defect in the dural substance, the incision in the dura, which is quite rigid at the clivus, does not allow for suture well; closure must be effected using muscle, fascia, and fibrin glue. We recommend that lumbar drainage of spinal fluid be maintained for three to four days following dural closure. The pharynx is closed in two layers, and the soft palate is closed in three layers to avoid dehiscence with disturbed phonation. The patient is fed for several days through a soft nasogastric tube, taking care to avoid pressure ulceration of the posterior pharyngeal wall.

Transcervical Approach
(Fig. CL 3a, b)

Introductory Remarks. Stevenson and Stoney in 1966 described the successful transcervical extirpation of a clivus chordoma. The authors desired to profit from the advantages of an oblique anterior approach while avoiding the high infection risk of the transoral procedure. Building on the preliminary work of White and Albin (1962), they performed extensive anatomical studies. Bartal and Heilbronn (1970) likewise removed a clivus chordoma transcervically, while Fox (1967) and Wissinger et al. (1967) successfully used the technique for the clipping of a basilar artery aneurysm.

The indications for transcervical exploration of the clivus and upper cervical spine correspond to those for the transoral approach. However, the transcervical route carries a lower infection risk when incision of the dura is required, because the pharyngeal cavity is not entered. The transcervical route also differs from the transoral in that the clivus is approached at a lower angle and from the side, rather than on the midline.

Operative Technique
(Fig. CL 3a, b)

The head is hyperextended and turned away from the surgeon. The skin incision extends from the mastoid tip along the anterior border of the sternocleidomastoid muscle to the level of the thyroid cartilage. The surgeon divides the superficial cervical fascia in front of the anterior sternocleidomastoid border dissecting between the vascular sheath and thyroid gland or pharyngeal tube toward the vertebral column. In the upper part of the field the superficial jugular vein is ligated, and the hypoglossal nerve crossing the vascular sheath is identified and retracted superolaterally. The inferior thyroid artery marks the inferior limit of the field. After dividing the pharyngeal muscles inserted on the superior horn of the thyroid cartilage and the stylohyoid muscles inserted on the hyoid bone, the surgeon mobilizes the larynx and pharyngeal tube so that these structures can be retracted anteromedially. Care is taken to avoid pressure from the retractor tip on the tracheoesophageal sulcus, which carries the recurrent nerve. The superior thyroid artery, the lingual artery, and if necessary the facial artery are identified along with their origins from the external carotid; they are ligated and divided to improve the access superiorly. The anterior surface of the cervical spine is reached by further dissection, and from that point the approach is easily extended cranially to reach the clivus.

On reaching the craniocervical junction, the surgeon splits the prevertebral fascia in the midline

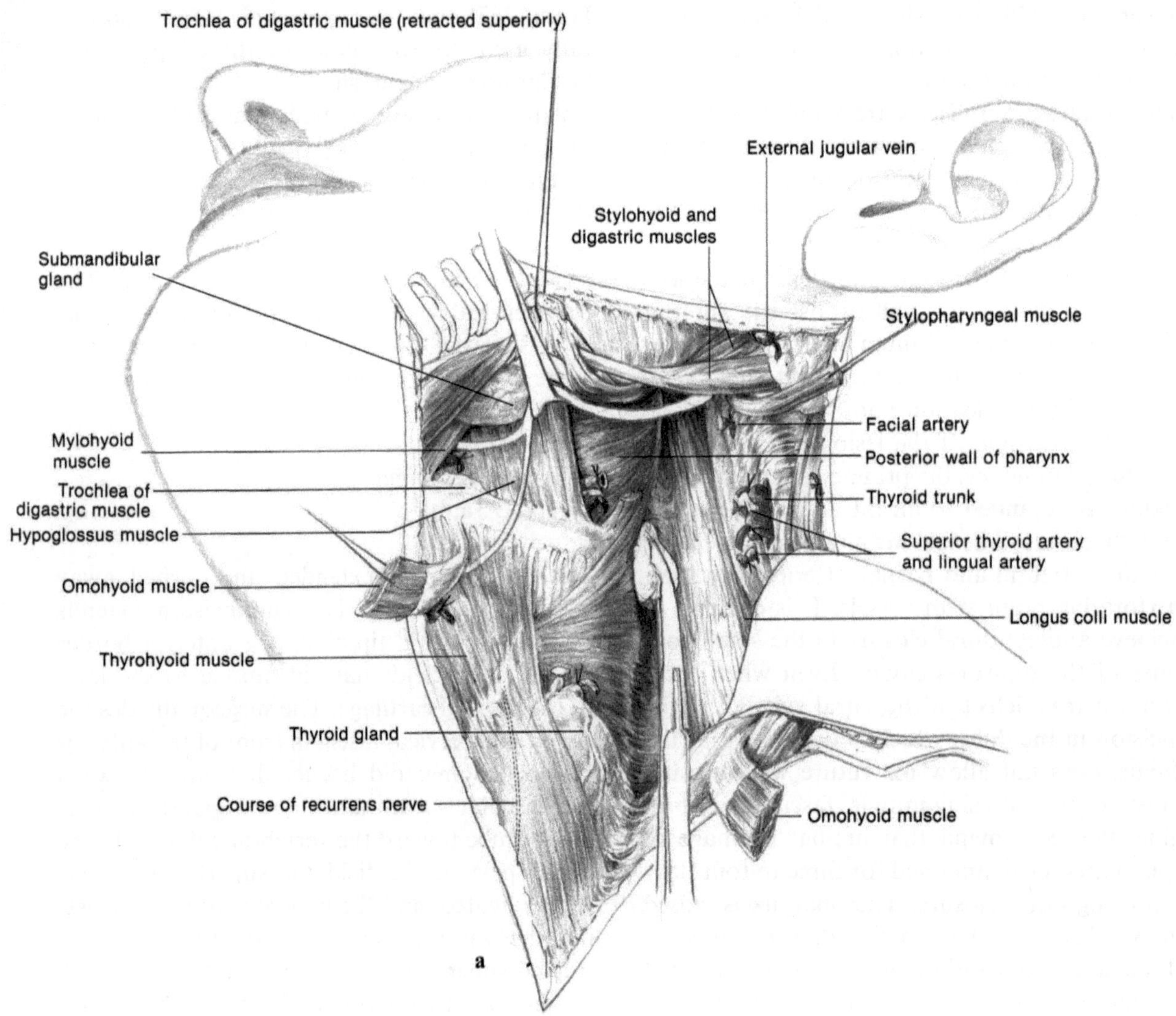

Trochlea of digastric muscle (retracted superiorly)
External jugular vein
Stylohyoid and digastric muscles
Submandibular gland
Stylopharyngeal muscle
Facial artery
Mylohyoid muscle
Posterior wall of pharynx
Trochlea of digastric muscle
Thyroid trunk
Hypoglossus muscle
Superior thyroid artery and lingual artery
Omohyoid muscle
Longus colli muscle
Thyrohyoid muscle
Thyroid gland
Course of recurrens nerve
Omohyoid muscle

a

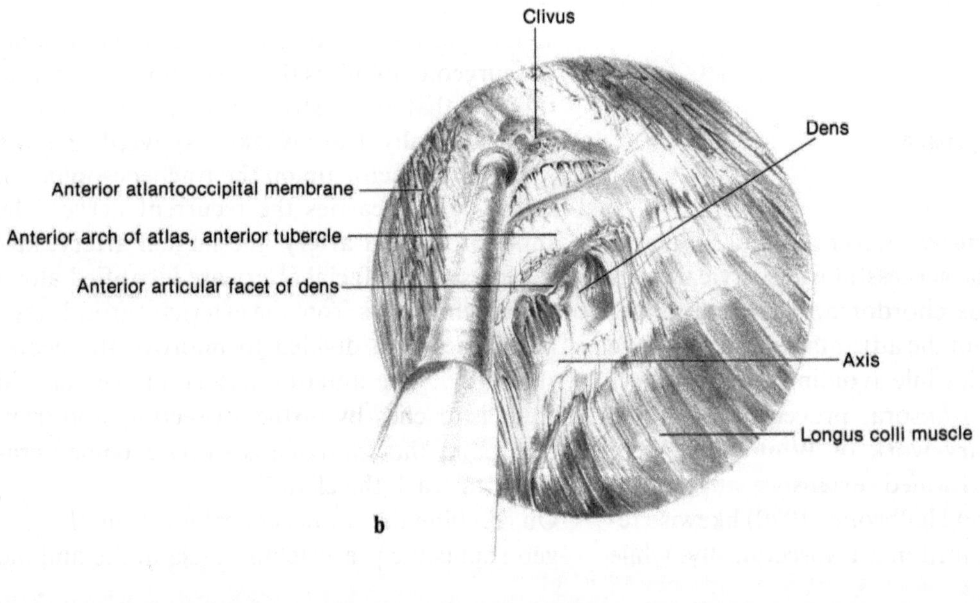

Clivus
Dens
Anterior atlantooccipital membrane
Anterior arch of atlas, anterior tubercle
Anterior articular facet of dens
Axis
Longus colli muscle

b

from the clivus to the level of C3 and then dissects the anterior cervical extensors to the transverse processes on the subperiosteal plane. At this stage the operative field on the outer skull base is bounded laterally by the entry of the internal carotid artery into the carotid canal. Anteriorly, the vomer should be palpable as the posterior component of the nasal septum. The pharyngeal tubercle of the clivus is identified on the midline approximately 2 cm from the anterior rim of the foramen magnum. Laterally, the soft tissues are mobilized as far as the pterygoid process. After the arch of the atlas and the dens have been drilled away, a bony window measuring 2.5 × 3 cm can be cut in the clivus. The limits of the inner skull base are formed by the internal carotid artery, the inferior petrosal sinus, the jugular tubercle medial to the hypoglossal canal, and the spheno-occipital suture. After the tumor has been removed or the aneurysm clipped, the dural defect is filled with muscle pieces and stored dura, and the wound is closed in multiple layers.

It should be noted that partial removal of the arch and dens of C1 and C2 can result in craniocervical instability, which may necessitate a second stabilizing procedure through a posterior approach.

Fig. CL 3a, b. Transcervical approach to the clivus.
a The head is hyperextended and turned to the opposite side. The skin incision extends from the mastoid tip along the anterior border of the sternocleidomastoid to the level of the upper border of the thyroid cartilage. Dissection is carried obliquely and medially in front of the anterior sternocleidomastoid border and vascular package. The superior thryoid artery and lingual artery are ligated (also the facial artery if necessary), and the stylohyoid muscles are divided. Then the hypoglossal nerve, thyroid gland, larynx, cervical esophagus, and pharynx are displaced anteromedially, and the vertebral column and soft-tissue mantle are exposed by blunt dissection. The upper limit of the operative field is formed by the hypoglossal nerve, retracted superiorly, and the lower limit by the inferior thyroid artery. Care is taken to avoid retractor injury to the recurrens nerve in the tracheoesophageal sulcus; it is not necessary to expose this nerve.
b The anterior arch of the atlas and the clivus are visualized. Both these structures and the dens are removed with the diamond burr to expose the dura of the posterior cranial fossa

Acute paraplegia with life-threatening complications is possible. If it occurs, it will usually do so during the interval between the successful clivus operation and the planned secondary cervical stabilization procedure (Bartal + Heilbronn 1970; DiLorenzo et al. 1982).

The operating microscope is routinely used for drilling away the arch of C1 and for the rest of the operation, so the depth of the field should not present serious difficulties.

Lateral Infratemporal Approach
(Fig. MS 4a–c, Fig. MS 32a, b)

The lateral part of the middle skull base can be widely exposed through this approach as far as the clivus. It involves removal of the zygomatic arch and may include partial mandibulectomy. This approach is indicated for clivus tumors that involve the skull base from below and whose main mass is in the infratemporal fossa, such as extensive tumors of the parotid gland, extensive soft-tissue tumors, etc. (see p. 300).

Posteroinferior Approach
(Fig. MS 33a–h, Fig. PS 35a–e)

The extracranial posteroinferior approach gives posterior access to the middle skull base between the mastoid process, the base of the zygomatic arch, and the condylar process of the mandible. It may involve opening the middle ear space, mastoidectomy, and removal of the styloid process. The pterygoid fossa and clivus can be reached by performing a mandibular condylectomy or marginal mandibulectomy. This approach is indicated for tumors in the area of the jugular foramen and carotid canal, such as neuromas or glomus tumors. Often mandibular resection is not required. An advantage of this approach is that it permits extension of the skull base resection back to the posterior cranial fossa for tumors at the junction of the middle and posterior fossae.

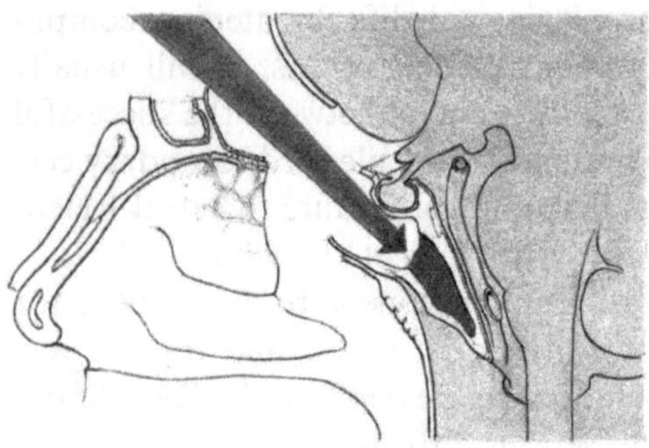

a

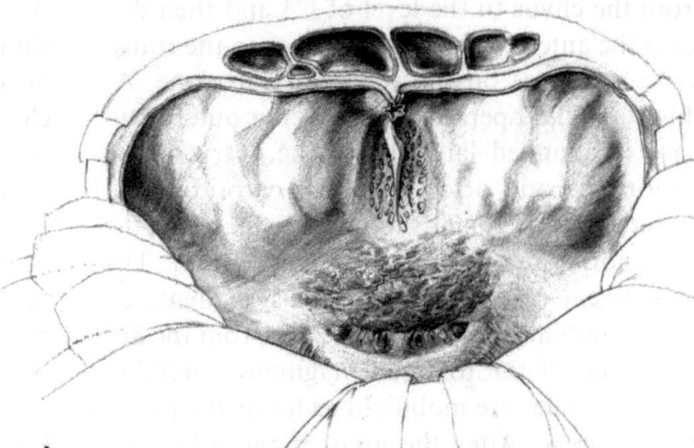

b

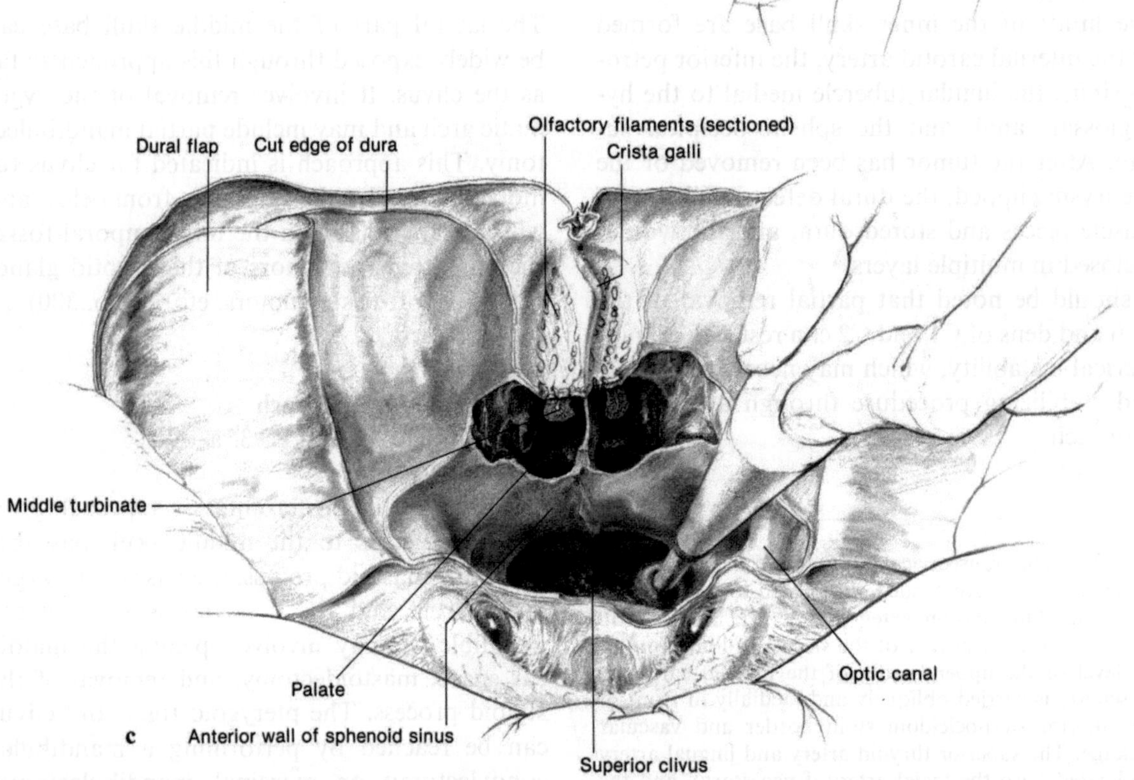

c

Fig. CL 4a–c. Transfrontal intradural approach to the clivus.
a Schematic lateral view of the route of approach.
b After bifrontal osteoplastic craniotomy and ligation of the superior sagittal sinus, the anterior skull base is exposed intradurally on both sides. The optic nerves and chiasm are visualized.
c After excision of the tumor-involved dura, bilateral dural flaps are created for later use as a viable tissue lining for the skull base. The middle and posterior ethmoid cells are exenterated, and the clivus is reached anterior to the sella through the widely opened sphenoid sinus. The optic canals can be exposed at this time for decompression of the optic nerves

Intracranial Approaches to the Clivus

Transfrontal Approach

(Fig. AS 21a, b, Fig. AS 22a, b, Fig. AS 37, 38, Fig. CL 4a–c)

The essentials of the transfrontal approach to the anterior skull base and its technical details were previously described (see p. 141). The transfrontal approach may be extradural or intradural, depending on the site of origin and maximal extent of the lesion. When the clivus is approached transfrontally, part of the operation is extracranial and involves clearing the posterior paranasal sinuses of tumor. After resection of the planum sphenoidale and part of the anterior wall of the sella, the clivus can be reached in continuity with the sphenoid sinus floor and cleared of disease almost to the rim of the foramen magnum.

The advantage of the transcranial approach to the clivus through the anterior skull base is that it can be extended to give access to all nearby intra- and extradural structures of importance, including the orbits, the lesser sphenoid wings (to the anterior clinoid processes), and the paranasal sinuses. In the middle skull base area, the internal carotid artery and the petrous apex can be reached laterally from the sphenoid sinus. The case presentations (Fig. AS 48a–r, Fig. MS 27a–e, see p. 289) illustrate the possibilities of this approach.

Frontotemporal, Subtemporal Approach to the Clivus

(Fig. MS 35a–h)

Yasargil (1976) recommended the standard frontotemporal approach for aneurysms of the carotid system and basilar bifurcation, and he has successfully used that approach in a slightly modified form for the removal of clivus meningiomas (Yasargil et al. 1980). Symon (1982) states that this approach is suitable for basilar bifurcation aneurysms in experienced hands but considers it too limiting for mass lesions of the superior clivus. Instead, he recommends an anterior temporal approach with resection of the temporal pole. Drake (1973) prefers the subtemporal approach which we have expanded. Essential elements are incision of the tentorium, coagulation and division of the superior petrosal sinus, and apical petrosectomy. Details were presented earlier. The possibilities of this approach are illustrated by case reports of petroclival meningiomas (see Fig. MS 48a–f, MS 49a–f, MS 50a–c) and by Figs. CL 5a f and CL 6a–f.

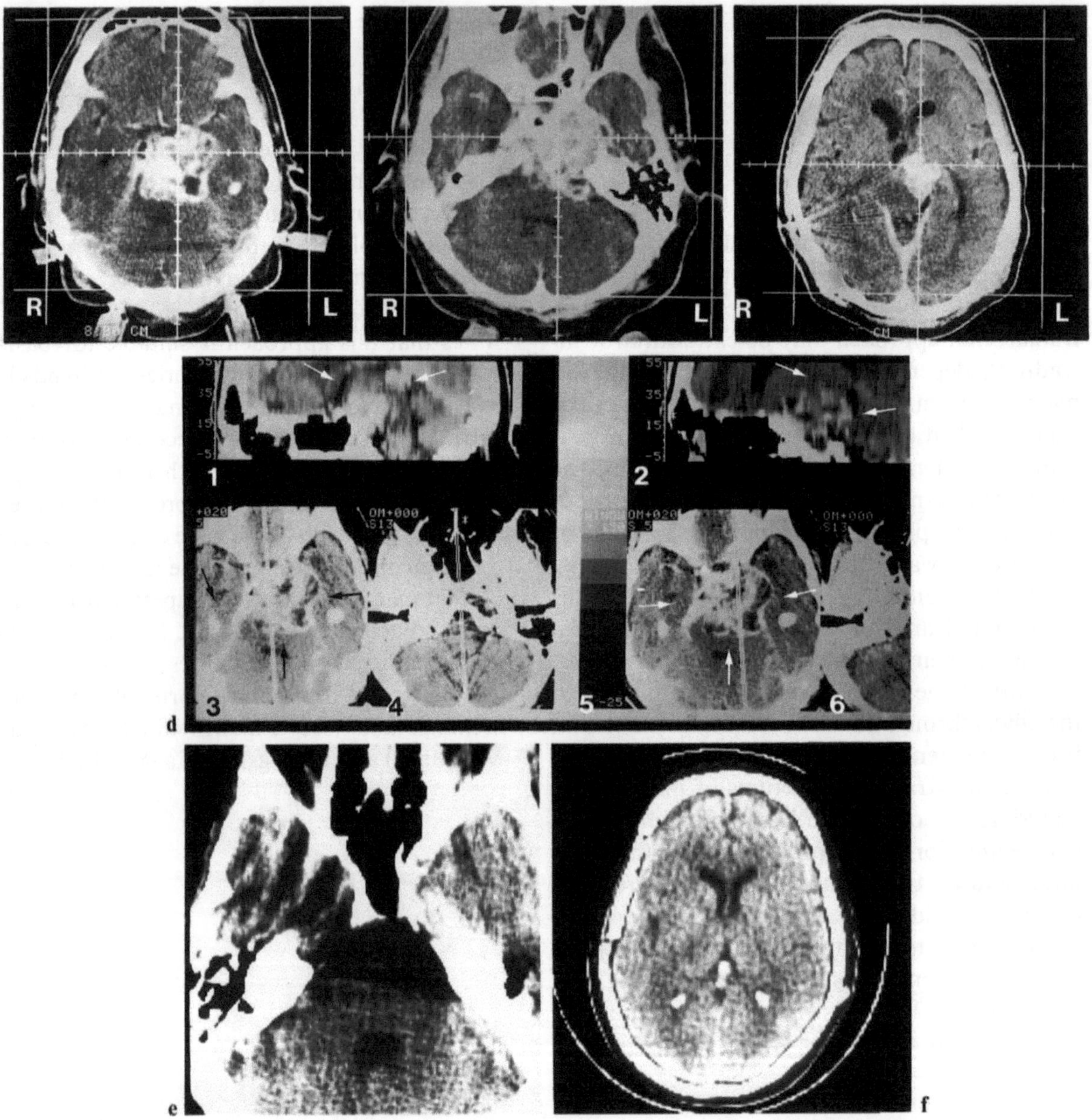

a, b c d e f

Fig. CL 5a–f. Extensive, predominantly right-sided meningioma of the middle and posterior cranial fossae in a 50-year-old man with left hemiparesis, trigeminal neuropathy, and a progressive psycho-organic syndrome. The tumor was totally removed through a right frontotemporal, transtentorial approach.

a–d Preoperative CT scans show the horizontal and vertical tumor extent with elevation of the brain stem and displacement of the third ventricle.

e, f Postoperative scans confirm total removal

a b c

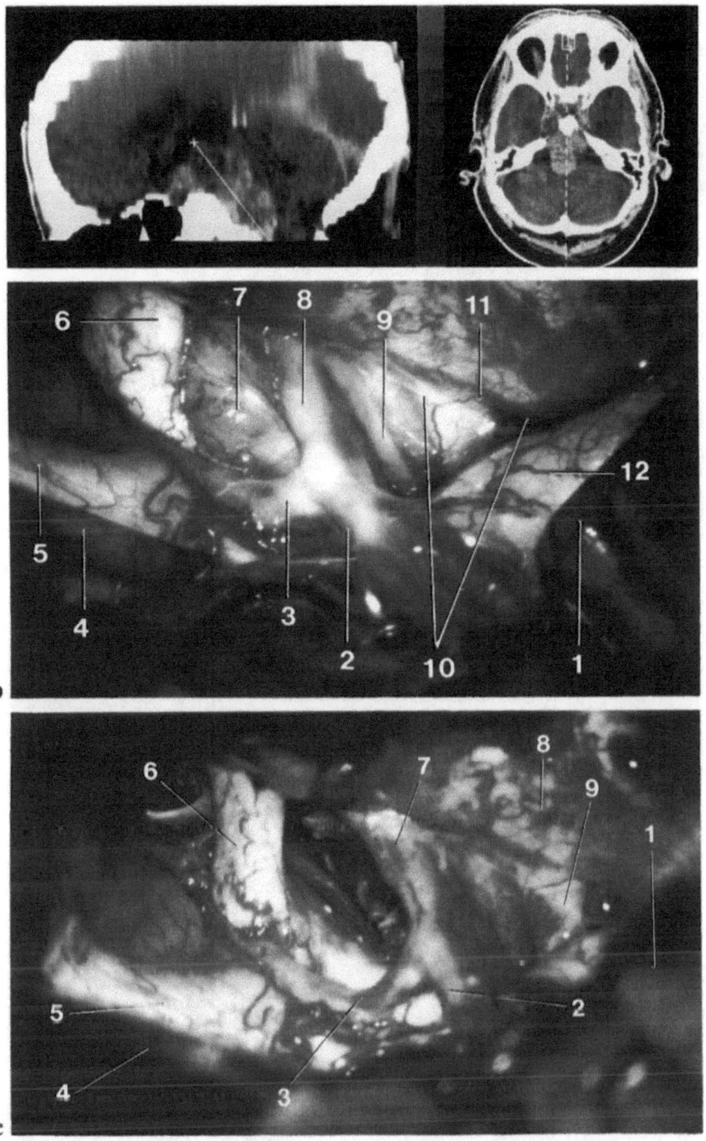

Fig. CL 6a–f. Supra- and infratentorial chordoma of the clivus and sellar region in a 55-year-old man whose major complaints were right hemiplegia, swallowing difficulties, and diplopia. Neurologic symptoms included papilledema and multiple cranial nerve deficits (VI, VII, IX, X, XI). He had bilateral pyramidal tract signs, more pronounced on the right side than on the left. The tumor was completely removed through a right frontotemporal approach.
a Axial CT scan and midsagittal reconstruction demonstrate a large clivus chordoma with suprasellar extension and compression of the third ventricle. The tumor has grown into the interpeduncular and prepontine cisterns.
b Through a frontotemporal craniotomy the dura was incised, the sylvian fissure was opened, and the frontal and temporal lobes were separated to expose the tumor and surrounding neurovascular structures along the minor sphenoid wing. (*1*) Posterior brain spatula, (*2*) middle cerebral artery, (*3*) anterior cerebral artery, (*4*) anterior brain spatula, (*5*) frontal lobe, (*6*) optic nerve, (*7*) suprasellar tumor component, (*8*) internal carotid artery, (*9*) posterior communicating artery, (*10*) tentorial margin, (*11*) oculomotor nerve, (*12*) temporal lobe.
c Surgical anatomy after removal of the suprasellar tumor component. (*1*) Posterior brain spatula, (*2*) middle cerebral artery, (*3*) anterior cerebral artery, (*4*) anterior brain spatula, (*5*) frontal lobe, (*6*) optic nerve, (*7*) internal carotid artery, (*8*) tentorial margin, (*9*) oculomotor nerve

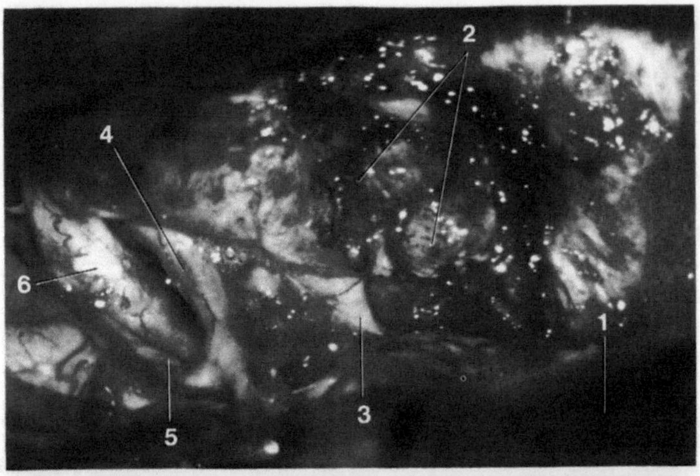

d

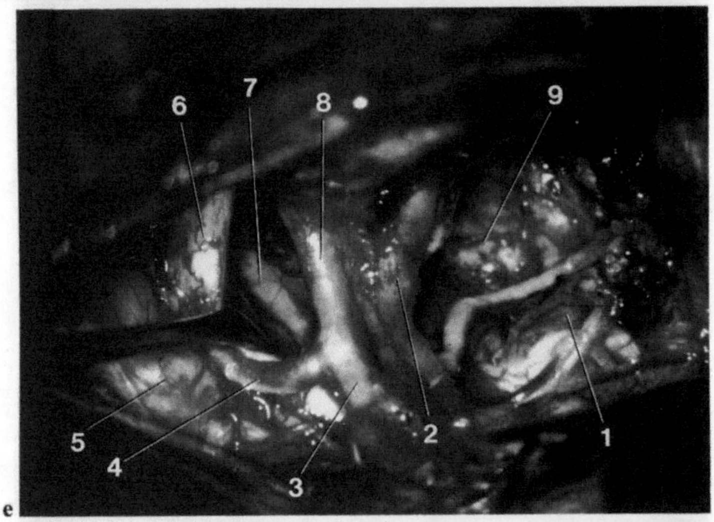

e

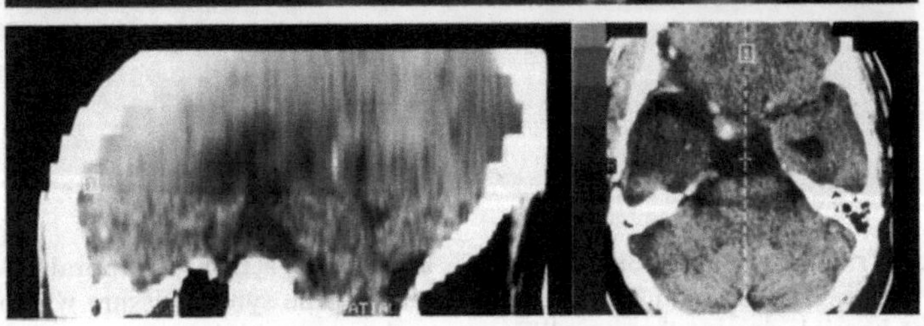

f

Fig. CL 6d–f.
d Extension of the operative field posteriorly. The tentorium is incised perpendicular to the petrous ridge behind the oculomotor nerve and is coagulated to gain access to the infratentorial tumor component. (*1*) Posterior brain spatula, (*2*) tumor, (*3*) oculomotor nerve, (*4*) internal carotid artery, (*5*) anterior cerebral artery, (*6*) optic nerve.

e View of the operative field after total removal of the suprasellar (*left*) and infratentorial (*right*) portions of the tumor. (*1*) Posterior cerebral artery, (*2*) oculomotor nerve, (*3*) middle cerebral artery, (*4*) anterior cerebral artery, (*5*) frontal lobe, (*6*) right optic nerve, (*7*) left optic nerve, (*8*) internal carotid artery, (*9*) brain stem.
f CT scan following complete tumor removal

Lateral Suboccipital Approach to the Clivus

In the early days of neurosurgery, it was common for surgeons to open the posterior cranial fossa bilaterally and extensively to achieve maximum decompression of inoperable cases or to obtain maximum freedom of movement, given the limitations of preoperative diagnosis (Cushing 1917). With later improvements in diagnostic and surgical techniques, the unilateral suboccipital approach was devised chiefly for the removal of cerebellopontine angle tumors (Dandy 1925). The development of modern anesthesia, microneurosurgery, and sophisticated imaging procedures (CT, MRI) has changed the panorama considerably. Today we are able to remove pathologic processes radically and atraumatically, without time pressure. We prefer the lateral suboccipital approach for clivus tumors that extend posteriorly to the cerebellopontine angle, displacing the brain stem posteriorly, laterally and superiorly. The tumor enlarges the narrow space between the cerebellopontine angle and clivus along the brain stem, making it possible to gain access to the clivus via the cerebellopontine angle without destroying important structures. This route is less suitable for clivus tumors that have grown laterally upward into the middle cranial fossa across the tentorial plane. It should be noted that some elevation of the tentorium is not a contraindication, but actually makes it easier to identify the subtentorial structures. It should be possible to visualize and preserve cranial nerves III–XII on the ipsilateral side while tumor debulking is carried out. The elevation of the brain stem and enlargement of the prepontine space also make it easier to identify and preserve the cranial nerves III–V on the contralateral side. Similarly, the vertebrobasilar vascular system can be visualized as far as the posterior communicating branch of the circle of Willis. This is an important advantage in terms of reducing postoperative morbidity.

The neural structures that course across the cerebellopontine angle define three surgical "corridors" for dissection in the clivus. The anterior rim of the foramen magnum and the inferior third of the clivus are reached by dissecting below the caudal cranial nerves after removal of the jugular tubercle (Fig. CL 8a–i). Another corridor exists between the vestibulocochlear nerve and the caudal cranial nerves and can be used to approach the middle clivus. Higher portions of the tumor are removed by dissecting between the vestibulocochlear nerve and trigeminal nerve. Finally, elevation of the tentorium by the neoplasm creates a sizable gap between the tentorium and trigeminal nerve that can be utilized for access to the tentorial incisure (Fig. CL 7a–i). This gap can be further enlarged by incising the tentorial margin laterally from its inferior aspect.

Some clivus tumors enlarge the tentorial incisure and expand the access to the cerebellopontine angle, and these tumors can be approached and completely removed through either the modified temporal intradural route or the lateral suboccipital route. In these cases we favor the lateral suboccipital technique on the side of the dominant hemisphere so that from the outset we can avoid damage to the temporal lobe with associated post operative speech disturbance.

The technique of the lateral suboccipital approach was previously described (see Fig. PS 1a, b, Fig. PS 16a–c, Fig. PS 20a–c).

Case Report. Chordoma of the middle and posterior cranial fossae (Fig. CL 8a–i). A girl 15 years of age first complained of severe headaches 2 years prior to operation. At that time she was diagnosed as having encephalitis, and her headaches ceased after 4 weeks' hospitalization. Two years later the headaches returned, accompanied by diplopia, paresthesias in the limbs, and imbalance. Initial cranial CT examination performed elsewhere was negative, but later scans showed an extensive mass lesion of the middle and posterior cranial fossae, predominantly on the right side. Stereotaxic needle biopsy identified the lesion as a chordoma. The patient was referred to us to be evaluated for operative treatment.

On admission the girl manifested an increasing tetraparesis with an unsteady gait and caudal cranial nerve deficits on the right side. A further neuroradiologic evaluation that included MRI showed an extensive, invasive mass lesion in the

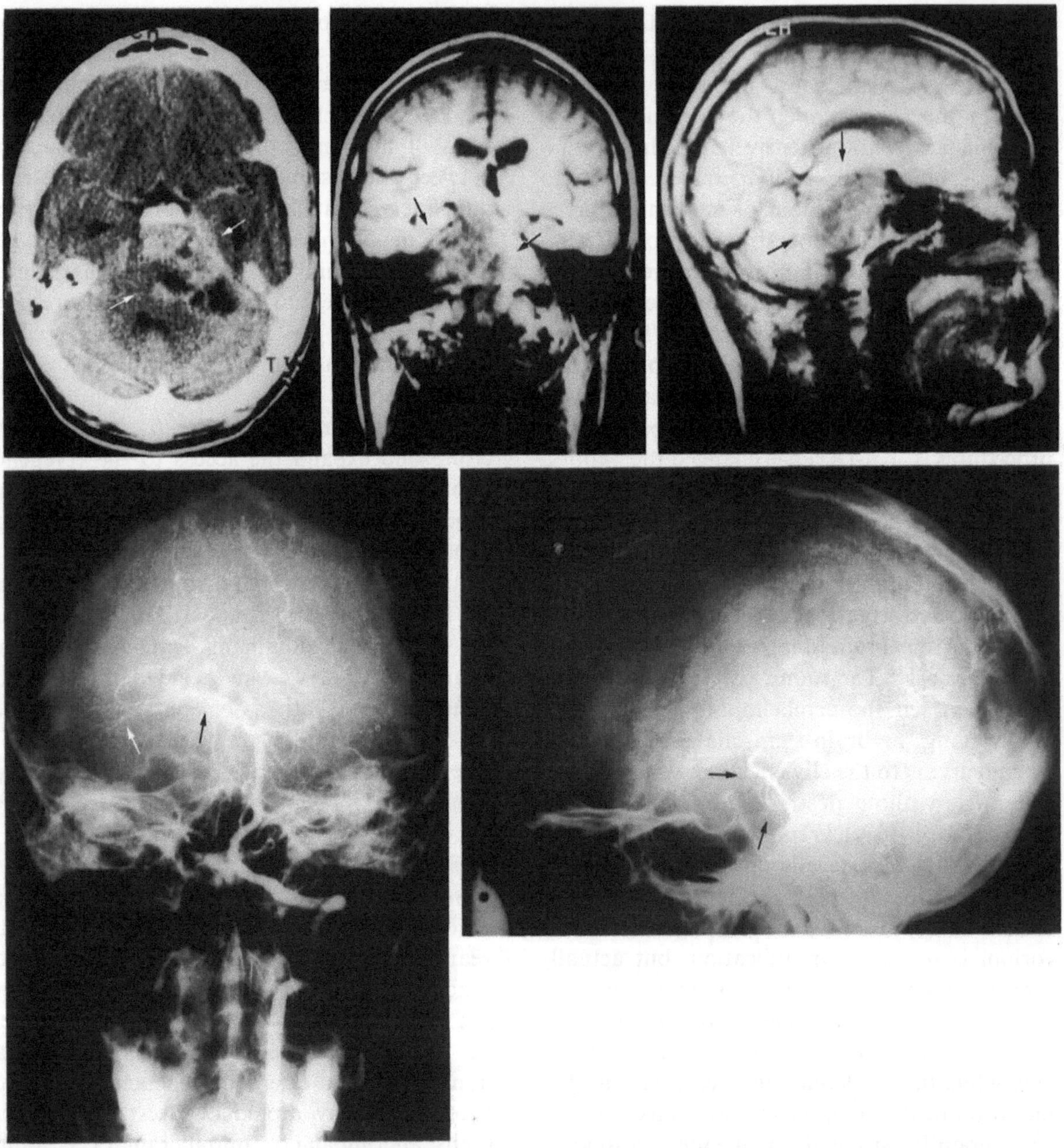

a, b c

d e

Fig. CL 7 a–i. Extensive neuroma arising from the trigeminal nerve and showing predominantly infratentorial extension from the clivus to the right cerebellopontine angle.

a Axial CT shows a partially cystic mass filling the prepontine space, displacing the brain stem posterolaterally, and extending into the cerebellopontine angle.

b Coronal MRI scan shows pronounced displacement of the brain stem and elevation of the third ventricle.

c Sagittal MRI scan shows the AP tumor extension and the displacement of brain-stem structures from the floor of the third ventricle through the cerebral aqueduct to the fourth ventricle.

d Left AP vertebral angiogram shows a displacement of the basilar artery toward the side opposite the tumor and an upward deflection of the posterior cerebral and superior cerebellar arteries.

e Lateral vertebral angiogram shows upward arching and posterior displacement of the basilar artery.

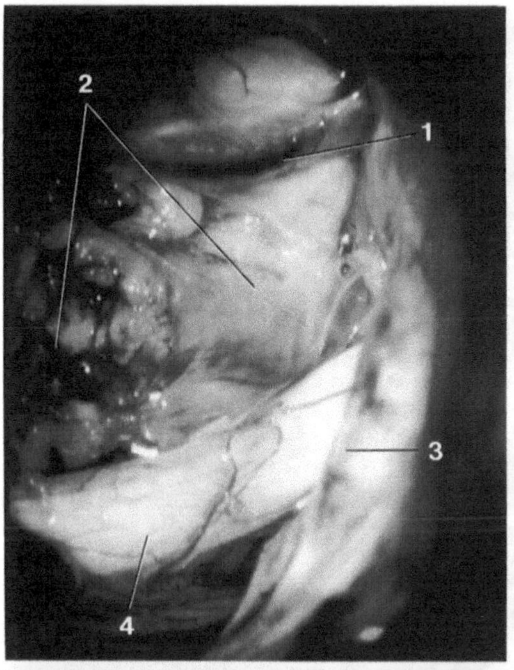

f

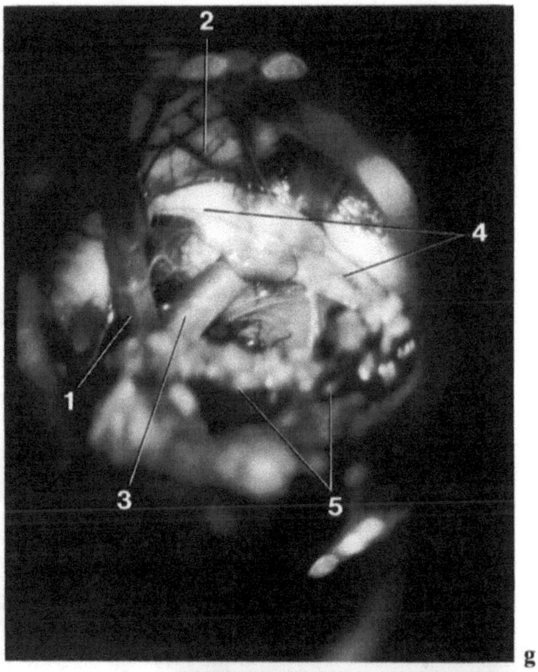

g

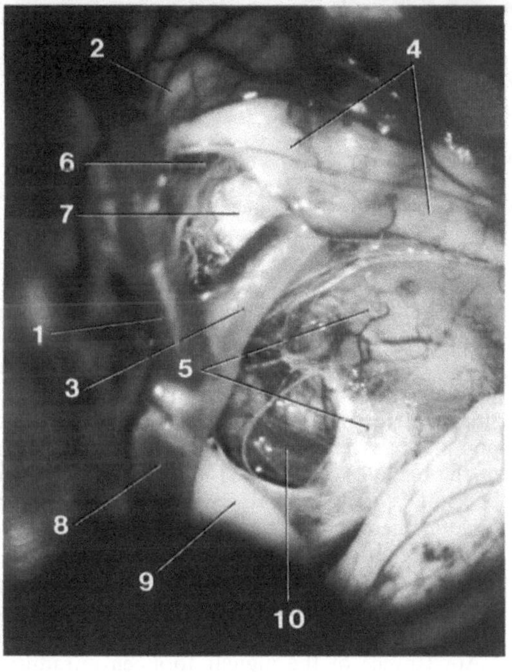

h

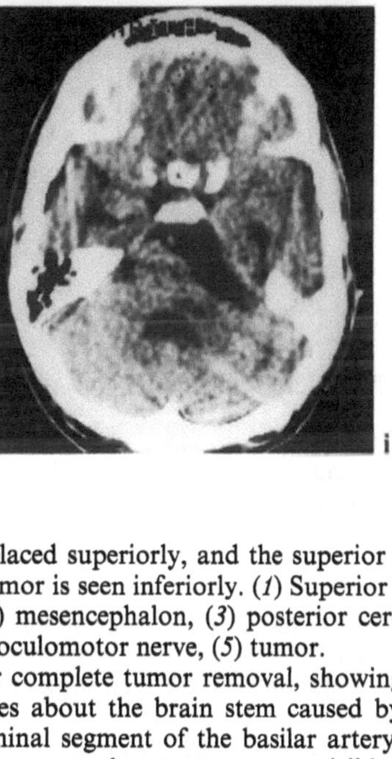

i

Fig. CL 7f–i.
f Surgical field following lateral suboccipital exposure of the cerebellopontine angle. The field is bounded inferiorly by the vestibulocochlear nerve. The petrosal vein courses superiorly, and below it is the large tumor, whose capsule has been incised. The porus of the internal auditory canal is visible. (*1*) Petrosal vein, (*2*) tumor, (*3*) porus acusticus, (*4*) vestibulocochlear nerve.
g View toward the tentorial incisure and brain stem after removal of the superior tumor component. The brain stem has been identified and elevated. The flattened oculomotor nerve appears between the posterior cerebral artery, also displaced superiorly, and the superior cerebellar artery. Tumor is seen inferiorly. (*1*) Superior cerebellar artery, (*2*) mesencephalon, (*3*) posterior cerebral artery, (*4*) right oculomotor nerve, (*5*) tumor.
h The field after complete tumor removal, showing the anatomic changes about the brain stem caused by the tumor. The terminal segment of the basilar artery and the ipsilateral neurovascular structures are visible, and on the opposite side the interpeduncular cistern and the superior cerebellar artery, trigeminal nerve, and left oculomotor nerve are visible through the prepontine space. (*1*) Right superior cerebellar artery, (*2*) mesencephalon, (*3*) right posterior cerebral artery, (*4*) right oculomotor nerve, (*5*) arachnoid, (*6*) left posterior cerebral artery, (*7*) left oculomotor nerve, (*8*) basilar artery, (*9*) left trigeminal nerve, (*10*) left superior cerebellar artery.
i Postoperative CT scan: The tumor is completely removed. The residual cavity with the basilar artery appears as a low-density zone from the clivus to the cerebellopontine angle

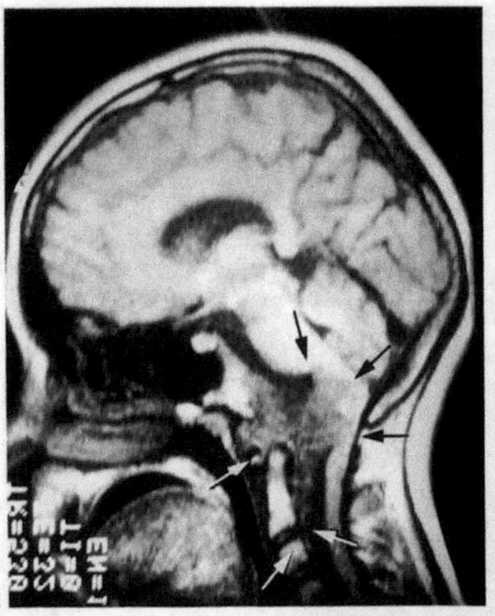

a

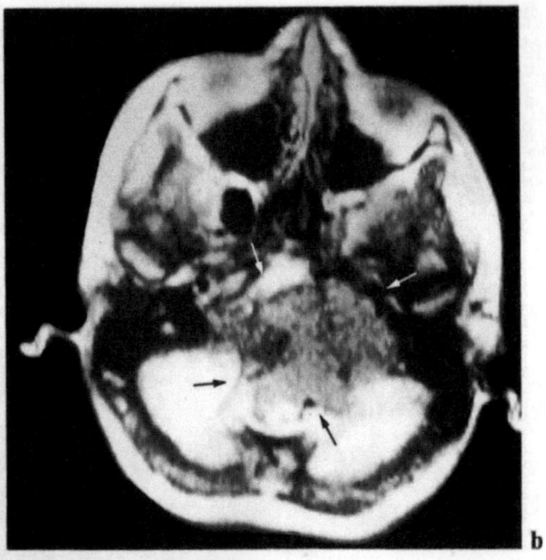

b

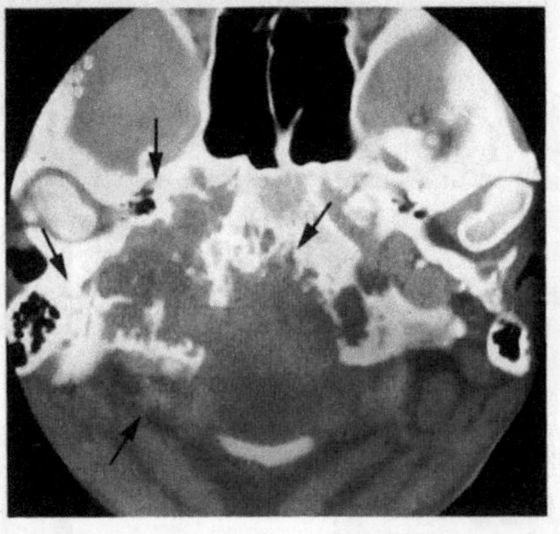

c

Fig. CL 8a–i. Predominantly left-sided chordoma of the middle and posterior cranial fossae. The tumor was totally removed through an extended left lateral suboccipital approach.
a Sagittal MRI scan, close to the midline, shows the tumor extent, the destruction of the lower clivus and anterior arch of C1, and the considerable compression of the brain stem and cord. The tumor extends through the spinal canal to the superior border of C3 (*arrows*).
b Axial MRI scan showing the tumor extent on the horizontal plane and in the posterior and middle cranial fossae (*arrows*).
c High-resolution axial CT scan shows the extreme bony destruction of the middle and posterior fossae, especially of the clivus and both petrous bones (*arrows*).
d The posterior fossa and craniocervical junction were exposed through an extended right-sided lateral suboccipital craniectomy. The relation of the posterior tumor component to the neurovascular structures of the craniocervical junction is demonstrated. (*1*) Medial dural margin, (*2*) tonsil of cerebellum, (*3*) vertebral artery, (*4*) tumor, (*5*) accessory nerve, (*6*) jugular tubercle, (*7*) dentate ligament, (*8*) C1 spinal root, (*9*) spinal cord.
e Operative field after removal of the intradural parts of the tumor. The medulla oblongata and cord are decompressed, and all major neurovascular structures are intact. Note the thinning of the spinal cord by prolonged tumor compression (*arrows*) and the expansion of the small cleft between the cerebellopontine angle and prepontine space caused by cord displacement and elevation of the medulla oblongata. This expansion provides suboccipital surgical access to the clivus region and petrous bone of the opposite side. (*1*) Medial cut edge of dura, (*2*) cerebellum, (*3*) medulla oblongata with perforating vessels, (*4*) lateral dural margin, (*5*) vertebral artery, (*6*) tumor in spinal canal, (*7*) cervical cord, (*8*) posterior inferior cerebellar artery, (*9*) accessory nerve.
f Appearance of the jugular foramen intradurally and extradurally after removal of the extradural tumor component in the petrous bone. The jugular tubercle has been removed. (*1*) Medial dural margin, (*2*) cerebellum, (*3*) jugular foramen, (*4*) glossopharyngeal nerve, (*5*) vagus nerve, (*6*) accessory nerve, (*7*) extradural lateral tumor resection cavity, (*8*) posterior inferior cerebellar artery, (*9*) cervical cord

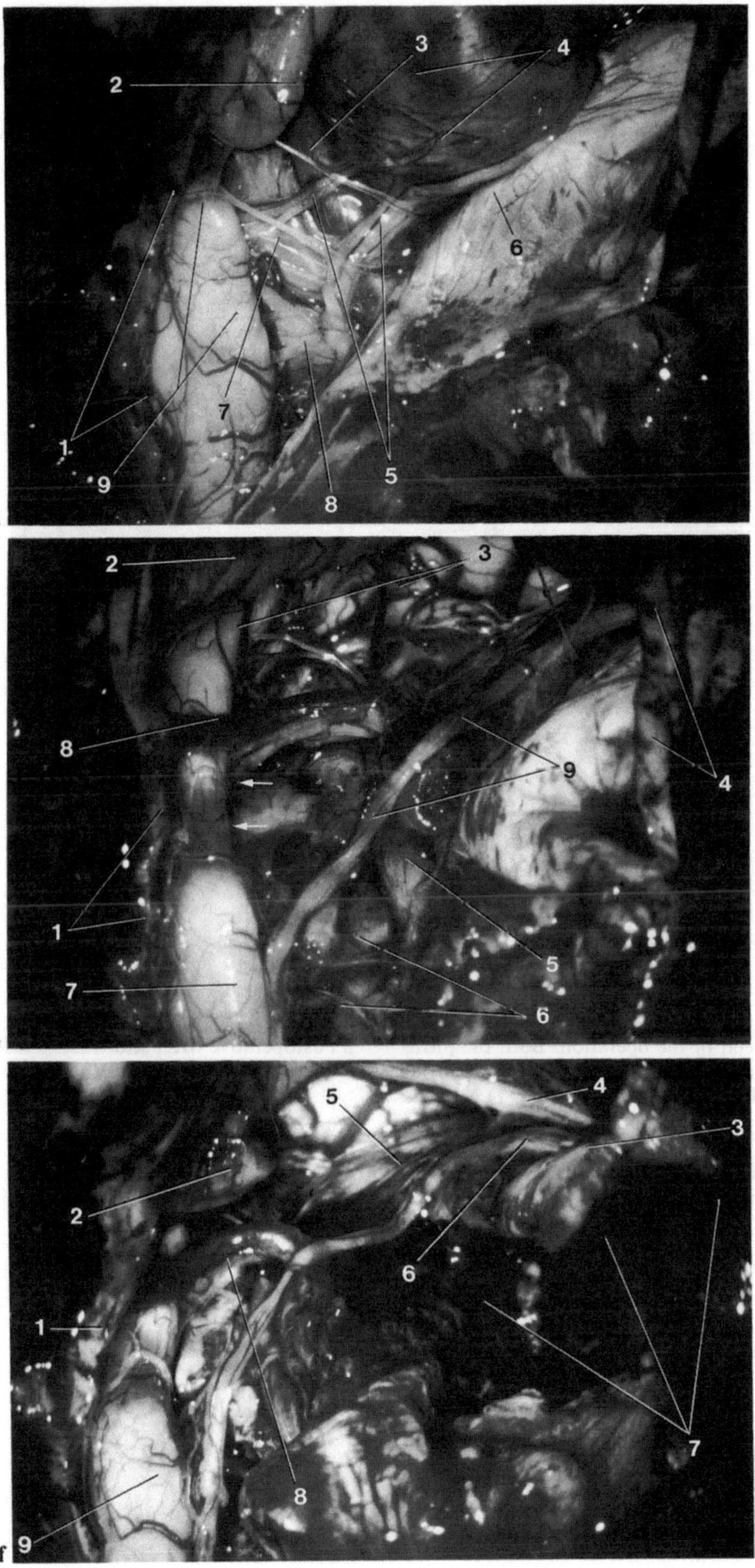

d e f

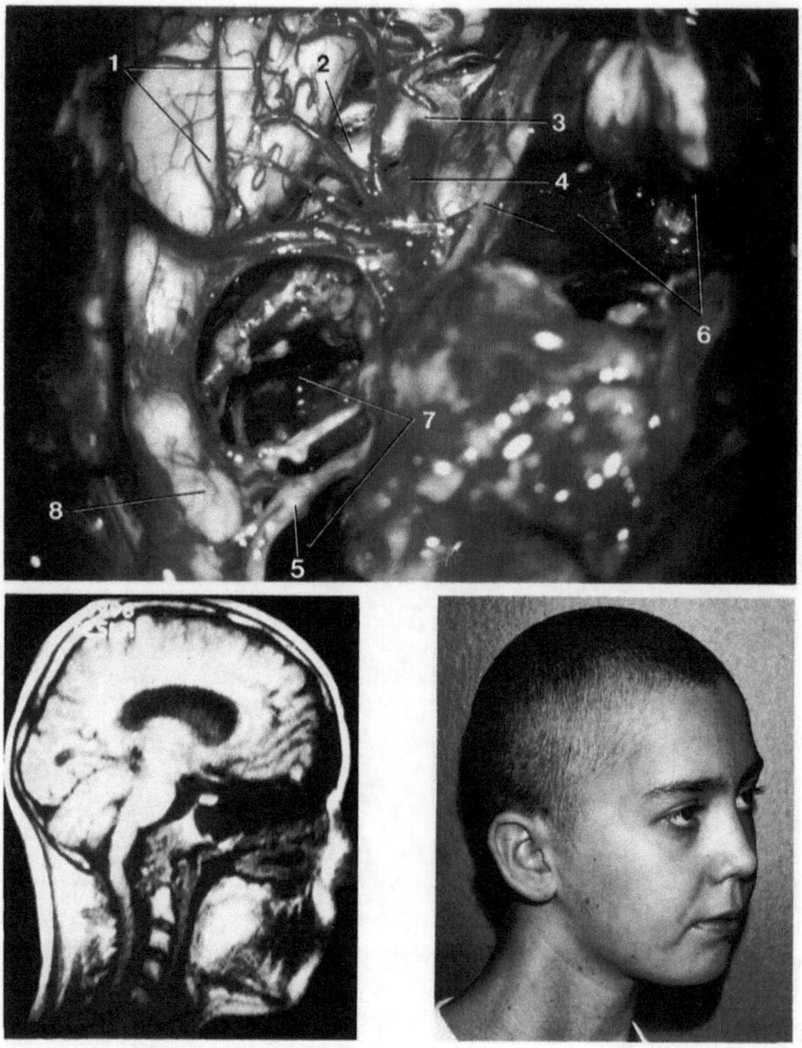

g

h

i

Fig. CL 8g–i.
g The field at the end of the operation. Both the intradural and extradural tumor components in the petrous bone and on the clivus have been removed. (*1*) Medulla oblongata with perforating rami, (*2*) left vertebral artery, (*3*) basilar artery, (*4*) right vertebral artery, (*5*) accessory nerve, (*6*) extradural tumor cavity in the petrous bone, (*7*) extradural tumor cavity at the craniocervical junction, (*8*) cervical cord.

h Postoperative MRI scan.
i The patient 14 days after surgery

region of the clivus, which extended down into the spinal canal to about the inferior border of C2 and was causing marked compression of the medulla and brain stem from the anterior side. Infiltration of the brain stem could not be excluded. The tumor extended forward to the posterior wall of the pharynx. There was destruction of the clivus, the anterior and lateral portions of the foramen magnum, and the right petrous bone. The fourth ventricle appeared compressed.

Starting from the vertical skin incision between the mastoid and midline, we performed a standard extended craniectomy of the right posterior fossa with exposure of the C1 and C2 arches. The arch of the atlas was removed on the right side to the midline. The craniectomy opening extended laterally to the mastoid and medially to the midline. The dura was opened with a curved incision and reflected down to C2. At that point the posterior surface of the tumor was visible in the foramen magnum. The spinal cord appeared thinned and was markedly constricted at the foramen magnum. The dentate ligament and the first cervical nerve root were sectioned on the right side. This enabled us to achieve more room and improve access to the inferior part of the tumor. The accessory nerve was displaced posterosuperiorly by the tumor and was adherent to it. We dissected the nerve free, opened the tumor capsule, and enucleated the tumor piecemeal to decompress the brain stem. The vertebral artery also was compressed and enveloped by the lesion, and we were able progressively to clear it of tumor. The tumor was well demarcated from the brain stem, caudal cranial nerves, vertebral artery, and basilar artery and could be removed piecemeal without much difficulty. Removal of the tumor on the right side gave us an unobstructed view of the left side anterior to the pons, and we proceeded to remove the tumor component in that area. Most of the dura of the clivus had to be sacrificed. Afterward we were able to remove the anterior part of the tumor at the arch of the atlas, at the dens, and at the inferior two-thirds of the clivus. The spinal extension also was removed with the surrounding dura. At that point we could see the elevated brain stem with the left vertebral artery and all the brain stem vessels arising from it. Removal of the tumor at the clivus and craniocervical junction created a huge cavity between the surface of the brain stem and the skull base. Removal of the jugular tubercle created a wide, lateral epidural access to the petrous bone and jugular foramen; this enabled us to remove the tumor in that area, which contained multiple bony septa. We were thus able to effect total gross removal of the extensive skull base tumor through a unilateral lateral suboccipital approach involving removal of the jugular tubercle and portions of the petrous bone and arch of the atlas on the right side. The petrous defect was obliterated with a piece of muscle attached with fibrin glue, then the wound was closed in layers.

The postoperative course was satisfactory. The unsteady gait and tetraparesis gradually improved, and there were no functional sequelae relating to the surgery.

Comments: This case involved a very extensive chordoma of the middle and posterior fossae with intra- and extradural growth, subtotal destruction of the bony clivus and petrous bone, and intraspinal extension to C3. The tumor had enlarged the communication between the cerebellopontine angle and prepontine space, enabling us to remove the lesion through a unilateral extended lateral suboccipital approach, working in the anterior and inferior directions and extending the dissection across the midline.

Medial Suboccipital Approach
(Fig. CJ 2a–d, Fig. CJ 3a–e)

The medial suboccipital approach is suitable for the removal of tumors of the inferior clivus that extend into the craniocervical junction and have spread to both sides from the midline. Lateral extension of the approach may be necessary on one or both sides. The skin is incised in the midline. Details regarding the operative technique are given in the chapter on the Craniocervical Junction (see p. 461).

Combined Supra- and Infratentorial Approach to the Clivus

Introductory Remarks. Tumors arising from the clivus can occasionally extend above the tentorium to the cavernous sinus and below the tentorium to the foramen magnum at the same time. Tumors of this kind cannot be completely removed through a supratentorial or infratentorial approach alone. Two surgical options are available:

1) A two-stage operation performed through a frontotemporal supratentorial approach and a lateral suboccipital infratentorial approach.
2) A combined supra- and infratentorial operation performed in one stage.

The major obstacles to developing a combined subtemporal-suboccipital approach are the transverse sinus and the sigmoid sinus with their important tributary vessel, the inferior anastomotic vein.

To decrease the amount of brain retraction needed in the subtemporal-transtentorial approaches and still obtain adequate exposure of the posterior surface of the petrous bone, the dorsum sellae, and the midline structures, the posterior subtemporal approach can be extended by a lateral craniectomy of the posterior cranial fossa (Bonnal et al. 1964; Luyendijk 1976; Malis 1985; Naffziger 1928; Pertuiset 1974; Verbrugghen 1952). This utilizes the advantages of both approaches and also provides additional space at the petrous bone. Hakuba described this interesting variant in 1977 for the removal of a clivus meningioma. He extended the translabyrinthine-transtentorial approach of Morrison and King (1973) for the removal of acoustic neuromas, using a suboccipital and subtemporal craniotomy. In 1977 Hakuba et al. reported on 6 clivus meningiomas removed by this technique, which he calls the transpetrosal-transtentorial approach. Recently he applied the approach for the removal of parasellar tumors (Hakuba et al. 1985). Complications relating to cerebral venous statis following ligation of the transverse sinus and sigmoid sinus can be avoided by confirming adequate venous drainage via the contralateral transverse and sigmoid sinuses on preoperative angiograms. Failure to confirm this is a contraindication for the combined approach *with* interruption of these large sinuses. In such cases it is necessary to preserve the continuity of the transverse and sigmoid sinuses when the supratentorial-infratentorial technique is employed. In borderline cases, one should select the approach that is most likely to provide access for total tumor removal, while allowing for extension to a combined approach.

The combined supratentorial-infratentorial approach is best suited for prepontine tumors (Symon 1982). The lesion is reached by dissection from the lateral side, and thus with minimal retraction of the temporal lobe and cerebellum. Vision is further improved by drilling away the lateral part of the petrous bone. When hearing is intact, we reject labyrinthectomy or petrosectomy merely to obtain a more favorable direction of entry.

Fig. CL 9a–i. The combined supratentorial-infratentorial approach to the clivus, indicated for clivus tumors with concomitant supratentorial extension to the cavernous sinus and infratentorial extension to the foramen magnum.

a Location of the skin incision and burr holes for the temporal craniotomy. The *shaded area* shows the possible extent of the suboccipital craniectomy. Major anatomic landmarks are the transverse and sigmoid sinuses and the inferior anastomotic vein.

b The scalp flap is reflected, and the temporal osteoplastic craniotomy is performed. Here the bone flap has been temporarily removed, but it also may be hinged on the temporal muscle. The extent of the occipital craniectomy is indicated. Both the temporal and the suboccipital dural flaps are based medially. The transverse sinus is ligated at its junction with the sigmoid.

c After division of the transverse sinus, the tentorium is incised a few millimeters medial to the superior petrosal sinus along the superior petrosal ridge to the tentorial notch.

d The supratentorial tumor component is exposed and debulked piecemeal, sometimes using an ultrasonic aspirator (e.g., CUSA).

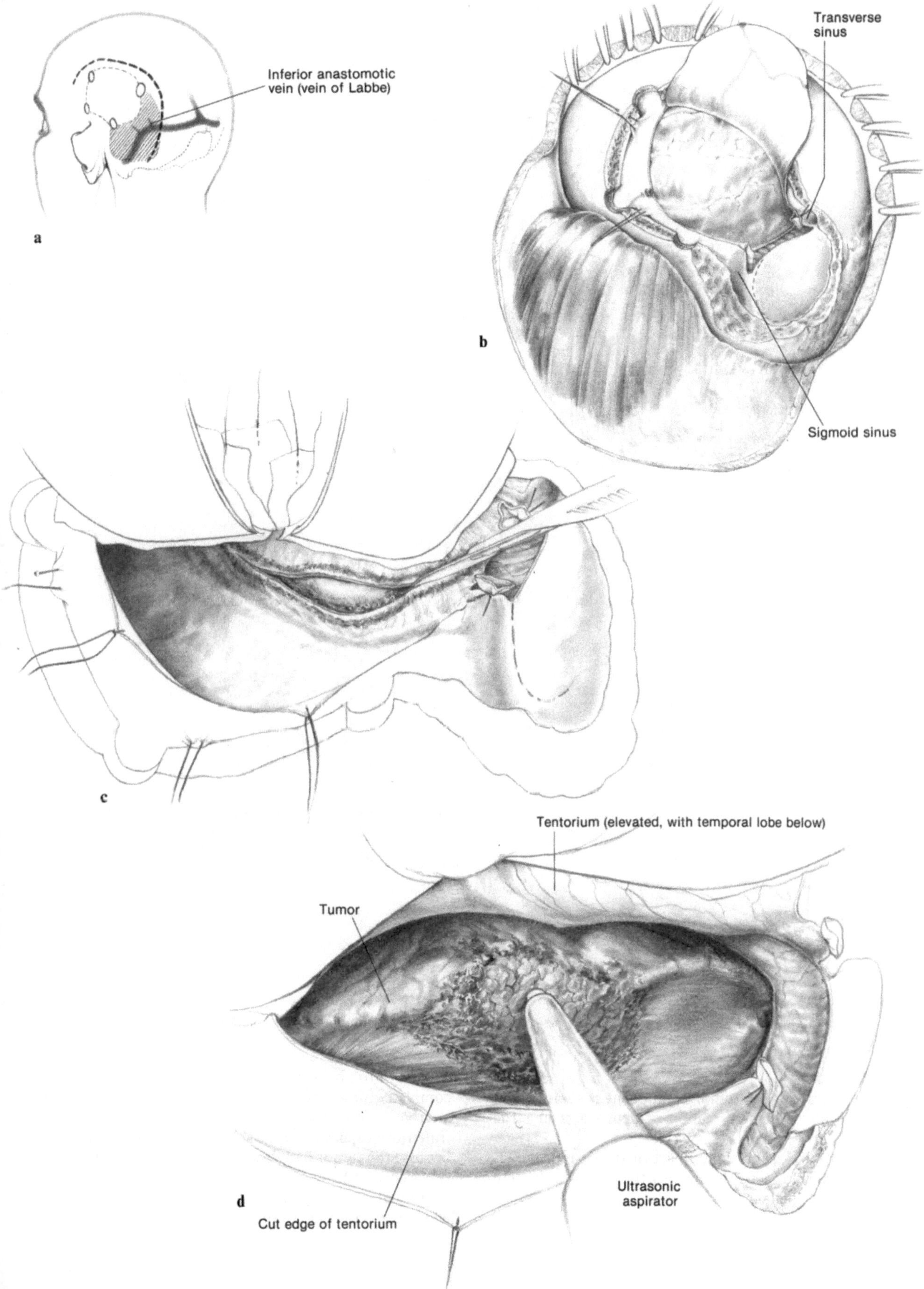
Inferior anastomotic vein (vein of Labbe)
a
Transverse sinus
b
Sigmoid sinus
c
Tentorium (elevated, with temporal lobe below)
Tumor
d
Cut edge of tentorium
Ultrasonic aspirator

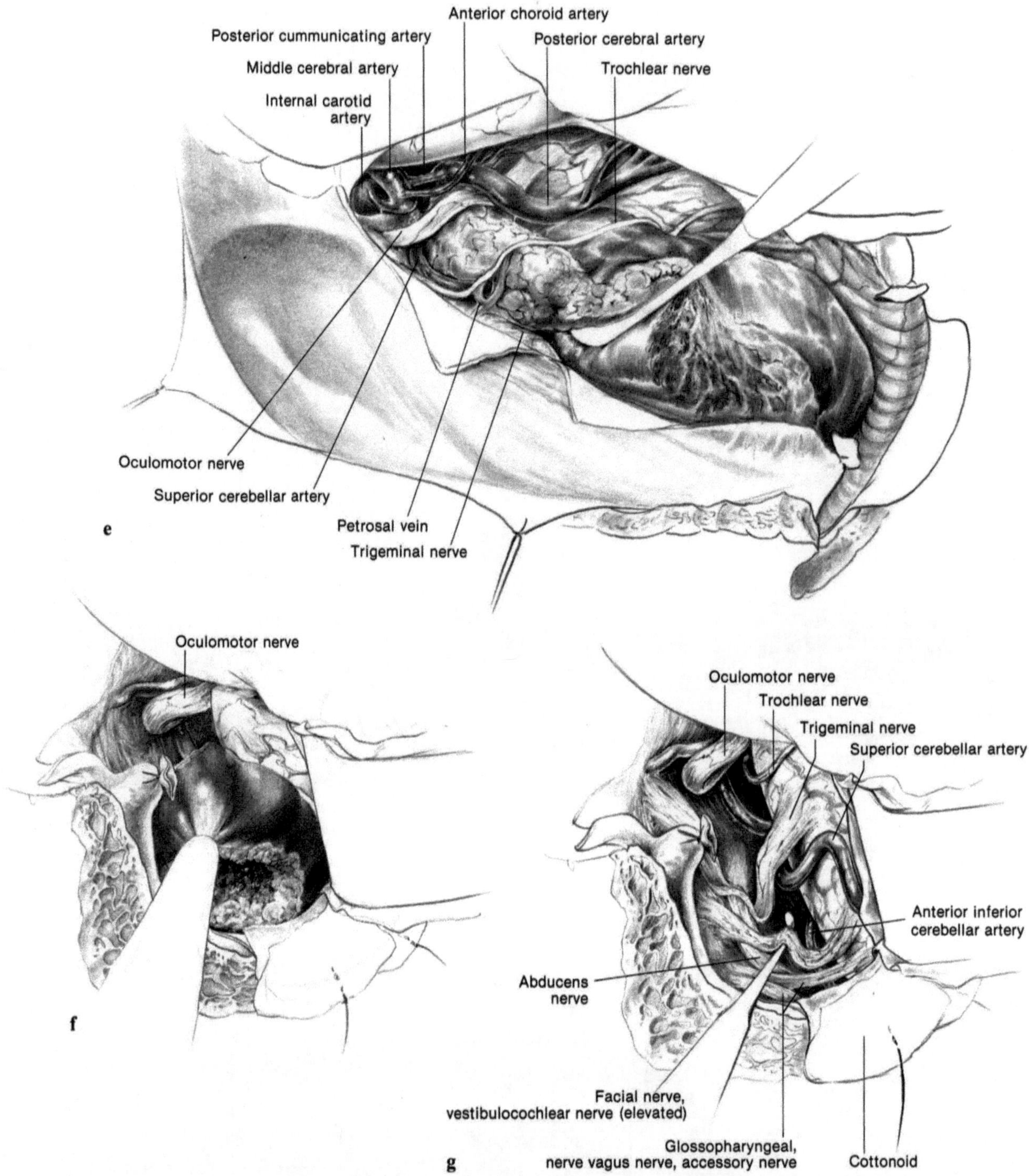

Fig. CL 9e–g.
e The supratentorial tumor component is removed microsurgically with preservation of neurovascular structures.
f Infratentorial, suboccipital part of the operation. The cerebellum is retracted to uncover the tumor in the cerebellopontine angle.
g View into the supra- and infratentorial space after complete tumor removal, showing the microsurgical anatomy. Concurrent visualization of the supra- and infratentorial space from the suboccipital aspect is possible because the tumor had displaced the brain stem posterosuperiorly and toward the opposite side. This produces a gradual stretching of the nerves and blood vessels, which may continue to function well

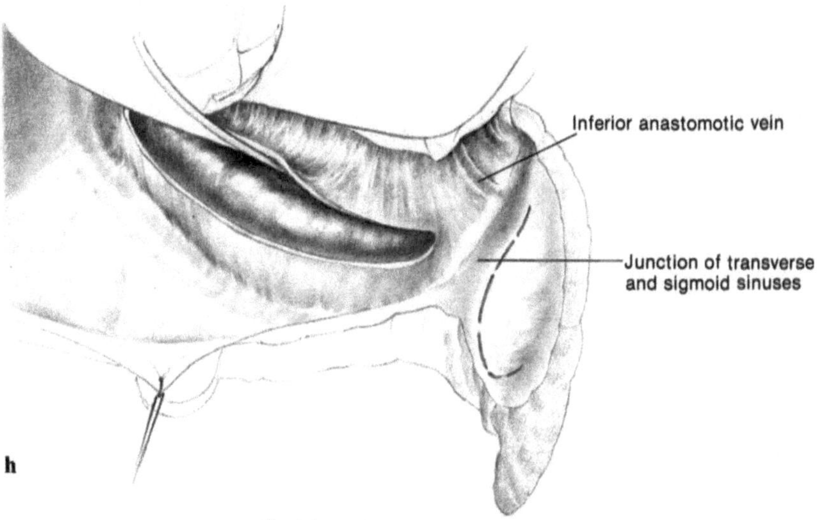

h

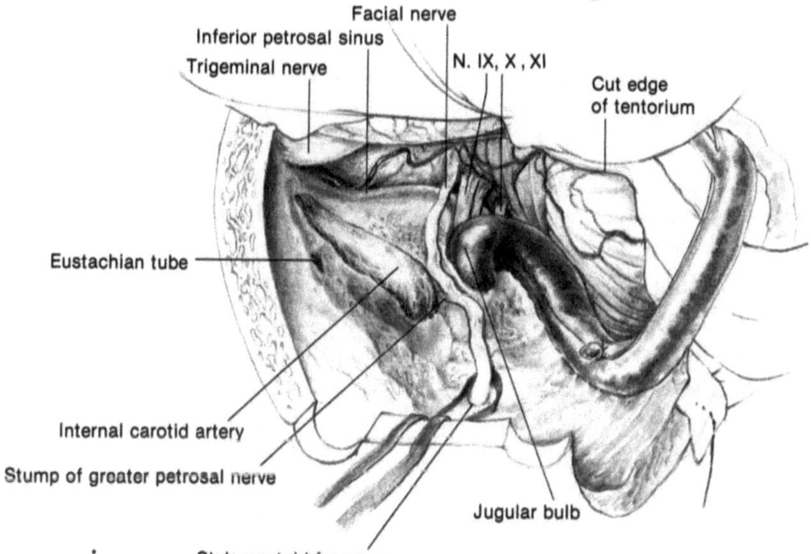

i

Fig. CL 9h, i.
h Combined supratentorial-infratentorial approach to the clivus with preservation of the transverse sinus. In this case the tentorium is divided anterior to the transverse or sigmoid sinus and medial to the superior petrosal sinus as fas as the tentorial incisure.

i If the tumor has invaded the petrous bone and destroyed the labyrinth, causing ipsilateral loss of vestibulocochlear function, the approach can be extended considerably by performing a subtotal petrosectomy, sparing the facial nerve. Generally this should not be done if hearing function exists

Operative Technique
(Fig. CL 9a–i)

The patient is placed in the "park bench" position with the head turned 30° downward. This will give the surgeon an equally good view of the posterior and middle cranial fossae. The viewing axis toward the clivus follows the posterior petrous ridge.

The skin incision is basically an extended retromastoid incision which curves upward and forward into the temporal area, roughly following the attachment of the temporal muscle. The temporal part of the craniotomy is performed first and must extend to the floor of the middle fossa. The craniotomy is extended over the sphenoid margin in the pterional direction for tumors with extension to the internal carotid artery, cavernous sinus, or optic nerve. The craniotomy flap may be temporarily removed, or it may be left attached to the temporal muscle and reflected frontally so that it will not interfere with the subtemporal dissection. The lateral suboccipital bone is removed by craniectomy. The posterior fossa is exposed past the transverse sinus to the posterolateral margin of the sigmoid sinus. The last bony structures over the sigmoid sinus are removed with a cutting burr. The extradural resection of the lateral part of the petrous ridge serves to extend further the operator's angle of vision.

The dura is opened in such a way so that the transverse sinus can be ligated and sectioned at its junction with the sigmoid sinus. When opening the supratentorial dura, care is taken to preserve the inferior anastomotic vein (vein of Labbé) as it enters the transverse sinus. The temporal lobe is elevated along with the transverse sinus and tentorium. The infratentorial dura is divided parallel and several millimeters posterior to the sigmoid sinus, leaving a margin sufficient for placing holding sutures. The infratentorial dura is incised far enough along the transverse sinus to permit elevation of the temporal lobe along with the transverse sinus and tentorium. The tentorium is incised along the petrous ridge close to its line of attachment. Sometimes the superior petrosal sinus will have to be coagulated. Before the tentorial incisure is reached, it must be considered that the trochlear nerve lies behind the dural margin and enters the dura in the area of the posterior petroclinoid fold. The trochlear nerve is most vulnerable at the site where it enters its dural pore. In the area of the ambient cistern, the nerve is protected by the arachnoid and can be mobilized with it. Because tumors of this region usually have reached the tentorial margin, the trochlear nerve is stretched laterally so that it crosses the surgical field and interferes with the dissection; that is why the nerve often cannot be salvaged. Fortunately, the functional sequelae of trochlear nerve section are minor.

Particular attention must be given to the oculomotor nerve, which generally is found in relation to the lateral superior circumference of the tumor. Left in its arachnoid sheath, it usually can be dissected free from the tumor without difficulty.

When the temporal lobe retractor is inserted or repositioned, care should be taken that the blade does not block drainage through the inferior anastomotic vein.

Slight retractor pressure on the sagging cerebellum should be sufficient to expose the cerebellopontine angle with cranial nerves VII and VIII running lateral to the tumor. Usually both nerves are easily separated from the tumor, as they are protected in a separate arachnoid pouch.

The trigeminal nerve may be displaced laterally by clivus meningiomas, but it is common for tumors to infiltrate between the nerve fibers, in which case it is no longer possible to preserve a useful degree of function.

The brain stem is reached by progressive debulking of the neoplasm. Dissection of the basilar artery is aided by preoperative angiograms showing the presence or absence of fluctuations in the vessel diameter. This study is helpful in determining whether the basilar artery and its major branches are enveloped by tumor. The location of the abducens nerve depends on the direction of tumor growth. The nerve may be located at the inferior, medial, or even lateral pole of the tumor. If identification of cranial nerves VII and VIII at the brain stem proves difficult, we recommend a progressive exposure of the nerves from the porus acusticus. If the brain stem is displaced posteriorly by the tumor, visualization of the contralateral porus acusticus may be possible after the neoplasm is removed.

Case Report. Extensive petroclival meningioma (Fig. CL 10a–h). A right hemiparesis and hypesthesia with left trigeminal neuropathy and obstructive hydrocephalus developed over a period of years in a woman who was 39 years of age at the time of her operation. The symptoms improved following placement of a ventriculoperitoneal shunt. Because of the location and extent of the meningioma, radical removal was not possible through the subtemporal-transtentorial or lateral suboccipital approach alone, so we undertook a combined supratentorial-infraten-

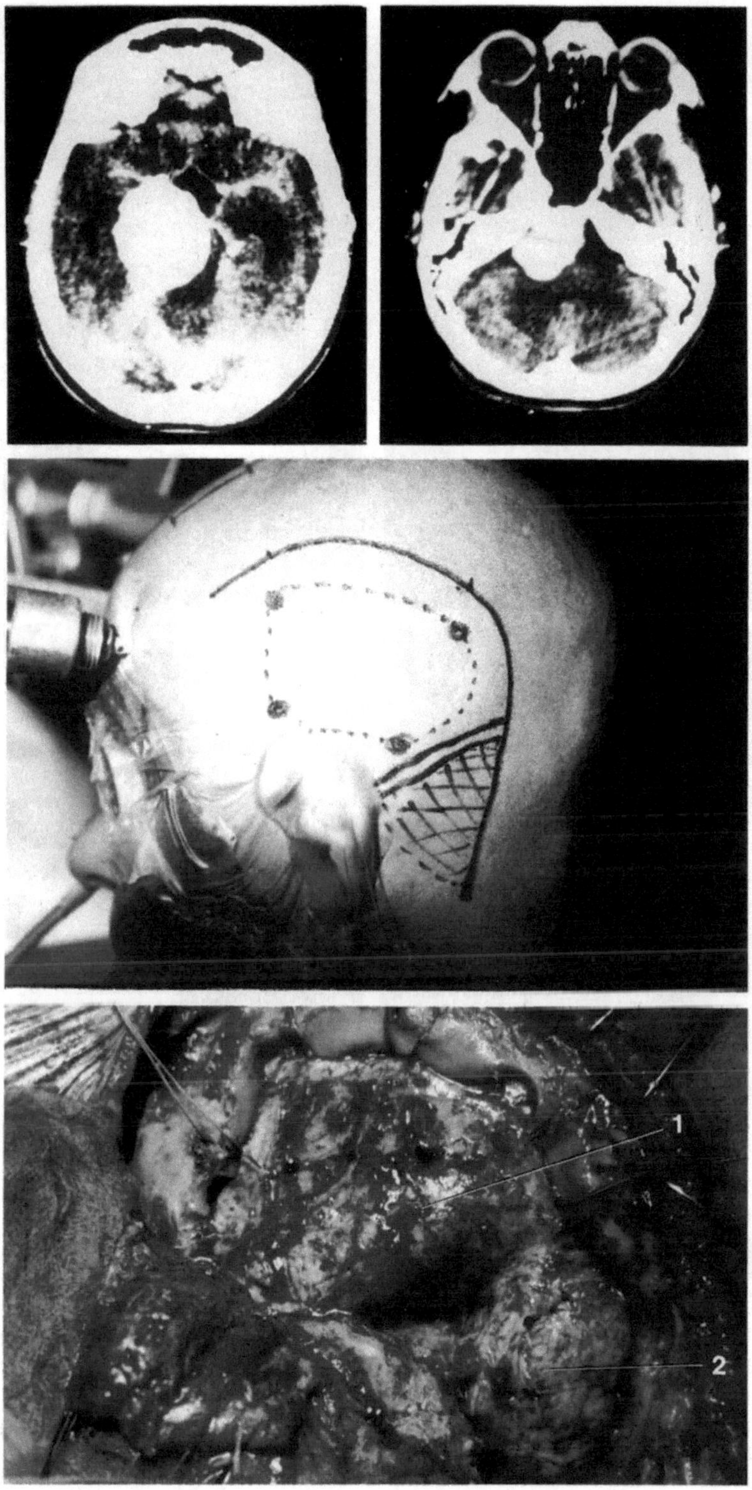

a b c d

Fig. CL 10a–h. Extensive petroclival meningioma removed through the combined supratentorial-infratentorial approach.
a, b Preoperative CT scans show tumor extension from the supratentorial region across the tentorial incisure to the cerebellopontine angle and clivus.
c Markings indicate the skin incision (——), the osteoplastic craniotomy (-----), and the craniectomy (*cross-hatched*). A *solid line* also marks the course of the transverse sinus.
d Status following temporal craniotomy and lateral suboccipital craniectomy. (*1*) Temporal dura, (*2*) cerebellar dura

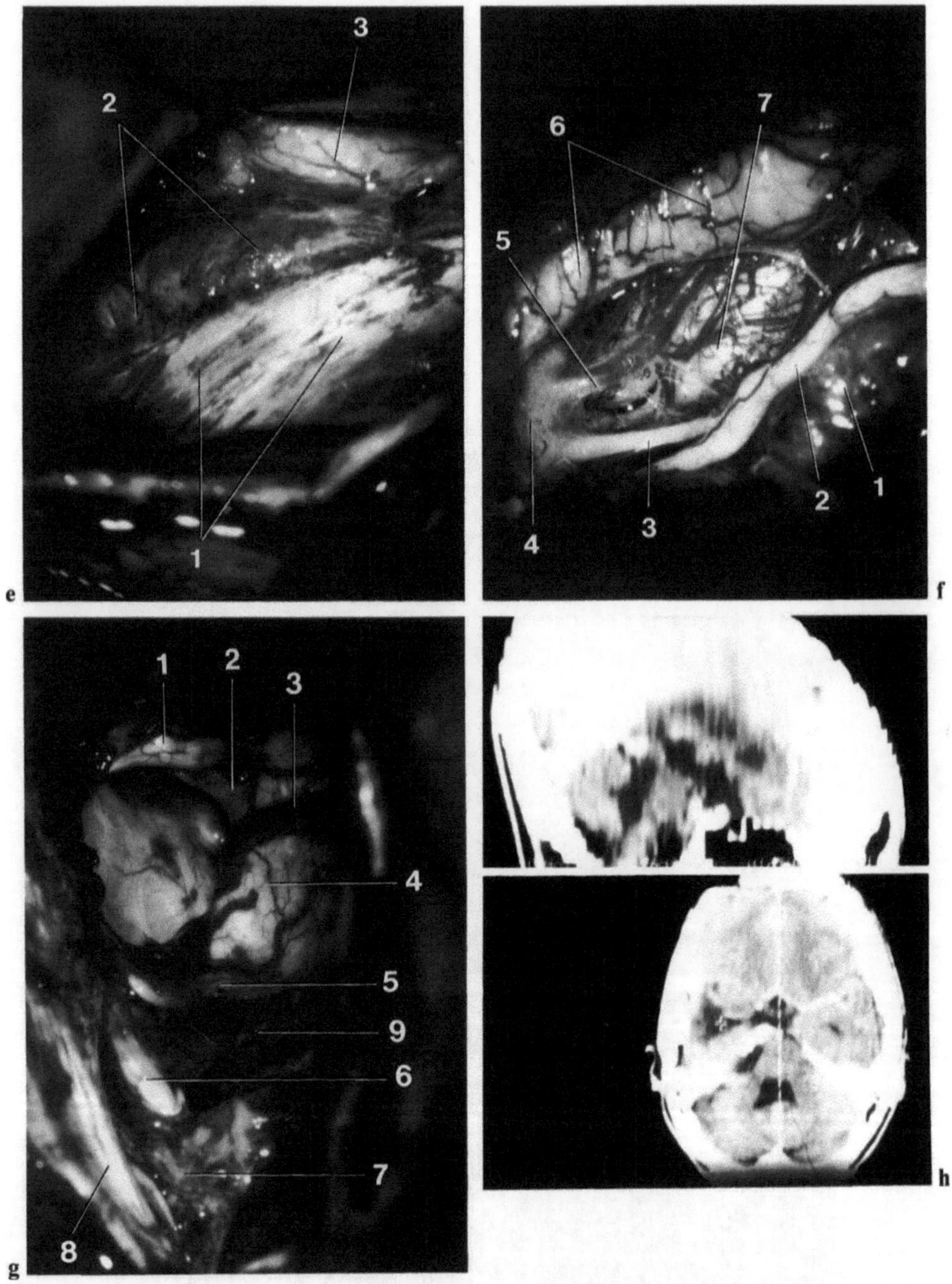

Fig. CL 10e–h.
e, f Supratentorial phase of the operation.
e The temporal lobe is retracted to expose the tentorium and the supratentorial tumor component. (*1*) Tentorium, (*2*) tumor, (*3*) temporal lobe.
f View of the brain stem after incision of the tentorium and removal of the supratentorial tumor. (*1*) Tumor, (*2*) oculomotor nerve, (*3*) posterior communicating artery, (*4*) internal carotid artery, (*5*) anterior choroid artery, (*6*) temporal lobe, (*7*) brain stem.
g Suboccipital phase of the operation: View through the cerebellopontine angle to the supratentorial space. (*1*) Oculomotor nerve, (*2*) posterior cerebral artery, (*3*) superior cerebellar artery, (*4*) brain stem, (*5*) trigeminal nerve, (*6*) nerves VII and VIII, (*7*) anterior inferior cerebellar artery, (*8*) caudal cranial nerves, (*9*) clivus.
h Follow-up CT scan 1 1/2 years postoperatively

torial approach without ligation of the transverse and sigmoid sinuses.

The right hemiparesis worsened to some degree in the immediate postoperative period, and a mild facial palsy was also present. The patient recovered well from the extensive surgery. She still had residual hemiparesis several months later. The trigeminal neuropathy did not improve, but the postoperative facial palsy regressed completely. Follow-up CT scans after 1 1/2 years showed no residual tumor.

Comments: A meningioma with supra- and infratentorial extension required the combined subtemporal-lateral suboccipital approach. The patency of the transverse sinus was preserved.

References

Bartal AD, Heilbronn YD (1970) Transcervical removal of a clivus chordoma in a 2-years old child. Reversal of quadriplegia and lumbar paralysis. Acta Neurochir 33:127–133

Bonnal J, Louis R, Combalbert A (1964) L'abord temporal transtentoriel de l'angle ponto-cerebelleux et du clivus. Neurochirurgie 10:3–12

Cushing H (1917) Tumors of the Nervus Acusticus and the syndrome of the Cerebellopontine Angle. Saunders WB, Philadelphia London

Dandy W (1925) An operation for the total removal of cerebellopontine (acoustic) tumors. Surg Gynecol Obstet 41:129–148

Decker RE, Malis LI (1970) Surgical approaches to midline lesions at the base of the skull: a review. Mount Sinai J Med NY 37:84–102

Delgado TE, Garrido E, Harwick R (1981) Labiomandibular, transoral approach to chordomas in the clivus and upper spine. Neurosurgery 8:675–679

Derome PJ, Guiot G (1979) Surgical approaches to the sphenoidal and clival area. In: Krayenbühl H (ed) Advanced and Technical standards in Neurosurgery, Vol. 6. Springer, Wien New York, pp 101–136

DiLorenzo N, Fortuna A, Guidetti B (1982) Craniovertebral junction malformations. Clinicoradiological findings, long term results and surgical indications in 63 cases. J Neurosurg 57:603–608

Drake CG (1969) The surgical treatment of vertebral basilar aneurysms. Clin Neurosurg 16:114–169

Drake CG (1973) Management of aneurysms of posterior circulation. In: Youmans JR (ed) Neurological Surgery, Vol. 2. Saunders, Philadelphia, pp 787–806

Drake CG (1978) Treatment of aneurysms of the posterior cranial fossa. Progr Neurol Surg 9:122–194

Fang HSY, Ong GB (1962) Direct anterior approach to the upper cervical spine. J Bone Joint Surg 44A:21588–1604

Fox JL (1967) Obliteration of midline vertebral artery aneurysm via basilar craniectomy. J Neurosurg 26:406–412

Gutkelch AN, Williams RG (1972) Anterior approach to recurrent chordomas of the clivus. Neurosurgery 36:670–672

Hakuba A, Nishimur S, Tanaka A, Kishi W, Nakamura T (1977) Clivus meningeoms: six cases of total removal. Neurol Med Chir (Tokyo) 17:63–77

Hakuba A, Nishimura S, Inoue V (1985) Transpetrosal, transtentorial approach and its application in the therapy of retrochiasmatic craniopharyngiomas. Surg Neurol 24:405–415

Hardy J (1977) L'abord transsphenoidal de tumeurs de clivus. Neurochirurgie 23:287–297

Krayenbühl H, Yasargil MG (1975) Chondromas. Progr Neurol Surg 6 (Basel: Karger):435–463

Laine E, Jomin M et al. (1977) Indications et possibilities. Neurochirurgie 23:249–314

Luyendijk W (1976) Operative approaches to the posterior fossa. In: Advances and Technical Standards in Neurosurgery. Krayenbühl H (ed) Vol II. Springer, New York, pp 81–101

Malis LI (1985) Surgical resection of tumors of the skull base. In: Wilkins RH, Rengashary SS (eds) Neurosurgery Vol. 1:1011–1021. McGraw Hill, New York

Morrison AW, King TT (1973) Experience with a translabyrinthine-transtentorial approach to the cerebello-pontine angle. J Neurosurg 38:382–390

Mullan S, Naunton R, Hekmat-Panach J, Vailati G (1966) The use of an anterior approach to ventrally placed tumors in the foramen magnum and vertebral column. J Neurosurg 24:536–543

Naffziger H (1928) Brain surgery with special reference to exposure of the brain stem and posterior fossa. Surg Gyn Obst 46:240–248

Pasztor E, Valda J, Piffko P, Horvath M, Horvath M, Gador I (1984) Transoral surgery for craniocervical occupying lesions. J Neurosurg 60:276–281

Peerless SJ, Drake CG (1987) Management of aneurysms of posterior circulation. In: Youmans JR (ed) Neurological Surgery Vol. 3. Saunders, Philadelphia, pp 1715–1763

Pertuiset B (1974) Supratentorial craniotomy. In: Krayenbühl H (ed) Advances and Technical Standards in Neurosurgery. Vol I. Springer, New York, pp 144–171

Pia HW, Lorenz R (1980) Transoral-Transpalatine-Transclival approaches to aneurysms of the vertebral and basilar artery. In: Grote et al (ed) Advances in Neurosurgery, vol 8. Springer, Berlin Heidelberg, pp 275–276

Rougerie J, Guiot G, Bouche J, Trigo JC (1967) Les voies d'abord du chordome du clivus. Neurochirurgie 13:559–570

Stevenson GC, Stoney RJ, Perkins RK (1966) A transcervical transclival approach to the ventral surface of the brain stem for removal of a clivus chordoma. J Neurosurg 24:544–551

Symon L (1982) Surgical approaches to the tentorial hiatus. In: Krayenbühl H (ed) Advances and technical standards No 9. Springer, Vienna New York
Verbiest H (1977) Lesions of the cervical spine: A critical review. International Congress Series No. 433. Neurological Surgery, Proceedings of the sixth International Congress of Neurological Surgery Sao Paulo, 1977. Excerpta Medica Amsterdam Oxford
Verbrugghen (1952) Paragasserian tumor. J Neurosurg 9:451–460
White RJ, Albin MS (1962) The technique of ligation of the basilar artery in monkeys. J Surg Rev 2:15–18
Wissinger JP, Danoff D, Wisiol ES, French LA (1967) Repair of an aneurysma of the basilar artery by a transclival approach: Case report. J Neurosurg 26:417–419
Wood BG, Sader ES, Levine HL, Dohn DF, Tucker HM (1980) Surgical problems of the base of the skull. An interdisciplinary approach. Arch Otolaryngol 106:1–5
Yasargil MG, Antic J, Lacigar (1976) Microsurgical pterional approach to aneurysms of the basilar bifurcation. Surg Neurol 6:83–91
Yasargil MG, Mortara RW, Curcic M (1980) Meningeomas of basal posterior cranial fossa. In: Krayenbühl H (ed) Advances and technical standards in Neurosurgery, Vol 7. Springer, Vienna New York

Surgery of the Craniocervical Junction (CJ)

Introductory Remarks. Surgical exposure of the region around the foramen magnum and the first two cervical vertebrae is necessary for lesions that threaten loss of stability and spinal cord compression, especially by the dens. Removal of the lesion may be combined with stabilization of the upper cervical spine in the same operation, or it may be best to do the stabilizing procedure in a second sitting. In other cases, clinical symptoms may require that a posterior fusion be performed first, followed later by an ablative procedure. Major recent contributions on this issue have been published by Brattström et al. (1973), Fang and Ong (1962), Stein et al. (1963), Gros et al. (1974, 1975), Verbiest (1961, 1969, 1977), Wayne and Robinson (1957) and Robinson et al. (1975).

Close interdisciplinary cooperation is valuable for patient selection and surgical management.

Indications for surgical procedures on the craniocervical junction include:

1) Basilar invagination (basilar impression).
2) Traumatic fracture-dislocation of the dens (Sherk 1975).
3) Dislocation of the dens secondary to rheumatoid disease (Brattström et al. 1973).
4) Tumors (cysts, osteoid-osteoma, osteochondroma, chordoma, plasmocytoma, etc.).

Basilar invagination and even benign tumors with minimal bone destruction can be adequately managed by removal of the dens, provided the cervical spine is sufficiently stable. Otherwise removal of the causative lesion must be combined with a stabilizing craniocervical fusion.

An essential part of the evaluation of these patients is a detailed *radiologic workup* that includes plain X-ray films in various projections and functional films, conventional tomograms, and CT scans. Special attention is given to Chamberlain's line, which connects the most posteromedial point of the hard palate with the posterior limit of the foramen magnum on the lateral cranial tomogram, as well as the "bimastoid line" (Fisch-Gold-Metzger line) on the AP tomogram (Fig. CJ 1a, b). Normally the dens

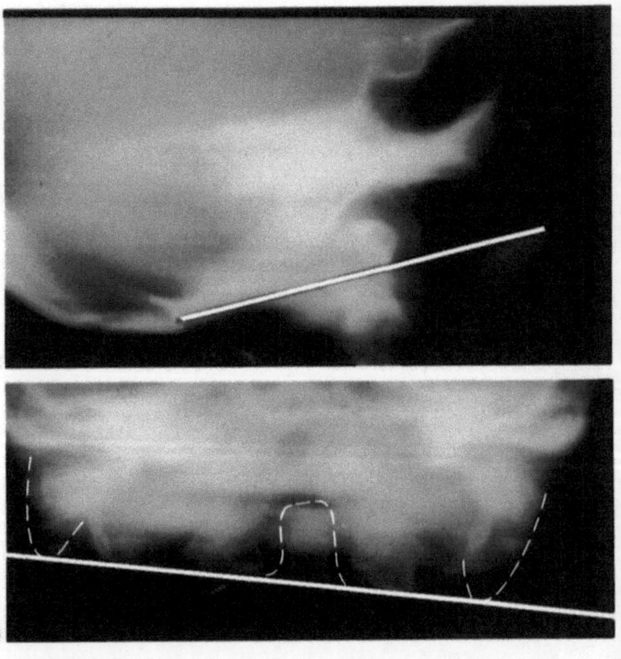

Fig. CJ 1a, b. Pronounced basilar impression in a 57-year-old female physician with multiple neurologic deficits (tetraparesis, sensory disturbances, vertigo) that were exacerbated by flexion of the neck.
a Chamberlain's line is drawn on the lateral tomogram from the posteriormost point of the hard palate to the posterior rim of the foramen magnum. The dens (-----) projects much more than 2 mm past Chamberlain's line.
b The bimastoid line (Fisch-Gold-Metzger line) is drawn on the AP tomogram of the skull base. Almost the entire dens (-----) projects past the bimastoid line

should project no more than 2 mm past both lines. If it projects farther cranially, and the patient manifests symptoms such as vertigo, tinnitus, paresis, and paresthesias that are exacerbated by flexion of the neck, one should suspect basilar impression.

Operative treatments consist of procedures for the *ablation* and/or correction of the pathological process and for the *stabilization* of the craniocervical junction.

Operative Technique

Ablative Procedures for Lesions of the Craniocervical Junction

Transoral Approach

Introductory Remarks. This technique provides good anterior exposure of C1 and C2 on the midline, and the surgical morbidity is low. The main disadvantage is the necessity of working through an unsterile area, which poses an increased risk of infection when incision of the dura is required. The approach is particularly suited for exposure of the dens (Verbiest 1961, 1977), dens fractures, and basilar invagination.

Technique for Exposing the Dens
(Fig. CL 2a–d)

This was previously described in the chapter on Surgery of the Clivus (see p. 432). The anterior arch of the atlas and the body of the axis are exposed, and two specula are inserted. The diamond burr is then used to drill away about two-thirds of the vertical height of the anterior arch of C1, working from below upward, until the anterior articular facet of the dens is visualized. This is followed laterally and superiorly to expose the apex of the dens and its lateral borders. Then the dens is reduced to its base with the diamond burr under constant irrigation. This is done with meticulous care to avoid spinal cord injury. The posterior articular facet of the dens and the transverse ligament of the atlas appear immediately anterior to the spinal cord. The last part of the dens is removed piecemeal using a burr and microelevators. The resulting cavity measuring 1 cm in depth, 1 cm in width, and 1.5 cm in height is filled with fibrin sponge before closure of the prevertebral soft tissues.

Transcervical Approach
(Fig. CL 3a, b)

The advantages and disadvantages of this approach and the operative technique were previously discussed (see p. 435). It provides excellent anterior exposure of the entire cervical spine. The anterior longitudinal ligament is approached somewhat obliquely, rather than from the front. The transcervical approach is suitable for the removal of anterior and anterolateral lesions of the cervical cord.

Medial Suboccipital Approach

Introductory Remarks. The medial suboccipital approach to the junction of the skull base and spine provides wide exposure of lesions that have spread from the posterior cranial fossa to involve the posterior or posterolateral portion of the cervical spinal canal. Posterior stabilization also can be accomplished through this approach.

Operative Technique
(Fig. CJ 2a–d, Fig. CJ 3a–e)

In the semisitting position, the skin is incised on the midline from the external occipital protuberance to the spinous process of C3, and the neck muscles are stripped aside bilaterally on the subperiosteal plane to expose the occipital bone and posterior arches of C1 and C2. Two paramedian burr holes are placed below the external occipital protuberance and are enlarged to a craniectomy that includes the posterior bony rim of the foramen magnum. Depending

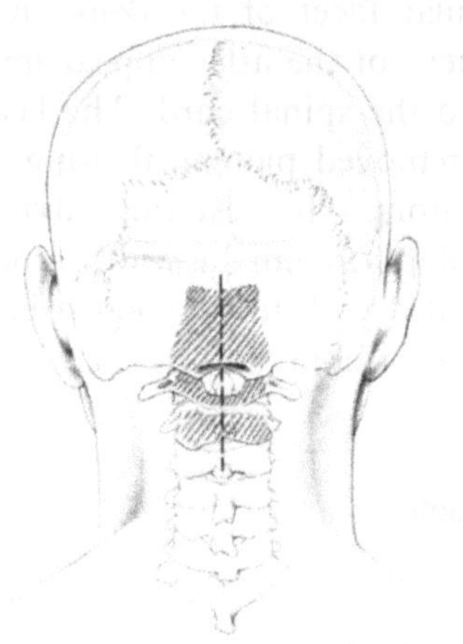

a

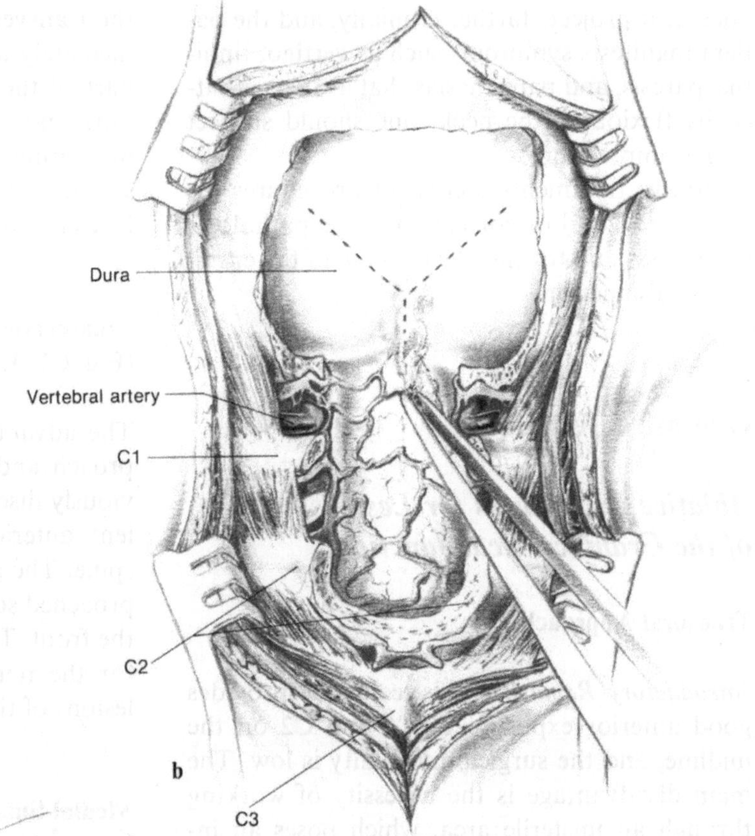
Dura
Vertebral artery
C1
C2
C3

b

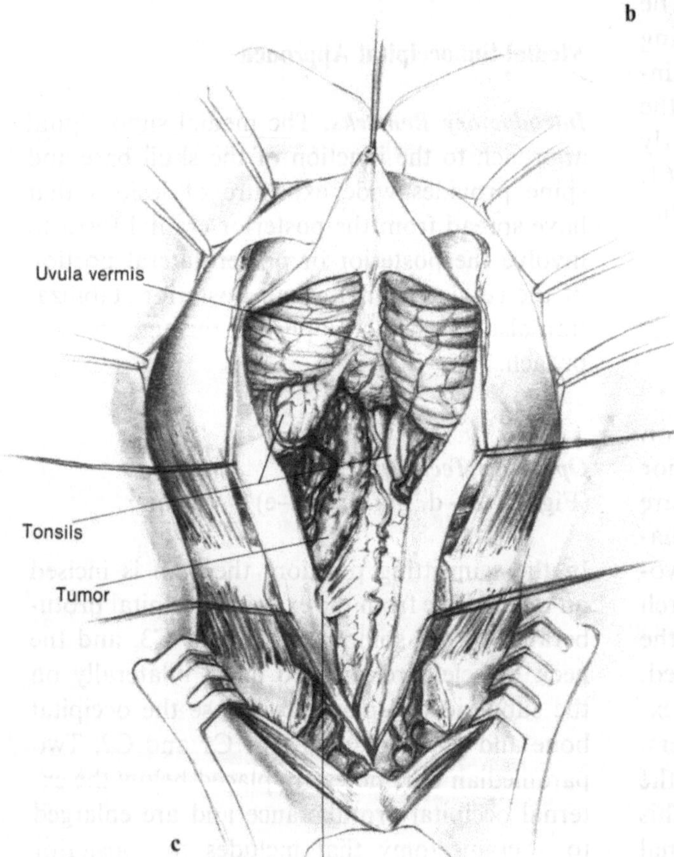
Uvula vermis
Tonsils
Tumor
N. CII

c

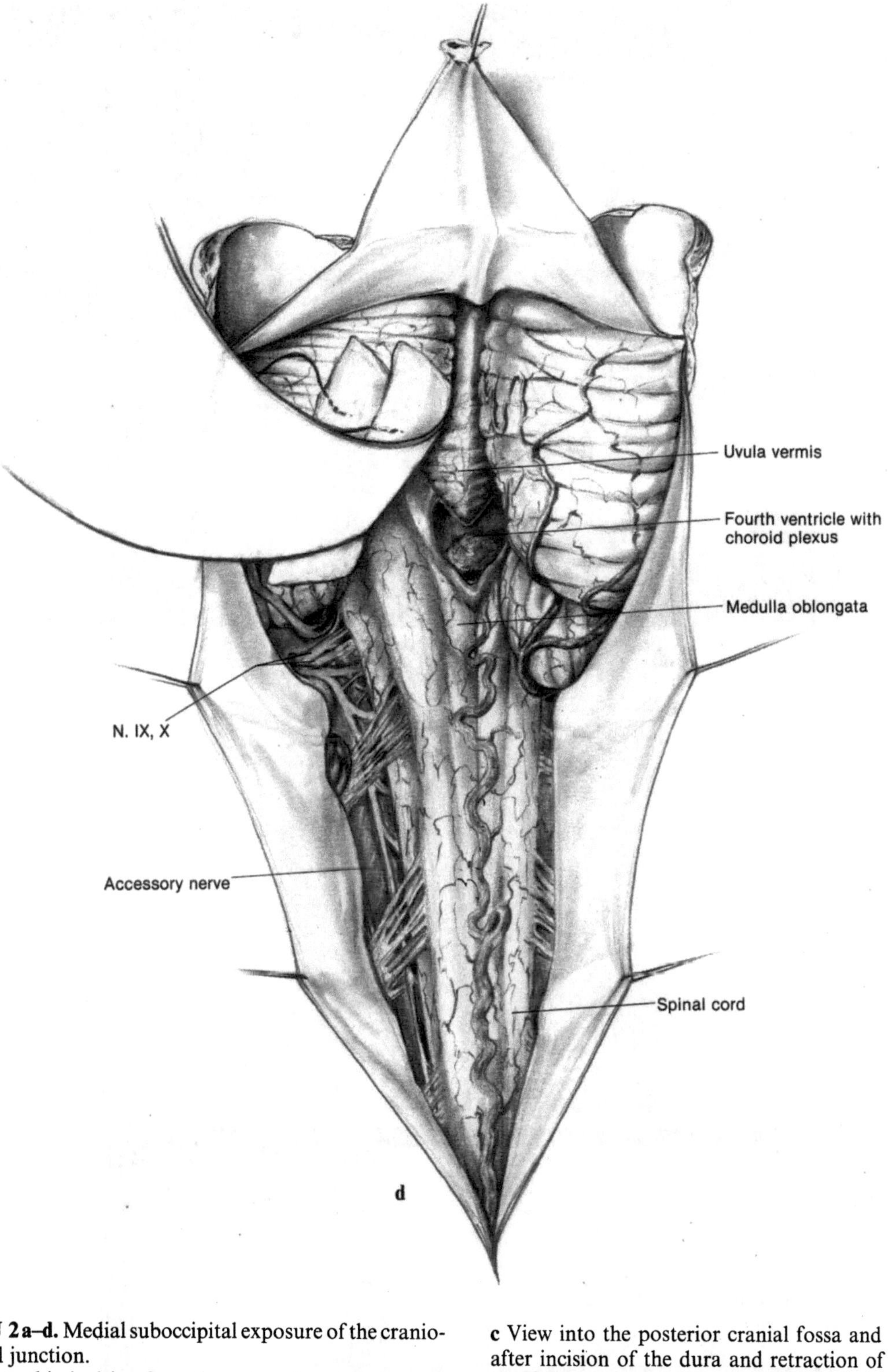

Fig. CJ 2a–d. Medial suboccipital exposure of the craniocervical junction.
a Midline skin incision from the external occipital protuberance to the spinous process of C3. The craniectomy is started with burr holes placed below the transverse sinus.
b Status following occipital craniectomy and atlantoaxial laminectomy. The Y-shaped dural incision line is shown.
c View into the posterior cranial fossa and spinal canal after incision of the dura and retraction of its margins. The tumor presents below the left cerebellar tonsil.
d View into the craniocervical junction and fourth ventricle following microsurgical tumor removal. The left cerebellar hemisphere, including the tonsil, is elevated with a spatula. The left caudal cranial nerves are visible

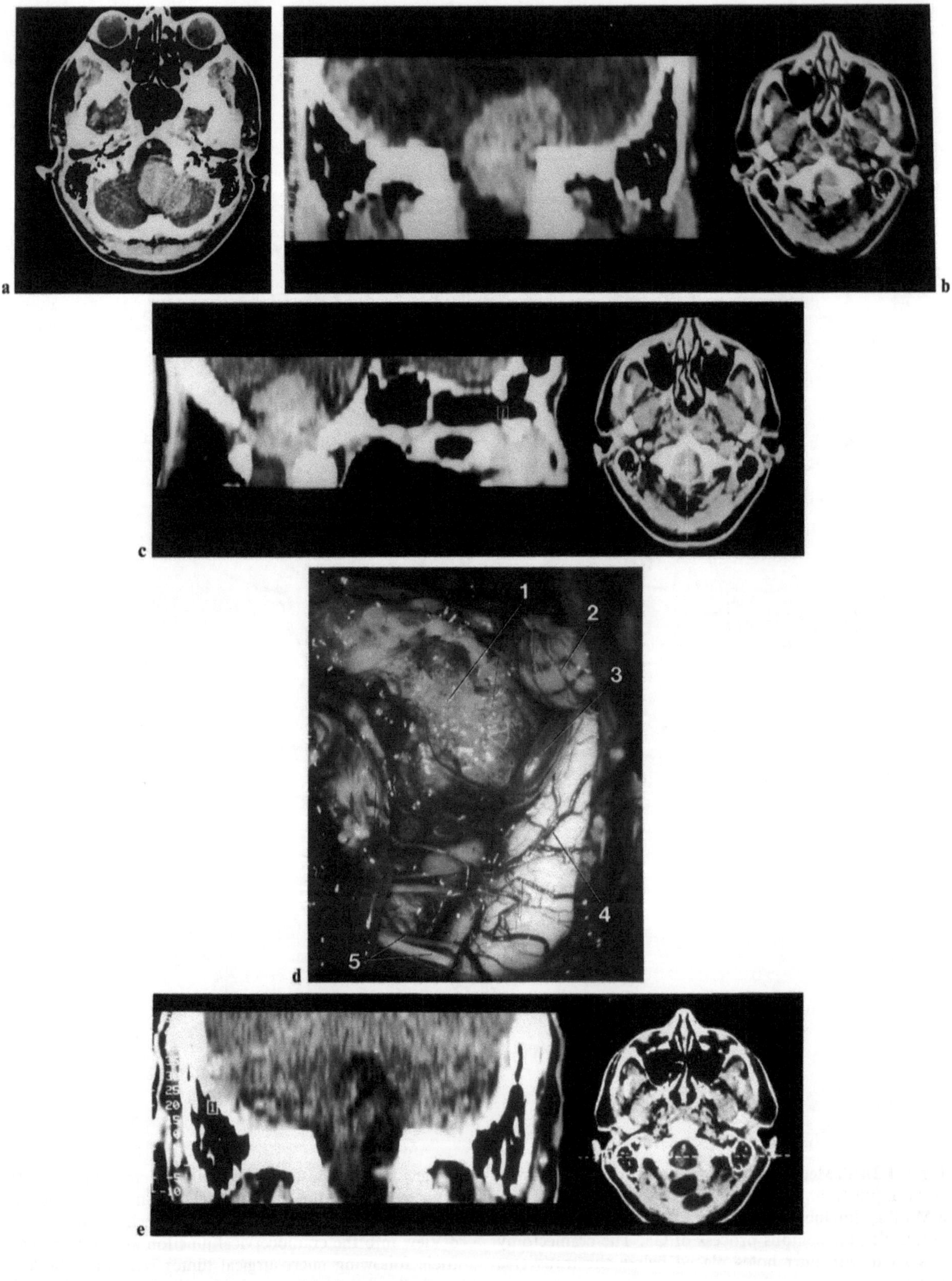
a
b
c
1
2
3
4
5
d
e

Fig. CJ 3a–e. Extensive meningioma at the left craniocervical junction in a 36-year-old man. The main clinical symptoms were hemihypoesthesia and hemihypalgesia, impaired thermal sensation on the right side, and unsteady gait.
a Axial CT scan covering the posterior fossa shows the large meningioma extending laterally into the cerebellopontine angle, anteriorly to the prepontine space, and posteriorly to the occiput. The tumor transgresses the midline.
b Axial CT with coronal reconstruction to demonstrate the foramen magnum: Half the tumor is in the posterior fossa and half in the spinal canal. The foramen magnum is greatly constricted.
c Axial CT scan with midsagittal reconstruction shows the relation of the tumor to the clivus, fourth ventricle, cisterna magna, and anterior arch of the atlas.
d Status following suboccipital craniocervical exposure and elevation of the cerebellum and tonsil. The tumor is displacing and compressing the brain stem; it impinges on the upper cervical nerve roots and the posterior inferior cerebellar artery. (*1*) Tumor, (*2*) cerebellar tonsil, (*3*) posterior inferior cerebellar artery, (*4*) medulla oblongata, (*5*) upper cervical nerve roots.
e Postoperative CT scans

on the extent of the lesion in the cervical canal, the posterior arch of C1 and the spinous process and posterior arch of C2 can then be removed. The vertebral artery is present at the lateral side in the field. The atlantooccipital ligament is sectioned to expose the posterior fossa dura and the upper cervical canal.

The dura is opened in a Y-shaped fashion to expose the cerebellar hemispheres and tonsils and the spinal cord. This provides access to all intradural processes at the craniocervical junction.

A space-occupying lesion will produce compression and displacement not only of the caudal cranial nerves, upper cervical roots, and the vertebral artery and its branches, but also of the medulla oblongata in the foramen magnum and of the cord. An extracerebral tumor can reach the fourth ventricle through the foramina of Luschka and Magendie and even determine an obstructive hydrocephalus by blocking the circulation of cerebrospinal fluid (Fig. CJ 3a–e).

The basic technique of benign tumor removal consists in the progressive, microsurgical reduction of the tumor bulk followed by dissection of the capsule from surrounding structures. While bipolar cautery is very useful throughout the operation, certain phases can be shortened by using an ultrasonic aspirator (CUSA) or a CO_2 laser. So far neither device has proven suitable for microsurgical dissection of the tumor capsule from the delicate cranial nerves and blood vessels or from the brain stem because of the high risk of injury to these structures.

A similar technique is employed for the exposure of vascular lesions close to the skull base, such as aneurysms and arteriovenous angiomas (Fig. CJ 4a–f).

After the ablative part of the surgery has been completed, the dura is closed in watertight fashion using simple interrupted sutures and continuous sutures. Reconstruction of the skull is not essential owing to the relatively powerful muscles in that region. Laminectomy of the atlas and axis alone does not necessitate further stabilizing measures. The muscles, superficial cervical fascia, and skin are reapproximated in three layers and provide stable coverage.

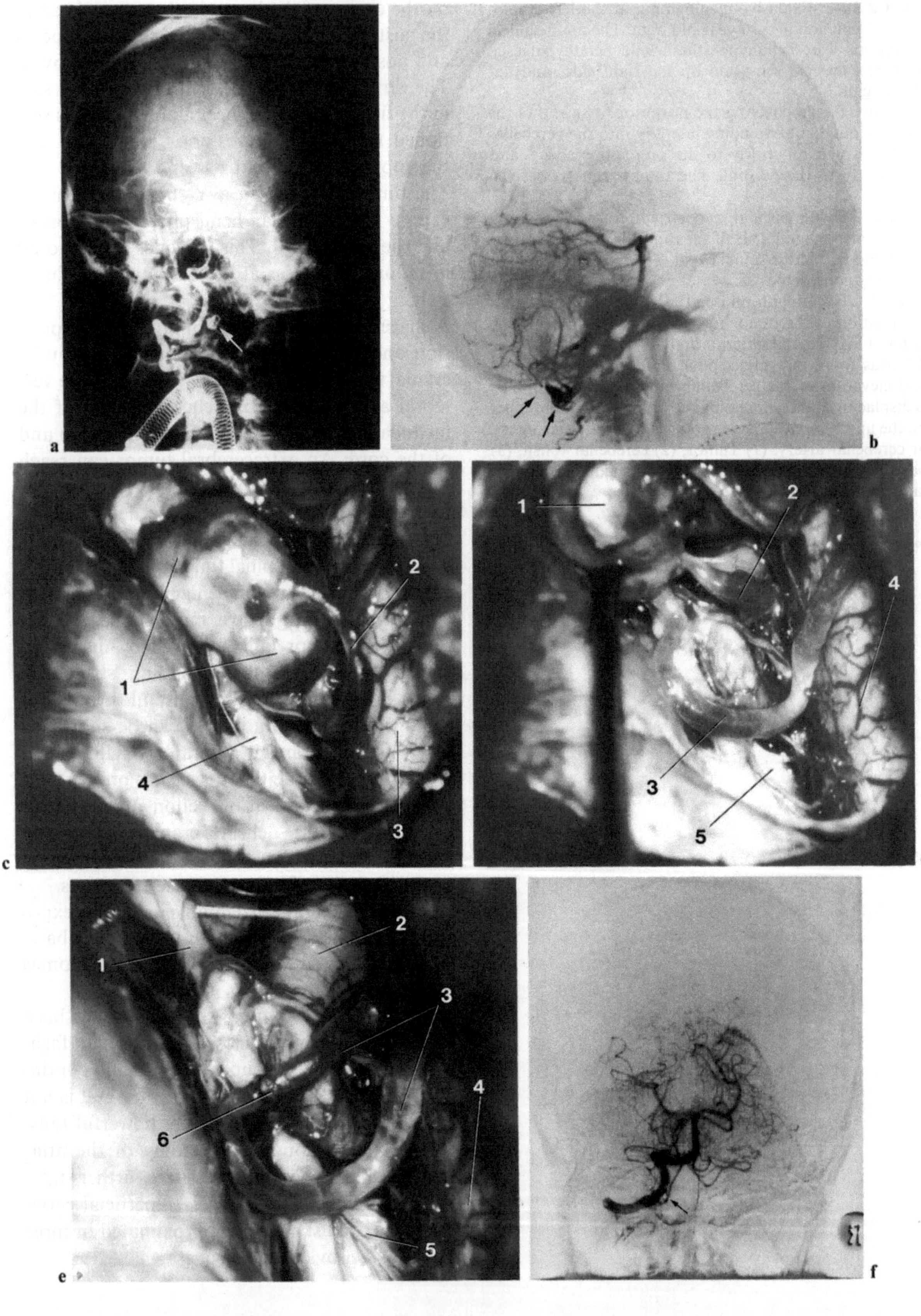
a
b
1
2
4
3
c
1
2
4
3
5
d
1
2
3
6
4
5
e
f

Fig. CJ 4a–f. Hypertensive woman 69 years of age referred to us in an unconscious state following a subarachnoid hemorrhage. A fusiform aneurysm of the vertebral artery was angiographically evidenced. At operation the lesion was identified as a fusiform aneurysm of the posterior inferior cerebellar artery. The involved segment was resected and the vessel repaired by end-to-end anastomosis.
a, b A left vertebral angiogram in the PA projection and lateral subtraction angiogram demonstrate the aneurysm with its afferent and efferent vascular supply (*arrows*).
c Surgical field after occipital craniectomy and resection of the arch of the atlas. The fusiform aneurysm and adjacent vascular segments are visible. (*1*) Aneurysm, (*2*) posterior inferior cerebellar artery, (*3*) medulla oblongata, (*4*) cervical roots of accessory nerve.
d After microsurgical dissection, the aneurysm is elevated with the dissector to get a better view of the afferent and efferent limbs of the posterior inferior cerebellar artery. The vertebral artery appears deep in the field. (*1*) Raised aneurysmal sac, (*2*) afferent vascular branch, (*3*) efferent vascular branch, (*4*) medulla oblongata, (*5*) cervical roots of accessory nerve.
e Status following resection of the aneurysm and end-to-end anastomosis of the vascular stumps. Both vascular segments are blood-filled. (*1*) Accessory nerve, (*2*) vertebral artery, (*3*) posterior inferior cerebellar artery, (*4*) medulla oblongata, (*5*) cervical roots of accessory nerve, (*6*) anastomosis.
f Postoperative angiogram in the AP projection confirms patency of the anastomosis

Procedures to Stabilize the Craniocervical Junction

Introductory Remarks. The *indications* for surgical stabilization are, in order of frequency:

1) Destruction of C1 and C2, especially of the dens and the body of the axis, by primary bone tumors or metastases, which may lead to severe displacement, pain, and cord compression (Sherk 1975).
2) *Pathologic* atlantoaxial *instabilities* and *subluxations* secondary to advanced rheumatoid arthritis (Schürmann 1979) or spinal anomalies such as Morquio's disease, which is associated with progressive tetraplegia.
3) Traumatic displacements such as atlantooccipital dislocation, certain nonunions of Jefferson burst fractures of the atlas, and traumatic displacement of the dens (Fig. CJ 5a–f).
4) Instability following bone resections in the area of C1 and C2.

Of the numerous surgical procedures available, we shall look at several that have given us good results when performed jointly by a neurosurgeon and orthopedic surgeon (Trentz and Samii 1982; Trentz et al. 1984).

Operative Techniques

Rigid Internal Fixation with a Tension Band and Bone Cement

Tension-band fixation may be accomplished with wire loops that are fixed through drill holes to the occiput, to the posterior arch of the atlas, and to the laminae or spinous processes of C2 or C3. After the dislocation is reduced and the alignment checked by image intensifier, the wire loops are tightened, and finally bone cement is applied to provide rigid internal fixation.
A modification of this technique employs a dacron mesh that is immersed in liquid bone cement and shaped into a figure-of-eight loop that is placed around the spinous process of C2 or C3. Its ends are inserted into two occipital drill holes. Fixation is accomplished with bone cement (Fig. CJ 6a, b).

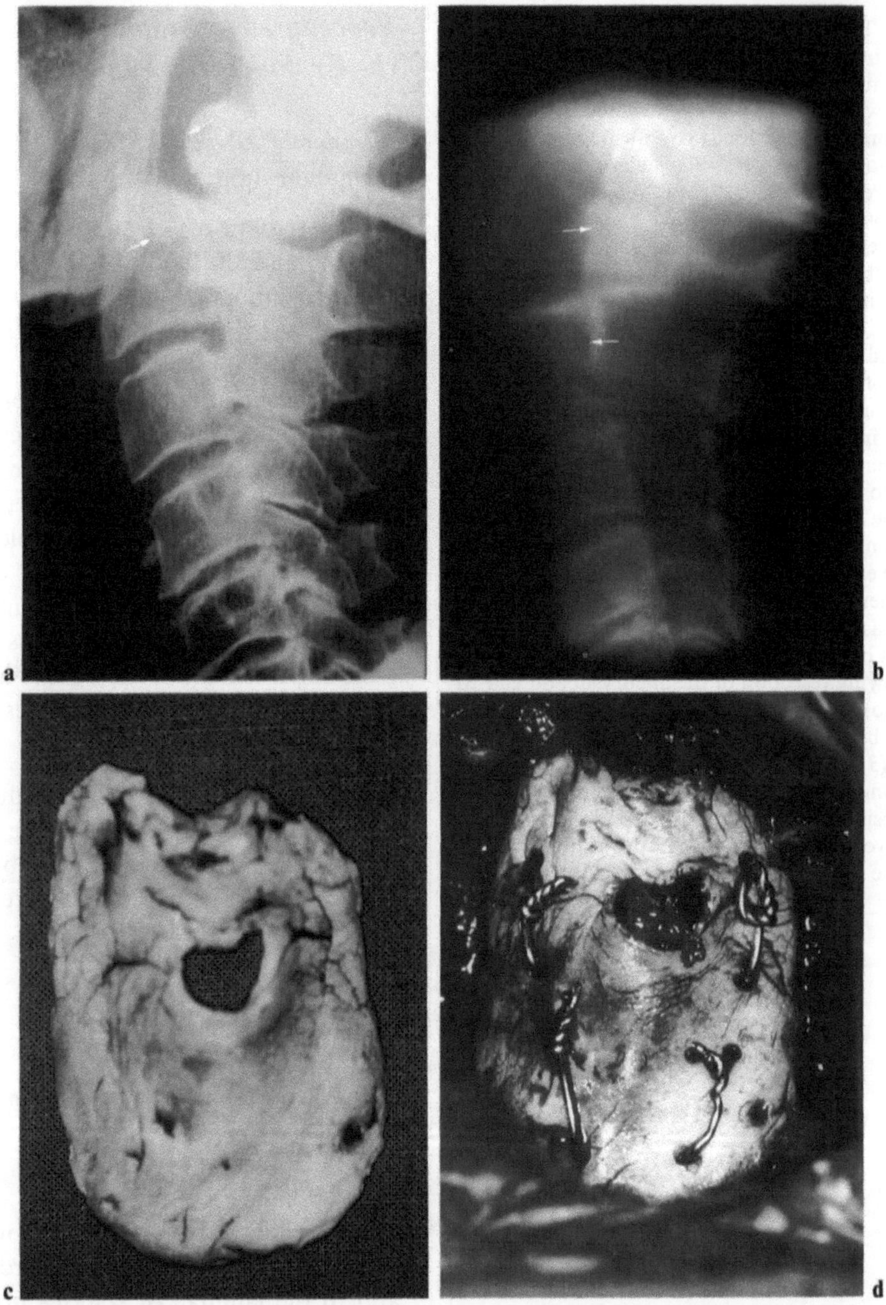

Fig. CJ 5a–f. Traumatic Anderson type III fracture of the dens in a woman 86 years of age. Because of the patient's advanced age, the fracture was treated in one stage by posterior fixation with methylmethacrylate and wire loops placed over the laminae of C1–C3.
a Lateral plain X-ray film of the upper cervical spine demonstrates a fracture of C2 with posterior displacement of the base of the dens.
b A lateral tomogram depicts the injury with even greater clarity.
c The premolded bone-cement plate used for atlantoaxial stabilization. The opening in the implant fits over the spinous process of C2.
d The plate spans the distance between the occiput and the spinous process of C3. The wire loops encircle the laminae and hold the plate securely against the first two cervical vertebrae.
e Postoperative lateral roentgenogram demonstrates the reduction of the fragments and the support of the upper cervical spine.
f The patient was mobilized from bed shortly after surgery

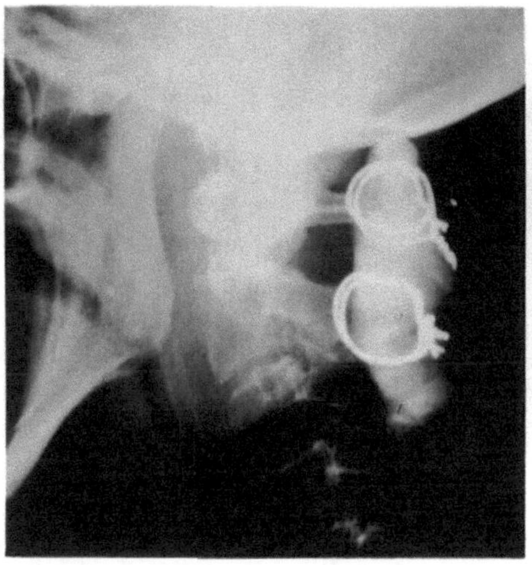
e

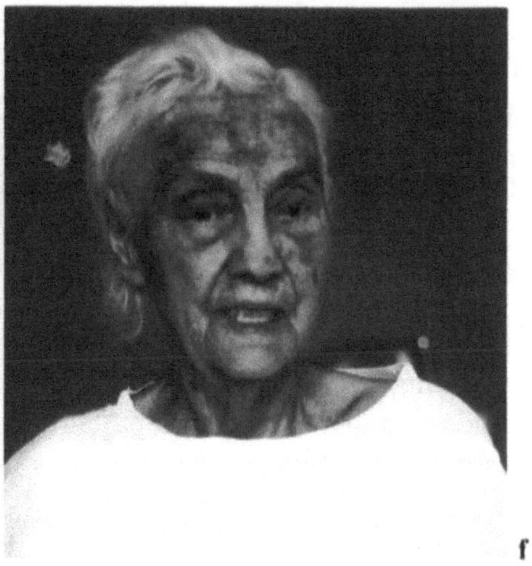
f

Fig. CJ 5e, f

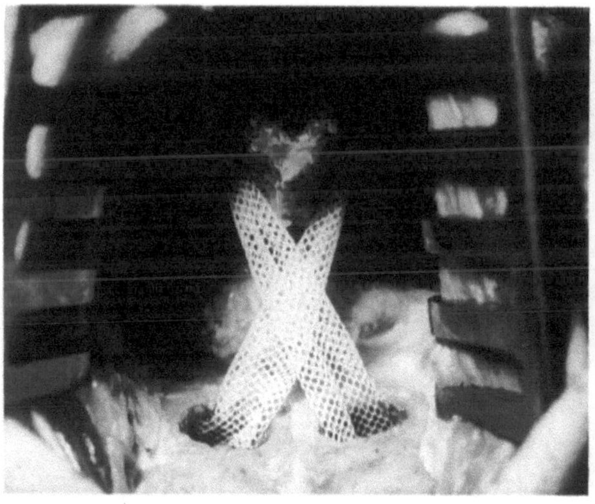
a

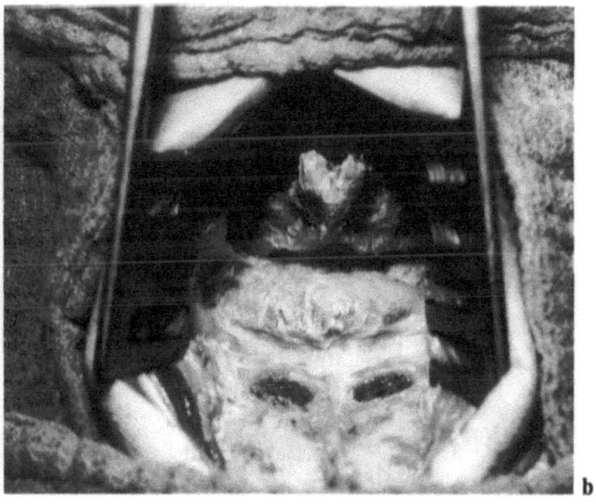
b

Fig. CJ 6a, b. Specimen illustrating the technique of rigid internal fixation with a dacron tension band and bone cement.
a The occiput is exposed and perforated with two burr holes next to the midline. The posterior atlantooccipital ligament, arch of the atlas, and the dens and posterior arch of the axis are visible.
b The dacron mesh is looped around the spinous process of C2 in figure-of-eight fashion. The ends of the loop are secured in the burr holes under tension with methylmethacrylate

Another option is rigid internal plating of the craniocervical junction. Gros et al. (1974, 1975) use an inverted Y-shaped metal plate that is attached with screws to the occiput, the stumps of C2, and the articular processes of C3 and C4.

We prefer rigid internal fixation as a palliative measure for incurable tumors associated with pain and spinal cord compression. It is also appropriate for traumatic and pathological displacements in elderly individuals and in patients who are poor surgical candidates.

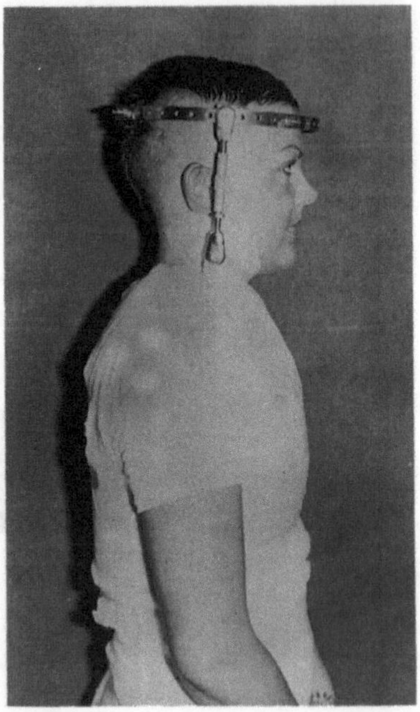

Fig. CJ 7. External fixation with a halo apparatus

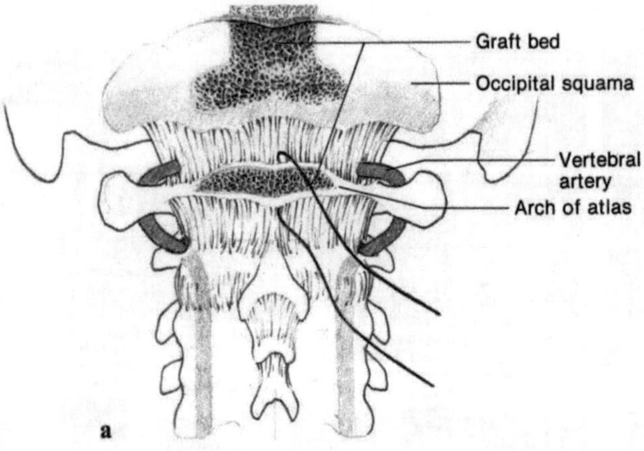

a

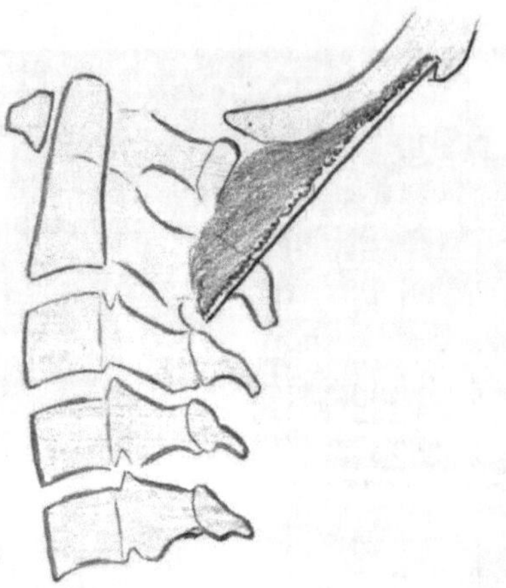

b

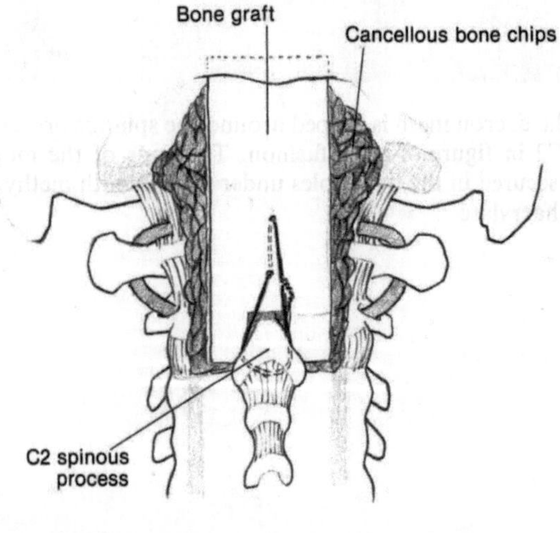

c

Fig. CJ 8a–c. Posterior stabilization of the craniocervical junction with a free iliac corticocancellous graft (*schematic drawing*).
a Posterior view of the craniocervical junction. A graft bed has been prepared in the occiput and arch of C1 with a cutting burr. A wire loop is passed through the posterior arch of the atlas.
b, c Lateral and posterior views after insertion of the iliac crest graft. The graft is wedged between the occiput superiorly and the arch of C1 and spinous process of C2 inferiorly. Spaces between the graft and recipient bed are filled with cancellous bone chips. The graft is secured with a wire loop

Stabilization by Bony Fusion and External Fixation with a Halo Apparatus (Fig. CJ 7) ***or Minerva Jacket***

Undoubtedly the best results can be achieved with autogenous bone grafts owing to their high osteogenic potential. Bony fusion also can be obtained with deep-frozen homologous grafts, though at a slower rate. Graft healing and osteoneogenesis are improved by decortication with a drill or osteotome. A layer of cancellous bone graft is applied over the opened haversian canals of the graft, and this is covered by a well-fitting cortical graft from the iliac crest supported at the base of the C2 spinous process and compressed with a wire loop (Figs. CJ 8 a–c, CJ 9). We prefer bony fusion using autogenous grafts and external stabilization with a halo apparatus.

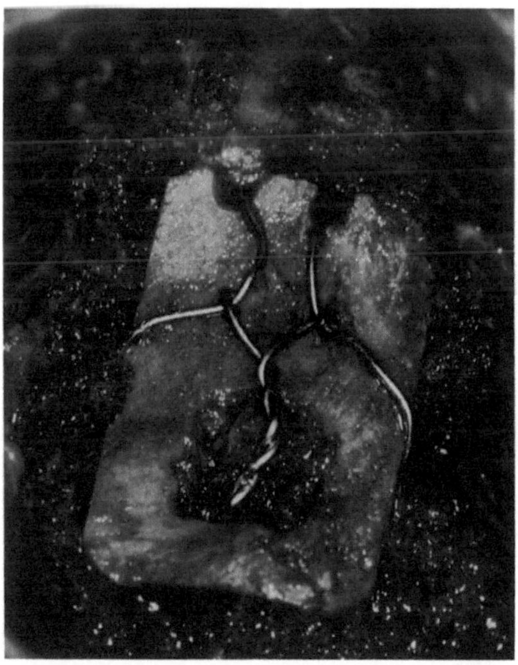

Fig. CJ 9. Posterior view of the upper cervical spine at operation. A wire loop encircles the laminae of the first two cervical vertebrae. A layer of cancellous bone was applied to C1 and C2 after decortication, and the cortical graft from the iliac crest was placed over it and compressed with a wire loop

Stabilization by Bony Fusion and Temporary Internal Fixation

The bone grafts are prepared and inserted as described above, but the wire fixation is reinforced with bone cement. After the bone grafts have become incorporated, the wire loops and bone cement may be removed. This technique should be considered when bony fusion is desired, but external stabilization is not possible.

Stabilization by Bony Fusion and Permanent Internal Fixation with a Compression Clamp

Roosen and coworkers (1982, 1983, 1984) have recently developed a *compression clamp* that can provide *permanent internal fixation* after bone grafts have been inserted for spinal fusion. Special clamps made of noncast steel are applied to the arches of C1, C2, or C3 on both sides of the corticocancellous grafts and tightened with a special wrench. Regardless of the type of bony injury and the degree of atlantoaxial instability, it may be necessary to apply additional anterior fixation with a plate or screws. Rosen et al. state that so far they have not found it necessary to remove the relatively small, bioinert implants.

References

Brattström H, Elner A, Granholm L (1973) Transoral surgery for myelopathy caused by rheumatoid arthritis of the cervical spine. Ann Rheum Dis 32:578–581

Fang HSY, Ong GB (1962) Direct anterior approach to the upper cervical spine. J Bone Joint Surgery 44:1588–1604

Gros C, Frerebeau Ph, Privat JM, Bazin M, Perez-Dominguez E (1974) Osteosynthese du rachis sons-occipital par plaques occipito-cervicales vissees. Montpellier-Chirurgical 20:269–274

Gros C, Privat JM, Frerebeau Ph, Bonnel F, Bazin VM, Benezech J (1975) Arthrodese du rachis spus-occipital par plaque occipito-cervicale vissee. Neurochirurgie (Paris) 21:231–238

Robinson RS, Lee H, Riley Jr (1975) Techniques of exposure and fusion of the cervical spine. Clin Orthop Rel Res 109:78–84

Roosen K, Grote W, Trauschel A (1982) Posterior atlanto-axial fusion. A new compression clamp for laminar osteosynthesis. Arch Orthop Traumat Surg 100:27–31

Roosen K, Grote W, Trauschel A (1983) Modern treatment of the symptomatic os odontoideum. Neurosurg Rev 6:223–229

Roosen K, Rauhut F, Maksoud M (1984) HWS-Verletzungen im Kindesalter. Neurochirurgia 27:1–5

Schürmann K (1979) Atlanto-axial dislocation in rheumatoid arthritis with cervical cord compression. Arch Neurosurgery 7:151–159

Sherk HH (1975) Lesions of the Atlas and Axis. Clin Orthop Rel Res 109:33–41

Stein BM, Leeds NE, Troveres IM, Pool JL (1963) Meningeomas of the Foramen magnum. J Neurosurg 20:740–751

Trentz O, Samii M (1982) Various techniques for the stabilisation of the occipito-cervical junction. Course on the surgery of the posterior skull base, March 17–20, Hannover

Trentz O, Flory P, Bühren V (1984) Verschiedene Techniken der occipito-cervikalen Fusion. Langenbeck Arch Chirurg 364:347–350

Verbiest H (1961) Anterior operative approach in cases of spinal cord compression by old irreducible displacement or fresh fracture of cervical spine. J Neurosurg 19:389–400

Verbiest H (1969) Anterolateral operations for fractures and dislocations in the middle and lower parts of the cervical spine. J Bone Joint Surgery 51a:1489–1530

Verbiest H (1977) Lesions of the cervical spine: A critical review. International Congress Series No. 433 Neurological Surgery. Proceedings of the Sixth International Congress of Neurological Surgery Sao Paulo. Excerpta Medica Amsterdam Oxford

Wayne O, Robinson RA (1957) Surgical approaches to the vertebral bodies in the cervical and lumbal regions. J Bone Joint Surgery 39:631–644

Facial Nerve and Skull Base Surgery (FN)

Introductory Remarks. The facial nerve has a special status among the cranial nerves because functional deficit may easily occur. This relates to its complicated anatomic course and to the very long facial nerve segment that transverses the bony skull base. Malformations, trauma, inflammations, and surgical procedures all are potential causes of facial nerve paralysis. The resulting functional disability and cosmetic deformity can be extremely distressful, and therefore every effort should be made to avoid facial nerve injury if possible, and to perform immediate, definitive repair of facial nerve lesions that are inflicted during an operation.

A variety of surgical procedures are available for the secondary treatment of facial paralysis, and their indications should be carefully considered on an individualized basis.

Patient selection for a reconstructive procedure and the timing of the operation are difficult issues of discussion, because it is not always easy to determine the extent of a post-traumatic or postsurgical facial nerve lesion.

From the standpoint of tumor surgery, it is relevant that the fibrous tissue sheath of the facial nerve is extremely delicate in the cerebellopontine angle and internal auditory canal and thins rapidly as the nerve courses peripherally from the geniculate ganglion. This means that mechanical irritation of the cerebellopontine and meatal segments of the facial nerve can have serious functional consequences even when the nerve is anatomically intact, and that recovery can be problematic. These cases require close, critical observation by the surgeon and the utilization of all diagnostic aids. Only in this way can the necessity of a direct or indirect nerve reconstruction be established promptly, before irreversible muscular changes have occurred. When facial palsy is due to inflammatory or neoplastic causes, elimination of the causative lesion often is sufficient to cure the palsy or at least is helpful in assessing the need for reconstruction.

It is known that the functional outcome of facial nerve reconstruction is related very definitely to the time at which the procedure is undertaken. On the other hand, we know from experimental and clinical findings in patients with unilateral division of the facial nerve that the paretic muscles can become partially reinnervated from the opposite side through collateral innervation (Fujita 1934). This mixed innervation extending across the facial midline may depend partly on congenital factors. In some cases the paralyzed muscles on the side where the nerve has been divided may receive fibers that sprout from the contralateral, intact facial nerve. Because the patient may continue to show the clinical manifestations of complete facial paralysis despite this collateral innervation, electromyographic testing is necessary when patients ask whether it is reasonable to attempt facial nerve reconstruction some years after the nerve lesion occurred.

Facial nerve surgery could not have attained its present status without the pioneering work of many authors, most notably Ballance (1909, 1932), Bonnel (1927), Cawthorne (1951, 1963, 1965), Clerc and Batisse (1954), Conley (1955, 1961, 1975), Dott (1958), Fisch (1969, 1972, 1973, 1976, 1977, 1979), W. F. House (1961, 1963), Jongkees (1958, 1961), Kettel (1957, 1959), Lathrop (1953, 1956, 1962), R. C. Martin (1930, 1931, 1936, 1955), Maxwell (1951, 1954), May (1986), Miehlke (1960, 1961, 1973, 1979), and Wullstein (1958, 1968).

General Operative Techniques

Surgical Approaches to the Different Facial Nerve Segments
(Fig. FN 1)

The surgical anatomy of the facial nerve is conveniently discussed in terms of four major segments (Draf 1980). From the center to the periphery, these are:

1) The cerebellopontine segment.
2) The internal auditory canal (meatal) segment.
3) The fallopian canal segment.
4) The extratemporal segment.

As it exits from the brain stem, the facial nerve is covered only by central glial cells for about the first 2 mm of its length. Afterward it is accompanied by Schwann cells. It is only in its fallopian and extratemporal course that the epineural and perineural fibrous tissue layers become thick enough to give significant protection against mechanical irritation. In the cerebellopontine angle and internal auditory canal, the facial nerve is exposed to rhythmic movements of the graft bed in the subarachnoid space. This compounds the difficulty of performing a successful anastomosis. The fallopian canal segment of the facial nerve is most favorable in terms of graft nutrition and anastomotic technique. The graft is immobile, and often an interposition graft can be placed without sutures. Graft nutrition also is very favorable in the extratemporal course of the nerve, although the motion factor in this area must be taken into account when determining the length of the graft. An overlapping exists in the surgical approaches to the various facial nerve segments. The cerebellopontine and meatal segments are accessible through the lateral suboccipital approach as well as through the transtemporal extradural and translabyrinthine routes. The initial labyrinthine portion of the fallopian canal about the geniculate ganglion can be reached by the transtemporal extradural route as well as transmastoidally. When pneumatization is poor, it may be necessary to dismantle the ossicular chain in order to reach the geniculate ganglion after mastoidectomy has been performed. With a low-lying dura, the geniculate ganglion may not be accessible by this route. The extratemporal segment is exposed either through preexisting soft-tissue injuries or through an incision like the one used for parotidectomy.

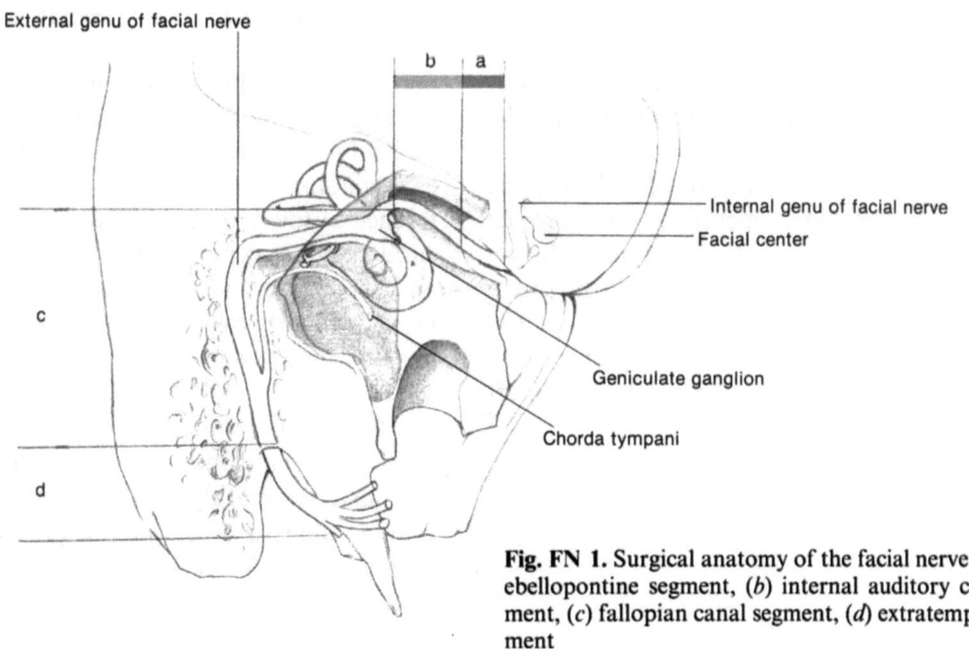

Fig. FN 1. Surgical anatomy of the facial nerve: (*a*) Cerebellopontine segment, (*b*) internal auditory canal segment, (*c*) fallopian canal segment, (*d*) extratemporal segment

Obtaining Grafts for Nerve Reconstruction

Introductory Remarks. Grafts for reconstruction of facial nerve continuity should have a diameter corresponding to that of the facial nerve *after* removal of the epineurium around the site of the anastomosis. Also, the graft must be available in sufficient length. A branching graft is frequently desirable for extratemporal grafting. Finally, removal of the graft should not create significant problems for the patient.

Branches of the cervical plexus, especially the greater auricular nerve, and the sural nerve are the most suitable donors of free grafts for facial nerve reconstruction. Their diameters approximate that of the facial nerve, branching segments can be obtained, and their proximity to the operative field has certain advantages. However, the maximum available graft length is only about 10 cm. In cases where a malignant tumor has been removed, the graft should be taken from the contralateral cervical plexus. The extra cervical incision should not be noticeable when good suturing technique is used, and the resulting sensory disturbances in the neck and auricle are well tolerated.

The sural nerve provides grafts up to 40 cm long with a diameter comparable to that of the facial nerve. Even branching grafts can be obtained in many cases. Removal of the nerve causes mild sensory loss on the side of the foot. Some experience is required for harvesting the graft. The substantial distance between the donor site and recipient bed has advantages and disadvantages. On the positive side, operating time can be shortened by performing the facial nerve dissection and graft removal concurrently; also, oncologic constraints are not a limiting factor. On the negative side, it is necessary to prepare and drape a separate area for an unplanned graft removal.

Operative Technique

Removal of a Cervical Plexus Graft (Fig. FN 2a)

In extracranial operations on the lateral skull base, it is usually possible to obtain a graft through the existing incision, or the incision may have to be extended inferiorly along the posterior border of the sternocleidomastoid muscle. If only a short graft is needed, a postauricular incision from the upper root of the auricle to the mastoid tip should suffice. The greater auricular nerve can be exposed just below the skin and dissected as far as Erb's point at the junction of the upper and middle thirds of the posterior sternocleidomastoid border, depending on the necessary length of the graft. A branched graft can be obtained if necessary by dissecting a branch of appropriate diameter, dividing it as centrally as possible, and removing it along with its peripheral branches, including the greater auricular nerve.

Removal of a Large Sural Nerve Graft (Fig. FN 2b,c)

The patient may be placed in the supine or prone position for removal of the sural nerve, although dissection is somewhat easier in the prone position. At the junction of the middle and anterior thirds of an imaginary line connecting the tip of the calcaneus with the lateral malleolus, the surgeon makes an anteriorly concave incision that parallels the posterior circumference of the malleolus. The main trunk of the sural nerve is generally found slightly anterior and medial to the small saphenous vein. The nerve is bluntly exposed along the course of the incision, and a small hemostatic forceps is inserted beneath it. By placing gentle traction on the hemostatic forceps and palpating for the nerve 10–15 cm above the lateral malleolus from the posterior midline of the lower leg, the surgeon is able to establish the proximal course of the nerve. A second, transverse incision is made at that level. Again the sural nerve is bluntly dissected and raised by a hemostatic for-

Fig. FN 2a–c. Free graft donor sites for facial nerve reconstruction.
a Anatomy of the cervical plexus as a donor site in the neck.
b Removal of a sural nerve graft from the leg. An anteriorly convex incision is made 1 cm behind the lateral malleolus, and the sural nerve is traced upwards by applying traction to the nerve and palpating its course. This is continued proximal by making a series of transverse incisions. The level at which the sural nerve disappears below the gastrocnemius muscle is variable. Branches of the sural nerve are most commonly found in its distal third.
c Topography of the sural nerve posterior to the lateral malleolus

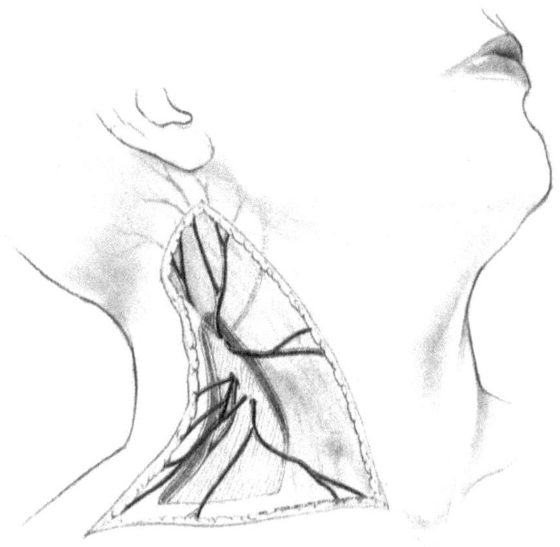

a

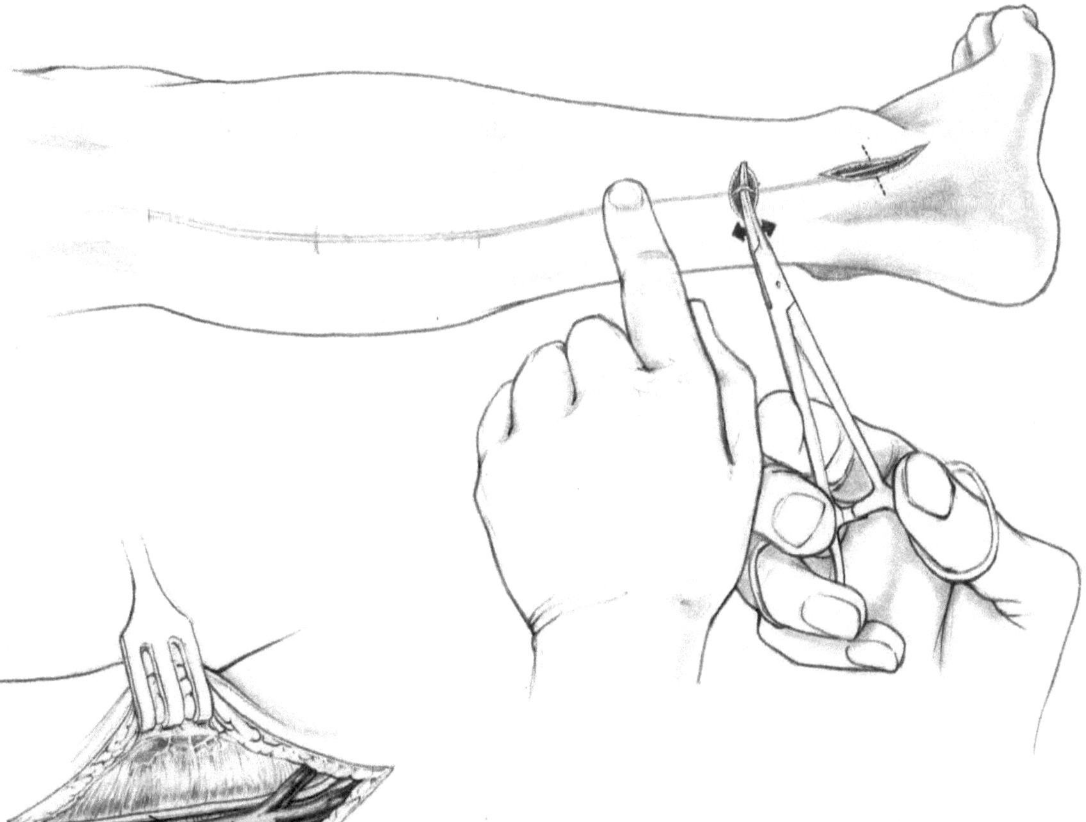

b

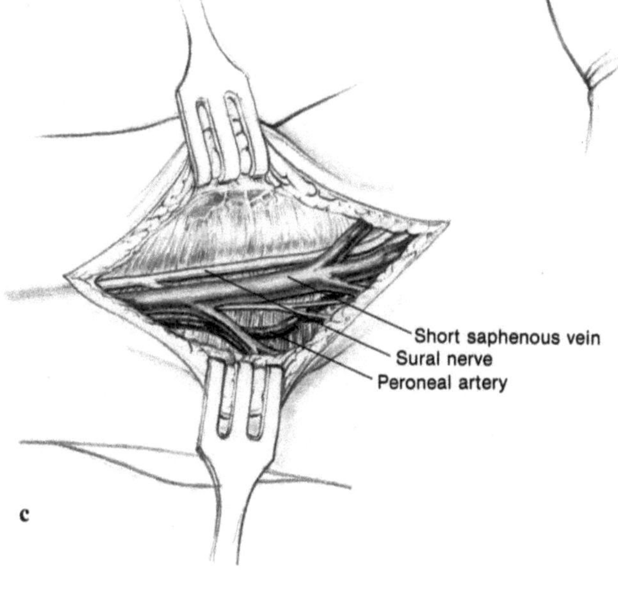

c

ceps placed beneath it, while gentle traction is placed on the distal forceps to confirm identification. The longitudinal fiber structure of the nerve readily distinguishes it from the small saphenous vein. One or two additional transverse incisions may be placed as far as the popliteal fossa, depending on the necessary length of the graft. The nerve is divided at that level and harvested by traction on the hemostatic forceps. If large branches exist in the midportion of the nerve, it may be necessary to expose them through additional transverse incisions and cut them from the main trunk so that the latter can be extracted with minimal injury. Finally the auxiliary incisions are closed in layers, and the lower portion of the leg is bandaged with a compressive elastic band.

Technique of Nerve Suture
(Fig. FN 3a–d)

Introductory Remarks. Three factors account for the superiority of the microsurgical technique (Samii 1975):

1) Precise determination of the extent of the nerve lesion.
2) Optimum approximation of the nerve ends.
3) Reduction of surgical trauma by the use of microinstruments and extremely fine suture material (10-0).

Before the introduction of the microsurgical nerve suture in peripheral nerve surgery, individual epineural sutures were used in an effort to obtain optimum approximation of the nerve ends. While this technique does give accurate approximation, it cannot prevent the overriding, kinking, or displacement of individual fascicles, and epineural fibrosis can greatly reduce the number of functioning peripheral axons (Fig. FN 3c, d).

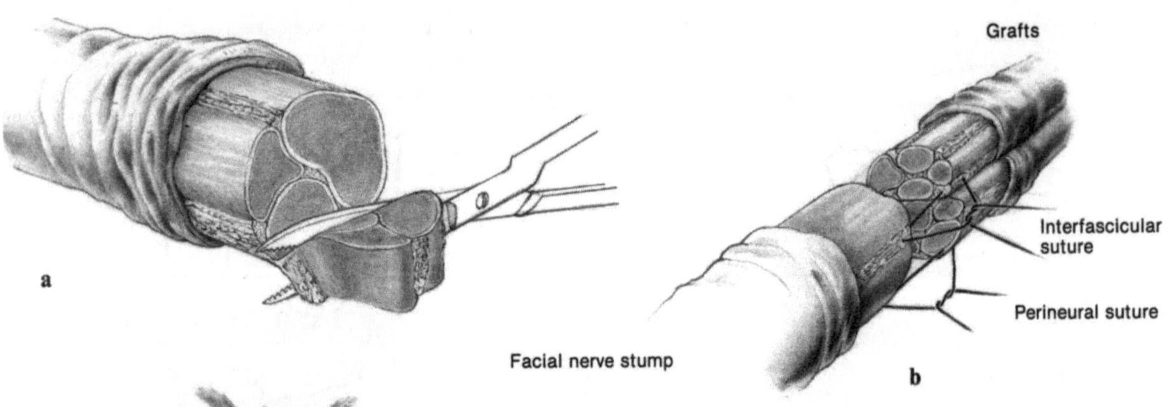

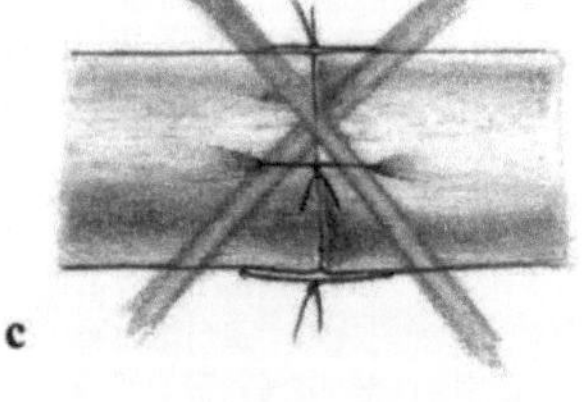

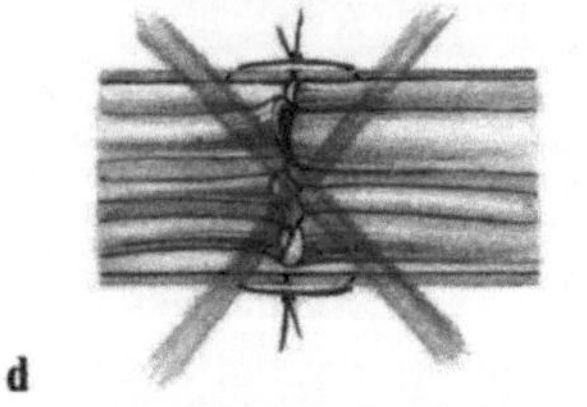

Fig. FN 3a–d. Technique of microsurgical perineural and interfascicular nerve suturing.
a Freshening the stump of the extratemporal facial nerve. The epineurium is stripped back, and the fascicles are freshened with scissors just before the anastomosis is performed.
b The nerve stumps are coapted with perineural and/or interfascicular sutures.
c, d With an epineural suture, the anastomosis may appear sound externally, but actually there is displacement and overriding of the nerve bundles within the epineural sheath

Before entering the stylomastoid foramen, the facial nerve consists microsurgically of a single nerve bundle, so splitting of the nerve should be avoided. This portion of the nerve is considered to have a monofascicular structure (Samii 1986). Opening and removing the epineurium at the nerve ends is crucial in preventing fibrosis at the suture site, which inhibits nerve regeneration. In its extratemporal course, the facial nerve consists of groups of fascicles that require interfascicular approximation. In the cerebellopontine and meatal segments of the nerve, the fibrous epineurium is so scant and has such little influence on nerve regeneration that it does not require removal.

Operative Technique

(Fig. FN 3a, b)

The first 1–2 mm of the epineurium is resected from the nerve stump and from the graft with microscissors. Smooth interfaces are created by cutting back the nerve fibers protruding from the fascicles. Then the perineural sutures are applied. We use 10-0 nonabsorbable monofilament for this purpose.

Besides precise approximation of the nerve stumps, a tension-free suture is crucial for a good functional result. In doubtful cases it is better to interpose an autogenous nerve graft and obtain two tension-free anastomotic sites than perform a single end-to-end anastomosis under tension (Samii 1975, 1980).

Special Operative Techniques

Introductory Remarks. Various techniques are available for the rehabilitation of facial paralysis, according to the site of the lesion and the timing of the intervention. These include decompressive procedures, methods of direct and indirect facial nerve reconstruction, and secondary plastic surgical measures for facial rehabilitation and reanimation. Direct or indirect facial nerve reconstructions may even be combined with secondary plastic procedures, depending on the nature of the lesion and the success of any prior reconstructive efforts. As a general rule, nerve decompression and direct facial nerve repairs produce the most satisfying results in terms of voluntary *and* emotional mimetic function. Techniques of indirect facial nerve reconstruction are regarded as methods of second choice, and secondary plastic surgical measures as methods of third choice. Various surgical options exist in each of these groups, and they differ markedly in their functional outcomes.

Decompression of the Facial Nerve

Introductory Remarks. Surgical decompression of the facial nerve is indicated after trauma, for Bell's palsy in rare cases, for inflammatory processes involving the petrous bone (especially certain forms of chronic otitis media), for cholesteatoma or necrotizing otitis externa, for tumor-related nerve compression, and for the treatment of hemifacial spasm caused by vascular compression at the brain stem. Even with modern diagnostic methods, it is not always possible to determine preoperatively whether it will be sufficient to expose the facial nerve, or whether reconstruction will be required. One should be prepared for the necessity of a nerve reconstruction whenever a decompressive procedure is undertaken. The techniques for simple exposure of the facial nerve after trauma (see p. 258), in inflammatory diseases (see p. 274), tumors (see p. 300), and for vascular decompression in hemifacial spasm (see p. 372) were previously described.

Bell's palsy represents a special case in terms of etiology and surgical management. The various names that have been given to the disease – idiopathic, rheumatoid, and ischemic facial paralysis – reflect the diversity of viewpoints concerning its etiology, which continues to be a topic of discussion. Hilger (1949) and several other authors attribute Bell's palsy to a spasm of the facial vessels arising from the external carotid artery. This spasm leads to nerve ischemia with capillary damage and consequent edema. The edema, in turn, compresses the nerve. A vicious cycle is established as this compression causes further obstruction of lymphatic and venous drainage, which in turn exacerbates the edema (Jongkees 1958, 1961). More recent investigations tend to minimize the importance of vascular dysregulation and point more to an allergic cause (McGovern 1977 a, b) or a viral etiology based on an acute, benign, cranial polyneuritis incited by a neurotropic herpes simplex virus (Adour 1977). Since Jannetta et al. (1978) achieved cures in six patients by exposing the cerebellopontine angle and relieving vascular nerve compression in that area, the sudden displacement of an arterial loop in the cerebellopontine angle with seventh nerve compression has been considered another potential cause of Bell's palsy. Idiopathic facial paralysis accounts for 58%–88% of all facial palsies (Adour 1975, 1976: 74%; Devriese 1977: 58%; Gomez 1977: 84%; Peitersen 1977: 70%). The attitude toward surgical decompression has changed markedly in the last decade. Formerly, when it was thought that Bell's palsy was caused by vascular dysregulation culminating in ischemia and nerve compression, chiefly in the bony fallopian canal, it was common to perform surgical decompression with neurolysis of the fallopian canal segment. But since the theories on an allergic or viral etiology became known, there has been much greater hesitancy to undertake decompression. This has also been due to various prospective studies showing that 70%–90% of patients display satisfactory recovery of facial nerve function with conservative treatment alone (Adour 1975, 1976, 1977; Peitersen 1977). Today surgical decompression of the facial nerve is rarely performed, and candidates are selected on the basis of various electrophysiologic studies such as electroneuronography and electromyography (Esslen 1973, 1977), the nerve excitability test (Jongkees 1977; Laumans and Jongkees 1963), and the minimal excitability test (May et al. 1971; May 1977).

Operative Technique

Transmastoid Facial Nerve Decompression
(Bonnel 1927, Wullstein 1958)

The operation may be performed under general anesthesia with postauricular injection of local anesthetic containing a vasoconstrictor, or local anesthesia and sedation may be employed. The operation begins with an extensive mastoidectomy in which the bone is removed to the dura of the middle cranial fossa and also posterolaterally to the sigmoid sinus. After locating the epitympanic recess with the incus and lateral semicircular canal, the surgeon identifies the bone overlying the mastoid facial nerve segment inferior to the tip of the short process of the incus. The more extensive the pneumatization, the thinner the bony coverage of the facial nerve. As the cutting burr approaches the facial canal, the nerve sheath will appear whitish through the bone when viewed with the microscope. A large accompanying blood vessel also will be visible as a reddish streak. The cutting drill is used with a constant up-and-down motion and gentle pressure while maintaining continuous irrigation to prevent thermal injury to the nerve. Occasionally the facial nerve may take an atypical course (Helms 1981). The bone over the nerve is exposed as far as the stylomastoid foramen, where it is removed somewhat more extensively. Next the bony shell in front of, above, and behind the facial nerve is thinned with the diamond burr until the bone can be elevated easily. After exposure of the mastoid fallopian canal, the angle between the chorda tympani and the facial nerve is drilled out to expose the incudostapedial joint and the tympanic facial nerve segment. With good pneumatization the geniculate ganglion, located medial to the long process of the incus, can be reached from above by dissecting along the floor of the middle cranial fossa with preservation of the ossicular chain. With only moderate pneumatization, it is necessary to disrupt the ossicular chain at the incudostapedial joint, extract the incus, and remove the head of the malleus with a punch rongeur. At the end of the operation a type III tympanoplasty is performed with elevation of the stapes, usually by the body of the incus. The geniculate ganglion lies in front of the anterior limb of the stapes at a distance equal to the distance between the stapedial limbs. After the bony shell has been thinned in the tympanic region, where mastoid dehiscence may occasionally be found, the bone overlying the entire facial nerve is progressively elevated with a small excavator. If a fracture is present, indriven bone fragments are removed. The operation concludes by incising the nerve sheath with a keratome knife or microscissors. The thick fibrous ring around the stylomastoid foramen is divided until the nerve fascicles are visualized. Trauma to the nerve bundles by the suction tip can be avoided by applying the suction indirectly through cotton. As the wound is closed in layers, the cutaneous auditory canal is retracted posteriorly to avoid stenosis of the introitus.

If hearing has been lost on the affected side, the mastoidectomy can be expanded to a labyrinthectomy to give access to the cerebellopontine portion of the facial nerve (see p. 257).

Transmeatal Decompression of the Geniculate Ganglion through the External Auditory Canal
(Helms 1976; Fig. FN 4a, b)

Various authors (Fisch and Esslen 1972; Fowler 1963; Helms 1976) believe that the causative lesion of idiopathic facial paralysis is located in the narrowest labyrinthine segment of the fallopian canal in more than 90% of cases. This view, if correct, provides a rationale for isolated surgical exposure of the geniculate ganglion (Helms 1976, 1982).

Building on the ideas of Cawthorne (1965a, 1965b, 1969), Helms began in 1971 to expose the geniculate ganglion through a transmeatal approach from the external auditory canal. Helms states that this approach is indicated when voluntary facial movements are not observed, and electrophysiologic tests show a reduction of excitability over a two-day period in the first two weeks. In Helms' series of over 40 patients with Bell's palsy, this approach was necessary in 8%. Recovery of nerve function was observed in all patients undergoing decompression, even those operated months or years after the onset of the palsy. Some amount of synkinesis was present in all cases, however.

The operation is generally performed under local anesthesia and sedation. Through an intra-aural auxiliary incision, a tympanomeatal flap based on the tympanic membrane is formed in the upper circumference of the auditory canal. The lateral wall of the attic is removed to expose the head of the malleus, the anterior sympathetic trunk (chorda tympani), and the attachment of the tensor tympani muscle. Directly anterior to the head of the malleus, the dissection is carried toward the medial wall of the tympanic cavity to the bone overlying the geniculate ganglion. Identification of the ganglion is facilitated by locating the greater petrosal nerve, which courses anteriorly. With good pneumatization, several smaller air cells will have to be opened before the ganglion can be identified.

The nerve sheath around the geniculate ganglion is incised. To conclude the operation, the tympanomeatal flap is turned back into position and splinted with two silicone strips, the external auditory canal is filled with sponge packing, and the intra-aural auxiliary incision is closed with sutures.

Our experience has been consistent with that of Helms. Compared with the transmastoid approach to the facial nerve, this operation is relatively simple for the experienced surgeon, takes little time, and is associated with low morbidity, especially with respect to the ossicular chain. When the bony skull base is situated low over the epitympanon, a contraindication exists to the transmeatal approach. This can be checked preoperatively by obtaining a Schüller X-ray view or a CT scan.

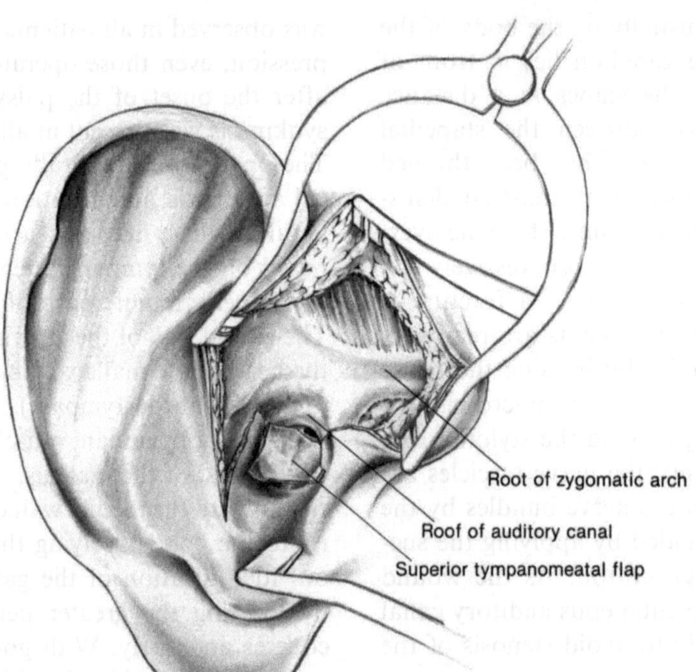

a

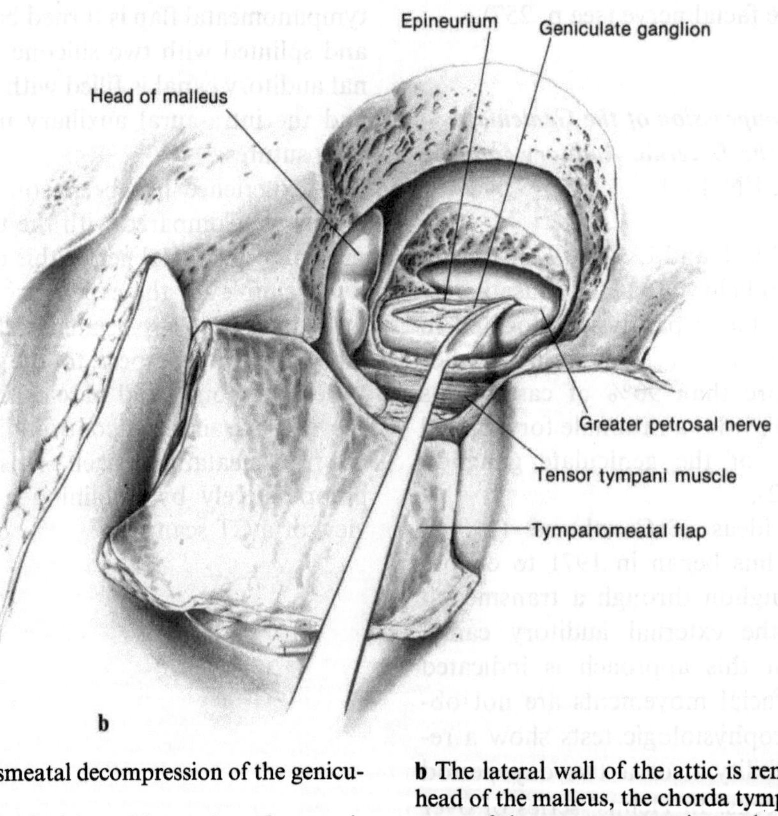

b

Fig. FN 4 a, b. Transmeatal decompression of the geniculate ganglion.
a Intra-aural auxiliary incision with creation of a superior tympanomeatal flap.
b The lateral wall of the attic is removed to expose the head of the malleus, the chorda tympani, and the attachment of the tensor tympani muscle. The geniculate ganglion has been exposed in the medial tympanic cavity. The nerve sheath is incised

Exposure of the Meatal, Labyrinthine, Tympanic, and Mastoid Segments of the Facial Nerve
(Fisch 1973, 1979; Fisch and Esslen 1972a, b)

Exposure of the facial nerve in the internal auditory canal and in the labyrinthine portion of the fallopian canal through the middle cranial fossa by the extradural, transtemporal route and of the tympanic and mastoid segments via a mastoidectomy in the same sitting is mainly indicated for extensive fractures of the petrous bone that have not destroyed hearing. In patients with Bell's palsy, Fisch exposes the facial nerve in the internal auditory canal and in the labyrinthine part of the fallopian canal. If the lesion can be objectively confirmed in this region by intraoperative neuronography, the procedure is concluded by slitting the epineurium at the geniculate ganglion. In 6% of patients this is not the case, according to Fisch, and it becomes necessary to perform a transmastoid exposure of the facial nerve in the same sitting. Fisch states that transtemporal exposure is sufficient in zoster oticus.

The technique of the transtemporal extradural approach to the lateral middle skull base (see p. 252) and the transmastoid approach to the facial nerve (see p. 257) have been previously described.

Methods of Direct Facial Nerve Reconstruction

End-to-End Anastomosis in the Cerebellopontine Angle (Fig. FN 5)

An end-to-end anastomosis of the facial nerve in the cerebellopontine angle may be necessary when the thinned nerve cannot be preserved during removal of a large cerebellopontine angle tumor through the suboccipital route. The elongated condition of the nerve makes end-to-end anastomosis feasible, provided the surgeon is able definitely to identify the proximal and distal nerve stumps using topographic criteria. An end-to-end suture can bridge a defect of approximately 1–1.5 cm in the stretched nerve without

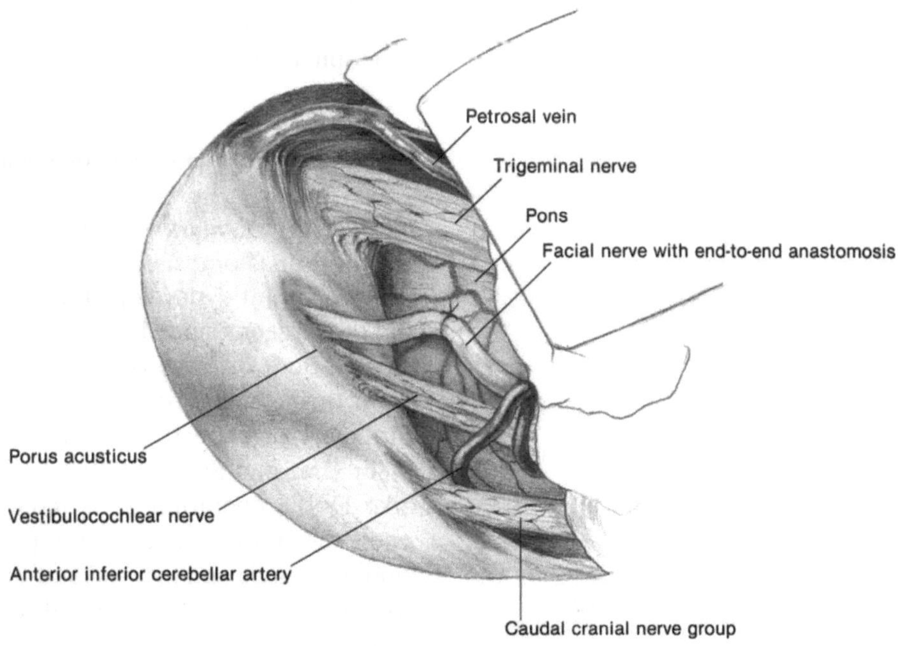

Fig. FN 5. End-to-end anastomosis of the facial nerve in the cerebellopontine angle. The site of the anastomosis is steadied against the brain stem

causing tension. The results of direct facial nerve repair in the cerebellopontine angle are encouraging (Drake 1973; Samii 1977, 1979, 1981). It is superior to all other reconstructive procedures and therefore worth attempting.

After the nerve ends have been freshened, they generally can be united with one or perhaps two sutures. Because of the pulsations in the cerebellopontine angle, it is good practice to place the anastomosis up against the brain stem or the porus of the internal auditory canal and support it temporarily with sponge packing. Larger nerve defects in the cerebellopontine angle may require the use of an interposition graft (Fig. FN 6).

Intracranial-Extracranial Anastomosis
(Dott 1958)

Introductory Remarks. Dott (1958) proposed a technique for bridging large facial nerve defects following acoustic neuroma surgery in which a long nerve graft is used to establish a communication between the central facial nerve stump in the cerebellopontine angle and the extratemporal main nerve trunk.

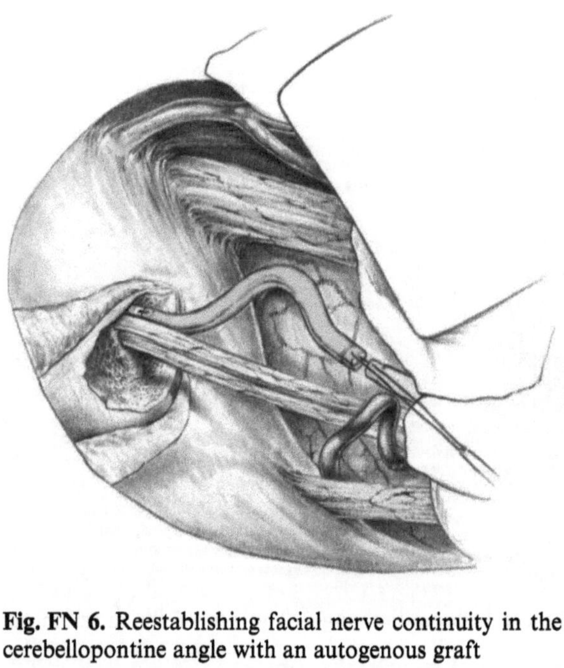

Fig. FN 6. Reestablishing facial nerve continuity in the cerebellopontine angle with an autogenous graft

Operative Technique
(Fig. FN 7a,b)

After removal of the tumor, a free autogenous sural nerve graft 15–20 cm long is harvested and anastomosed to the central facial nerve stump at the brain stem. The donor nerve is brought out over the edge of the craniectomy and pulled down between the sternocleidomastoid and splenius capitis muscles through a subcutaneous tunnel below the mastoid. The distal end of the graft is marked with a silver clip and fixed in the retromandibular fossa. In a second operation approximately three months later, the distal end of the graft is located and anastomosed to the peripheral main facial nerve trunk distal to the stylomastoid foramen. Despite reports of good to excellent results (Drake 1960; Loew 1961; Miehlke 1960, 1967), we know of only seven cases that have been published since Dott first described the operation. The most likely reason for this is the difficulty of identifying the facial nerve at the brain stem without benefit of the operating microscope.

It is best to route the nerve graft out of the cranium through a separate incision made obliquely through the dural layers, rather than through the dural suture, as this lessens the danger of secondary graft compression and cerebrospinal fluid leakage.

Intracranial-Intratemporal Anastomosis

Introductory Remarks. The intracranial-intratemporal anastomosis is a new procedure that has been jointly developed by neurosurgeons and otosurgeons since 1975 in an effort to make preservation or reconstruction of the facial nerve through microsurgical technique a standard part of acoustic neuroma surgery (Draf 1980; Draf and Samii 1982; Samii 1979, 1981). Like Dott's operation, it is indicated in cases where the peripheral nerve stump in the cerebellopontine angle and internal auditory canal does not appear to be suitable for a direct reconstruction.

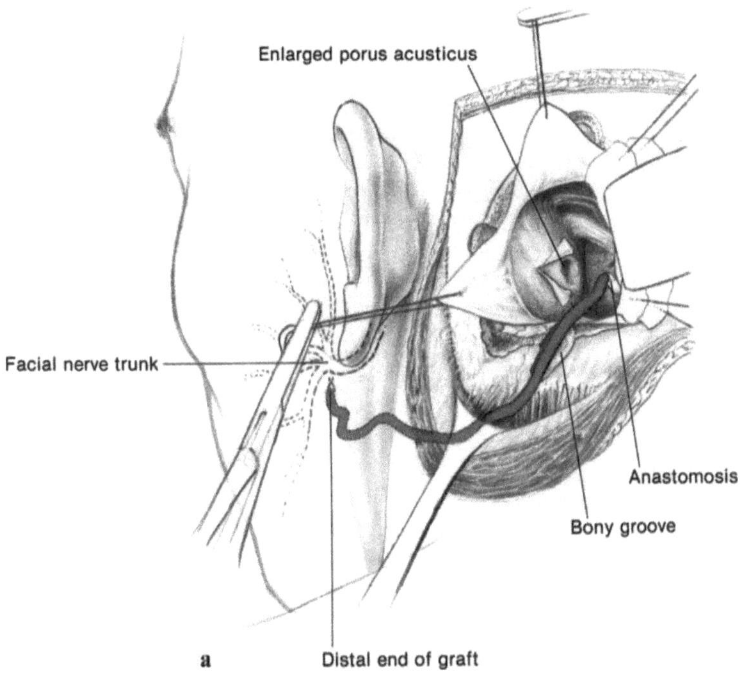

a

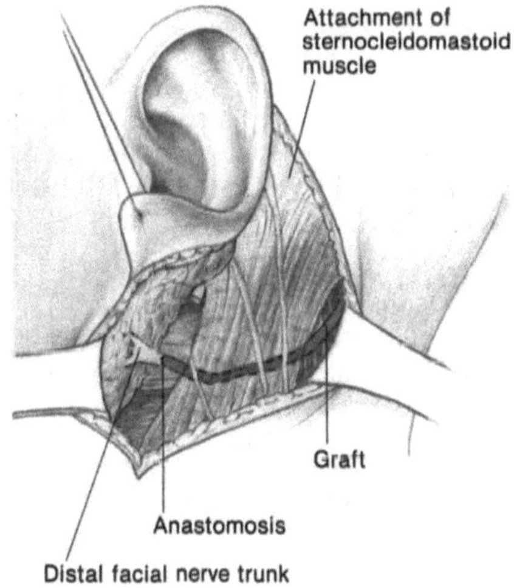

b

Fig. FN 7 a, b. Dott's operation.
a After the graft is united to the facial nerve stump in the cerebellopontine angle, it is brought out through a bony groove in the inferior edge of the suboccipital craniectomy, and the distal stump is marked with a thread and delivered to a point near the stylomastoid foramen. Then the dura of the suboccipital approach is closed.
b In a second operation several weeks or months later, the distal end of the graft is anastomosed to the distal stump of the main facial nerve trunk, which is divided at the stylomastoid foramen

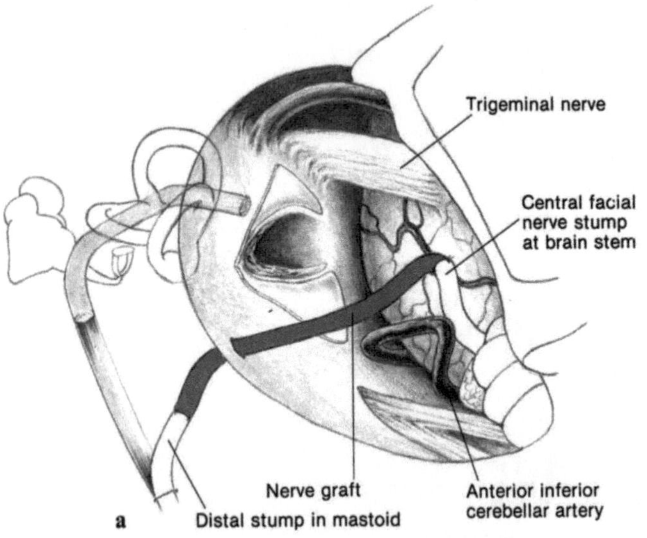

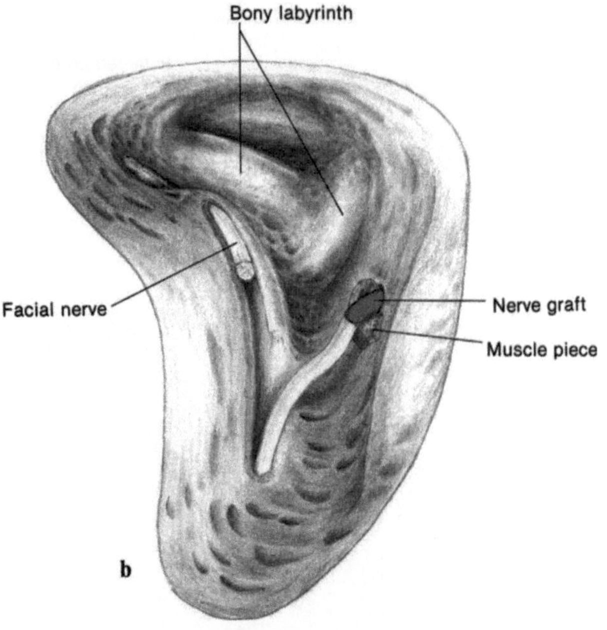

Fig. FN 8 a, b. The intracranial-intratemporal anastomosis.
a Cerebellopontine angle and petrous bone with mastoid (*semischematic view*). The intracranial anastomosis between the facial nerve stump and a sural nerve graft is performed so that the anastomotic site rests against the brain stem and is stabilized by it. Following mastoidectomy, the graft is brought out through a small dural incision behind the porus acusticus and delivered into the mastoid process.
b View into the mastoid after completion of the intratemporal anastomosis. The facial nerve has been divided below the lateral semicircular canal and the distal part transposed posteriorly

Operative Technique

(Fig. FN 8a, b; Fig. FN 9a–c; Fig. FN 10a–c)

Even after removal of a large acoustic tumor, it is usually possible to preserve 1–1.5 cm of the central facial nerve stump at the brain stem. An autogenous nerve graft approximately 5 cm long is taken from the sural nerve and united with 1 or 2 sutures to the central facial nerve stump at the brain stem. Initially we routed the distal end of the graft into the internal auditory canal and pulled it through into the mastoid following a transmastoid-translabyrinthine exposure. We have found it more appropriate to bring the graft out of the cerebellopontine angle into the mastoid through an oblique dural incision after removing some of the posterior surface of the petrous bone at the sinodural angle. This obviates the need for a time-consuming labyrinthectomy. In the same sitting the otosurgeon performs a mastoidectomy through a separate postauricular incision. The mastoid segment of the facial nerve is exposed, sectioned below the lateral semicircular canal, and transposed posteriorly toward the sinodural angle along a new bony groove for anastomosis to the distal end of the graft. Sponge is packed around the site of entry of the graft into the mastoid to prevent cerebrospinal fluid leak. The operation concludes with closure of the suboccipital dura and soft tissues. This measure increases the total operating time in no more than about one hour with proper organization. We feel that this is more than justified by the excellent results that we have achieved to date in 12 patients (Samii 1984).

Fig. FN 10. Patient who underwent removal of a large acoustic neuroma and intracranial-intratemporal nerve grafting, in the early postoperative period (**a**) and 15 months after facial nerve reconstruction (**b, c**) with satisfactory function

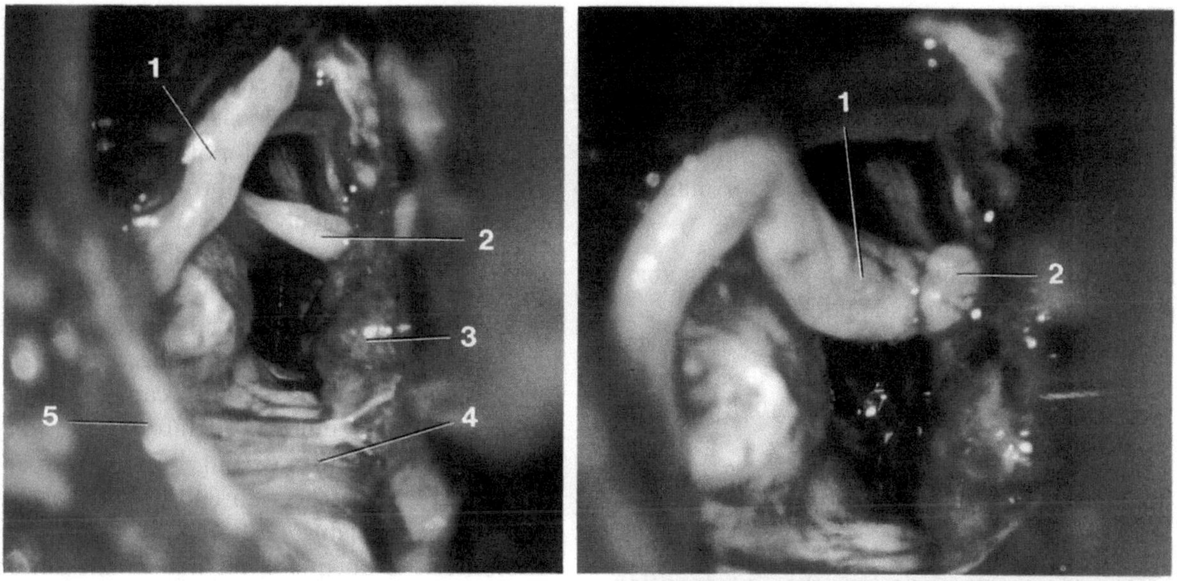

a b

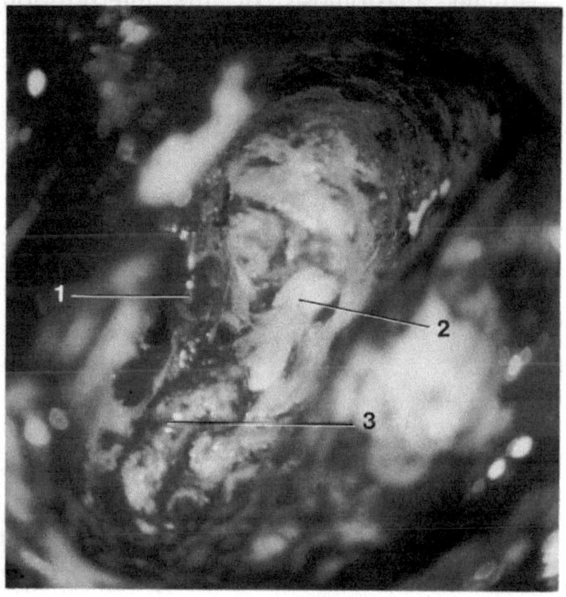

c

Fig. FN 9a–c. Example of an intracranial-intratemporal facial nerve graft.
a View into the left cerebellopontine angle. The central facial nerve stump is exposed, and a nerve graft has already been routed from the cerebellopontine angle to the mastoid. (*1*) Graft, (*2*) central facial nerve stump, (*3*) flocculus, (*4*) caudal cranial nerves, (*5*) dural margin.
b The central anastomosis is completed. (*1*) Nerve graft, (*2*) central facial nerve stump.
c Mastoid part of the operation, showing the anastomosis between the peripheral main trunk of the facial nerve and the distal end of the graft. (*1*) Posterior wall of auditory canal, (*2*) graft from the posterior cranial fossa, (*3*) facial nerve (peripheral)

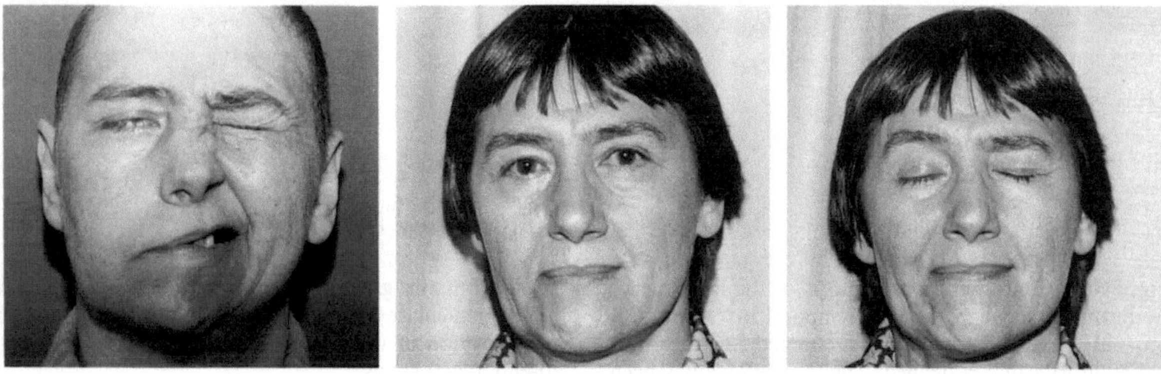

a, b c

Meatal Anastomosis

Introductory Remarks. In the transtemporal or translabyrinthine approach for the treatment of skull base fractures or removal of tumors, any of several techniques can be used for management of the facial nerve:

1) For nerve stretching, simple end-to-end anastomosis in the internal auditory canal.
2) For defects up to 1 cm, rerouting and end-to-end anastomosis of the facial nerve stumps (Bonnel 1927; Fisch 1969, 1970; Martin 1930, 1931, 1936).
3) Use of an interposition graft. In all cases there must be no tension at the anastomotic site. With proper technique, using the end-to-end anastomosis or the interposition graft, comparable functional results can be achieved.

Operative Technique

The technique of end-to-end anastomosis in the internal auditory canal is basically the same as that used in the cerebellopontine angle (see p. 483). In both areas the fibrous tissue sheath of the nerve is extremely thin.

For rerouting via the transtemporal extradural approach to the internal auditory canal (Fisch 1969, 1970), the central facial nerve stump is identified from above and mobilized from the labyrinthine part of the fallopian canal, the tympanic segment is mobilized, and a new bony canal is created with a cutting burr to gain enough length to perform an end-to-end anastomosis of the segments. Occasionally a sutureless anastomosis is adequate, relying on the action of endogenous fibrin to provide adherence between the nerve ends (Fig. FN 11). If the defect cannot be bridged by rerouting, an autogenous nerve graft is interposed (Fig. FN 12).

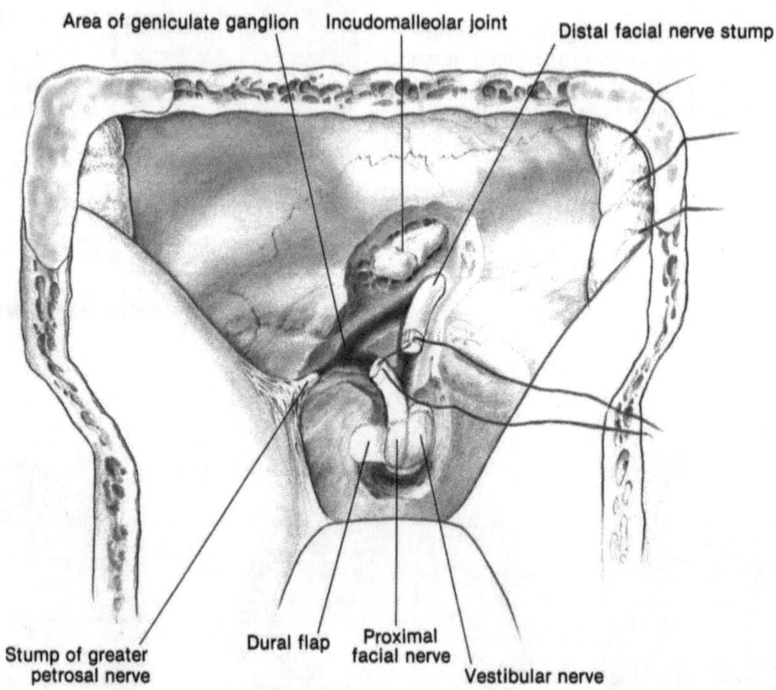

Fig. FN 11. End-to-end anastomosis of the facial nerve by rerouting through the transtemporal extradural approach. The middle fossa dura is retracted, and the internal auditory canal is opened. The facial nerve has been freed from the greater petrosal nerve. A short defect at the geniculate ganglion can be bridged by posterior transposition of the stumps and their tension-free end-to-end anastomosis

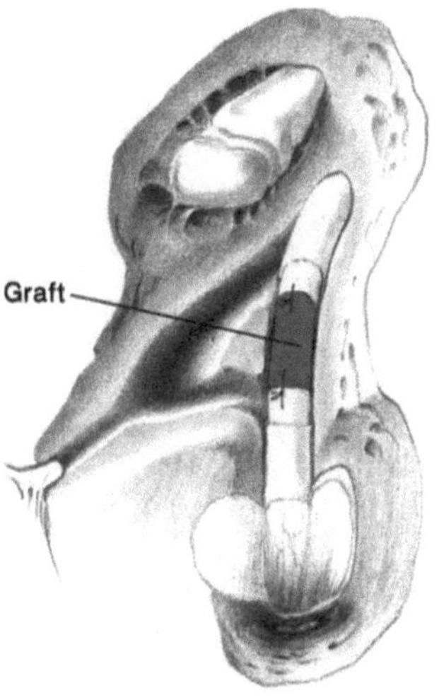

Fig. FN 12. Bridging a defect at the start of the fallopian canal through the transtemporal extradural approach. The junction of the internal auditory canal and fallopian canal is demonstrated. An autogenous nerve graft is interpolated to bridge the gap

The procedure is basically similar in cases where the internal auditory canal has been entered by the translabyrinthine route. After the central facial nerve stump has been identified, the peripheral end of the nerve is divided from the greater petrosal nerve at the geniculate ganglion, mobilized posteriorly, and united to the central stump in the internal acoustic meatus (Fig. FN 13a, b). The peripheral part of the nerve is easier to mobilize by dismantling the ossicular chain, leaving the stapes in place.

If rerouting is not possible, a free nerve graft is interpolated between the nerve ends. Suturing is necessary in the mobile graft bed within the internal auditory canal, but sutureless approximation of the nerve stumps is often adequate in the stable bony mastoid. The internal auditory canal must be sealed off from the mastoid with a piece of fascia or stored dura attached with adhesive. The mastoid process is freed of mucosa and obliterated with freshly obtained pieces of abdominal fat as a precaution against cerebrospinal rhinorrhea.

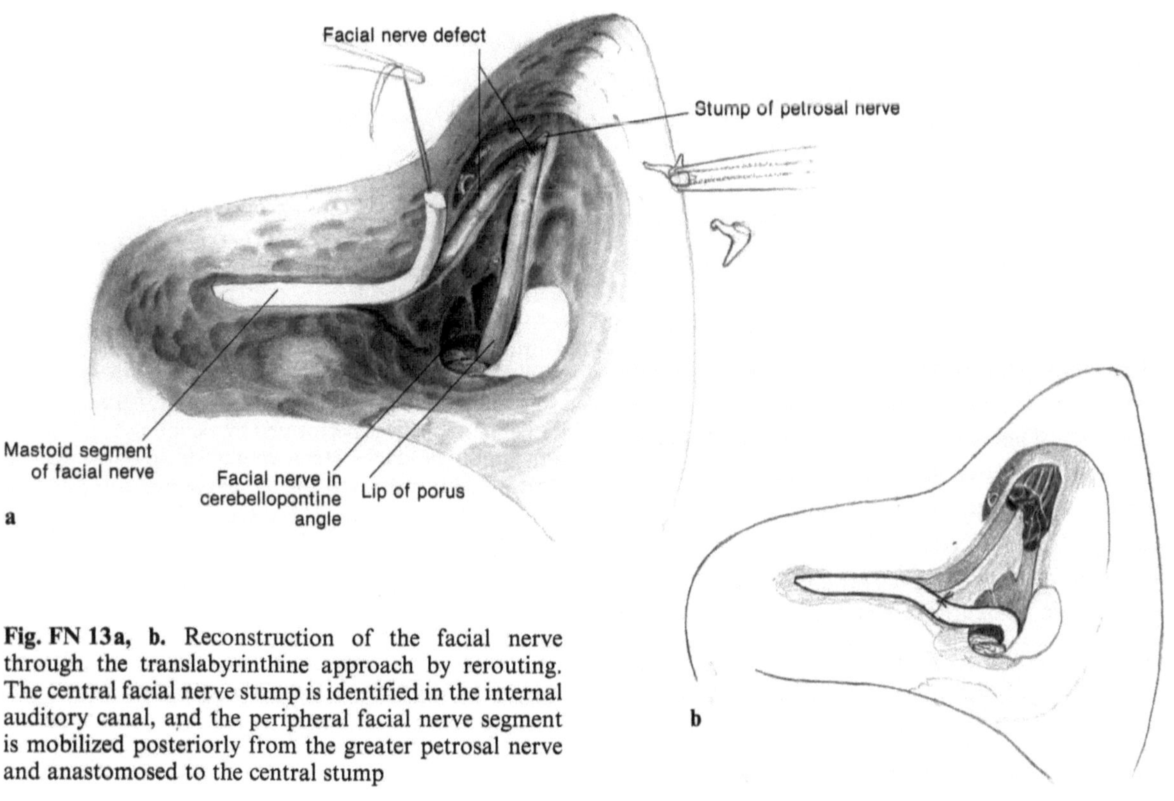

Fig. FN 13a, b. Reconstruction of the facial nerve through the translabyrinthine approach by rerouting. The central facial nerve stump is identified in the internal auditory canal, and the peripheral facial nerve segment is mobilized posteriorly from the greater petrosal nerve and anastomosed to the central stump

Tympano-Mastoid Reconstruction
(Fig. FN 14a, b)

Comminuted fractures of the petrous bone can severely damage the facial nerve in its tympanic and mastoid course. This is frequently accompanied by a dislocation of the ossicular chain and a dural defect. Besides repairing the cerebrospinal fluid fistula with a dural graft, it is necessary to expose the nerve defect and bridge it with a graft. Sutures are often unnecessary in this portion of the nerve. The ossicular chain is reconstructed if inner ear function is intact.

Intratemporal-Extratemporal Reconstruction

Introductory Remarks. Reconstruction of the main facial nerve trunk may present difficulties if the lesion extends into the stylomastoid foramen from above, from below, or from the mastoid aspect. This is especially true if the surgeon is not familiar with the intramastoid and extratemporal topographic anatomy of the facial nerve. In these cases interdisciplinary cooperation is strongly advised. Problems of nerve access or identification in the area of the stylomastoid foramen should never be the cause of an insufficient anastomosis in cases where the surgeon has been unable to obtain normal-appearing central and distal nerve stumps.

Operative Technique
(Fig. FN 15a–c)

If the main traumatic or tumor-related facial nerve lesion is extratemporal, this region is exposed first. The skin may be incised along preexisting scars or opened with an incision like that used for parotidectomy. We use an incision extending from the upper border of the tragus along the auricle to the base of the lobule of the ear. We then angle the incision 90° downward and carry it along the anterior border of the sternocleidomastoid to the junction of the superior and middle portions of the muscle. Our preferred landmarks for extratemporal identification of the facial nerve trunk are the anterior

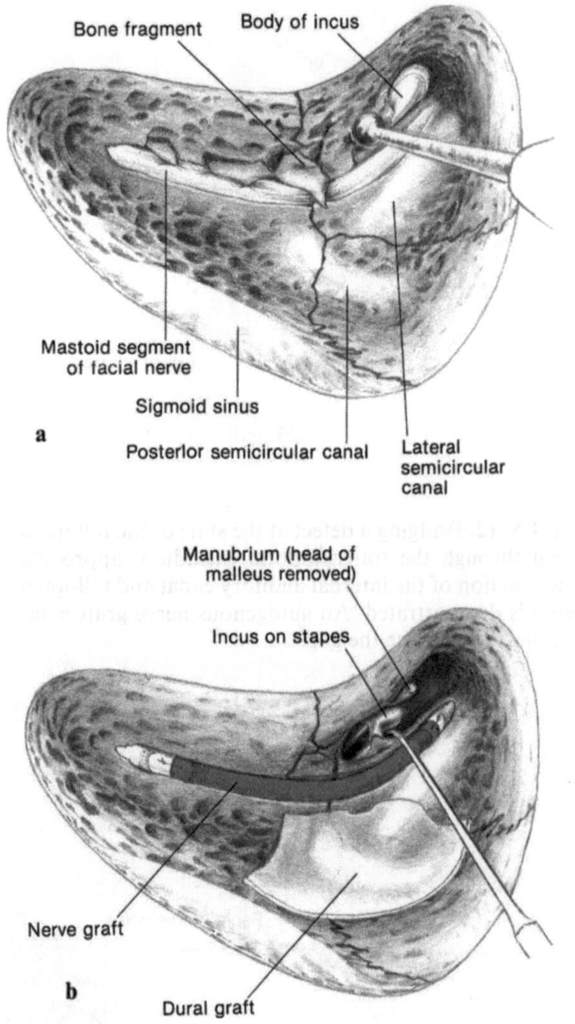

Fig. FN 14a, b. Facial nerve reconstruction with an autogenous graft in the tympanic and mastoid segments.
a A comminuted fracture has destroyed a significant portion of the facial nerve in its tympanic and mastoid course.
b After sealing the fracture lines with a dural graft and debriding the facial canal, the nerve defect is bridged with a graft. Sutures are not always necessary in the tympanic and mastoid segments of the nerve. A type III tympanoplasty is performed by elevating the dislocated incus on the stapes. Removing the head of the malleus creates additional room for the nerve anastomosis near the geniculate ganglion. This is especially necessary when pneumatization is poor

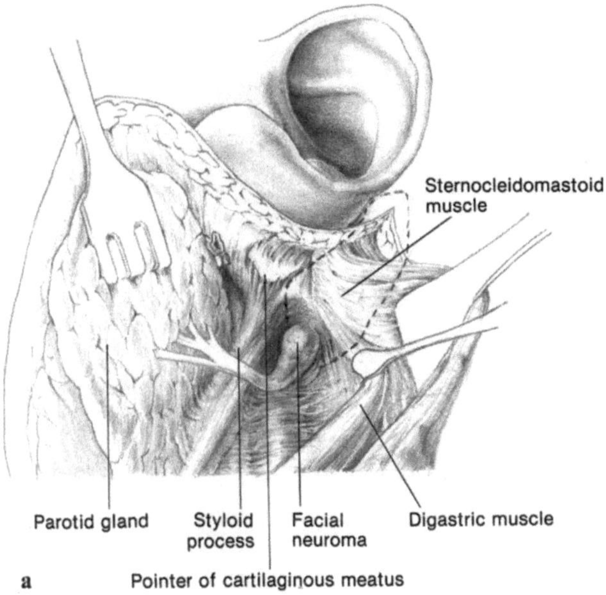

a

Fig. FN 15a–c. Intratemporal-extratemporal facial nerve reconstruction with an autogenous graft.

a The facial nerve is exposed from the stylomastoid foramen to its first branches in the parotid gland. There is neuromatous thickening of the nerve at the stylomastoid foramen. The landmarks for locating the facial nerve are shown: the styloid process, the "pointer" of the cartilaginous auditory canal, the attachment of the posterior portion of the digastric muscle, and the sternocleidomastoid attachment.

b The mastoid tip is removed to expose a significant length of healthy nerve proximal to the neuroma. The pathological nerve segment is excised.

c After the nerve stumps have been freshened, a graft is interposed and fixed with sutures

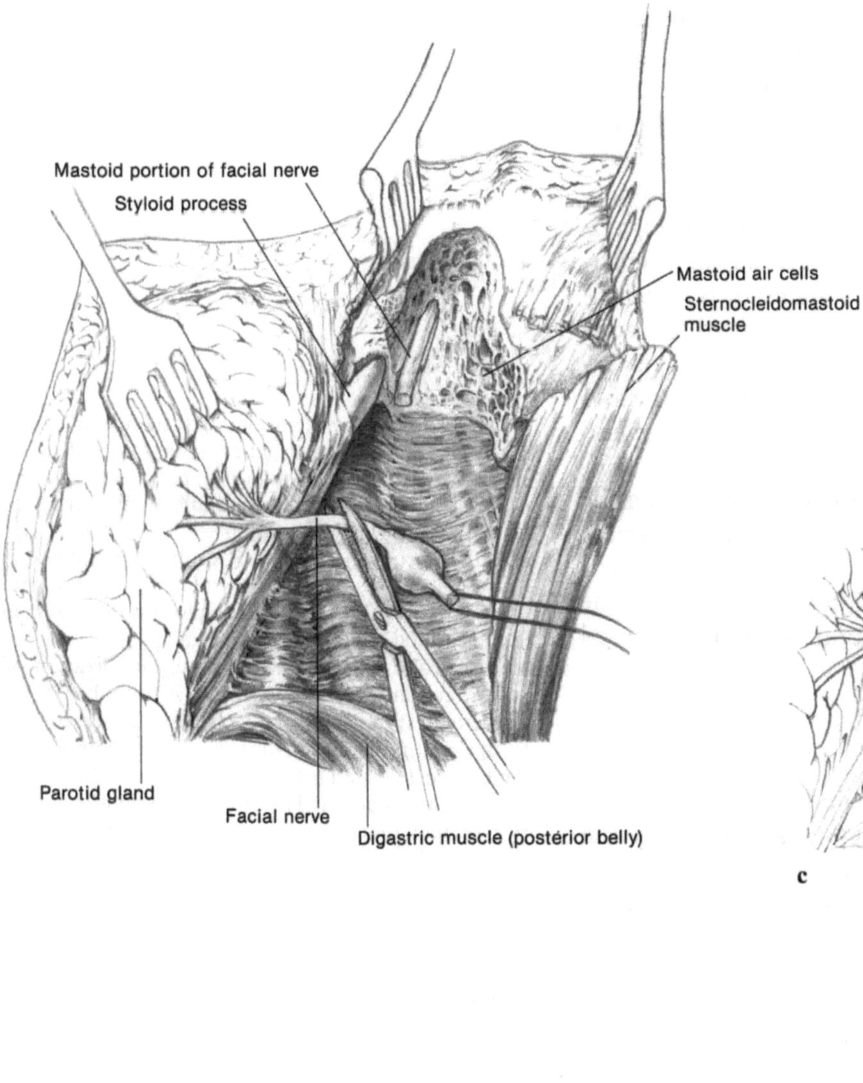

b

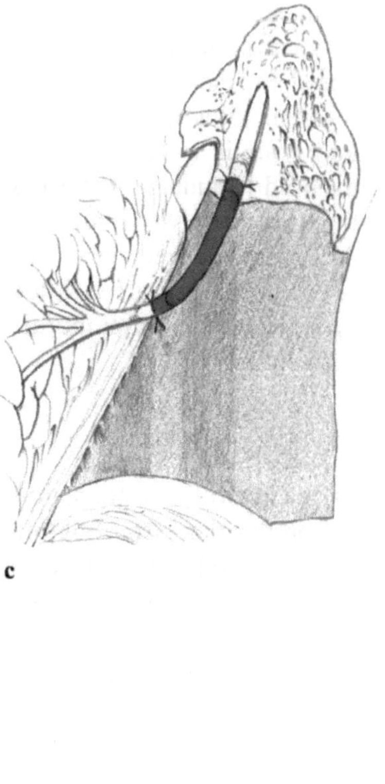

c

attachment of the sternocleidomastoid muscle, the attachment of the posterior portion of the digastric on the mastoid, and the "pointer" of the cartilaginous auditory canal (Conley 1975). The main facial nerve trunk is located just superior to the muscular attachments, medial to the posterior portion of the digastric, and, with the auricle reflected upward, approximately 10 mm medial to the cartilaginous "pointer." Wide exposure is obtained by separating the connective tissue fibers leading from the cartilaginous auditory canal to the parotid capsule as far as the muscle attachments. Once the main nerve trunk has been exposed, it is dissected free to its site of division or even farther peripherally if necessary, in which case the superficial lobe of the parotid gland is also removed. Next the nerve is inspected with the microscope, especially if the continuity of the nerve is grossly intact but the nerve appears thickened. If pathology is found that extends into the stylomastoid foramen, two options exist: The main nerve trunk can be traced farther cranially by progressive bone removal from the stylomastoid foramen, which can be difficult because of the tough connective tissue ring around the foramen. The better option is to perform a standard postauricular mastoidectomy similar to that used for facial nerve decompression. The facial nerve is exposed and isolated in the area where the mastoid segment joins with the extratemporal segment, and bone is widely removed around the stylomastoid foramen. This necessitates dividing the thick connective tissue ring in the foramen. After the lesioned nerve segment has been excised, a nerve graft is interposed between the mastoid and extratemporal trunk and secured with sutures.

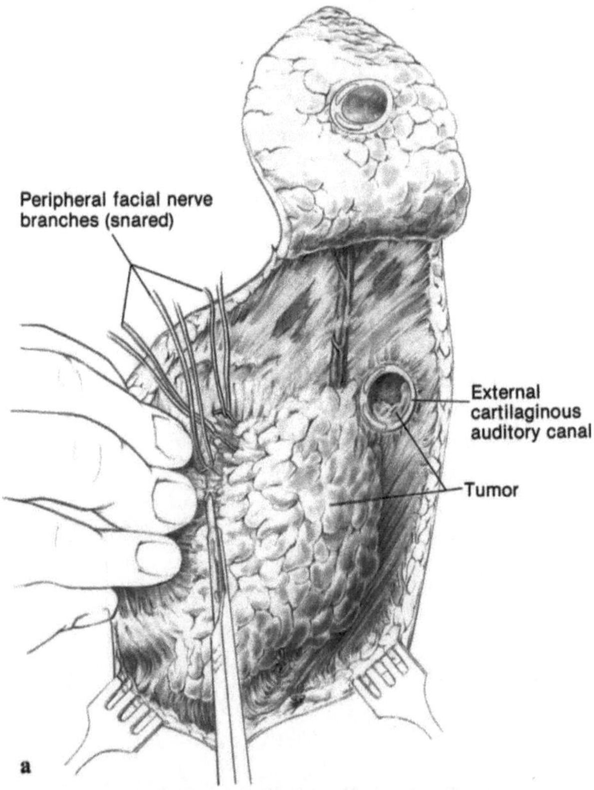

Fig. FN 16a–d. Intratemporal-extratemporal autogenous facial nerve reconstruction after removal of an ear canal carcinoma with subtotal petrosectomy, radical parotidectomy, partial mandibulectomy, and radical neck dissection.
a At the start of the operation, as many peripheral facial nerve branches as possible are isolated along the anterior edge of the parotid capsule. The parotid itself is included in the en bloc resection.
b Status following almost complete mobilization of the tumor specimen. A subtotal petrosectomy has been performed. A stump of facial nerve is still present central to the internal auditory meatus. The remaining part of the bony eustachian tube is occluded with the incus after inverting the mucosa. The dura of the middle and posterior cranial fossae is exposed. The sigmoid sinus still retains its bony coverage. The horizontal portion of the carotid artery and the jugular bulb are isolated. The field is limited in depth by the transverse process of the atlas. The accessory nerve is resected; the glossopharyngeal and hypoglossal nerves are spared. The head of the mandible and part of the vertical ramus have been resected. The peripheral facial nerve stumps overlie the masseter muscle

Intratemporal-Extratemporal Facial Nerve Reconstruction After Subtotal Petrosectomy and Total Parotidectomy Including Facial Nerve Resection (Conley 1955, 1975; Denecke 1958)

Introductory Remarks. Malignancies and large benign tumors of the parotid gland and petrous bone may necessitate an en bloc resection of

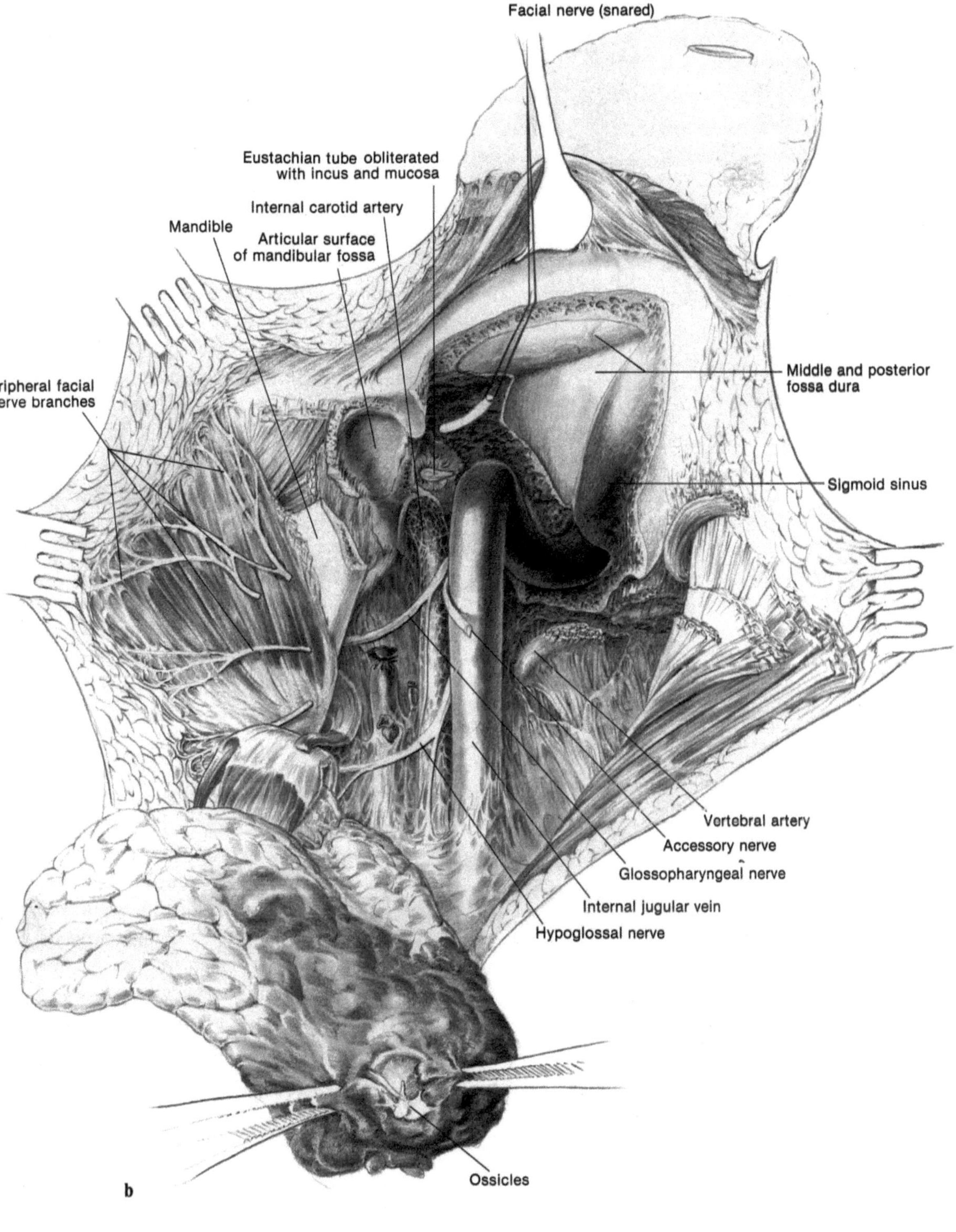
Facial nerve (snared)
Eustachian tube obliterated with incus and mucosa
Internal carotid artery
Mandible
Articular surface of mandibular fossa
Peripheral facial nerve branches
Middle and posterior fossa dura
Sigmoid sinus
Vertebral artery
Accessory nerve
Glossopharyngeal nerve
Internal jugular vein
Hypoglossal nerve
Ossicles

b

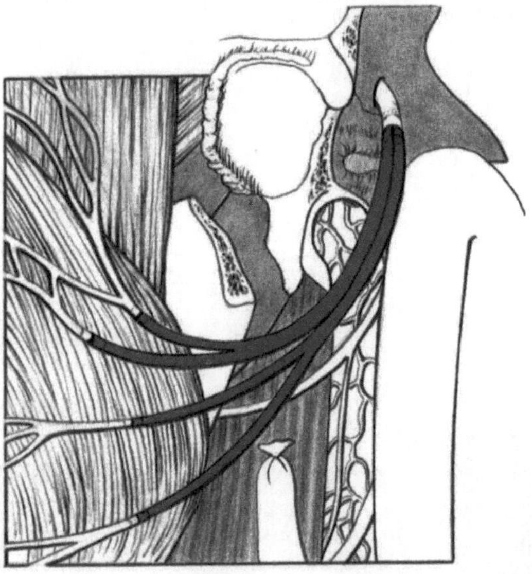

c

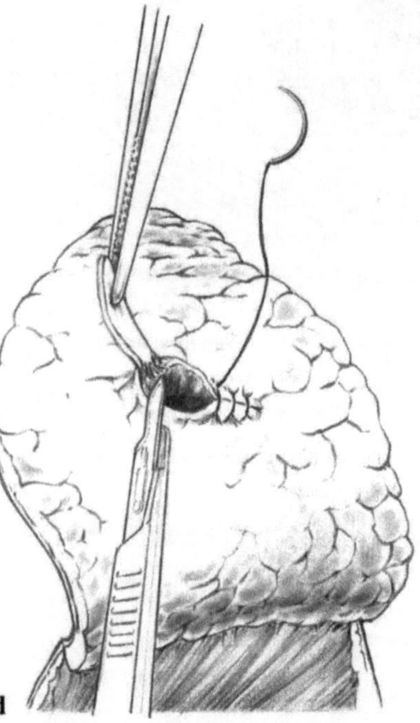

d

Fig. FN 16c, d.
c Two autogenous sural nerve grafts are anastomosed to the proximal facial nerve stump. Each graft is split peripherally and anastomosed to the peripheral facial nerve stumps. The deep surgical cavity can be partially ablated with a temporal muscle rotation flap.
d Before the auricle is turned down and sutured over the temporal muscle, the rest of the auditory canal inlet should be well sealed to prevent infection. This can be done by everting and suturing the meatal flaps after resecting the remaining cartilage of the auditory canal

the petrous bone and parotid gland and a neck dissection with concomitant removal of the facial nerve. Primary reconstruction of the facial nerve should be incorporated into the plan of operation if at all possible.

Operative Technique
(Fig. FN 16a–d)

For oncologic reasons, the distal extratemporal facial nerve branches are identified at the anterior border of the parotid capsule in these cases. By placing tension on the parotid capsule and its junction with the buccal fat and by careful dissection of the connective tissue fibers with the aid of a binocular loupe, the surgeon should be able to identify the peripheral facial nerve branches and expose them without injury. Usually four or five larger divisions can be identified, and these are tagged with dark threads. The extent of the pathological process may require that the facial nerve trunk be identified centrally in the mastoid or in the tympanic cavity at the geniculate ganglion. Less frequently it may be necessary to open the intradural space in the internal auditory canal. Following the en bloc tumor removal, it is best to obtain a branched sural nerve graft because of the length of the defect to be bridged. If a branched graft is not available, part of the sural nerve may be split into fascicular bundles for the distal anastomosis. The graft should be of sufficient length so that all parts lie against the tissue in the wound bed. No parts of the graft should pass freely through the surgical cavity, as this might cause trophic problems. Generally we first anastomose the central stump with two or three sutures before proceeding with the peripheral anastomoses. If possible we try to obliterate the surgical cavity with muscle (sternocleidomastoid or temporal) to prevent seroma formation. When the suction drain is inserted after facial nerve grafting, care is taken to place it well away from the anastomotic sites and to fix it securely. The cartilaginous auditory canal is closed in two layers to avoid wound healing problems. Circumferential cartilage resection makes it easier to obtain a tension-free skin closure.

Extratemporal Facial Nerve Reconstruction
(Fig. FN 17a, b)

When injury has occurred to the extratemporal portion of the facial nerve, parotidectomy is necessary for exposing the nerve trunk due to the great variability in its ramification. The primary repair of nerve divisions in this region is strongly recommended, before scar tissue has had time to form. If extensive scar formation has already occurred, an attempt is made to identify nerve branches peripherally or at the stylomastoid foramen in an anatomically normal area and follow them to the site of the lesion. If the continuity of the nerve branches is intact, a microsurgical fascicular neurolysis is performed. If the surgeon is unable to follow the nerve branches in the scar tissue, he should assume that the nerve continuity is disrupted and proceed by resecting the scars and bridging the defects with grafts. Experience has shown that the functional results of reconstructions peripheral to the main nerve trunk are quite good and are rarely associated with mass movements and synkinesis.

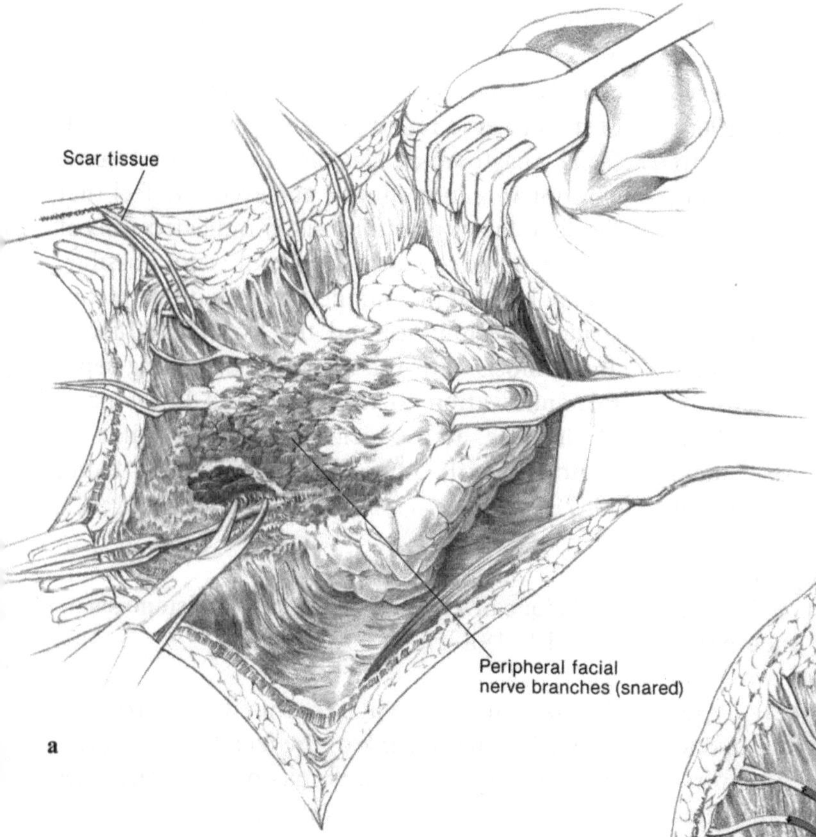

a

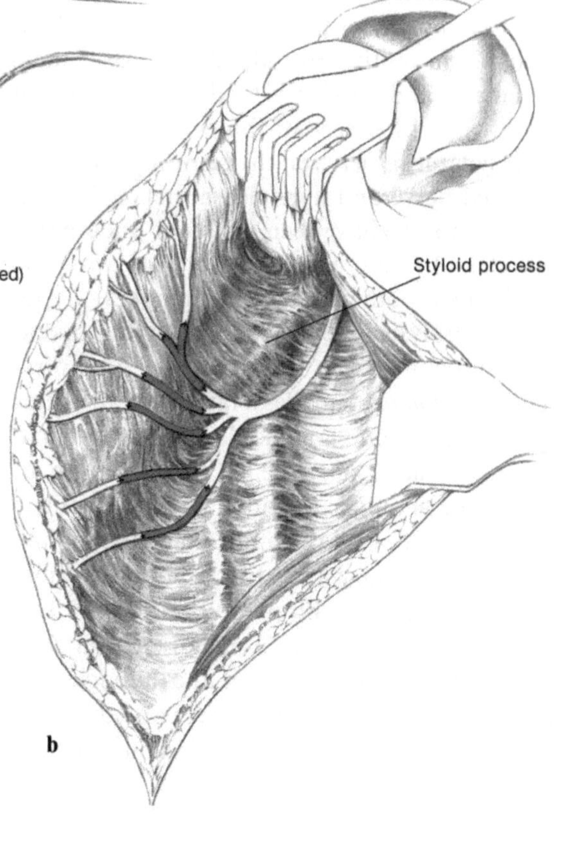

b

Fig. FN 17a, b. Autogenous peripheral facial nerve reconstruction after removal of scar tissue encompassing the nerve branches.
a The facial nerve branches are isolated from the periphery toward the center, as far into the scar tissue mass as possible.
b After the central, ramifying facial nerve stump has been identified and the scar tissue excised, multiple autogenous nerve grafts are used to restore the continuity of the peripheral branches

Methods of Indirect Facial Nerve Reconstruction

Introductory Remarks. An indirect facial nerve reconstruction relies on the sprouting of fibers from a different cranial nerve or from the contralateral facial nerve into the peripheral facial nerve branches of the affected side. As early as 1879, Drobnik successfully established a communication between the external branch of the accessory nerve and the peripheral, extratemporal facial nerve stump. The first hypoglossal-facial nerve anastomosis was performed by Körte (1903). Although the glossopharyngeal nerve (Ballance 1924; Watson-Williams 1927) and the phrenic nerve (Hardy et al. 1957) have also been used as donors, the hypoglossal nerve is preferred (Kautzky 1956; Metelka 1966; Miehlke 1973, 1979). Our own experience is consistent with the findings of an interesting study by Stennert (1979): The hypoglossal-facial anastomosis provides a very good resting tone and good voluntary motor function around the mouth; movement around the eyes is somewhat less satisfactory. With appropriate training, very good voluntary facial reinnervation can be achieved in younger patients as well as in older, especially in motivated individuals. Also, mass movements and synkinesis tend to decrease after several years. Stennert attributes this to a preexisting synergism between the central portions of the facial nerve and hypoglossal nerve. Neither Stennert nor we have seen a patient undergoing hypoglossal-facial anastomosis who was still significantly bothered by the unilateral hypoglossal paralysis several weeks after the operation. By comparison, the results of *accessory-facial anastomosis* are less favorable in terms of facial nerve function and donor nerve deficit. Synkinetic facial movements during lifting of the arm or shoulder continue to be a problem even years after surgery, and some patients find the loss of accessory nerve function to be permanently troublesome and painful (Behrens 1979; Stennert 1979). That is a major reason why Stennert (1979) incorporated the hypoglossal-facial anastomosis into his concept of the combined extratemporal facial nerve reconstruction.

The technique of the *faciofacial anastomosis* (cross-facial grafting), in which facial nerve branches on the healthy side are anastomosed to peripheral nerve branches on the affected side via a long subcutaneous graft, was first described by Scaramella at the Second International Symposium on Facial Nerve Surgery in 1970 (Scaramella 1971). The following year Smith described three cases that he had treated using a similar procedure. Other authors introduced modifications of the technique (Anderl 1973; Pialoux et al. 1976; Samii 1975). Based on our own results in 62 patients followed for several years (Samii 1981), we believe that cross-facial grafting represents an important advance in the rehabilitation of facial paralysis. For numerical reasons, however, the results of faciofacial grafting alone cannot compete with those of direct nerve repairs or even the hypoglossal-facial anastomosis, despite the fact that some emotional reanimation is achieved. We feel that the faciofacial anastomosis is indicated only if a direct nerve repair has failed or is not possible. It may be used in conjunction with direct reconstructive techniques and the hypoglossal-facial anastomosis with the object of providing separate innervation to the upper and lower parts of the face. Cross-facial grafting can also be combined with other surgical measures (Samii 1981).

Technique of Hypoglossal-Facial Anastomosis (Fig. FN 18a–c)

The skin incision is like that used for parotidectomy. The main trunk of the facial nerve is identified distal to the stylomastoid foramen (see p. 491) and traced to its bifurcation by elevating the superficial parotid lobe. Next the hypoglossal nerve is identified lateral or medial to the internal jugular vein in the angle between the lower border of the posterior digastric portion and the anterior border of the sternocleidomastoid. The hypoglossal nerve crosses the carotid bifurcation. It is traced as far distally as possible, past the origin of the descending ramus, and divided. Medial to the posterior portion of the digastric, the hypoglossal nerve trunk is

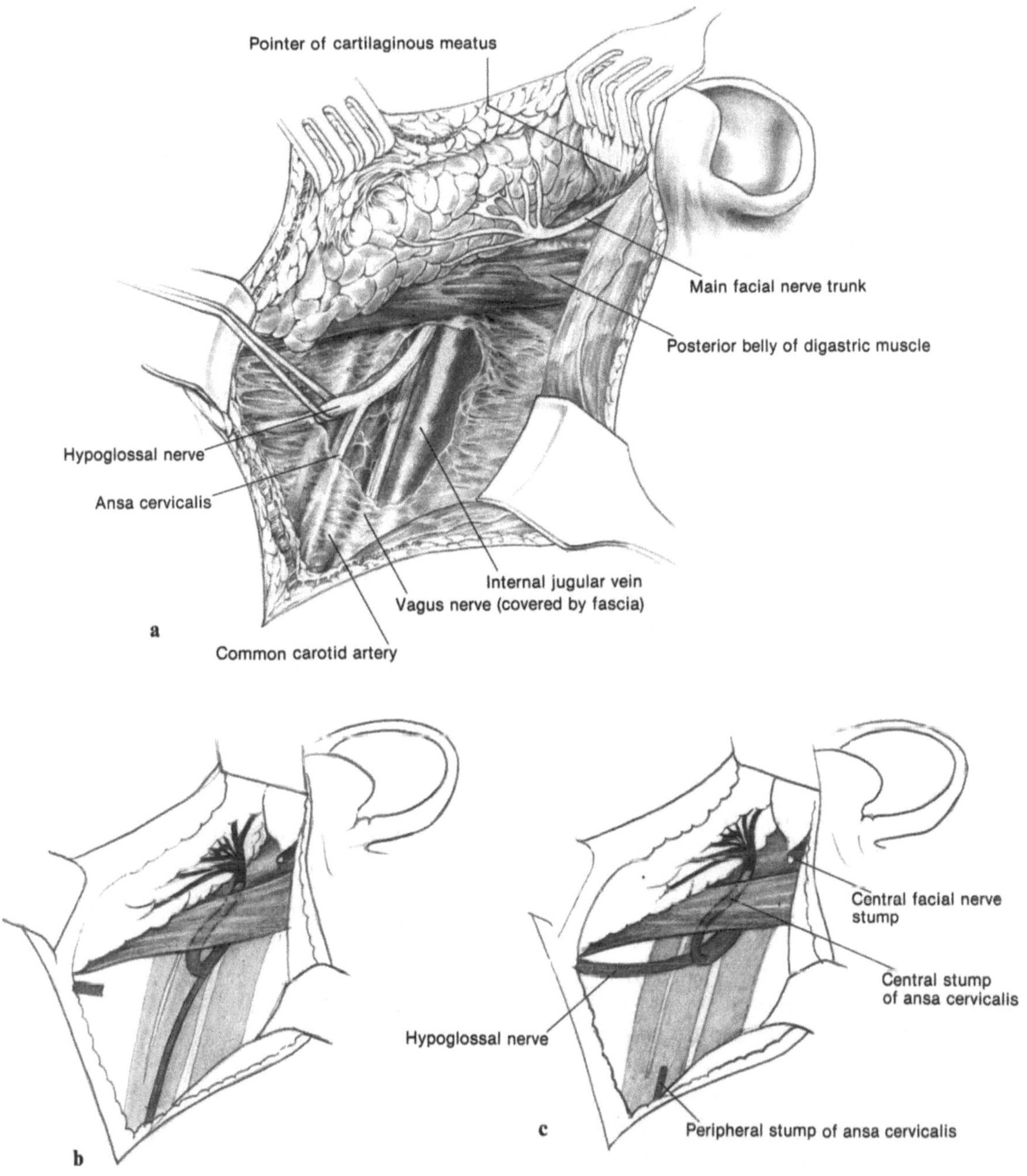

Fig. FN 18a–c. Technique of hypoglossal-facial anastomosis.
a The main trunk of the facial nerve is exposed through a parotidectomy-type incision curving down from the tragus along the anterior border of the sternocleidomastoid muscle. The major landmarks are the anterior borders of the posterior digastric muscle portion and the sternocleidomastoid muscle and the "pointer" of the cartilaginous auditory canal. The vascular package with the jugular vein, vagus nerve, and carotid artery is opened below the inferior border of the posterior portion of the digastric muscle. The hypoglossal nerve courses obliquely down over the carotid bifurcation. It is best to dissect the hypoglossal nerve with the ansa hypoglossi as far peripherally as possible so that the anastomosis can be effected without tension. Additional length can be gained by pulling the central stump of the hypoglossal nerve upward medial to the posterior digastric muscle portion.
b The main hypoglossal nerve trunk is employed for the anastomosis, preserving the ansa cervicalis. The trunk is reflected upward medial to the posterior digastric muscle portion.
c Occasionally the ansa cervicalis has a diameter sufficient to qualify it as a substitute for the hypoglossal nerve trunk

brought up in front of the stylomastoid foramen and anastomosed without tension to the peripheral facial nerve stump. Additional length is gained in the hypoglossal nerve by first dividing the descending ramus. Occasionally it may be possible to graft the descending limb of the hypoglossal nerve (the ansa cervicalis) to the facial nerve in cases where the ansa cervicalis is very well developed. This spares the hypoglossal nerve and preserves tongue mobility.

Technique of Faciofacial Anastomosis
(Fig. FN 19a–c)

The principle of the faciofacial anastomosis is based on the fact that the facial nerve branches form a kind of plexus (pes anserinus) in the face, and a portion of this plexus can be divided without causing a clinically apparent deficit. The sural nerve makes the best donor. The course of the peripheral branches of the facial nerve is highly variable. Also, discrepancies may exist between the two facial halves in the same individual (Davis et al. 1956; Fujita 1934; Krmpotic-Nemanic et al. 1988; McCormack et al. 1945; Miehlke 1973). Because of this variability in the peripheral branching of the facial nerve, great importance is placed on intraoperative electrostimulation with determination of the areas innervated by the different facial nerve branches. The "key" peripheral branch is the zygomatic. Electrostimulation of this branch elicits contraction of the orbicularis oculi and orbicularis oris muscles. Even with complete division of this branch, there will be no clinically apparent paralysis on the donor side, because the adjacent branches take over its function completely. Prompted by this clinical observation, we made microscopic counts of the nerve fibers of the zygomatic branch in cadaveric specimens and found that this branch contained as much as 40% of all the facial nerve fibers. Initially we performed faciofacial anastomosis by joining the individual branches, including the temporal branch, to the analogous branches of the paralyzed side. However, long-term observations showed that there was no case in which reinnervation of the frontal branch was achieved. We

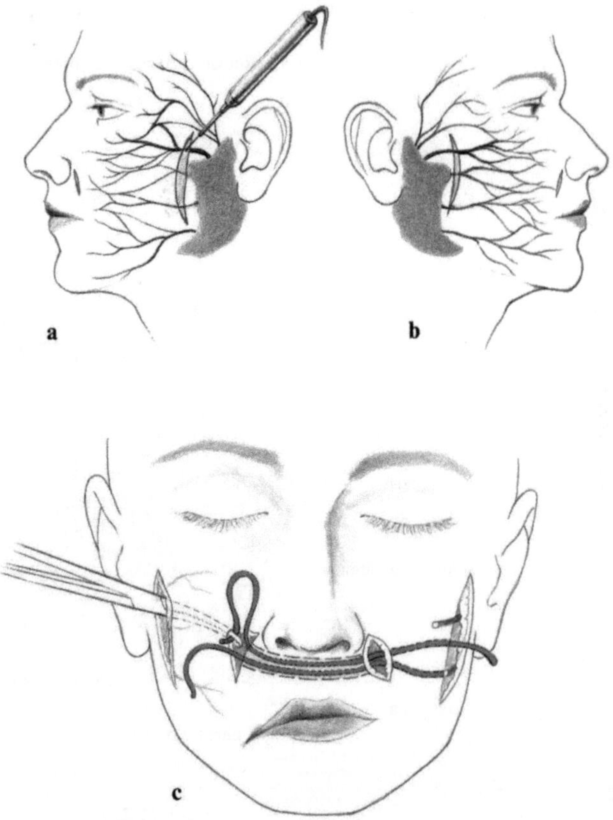

Fig. FN 19a–c. Technique of the faciofacial anastomosis (cross-facial grafting).
a Location of suitable donor nerves on the contralateral side. The anterior border of the masseter muscle is palpated, and a vertical preauricular skin incision, about 4 cm long and slightly concave anteriorly, is made down along the masseter border from the zygomatic arch. Usually two facial nerve branches of substantial size can be identified in the angle between the zygomatic arch and anterior masseter border at the anterior edge of the parotid capsule. Electrical stimulation is used to identify the areas innervated by the nerve branches. The central stumps used for the anastomosis are drawn in *heavy ink*.
b A similar incision is made on the paralyzed side, and two facial nerve branches of equal caliber are identified in the angle between the zygomatic arch and anterior masseter border. The peripheral stumps used for the anastomosis are drawn in *heavy ink*.
c Before the nerve stumps are prepared for anastomosis, additional incisions are placed in the nasolabial folds, the facial soft tissues and upper lip are undermined, and the sural nerve grafts are pulled through with a curved hemostat. At that point the designated facial nerve branches are sectioned, and the stumps are prepared and anastomosed to the graft ends on both sides

simplified the technique, therefore, by no longer exposing all the peripheral facial nerve branches, and simply exposing the two or three zygomatic branches on both sides. Using auxiliary skin incisions in the nasolabial folds, the zygomatic branches are interconnected by means of a sural nerve graft. Bleeding is minimized by using atraumatic technique when preparing the supralabial tunnel for the graft. Care is also taken to preserve the orbicular muscle.

Secondary Plastic Surgery Measures for Facial Rehabilitation

Introductory Remarks. These procedures represent rehabilitative measures of third choice. They are appropriate only if it is not possible to reconstruct the paralyzed nerve directly or indirectly by any of the techniques already described. They may also be used to supplement direct or indirect reconstructions that have been only partially successful. Secondary plastic surgical measures should be performed only when the result of a direct or indirect nerve reconstruction may be considered definitive after some years have passed. However, there is no strict time limit beyond which the use of secondary rehabilitative procedures would definitely be indicated, or a direct or indirect nerve reconstruction would no longer be appropriate without extensive electrophysiologic testing. The procedures may be classified as static (suspensory) or dynamic, depending on whether the intent is to reestablish facial symmetry alone or additionally to restore facial movement. The selection of a particular method is governed in each case by the degree of the paralysis or the degree of functional recovery following treatment. Each individual muscle region must be separately examined and evaluated using clinical and electrophysiologic techniques. Numerous surgical procedures have been devised. Here we shall describe only a few that are not too complicated technically and have demonstrated their value in clinical practice. The *static procedures* include tarsorrhaphy, lifting the sagging corner of the mouth with a fascial sling attached to the zygomatic arch or temporal muscle (McLaughlin 1953) or by an elliptical or parabolic excision of soft tissue at the nasolabial fold (Vogel 1953–1954; Kapovits 1961), closure of the eyelids by means of two small implanted magnets (Mühlbauer et al. 1973), and the various types of "face-lifting" procedure.

The *dynamic* rehabilitative procedures attempt to reanimate the paralyzed side of the face by transposing the two masticatory muscles supplied by the trigeminal nerve, the temporal and masseter muscles, into the paralyzed muscles (Rosenthal 1916, 1956), or by the free transplantation of autologous muscles or muscles and nerves (Freilinger 1975; Millesi and Samii 1975; Thompson 1971) or muscle-nerve-vascular units (Harii 1976 and 1977).

Operative Techniques

Tarsorrhaphy

Tarsorrhaphy is an important primary measure in patients with pronounced laxity of the lower eyelid in order to prevent corneal damage and troublesome conjunctivitis. Numerous methods have been reported. The simplest involves de-epithelializing the lateral canthus and closing it with mattress sutures. The sutures are removed after eight days.

Excision of Nasolabial Soft Tissue

(Kapovits 1961; Vogel 1953) (Fig. FN 20a, b)

One way to correct sagging of facial tissues about the mouth is by excising an elliptical piece of skin 4 cm wide, along with the attached subcutaneous fat, at the nasolabial fold. The lifting effect is maximized by approximating the wound edges without mobilizing the skin. Insertion of a mini suction drain is advised.

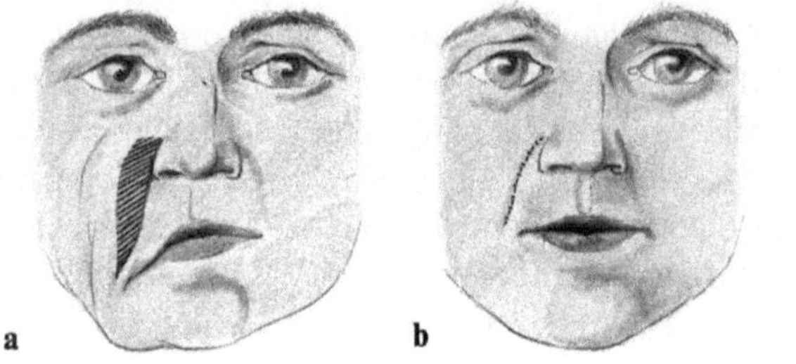
a b

Fig. FN 20a, b. Simple excision of nasolabial soft tissue for the static correction of facial paralysis.
a The excised strip of skin and fat is elliptical and up to 4 cm wide, depending on the amount of lift required.
b The wound margins are approximated in layers

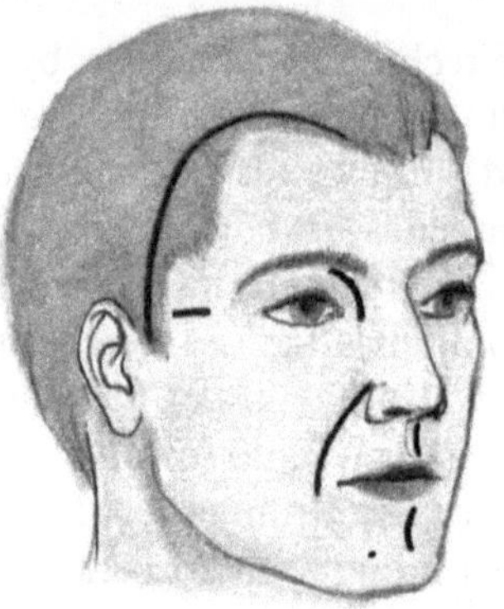

Fig. FN 21. Incisions for secondary plastic surgical rehabilitation of facial paralysis using a fascial sling or muscle transfer

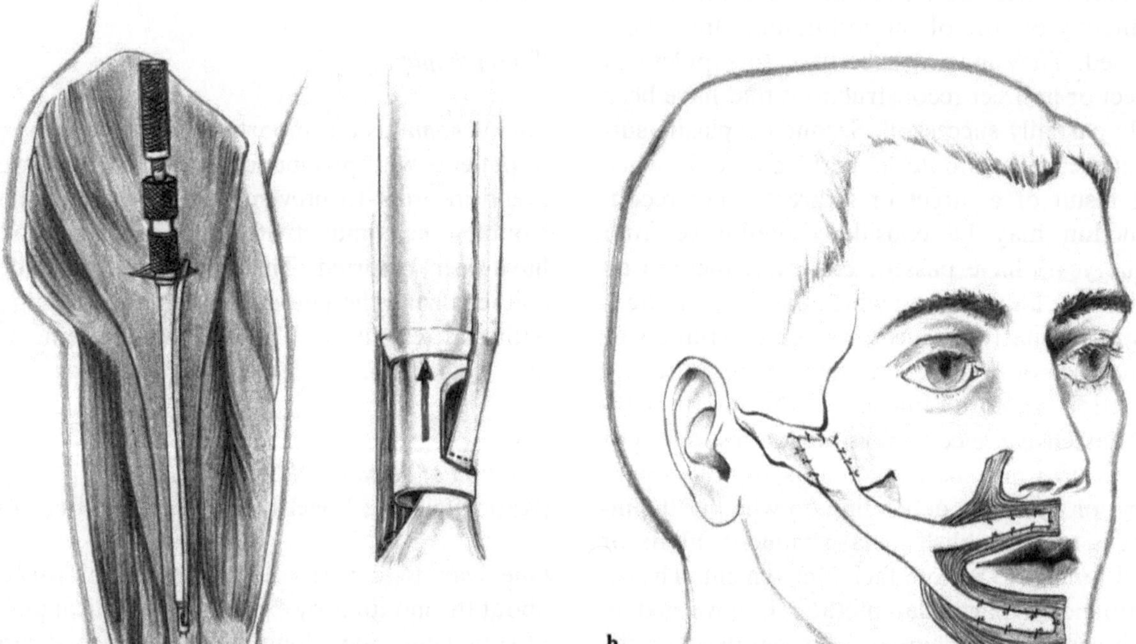
a b

Fig. FN 22a, b. Fascial sling procedure for the static correction of facial paralysis.
a Stripping instrument of Blair (1926) for obtaining fascia lata.
b The distal ends of a split fascial strip are secured to the orbicularis oris muscle with buried sutures through a nasolabial incision and auxiliary incisions extending to the midline of the upper and lower lip. The fascial sling is fixed superiorly to the periosteum of the body of the zygomatic arch

Fascial Sling Procedure
(Blair 1926; Stein 1913) (Fig. FN 21, Fig. FN 22a, b)

Fascia lata is taken with the Blair fascial stripper through a small skin incision just below and anterior to the greater trochanter of the ipsilateral thigh. One or even two fascial strips up to 25 cm in length can be obtained without difficulty. Next the circumference of the orbicularis oris muscle is exposed through a nasolabial incision. Bleeding during dissection can be reduced by injecting a local anesthetic containing a vasoconstrictor. The distal end of a split fascial strip is tacked onto the orbicularis oris with buried, nonabsorbable interrupted sutures through auxiliary radial incisions placed in the philtrum of the upper lip and the middle of the lower lip. The proximal end of the fascial sling is fixed to the periosteum of the zygomatic arch through a small skin incision to suspend the corner of the mouth. Slight overcorrection is desirable to compensate the sagging that occurs during the first postoperative weeks or months. Lifting the corner of the mouth creates redundant nasolabial skin, which is resected before nasolabial wound closure.

Temporal and Masseter Muscle Transfers
(Lexer 1908, 1919; Lexer and Eden 1911)

Introductory Remarks. Muscle transfers involve the transposition of a muscle possessing an adequate blood and nerve supply. Combined transfer of the temporal and masseter muscles is a procedure dating back to Lexer. The author, along with Eden, developed the theory of muscle neurotization, which was confirmed experimentally by Erlacher (1914, 1915). Although recent evidence (Miehlke 1973) casts doubt on the possibility of trigeminal nerve fiber growth from the transposed muscles into the paralyzed muscles, transfer of the temporal and masseter muscles is nevertheless valuable in that it gives mechanical support to sagging facial tissues and also restores some degree of voluntary facial movement. The utilization of one or both of these muscles depends on the degree of the paralysis. If eye closure is satisfactory and there is no appreciable asymmetry of the cheeks, it is sufficient to perform a masseter transfer to lift the corner of the mouth and give it mobility. If ocular symptoms are predominant, it is sufficient to transpose the anterior portion of the temporal muscle. Two options exist for total paralysis: Multiple slips from the temporal muscle may be transferred to the eye, cheek, and corner of the mouth (Fig. FN 23), or the upper face may be reanimated with the temporal muscle by the original Lexer method while the masseter muscle is used to raise the angle of the mouth.

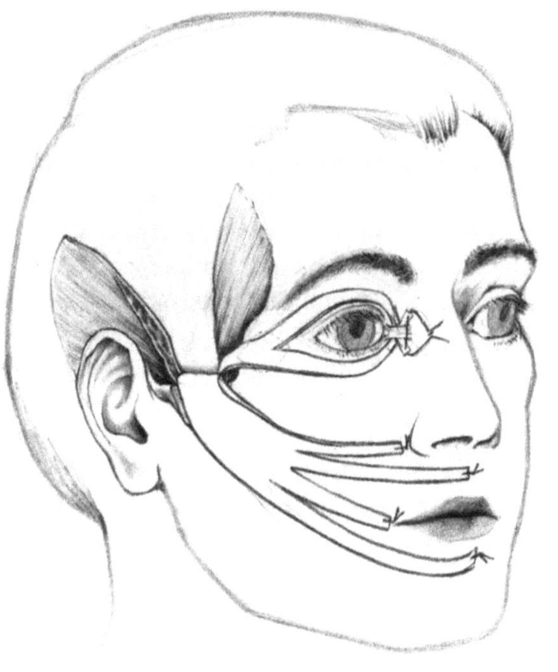

Fig. FN 23. Temporal muscle transfer to the eyelids, cheek, and corner of the mouth (Lexer 1919)

Operative Techniques

1) Temporal Muscle Transfer (Figs. FN 21 and 23). The *temporal muscle* is exposed through a curved, almost vertical incision placed behind the hairline and approximately over the center of the muscle. The incision is extended inferiorly to the tragus. The muscle is dissected free subcutaneously, sparing the outer fascial layer, and the zygomatic arch is exposed. Further dissection depends upon the number of muscle-fascia slips desired. For total hemifacial paralysis, almost the entire temporal muscle will be needed. Before dissecting the muscle itself, we inject and undermine the facial skin from the temporal incision to the eye and also to the cheek and corner of the mouth. Undermining at the corner of the mouth is completed through a nasolabial auxiliary incision and through radial incisions placed close to the midline in the upper and lower lip. A horizontal incision is made toward the eye, and auxiliary incisions are placed at the medial canthus and if necessary in the upper and lower lids. Bleeding is reduced by undermining the skin on the plane between the subcutaneous fat and muscle, as in face-lift operations. The transfer itself is carried out as follows:

First the fatty layer overlying the temporal muscle above the zygomatic arch and extending from the lateral orbital margin to the auricle is dissected off the muscle in an anterior-to-posterior fashion, creating a fat flap based near the root of the auricle. Care is taken to spare the superficial temporal artery branches that supply the flap. Usually this fatty layer and the temporal fascia are separated by a loose layer of connective tissue that provides a good plane of dissection. Mobilizing the fat flap ensures that the muscle, when reflected inferiorly, does not create an excessive bulge in the temporal area. Also, the flap can later be transposed into the muscle defect to partially obliterate it. As the flap is mobilized, great care is taken to preserve the layer of fascia and pericranium that covers the temporal muscle and extends upward from it. That layer will be used to form the muscle-fascia slips. The necessary lengths of the slips can be determined with a measuring tape held at the zygomatic arch. The slips for the eye and lower facial areas are successively mobilized by sharp dissection, starting anteriorly with the two slips for the upper and lower lids. The length of the slips equals the distance from the anterior zygomatic arch to the medial canthus of the eye. Both slips should have sufficient fascial or pericranial tissue at their ends to permit secure fixation to the medial palpebral ligament. The surgeon must be careful not to mobilize the muscle too far; otherwise the slip will be too long and too lax for effective lid closure. Shortening the slip then becomes a problem, because it may be necessary to resect the slip back into muscle tissue, which is apt to tear loose from the medial palpebral ligament. It is necessary in such cases to suture a loop of fascia around the distal, muscular end of the slip so that stable sutures can be placed in the medial canthus area. The slips for the lower face are prepared in analogous fashion. As many as eight separate slips can be formed if necessary – two for the eye, two for the upper cheek, and the rest for the mouth (orbicularis oris). Several points should be noted with regard to dissection around the eyelids: The palpebral skin is undermined directly along the lid margins, preferably using a fine, sharp scissors. If this proves difficult, a small auxiliary incision may be made at the center of the lid. The width of the tunnel should correspond to the width of the fascial slip. During dissection in the medial canthus, the medial palpebral ligament is widely exposed and is undermined with a small hemostat, preserving its attachments. The posterior situation of the lacrimal ducts should protect them from injury if the dissection is done carefully. Pulling through of the fascial slip is made easier by placing a heavy thread at the distal end of the slip and pulling it through with a hemostat. It is fixed to the medial palpebral ligament with two nonabsorbable sutures. Next one or two fascial strips are sutured to the oblique muscles coursing between the orbicularis oculi and orbicularis oris muscles, again using nonabsorbable threads. Finally the remaining four muscle-fascia slips are sutured to the orbicularis oris muscle. The skin of the upper and lower lips is undermined to a point very close to the midline, where a number of buried mattress sutures are placed to create a broad area of attachment between the fascial slip and muscle. It is especially important to support the lower lip with one wide slip or two narrow slips, attaching one slip directly to the angle of the mouth. All the slips should be sufficiently taut, and the tension should be evenly distributed so that one area is not raised more than another. Slight overcor-

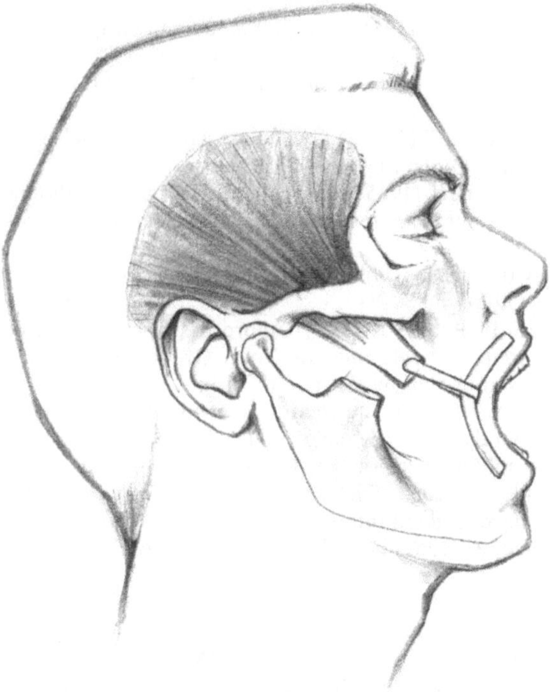

Fig. FN 24. Transfer of the temporal tendon of insertion by osteotomy of the coronoid process to raise the corner of the mouth (McLaughlin 1953)

rection is recommended in the recumbent patient to allow for later gravitational sagging. At the end of the operation hemostasis is rechecked, and the wounds are closed in two layers.

2) Transfer of the Temporal Tendon Inserted to the Coronoid Process to Raise the Corner of the Mouth (McLaughlin 1953, Fig. FN 24). Through an intraoral incision, the coronoid process of the vertical ramus of the mandible is osteotomized, taking with it the tendon of insertion of the temporalis muscle. A loop of fascia is sutured to the ipsilateral orbicularis oris muscle, its ends extending to the midline of the upper and lower lip, and a second loop is sutured to the initial loop and passed through a drill hole in the coronoid process, creating a link that suspends the corner of the mouth from the mobilized temporal tendon. The drill hole should be placed relatively close to the temporal insertion to lessen the danger of eventual ripping of the fascial loop.

3) Masseter Muscle Transfer (Fig. FN 25a, b). Transfer of the masseter muscle can be performed externally through an incision in the nasolabial fold.

In the intraoral approach, the operative area is widely injected with a local anesthesia and hemostasic, and two vertical mucosal incisions are made, one 2 mm posterior and parallel to the lateral angle of the mouth, and one directly

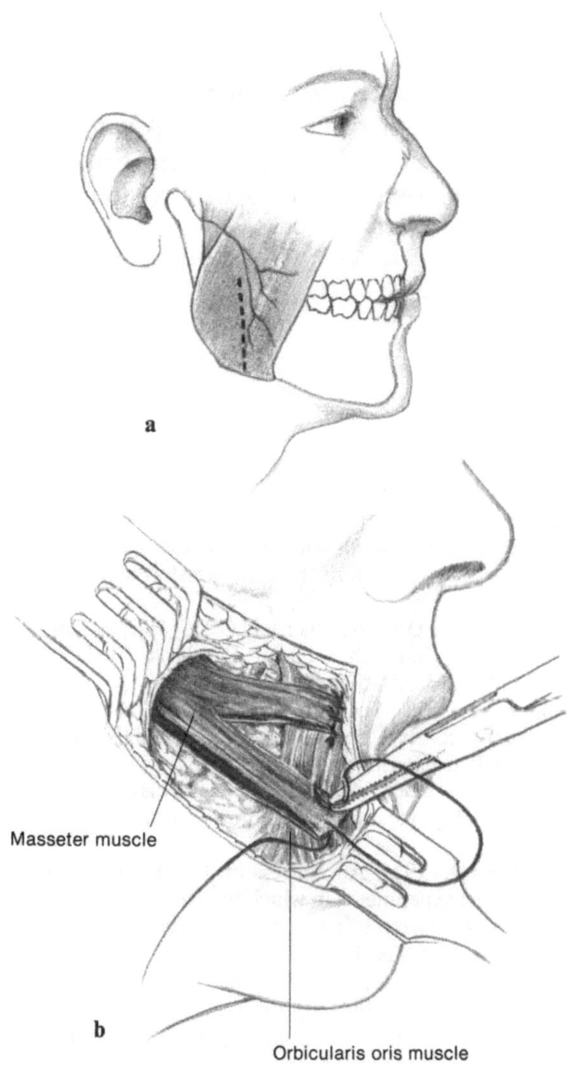

Fig. FN 25a, b. Transfer of the masseter muscle to the corner of the mouth.

a The *dashed line* indicates the correct incision of the masseter muscle, parallel to the motor branches of the trigeminal nerve.

b The masseter muscle is split distally and fixed to the orbicularis oris muscle of the upper and lower lip with nonabsorbable sutures anterior to the vertical ramus of the mandible extending from the zygomatic arch to the horizontal ramus. The oral mucosa is undermined, and the anterior border and medial surface of the masseter muscle are exposed along with the insertion of the muscle at the angle of the mandible. The insertion is sharply mobilized with a margin of periosteum to the middle of the muscle, and then the muscle is split obliquely upward, avoiding the nerve branches coursing in that direction. The masseter muscle is now delivered through the mucosal tunnel to the orbicularis oris muscle and sutured to it over a wide area (!) chiefly in the upper labial portion and at the corner of the mouth. Again, some overcorrection is desirable. Excess nasolabial skin is removed by an elliptical excision in the nasolabial fold.

References

Adour K (1976) Cranial Polyneuritis and Bell Palsy. Arch Otolaryng 102:262–264

Adour K (1977) Etiology and Pathogenesis of Bell's Palsy. Panel Discussion No. 10. In: Fisch U (ed) Facial Nerve Surgery. Kugler, Amstelveen, pp 371–381

Adour K, Bell DN, Hilsinger RD (1975) Herpes Simplex Virus in Idiopathic Facial Paralysis (Bell Palsy) JAMA 233:527–530

Anderl H (1973) Reconstruction of the face through cross-face-nerve transplantation in facial paralysis. Chir Plast (Berlin) 2:17–46

Ballance CA (1909) A Case of Facial Palsy Treated by Facio-Hypoglossal Anastomosis. Lancet 1:1675–1677

Ballance CA (1924) An address on the results obtained in some experiments in which the facial and recurrent laryngeal nerves were anastomosed with other nerves. Brit Med J 2:349–354

Ballance CA, Duel AS (1932) The operative treatment of facial palsy; by the introduction of nerve grafts into the fallopian canal and by other intratemporal methods.Arch Otolaryng 15:1–70

Behrens H (1979) Der N. facialis und seine chirurgische Behandlung unter besonderer Berücksichtigung des Kleinhirnbrückenwinkels. Univ Mainz 1979

Blair VP (1926) Notes on the operative correction of the facial palsy. South Med J 19:116

Bonnel S (1927) Suture of facial nerve within the temporal bone with the report of first successful case. Surg Gynec Obstet 45:780–785

Cawthorne T (1951) The pathology and surgical treatment of Bell's palsy. J Laryng 65:792–798

Cawthorne T (1963) Bell's Palsies. Ann Otol (St Louis) 72:774

Cawthorne T (1965a) Geniculate ganglion facial palsy. Arch Otolaryng 81:502–503

Cawthorne T (1965b) Idiopathic facial palsy: Pathology and surgical treatment. Arch Otolaryngol 81:494–496

Cawthorne T (1969) Intratemporal facial palsy. Arch Otolaryng 80:789

Clerc P, Batisse R (1954) Abord des organes intra-petreux par vole endocranienne (Greffe du nerf facial) Ann Otolaryng (Paris) 71:20–38

Conley J (1975) The treatment of long standing facial paralysis: a new concept. Trans Am Acad Ophthalmol Otolaryngol 78:386–392

Conley JJ (1955) Facial nerven grafting in treatment of parotic gland tumors. Arch Surg 70:359–366

Conley JJ (1961) Facialis nerve grafting. Arch Otolaryng 73:322–327

Conley JJ (1975) Salivary glands and the facial nerve. Thieme, Stuttgart

Davis RA, Anason BJ, Budinger JM et al (1956) Surgical anatomy of the facial nerve and parotid gland based upon a study of 350 cervicofacial halves. Surg Gynec Obstet 102:305–412

Denecke HJ (1958) Zur Chirurgie der Parotiserkrankungen unter Berücksichtigung des N. facialis. Laryngol Rhinol Otol (Stuttg) 37:403

Devriese PP (1977) Treatment of facial palsy of infectious origin. Panel Discussion No. 12. In: Fisch U (ed) Facial Nerve Surgery. Kugler, Amstelveen, The Netherlands, 419–424

Dott NM (1958) Facial paralysis. Restitution by extrapetrous nerve graft. Proc R Soc Med 51:900–902

Draf W (1980) Zur Bedeutung des Transplantatlagers bei der autogenen Nerventransplantation im HNO-Bereich. In: Hierholzer G, Zilch H (eds) Transplantatlager und Implantatlager bei verschiedenen Operationsverfahren. Springer, Berlin Heidelberg New York, pp 147ff

Draf W, Samii M (1982) Intracranial-intratemporal Anastomosis of the Facial Nerve after Cerebellopontine Angle Tumor Surgery. In: Graham MD, House WF (Ed) Disorders of the Facial Nerve. Raven, New York, pp 441–449

Drake CG (1960) Acoustic neurinoma. Repair of facial nerve with autogenous graft. J Neurosurg 17:836–842

Drake CG (1973) Experiences and results with posterior approaches. In: Schürmann K, Brock M, Reulen HJ et al. Brain Edema – Cerebello Pontine Angle Tumors. Adv in Neurosurg. Springer, Berlin Heidelberg New York, pp 240–241

Drobnik T (1879) Facial palsy. Würtzburg JM Richter

Erlacher P (1914) Über die motorischen Nerven. Z Orthop Chir 34:561

Erlacher P (1915) Direct and muscular neurotization of paralyzed muscles. Experimental research. Am J Orthop Surg 13:22

Esslen E (1973) Electrodiagnosis of facial palsy. In: Miehlke A (ed) Surgery of the Facial Nerve. Urban & Schwarzenberg, München and Saunders, Philadelphia

Esslen E (1977) Electromyography and electroneurography. In: Fisch U (Ed) Facial nerve surgery. Kugler, Amstelveen and Aesculapius Birmingham AL, p 93

Fisch U (1969) Die transtemporale, extralabyrinthäre Chirurgie des inneren Gehörganges. Arch Klin Exp Ohren-, Nasen- und Kehlkopfheilk 194:232–243

Fisch U (1970) Transtemporal surgery of the internal auditory canal. Report of 92 cases, technique, indications and results. Adv Otorhinolaryngol 17:203

Fisch U (1973) Operations on the Facial Nerve in its Labyrinthine and Meatal Course. In: Miehlke A (ed) Surgery of the Facial Nerve. Urban & Schwarzenberg, München, pp 175–205

Fisch U (1976) Richtlinien zur Versorgung traumatischer Verletzungen des N. facialis. ORL 38:42-29

Fisch U (ed) (1977) Facial Nerve Surgery. Kugler, Amstelveen, The Netherlands

Fisch U (1979) Klinik und Therapie der häufigsten Fazialislähmungen im labyrinthären, meatalen und intrakraniellen Bereich. In: Berendes J, Link R, Zöllner F (eds) Hals-Nasen-Ohrenheilkunde in Praxis und Klinik. Thieme, Stuttgart

Fisch U (1979) Surgery for Bell's Palsy and Herpes zoster oticus. Proc Symp Neurological Surgery of the ear, Sarasota

Fisch U, Esslen E (1972) The surgical treatment of facial hyperkinesis. Arch Otolaryngol 95:400–405

Fisch U, Esslen E (1972) Total intratemporal exposure of the facial nerve. Arch otolaryng 95:335

Fowler EP Jr (1963) The pathologic findings in a case of facialis paralysis. Trans Amer Acad Ophthal Otolaryng 67:187

Freilinger G (1975) A new technique to correct facial paralysis. Plast Reconstr Surg 56:44–48

Fujita T (1934) Über die periphere Ausbreitung des N. facialis beim Menschen. Gegenbaucrs Morph Jahrb 73:578–614

Gomez JG (1977) Incidence and Management of Bell's Palsy According to Geographic Distribution. In: Fisch U (ed) Facial Nerve Surgery Kugler, Amstelveen, The Netherlands, pp 319–336

Hardy RC, Perret G, Meyers R (1957) Phrenicofacial nerve anastomosis for facial paralysis. J Neurosurg 14:400–404

Harii K (1977) New Concepts in Rehabilitation of the Long Standing Facial Paralysis. Panel Discussion No. 7. In: Fisch U (ed) Facial Nerve Surgery. Kugler, Amstelveen, The Netherlands, pp 251–284

Harii K, Ohmori K, Torii S (1976) Free gracilis muscle transplantation with microneurovascular anastomosis for the treatment of facial paralysis. A preliminary report. Plast Reconstr Surg 57:133–143

Helms J (1976) The transmeatal approach to the geniculate ganglion. Acta Otorhinolaryng Belg 30:84–89

Helms J (1981) Variations of the course of the facial nerve in the middle ear and mastoid. In: Samii M, Jannetta P (eds) The cranial nerves. Springer, Berlin Heidelberg New York, p 391

Helms J (1982) Surgery and Bell's Palsy. In: Granam MD, House WF (eds) Disorders of the facial nerve. Raven New York, p 287

Hilger JA (1949) The nature of Bell's palsy. Laryngoscope 59:228–235

House WF (1961) Surgical exposure of the internal auditory canal and its contents through the middle cranial fossa. Laryngoscope 71:1363–1385

House WF (1963) Middle cranial fossa approach to the petrous pyramid. Arch Otolaryng 78:460–469

Jannetta PJ, Bissonette DJ (1978) Bell's palsy: a theory as to etiology. Observations in six patients. Laryngoscope 88:849–854

Jongkees LBW (1958) Die chirurgische Behandlung der intratemporalen Fazialislähmung. Dtsch Med Wschr 83:865–869

Jongkees LBW (1961) Über die intratemporale Fazialislähmung und ihre chirurgische Behandlung. Z Laryng Rhinol 40:319–336

Jongkees LBW (1977) Nerve excitability test. In: Fisch U (ed) Facial nerve surgery. Kugler, Amstelveen, The Netherlands and Aesculapius Birmingham AL, p 83

Kapovits M (1961) Indikation und Technik der Gesichtshautstraffung. Arch Klin Chirurgie 298:950

Kautzky R (1956) Die periphere Fazialislähmung und ihre Behandlung mittels Nervenpfropfung. Fortschr Kiefer Gesichtschir 2:119–126

Kettel K (1957) Repair of the facial nerve in traumatic facial palsies. Results of decompression, nerve suture and nerve grafting in onehundred twentyseven cases. Arch Otolaryng 66:634–672

Kettel K (1959) Peripheral Facial Palsy, Pathology and Surgery. Munksgaard, Copenhagen

Körte W (1903) Ein Fall von Nervenpfropfung des N. facialis auf den N. hypoglossus. Dtsch Med Wschr 29:293–295

Krmpotic-Nemanic J, Draf W, Helms J (1988) Surgical Anatomy of Head and Neck. Springer, Berlin Heidelberg New York

Lathrop FD (1953) The facial nerve: technique of exposure and repair. Surg Clin N Amer 33:909–926

Lathrop FD (1956) Surgical repair of facial nerve: technique. Surg Clin N Amer 36:583–588

Lathrop FD (1962) Management of the facial nerve during operations on parotid gland. Ann Otol (St. Louis) 72:780–801

Laumann EPJ, Jongkees LBW (1963) On the prognosis of peripheral facialis paralysis of endotemporal origin. Ann Otol (St Louis) 72:307

Lexer E (1908) General Surgery: A Presentation of the Scientific Principles upon which the Practise of Modern Surgery is based. Appleton, New York

Lexer E (1919) Die freien Transplantationen. Neue Deutsche Chirurgie, 548

Lexer E, Eden R (1911) Über die chirurgische Behandlung der peripheren Fazialislähmung. Beitr Klin Chir 73:116

Loew F (1961) Die kombinierte intrakranielle-extratemporale Fazialisplastik nach DOTT. Langenbecks Arch Kli Chir 298:934–935
Martin RC (1930) Intratemporal Suture of the Facial Nerve. Trans Pacific Coast Oto Ophth Soc 119–129
Martin RC (1931) Intratemporal Suture of the Facialis Nerve. Arch Otolaryng 13:259–264
Martin RC (1936) Surgical Repair of the Facial Nerve. Arch Otolaryng 23:458–468
Martin RC (1955) Late Results of Facial Nerve Repair. Anal of Otology 64:659–669
Maxwell JH (1951) Extratemporal Repair of the Facial Nerve. Ann Otol 60:1114–1133
Maxwell JH (1954) Repair of the Facial Nerve after Facial Lacerations. Trans Amer Acad Ophthal Otolaryng 58:733–740
May M (1986) The facial nerve. Thieme, New York
May M (1977) Maximal excitability test. In: Fisch U (Ed) Facial nerve surgery. Kugler, Amstelveen and Aesculapius, Birmingham, pp 87
May M et al. (1971) The prognostic accuracy of the maximal stimulation compared with that of the nerve excitability test in Bell's palsy. Laryngoscope 81:931–938
McCormack LJ, Cauldwell EW, Anson BJ (1945) The surgical anatomy of the facial nerve. "With special reference to the parotid gland" Surg Gynec Obstet 80:620–630
McGovern FH (1977a) Etiology and Pathogenesis of Bell's Palsy. Panel Discussion No. 10. In: Fisch U (ed) Facial Nerve Surgery. Kugler, Amstelveen, The Netherlands, pp 371–381
McGovern FH, Estevez J, Jackson R (1977b) Immunological concept for Bell's Palsy. Ann Otol Rhinol Laryngol 86:300–305
McLaughlin CR (1953) Permanent facialis paralysis. Lancet 2:647
McLaughlin CR (1953) Surgical support in permanent facialis paralysis. Plast Reconstr Surg 11:302
Metelka M (1966) Anastomoza N VII N XII lepenim Plazmou. Cesk Neurol 29:305–310
Miehlke A (1960) Die Chirurgie des N. facialis. Urban & Schwarzenberg, Munich
Miehlke A (1960) Über den chirurgischen Wiederaufbau des Gesichtsnerven nach extratemporalen Läsionen. Dtsch Med Wochenschr 85:506–510
Miehlke A (1961) Extratemporale Fazialischirurgie. Z Laryng Rhinol 40:338–358
Miehlke A (1973) Surgery of the Facial Nerve, vol 2. Urban & Schwarzenberg, Munich
Miehlke A (1979) Fazialislähmungen. In: Berendes J, Link R, Zöllner F (eds) Hals-Nasen-Ohrenheilkunde in Praxis und Klinik. Thieme, Stuttgart
Miehlke A, Bushe KA (1967) Die operative Freilegung der mittleren Schädelgrube und des Porus acusticus internus zur Behandlung intralabyrinthärer Läsionen des N. facialis. Chir Plast Reconstr 3:37
Miehlke A, Stennert E, Arold R, Chilla R, Penzholz H, Kühner A, Sturm V, Haubrich J (1981) Surgery of the Nerves of the Neck, Nose and Ear Region (Except Nn stato-acusticus and olfactorius). Arch Otorhinolaryngol 231:89–449
Millesi H, Samii M (1975) Erfahrungen mit verschiedenen Wiederherstellungsoperationen am N. facialis. In: Höhler H (ed) Plastische- und Wiederherstellungschirurgie. Fischer, Stuttgart, pp 111–127
Mühlbauer W, Segeth H, Viessmann A (1973) Restoration of Lid Function in Facial Palsy with Permanent Magnets. Chir Plast (Berl) 1:295–304
Peitersen E (1977) Spontaneous Course of Bell's Palsy. In: Fisch U (ed) Facial Nerve Surgery. Kugler, Amstelveen, The Netherlands, pp 337–343
Pialoux P, Jost G, Freyss G, Rey A, Cophignon J (1976) Notre technique d'anastomose facio-faciale hetirolatiraleger autograffe nerveuse dans le traitment des paralysies faciales peripheriques definitives. Ann Oto Laryng (Paris) 93:471–486
Rosenthal W (1916) Über muskuläre Neurotisation bei Fazialislähmung. Zbl Chir 24:489–491
Rosenthal W (1956) Die muskuläre Neurotisation. Fortschr Kiefer Gesichtschir 2:139–140
Samii M (1975) Modern aspects of peripheral and cranial nerve surgery. In: Krayenbühl H (Ed) Advances and Technical Standards in Neurosurgery Vol 2. Springer, Vienna New York
Samii M (1977) Panel discussion Management of facial nerve in intracranial tumors. In: Fisch U (Ed) Facial nerve surgery. Kugler, Amstelveen, The Netherlands and Aesculapius, Birmingham AL p 475
Samii M (1979) Operative treatment of cerebellopontine angle tumors with special consideration of the facial and acoustic nerve. Advances in Neurosurgery 7:138–145
Samii M (1979) Neurochirurgische Behandlung der Akustikusneurinome mit besonderer Berücksichtigung des N. facialis. Laryngol Rhinol Otol (Stuttg) 58, 97–106
Samii M (1980) Nerves of the head and neck. In: Omer GE, Spinner M (Ed) Management of peripheral nerve problems. Saunders, Philadelphia London Toronto, p 507–547
Samii M (1981) Preservation and reconstruction of the facial nerve in the cerebellopontine angle. In: Samii M, Jannetta P (Ed) The cranial nerves. Springer, Berlin Heidelberg New York, p 438
Samii M (1981) Facio-Facial Anastomosis. In: Samii M, Jannetta P (Ed) The cranial nerves. Springer, Berlin Heidelberg New York, p 515
Samii M (1981) Zur Indikation, Technik und zu den Ergebnissen der fazio-fazialen Anastomose. Neurochirurgia 24:90–93
Samii M (1984) Facial Nerve Grafting in Acoustic Neurinoma. Clin Plast Surg 11:221–225
Samii M (1986) Allgemeine Hinweise zur chirurgischen Therapie und Technik in Neurologie, Praxis und Klinik. In: Hopf H Ch, Poersk K, Schliack H (eds) Neurologie, Praxis und Klinik, vol 3, pp 28–34. Thieme, Stuttgart
Scaramella L (1971) L'anastomosi tra i due nervi faciali. Arch Ital Otol 82:209–215
Smith JW (1971) A new technique of facial animation. Transaction of the Vth International Congress of Plastic and Reconstructive surgery, Melbourne Feb 1971, London, p 83–84

Stein AE (1913) Die kosmetische Korrektur der Fazialislähmung durch freie Faszienplastik. Münch Med Wschr 60:1370

Stennert E (1979) Combined approach in extratemporal facial nerve reconstruction. Clin Plast Surg 6, 481–486

Thompson N (1971) Treatment of facial paralysis by free skeletal muscle grafts. Transaction of the Vth Internation Congress of Plastic and Reconstructive Surgery, Melbourne Feb 1971, London, p 66–82

Vogel K (1953/1954) Zur Gesichtskorrektur bei Fazialislähmung. HNO 4:344

Watson-Williams E (1927) Glossopharyngeal Facial Nerve Anastomosis. Proc Roy Soc Med 20:1439–1442

Wullstein H (1958) Die Methode der Dekompression des N. facialis vom Austritt aus dem Labyrinth bis zum Foramen stylomastoideum ohne Beeinträchtigung des Mittelohres. Arch Ohr-, Nas- u. Kehlkopf Heilk 172:582

Wullstein H (1968) Operationen zur Verbesserung des Gehörs. Thieme, Stuttgart (1968)

Subject Index

P

U

V

Z

MIX
Papier aus verantwortungsvollen Quellen
Paper from responsible sources
FSC® C105338

If you have any concerns about our products,
you can contact us on
ProductSafety@springernature.com

In case Publisher is established outside the EU,
the EU authorized representative is:
Springer Nature Customer Service Center GmbH
Europaplatz 3, 69115 Heidelberg, Germany

Printed by Libri Plureos GmbH
in Hamburg, Germany